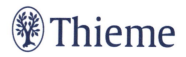

Foot and Ankle Surgery

Tricks of the Trade

Steven M. Raikin, MD
Director
Foot and Ankle Services
Rothman Institute
Professor of Orthopaedic Surgery
Thomas Jefferson Medical College
Philadelphia, Pennsylvania

457 illustrations

Thieme
New York • Stuttgart • Delhi • Rio de Janeiro

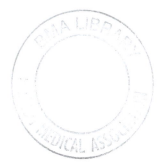

Executive Editor: William Lamsback
Managing Editor: Sarah Landis
Director, Editorial Services: Mary Jo Casey
Assistant Managing Editor: Nikole Connors
Production Editor: Naamah Schwartz
International Production Director: Andreas Schabert
Editorial Director: Sue Hodgson
International Marketing Director: Fiona Henderson
International Sales Director: Louisa Turrell
Director of Institutional Sales: Adam Bernacki
Senior Vice President and Chief Operating
Officer: Sarah Vanderbilt
President: Brian D. Scanlan

Illustrations by Andrea Hines

Library of Congress Cataloging-in-Publication Data

Names: Raikin, Steven M., editor.
Title: Foot and ankle surgery : tricks of the trade / [edited by]
Steven M.   Raikin.
Other titles: Foot and ankle surgery (Raikin)
Description: New York : Thieme, [2018] | Includes bibliographical references.
Identifiers: LCCN 2017058035| ISBN 9781626234918 (print) |
ISBN 9781626234925
(ebook)
Subjects: | MESH: Foot–surgery | Foot Deformities–surgery | Foot
Injuries–surgery | Ankle–surgery | Ankle Injuries–surgery | Foot
Joints–surgery
Classification: LCC RD563 | NLM WE 880 | DDC 617.5/85059–
dc23 LC record available at https://lccn.loc.gov/2017058035

© 2018 Thieme Medical Publishers, Inc.

Thieme Publishers New York
333 Seventh Avenue, New York, NY 10001 USA
+1 800 782 3488, customerservice@thieme.com

Thieme Publishers Stuttgart
Rüdigerstrasse 14, 70469 Stuttgart, Germany
+49 [0]711 8931 421, customerservice@thieme.de

Thieme Publishers Delhi
A-12, Second Floor, Sector-2, Noida-201301
Uttar Pradesh, India
+91 120 45 566 00, customerservice@thieme.in

Thieme Publishers Rio de Janeiro, Thieme Publicações Ltda.
Edifício Rodolpho de Paoli, 25º andar
Av. Nilo Peçanha, 50 – Sala 2508,
Rio de Janeiro 20020-906 Brasil
+55 21 3172-2297 / +55 21 3172-1896

Cover design: Thieme Publishing Group
Typesetting by DiTech Process Solutions

Printed in The United States of America by
King Printing Company, Inc.   5 4 3 2 1

ISBN 978-1-62623-491-8

Also available as an e-book:
eISBN 978-1-62623-492-5

Important note: Medicine is an ever-changing science undergoing continual development. Research and clinical experience are continually expanding our knowledge, in particular our knowledge of proper treatment and drug therapy. Insofar as this book mentions any dosage or application, readers may rest assured that the authors, editors, and publishers have made every effort to ensure that such references are in accordance with **the state of knowledge at the time of production of the book.**

Nevertheless, this does not involve, imply, or express any guarantee or responsibility on the part of the publishers in respect to any dosage instructions and forms of applications stated in the book. **Every user is requested to examine carefully** the manufacturers' leaflets accompanying each drug and to check, if necessary in consultation with a physician or specialist, whether the dosage schedules mentioned therein or the contraindications stated by the manufacturers differ from the statements made in the present book. Such examination is particularly important with drugs that are either rarely used or have been newly released on the market. Every dosage schedule or every form of application used is entirely at the user's own risk and responsibility. The authors and publishers request every user to report to the publishers any discrepancies or inaccuracies noticed. If errors in this work are found after publication, errata will be posted at www.thieme.com on the product description page.

Some of the product names, patents, and registered designs referred to in this book are in fact registered trademarks or proprietary names even though specific reference to this fact is not always made in the text. Therefore, the appearance of a name without designation as proprietary is not to be construed as a representation by the publisher that it is in the public domain.

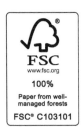

Contents

Contents

Contents

Foreword

This book provides a very utilitarian approach to guiding both the novice and the more advanced surgeon through the steps of a plethora of surgical procedures. I appreciate the standardized organization of each chapter that facilitates reading and seeking out a particular technique in which one has a specific interest. This step-by-step format also makes it easy to skim through a topic and find a specific aspect of the procedure that the reader wants to review, and the book is very well illustrated throughout.

Chapters are written by experts in that particular procedure and those who have developed a specific technique or who have popularized the surgery through innovation and their own research. This adds not only to the credibility of the material, but consistently brings to the reader a current and authoritative view of the topic. This is particularly notable with the various chapters on ankle replacement, which are written by one of the designers of that prosthesis; the reader benefits immensely by having a senior surgeon who was involved in the design process write their technique and tips that are essential to anyone using that prosthesis.

Books written in this consistent style enable the reader to learn about a particular technique, but perhaps without an in depth understanding of why that procedure works for the surgeon-author. To some extent, this is overcome by having multiple chapters on a similar topic, for example chronic ankle instability which includes both arthroscopic and open techniques as well as the simpler and augmented approaches. This style is especially useful for the surgeon who knows what he or she wants to do, and needs further clarification of the technical approach. Occasionally, however, one might want to know more about variations on a procedure rather than the author's own approach. This does not in any way detract from the success of the very comprehensive, detailed perspective on a particular technique which the reader will find most useful. I congratulate Dr. Raikin on a very well-thought-out book which has been written in a consistent style, focusing on techniques and tips by leaders in the field.

Mark Myerson, MD
Medical Director
Step by Step
The Foot and Ankle Association
Baltimore, Maryland

Preface

The field of foot and ankle corrective surgery continues to rapidly evolve in understanding and management. Through better understanding of the biomechanics of the foot and ankle and improved outcome research, our surgical techniques have advanced exponentially to give our patients superior results and improved functional outcomes. With these advancements have come new procedures and refined techniques, each with specific nuances honed by experts who have developed and improved these techniques through experience and study.

There are numerous textbooks on foot and ankle surgery and most of these expound in detail the historic understanding of the pathology, clinical evaluation, diagnostic options and varied treatment options. These, however, are literature-based and often do not direct the reader to what the expert author feels is the best surgical choice. Other surgical technique guides expand into the "how to do it," yet may lack specific tricks that the author surgeons themselves use to optimize their own results.

This *Tricks of the Trade* book invites experts in the field to share step-by-step ways to perform specific common foot and ankle procedures in a concise, easy-to-read, and well-illustrated format. This is aimed to assist the novice or less experienced foot and ankle surgeon to easily review and feel more comfortable in performing common foot and ankle procedures. Additionally, each author has shared their tricks and pearls in optimizing the performance of the procedure, in addition to offering suggestions to avoid or troubleshoot problems should they occur intraoperatively. Each succinct chapter takes the reader from patient assessment through pertinent diagnostic evaluations, patient selection, surgical planning/positioning, the procedure itself, and the postoperative management.

The book is divided into forefoot, midfoot, hindfoot and ankle pathologies – including commonly performed reconstructive and traumatic procedures. Experts share different techniques for similar pathologies, such as different chapters on open and arthroscopic lateral ankle ligament reconstruction, as well as augmentation options utilizing tendon allograft or an Internal Brace. The book also includes detailed techniques outlining the advantages of six different total ankle replacement systems, many written by the designers of the system themselves, offering the reader the option of choosing which system they would like to use while still becoming comfortable in the specific distinctions of each technique.

Another specific goal of this text is that every chapter was written according to an identical outline, making it easy for the reader to find the pertinent portion of a chapter they may wish to reference.

Each chapter begins with a brief summary followed by the text itself, starting with an introduction in point form outlining the following:
• **Indications**
• **Pathology**
• **Clinical Evaluation**
• **Radiographic Evaluation**
• **Nonoperative Options**
• **Contraindications**

This is followed by a point form outline of the following:
• **Goals of Surgical Procedure**
• **Advantages of Surgical Procedure**
• **Key Principles**

The next section on operative technique is the meat of the chapter where the author explains the following:
• **Preoperative Preparation and Patient Positioning**
• **Operative Technique**
• **Tips and Pearls**
• **Hazards and Pitfalls**
• **Complications/Bailout/Salvage**
• **Postoperative Care**

Chapters end with a brief report of outcomes with references, and each chapter is punctuated with a combination of artist-drawn illustrations and intraoperative photographs demonstrating the details of the procedure.

I have recruited an assembly of experts from around the world, representing 12 different countries and every field of foot and ankle surgery, to contribute their expert suggestions and pearls of management. There is input from 93 contributing authors, whose expertise and wealth of knowledge and experience in performing foot and ankle surgery has been condensed down to the essentials needed by every surgeon to successfully perform the surgical procedures included in this book. It is our hope that the quality of information and the format used will assist foot and ankle surgeons in optimally treating patients and alleviate any anxiety often faced in performing many of these procedures.

Steven M. Raikin, MD

Acknowledgments

Any text is only as good as the efforts of the participating authors. I invited exclusively senior and experienced surgeons to participate in writing chapters for this book, all of whom have busy clinical practices and a myriad of academic responsibilities and commitments. It is because of their enthusiastic involvement and commitment to this project that the book was able to be completed and offer such high-quality information. I thank each of the authors for their time, dedication to quality, and willingness to share their expertise and knowledge which they have taken so many years to perfect. Most authors wrote their chapters in the evenings and on weekends. This has required a personal sacrifice by them, and even more so by their spouses and families – and I thank each of them for allowing the chapters to be written and the book completed.

This project would also not have been possible without the support from the dedicated team at Thieme: Bill Lamsback (Execute Editor), Sarah Landis (Managing Editor), and Andrea Hines (medical illustrator).

On a personal note, I would like to acknowledge my wife Belinda, my rock and compass in life, and my three special children Daniel, Jared, and Talia. They forfeited the most of my time and attention, while never wavering from their support of my endeavor to create this text. I would also like to acknowledge my greatest fans and supporters, my parents Harold and Irma Raikin, and my in-laws Julian and Eileen Tankin, for their support and encouragement over the years without which I would never be where I am today. Finally, I would like to thank my mentors in the field of foot and ankle surgery, all of whom have inspired me to be the best physician I can be.

Steven M. Raikin, MD

Contributors

Jorge I. Acevedo, MD
Director
Foot and Ankle Center of Excellence
Southeast Orthopedic Specialists
Jacksonville, Florida

Samuel B. Adams, MD
Department of Orthopaedic Surgery
Duke University Medical Center
Durham, North Carolina

Meshal Alhadhoud, MBBCh, SB-Orth
Orthopaedic Surgeon
Dalhousie University
Queen Elizabeth II Health Sciences Center, Halifax Infirmary
Halifax, Nova Scotia, Canada

Robert B. Anderson, MD
Founder, Foot and Ankle
OrthoCarolina
Charlotte, North Carolina
Director, Foot and Ankle
Titletown Sport Medicine and Orthopaedics
Green Bay, Wisconsin

Mauricio P. Barbosa, MD
Northwestern University-Feinberg School of Medicine
Department of Orthopedic Surgery
Northwestern Memorial Hospital
Evanston, Illinois

**Andrew D. Beischer, MD, MBBS, FRACS, FAOrthA,
Dip Anat, Dip Bus (Gov)**
Consultant Orthopaedic Foot & Ankle Surgeon
Victorian Orthopaedic Foot & Ankle Clinic
Melbourne, Victoria, Australia

Gregory C. Berlet, MD, FRCS(C), FAOA
Orthopedic Foot and Ankle Center
Columbus, Ohio

Michael Brage, MD
Associate Professor
Department of Orthopaedics
University of Washington
Seattle, Washington

James W. Brodsky, MD
Clinical Professor of Orthopaedic Surgery
University of Texas Southwestern Medical School
Professor of Surgery, Orthopaedics
Texas A & M HSC College of Medicine
Director, Foot and Ankle Surgery Fellowship Program
Baylor University Medical Center
Dallas, Texas

James D.F. Calder, MD, PhD, FRCS(Tr & Orth), FFSEM(UK)
Consultant Orthopaedic Surgeon and Visiting Professor
Fortius Clinic and Imperial College
London, United Kingdom

John Campbell, MD
Foot and Ankle Orthopaedic Surgeon
Mercy Medical Center
Baltimore, Maryland

Christopher P. Chiodo, MD
Foot and Ankle Division Chief
Department of Orthopaedic Surgery
Brigham and Women's Hospital
Harvard Medical School
Boston, Massachusetts

Elizabeth A. Cody, MD
Fellow
Orthopaedic Foot and Ankle Surgery
Duke University
Durham, North Carolina

J. Chris Coetzee, MD
Twin Cities Orthopedics
Minneapolis, Minnesota

Elizabeth H. Coughlin, NP-C
Orthopaedic Nurse Practitioner
Saint Alphonsus Regional
Medical Center Coughlin Clinic
Boise, Idaho

Michael J. Coughlin, MD
Director
Coughlin Foot and Ankle Clinic
Saint Alphonsus Hospital
Boise, Idaho
Clinical Professor of Orthopaedic Surgery
University of California San Francisco
San Francisco, California

Joseph N. Daniel, DO
Orthopedic Surgeon
Rothman Institute
Sewell, New Jersey

Timothy R. Daniels, MD, FRCS(C)
Head
Division of Orthopaedic Surgery
St. Michael's Hospital
Professor
University of Toronto
Head, Foot, & Ankle Program
Toronto, Ontario, Canada

W. Hodges Davis, MD
Medical Director
OrthoCarolina Foot and Ankle Institute
Charlotte, North Carolina

Jonathan Deland, MD
Attending Orthopaedic Surgeon
Hospital for Special Surgery
Professor of Clinical Orthopaedic Surgery
Weill Cornell Medical College
New York, New York

Vincenzo Denaro, MD
Department of Orthopedic and Trauma Surgery
Campus Biomedico University of Rome
Rome, Italy

Sheryl de Waard, MD
PhD Candidate
Slotervaart Centre of Orthopedic Research and Education (SCORE)
Amsterdam, The Netherlands

Christopher Diefenbach, MD
Foot & Ankle Surgery Service
Department of Orthopaedics
University of California, Davis
Sacramento, California

Mark E. Easley, MD
Associate Professor
Department of Orthopaedic Surgery
Duke University Medical Center
Durham, North Carolina

Scott J. Ellis, MD
Associate Professor
Orthopaedic Foot and Ankle Surgery
The Hospital for Special Surgery
New York, New York

Cesare Faldini, MD
Professor
Bologna University
Clinical Orthopaedic and Traumatology
Rizzoli Orthopaedic Institute
Bologna, Italy

Eric I. Ferkel, MD
Orthopaedic Surgeon
Southern California Orthopedic Institute
Los Angeles, California

Richard D. Ferkel, MD
Director of the Sports Medicine Fellowship Program
Southern California Orthopedic Institute
Los Angeles, California

Wesley W. Flint, MD
Orthopaedic Surgeon
Coughlin Clinic, Saint Alphonsus Medical Group
Boise, Idaho

Joyce Fu, MD, MSc
Orthopaedic Surgery
University of Toronto
Toronto, Ontario, Canada

David N. Garras, MD
Orthopaedic Foot and Ankle Surgeon
Midwest Orthopaedic Consultants
Orland Park, Illinois
Assistant Professor
Department of Orthopaedic Surgery
University of Illinois at Chicago
Chicago, Illinois

Taggart T. Gauvain, MD
Assistant Professor of Orthopaedic Surgery
UT Physicians Department of Orthopaedics
University of Texas McGovern Medical School
Houston, Texas

Sandro Giannini, MD
Professor
Bologna University
Clinical Orthopaedic and Traumatology
Rizzoli Orthopaedic Institute
Bologna, Italy

Eric Giza, MD
Foot & Ankle Surgery Service
Department of Orthopaedics
University of California, Davis
Sacramento, California

Mark Glazebrook, MSc, PhD, MD, FRCS (C)
Professor of Surgery
Dalhousie University & Queen Elizabeth II Health Sciences
Center
Halifax, Nova Scotia, Canada

Gregory P. Guyton, MD
Department of Orthopaedic Surgery
MedStar Union Memorial Hospital
Baltimore, Maryland

Steven L. Haddad, MD
Senior Attending Physician
Illinois Bone and Joint Institute, LLC
Glenview, Illinois

Andrew Harston, MD
Orthopedic Surgeon
Norton Orthopedic Specialists
Louisville, Kentucky

Daniel Haverkamp, MD, PhD
Orthopedic Surgeon
Slotervaart Centre of Orthopedic Research and
Education (SCORE)
Amsterdam, The Netherlands

Ben Hickey, BM, MRCS, MSc, FRCS, MD
Trauma and Orthopaedic Registrar
Morriston Hospital
Swansea, Wales, United Kingdom

Beat Hintermann, MD
Clinic for Orthopedic and Trauma Surgery
Kantonsspital Baselland
Switzerland

Clifford L. Jeng, MD
Medical Director
Institute for Foot and Ankle Reconstruction
Mercy Medical Center
Baltimore, Maryland

Carroll P. Jones, MD
Director, Foot and Ankle Fellowship
OrthoCarolina
Charlotte, North Carolina

Mackenzie Jones, BA
Medical Student
University of Miami Miller School of Medicine
Miami, Florida

Anish R. Kadakia, MD
Northwestern University-Feinberg School of Medicine
Department of Orthopedic Surgery
Northwestern Memorial Hospital
Evanston, Illinois

John G. Kennedy, MD, MCh, FRCS
Hospital for Special Surgery
New York, New York

Christopher Kreulen, MD
Foot & Ankle Surgery Service
Department of Orthopaedics
University of California, Davis
Sacramento, California

James C. Krieg, MD
Professor and Chief of Orthopaedic Surgery
Rothman Institute at Thomas Jefferson University
Philadelphia, Pennsylvania

Trapper A.J. Lalli, MD
Assistant Professor
Department of Orthopaedic Surgery
University of Texas Southwestern Medical Center
Dallas, Texas

Johnny T.C. Lau, MD, MSc, FRCSC
Assistant Professor
Department of Orthopaedic Surgery
University of Toronto
Toronto, Ontario, Canada

David J. Love, MD
Resident Physician
Department of Orthopaedic Surgery
MedStar Georgetown University Hospital
Washington, DC

Gordon M. Mackay, BSc, FRCS(Orth), FFSEM(UK), MD
Professor
University of Stirling
Stirling, Scotland

Nicola Maffulli, MD, MS, PhD, FRCP, FRCS (Orth)
Department of Musculoskeletal Disorders
Faculty of Medicine and Surgery
University of Salerno
Centre for Sports and Exercise Medicine
Barts and the London School of Medicine and Dentistry
Mile End Hospital
London, England
Salerno, Italy

Peter G. Mangone, MD
Co-Director
Fook and Ankle Center of Excellence
Blue Ridge Bone & Joint
Division of Emergeortho
Arden, North Carolina

Richard M. Marks, MD, FACS
Professor
Department of Orthopaedic Surgery
Director
Division of Foot and Ankle Surgery
Medical College of Wisconsin
Milwaukee, Wisconsin

Lyndon Mason, MB BCh, MRCS, FRCS (Tr&Orth)
Consultant Orthopaedic Surgeon
University Hospital Aintree
Honorary Clinical Senior Lecturer
Liverpool, United Kingdom

Graham McCollum, MBChB (UCT), FC Orth (SA), MMED (UCT)
Orthopaedic Surgeon
Department of Orthopaedics
University of Cape Town
Cape Town, Western Cape, South Africa

William C. McGarvey, MD
Associate Professor
Residency Program Director
Fellowship Program Director
McGovern Medical School at the University of Texas Health
Science Center- Houston
Houston, Texas

Adam G. Miller, MD
Orthopaedic Surgeon
Foot and Ankle Specialist
Beacon Orthopaedics and Sports Medicine
Cincinnati, Ohio

Andy Molloy, MBChB, MRCS, FRCS Tr & Orth
Consultant Orthopaedic Surgeon
University Hospital Aintree
Honorary Clinical Senior Lecturer
Liverpool, United Kingdom

Alireza Mousavian, MD
Assistant Professor
Department of Orthopedics
Mashhad University of Medical Sciences
Iran

Steven K. Neufeld, MD
Foot & Ankle Orthopedic Surgeon
Orthopaedic Foot & Ankle Center of Washington
Falls Church, Virginia

Martin J. O'Malley, MD
Attending Orthopaedic Surgeon
Hospital for Special Surgery
Associate Professor of Orthopaedics
Weill Medical College of Cornell University Team
Physician, Brooklyn Nets
New York, New York

Rocco Papalia, MD, PhD
Department of Orthopedic and Trauma Surgery
Campus Biomedico University of Rome
Rome, Italy

Selene G. Parekh, MD, MBA, FAOA
Co-Chief Foot and Ankle Division
Professor, Department of Orthopaedic Surgery
Partner, North Carolina Orthopaedic Clinic
Adjunct Faculty, Fuqua Business School
Duke University
Durham, North Carolina

Milap S. Patel, DO
Northwestern University-Feinberg School of Medicine
Department of Orthopedic Surgery
Northwestern Memorial Hospital
Evanston, Illinois

David I. Pedowitz, MS, MD
Associate Professor
Department of Orthopaedic Surgery
Thomas Jefferson University
Foot and Ankle Division
The Rothman Institute
Philadelphia, Pennsylvania

Walter J. Pedowitz, MD
Clinical Professor
Department of Orthopaedic Surgery
Columbia University
College of Physicians & Surgeons
Union County Orthopedic Group
New York, New York

Anthony M.N.S. Perera, MBChB, FRCS(Orth)
Consultant Orthopaedic Foot and Ankle Surgeon
University Hospital of Wales, Cardiff
Cardiff, United Kingdom

Rupesh Puna, MBChB, FRACS (Orth)
Clinical Orthopaedic Fellow
Dalhousie University
Queen Elizabeth II Health Sciences Centre, Halifax
Infirmary Site
Halifax, Nova Scotia, Canada

Omar F. Rahman, MD, MBA
Resident Physician
Department of Orthopaedic Surgery
Lenox Hill Hospital - Northwell Health
New York, New York

Steven M. Raikin, MD
Director
Foot and Ankle Services
Rothman Institute
Professor of Orthopaedic Surgery
Thomas Jefferson Medical College
Philadelphia, Pennsylvania

Christopher W. Reb, DO
Orthopaedic Surgeon
University of Florida Orthopaedic and Sports Medicine
Institute
Gainesville, Florida

William J. Ribbans, PhD, FRCS(Orth), FFSEM(UK)
Professor
University of Northampton
Northampton, England, United Kingdom

David R. Richardson, MD
Associate Professor
Department of Orthopaedic Surgery
University of Tennessee-Campbell Clinic
Memphis, Tennessee

Andrew W. Ross, BA
Hospital for Special Surgery
New York, New York

Roxa Ruiz, MD
Clinic for Orthopedic and Trauma Surgery
Kantonsspital Baselland
Switzerland

Jefferson Sabatini, MD
Foot and Ankle Attending Surgeon
OrthoCarolina Foot and Ankle Institute
Charlotte, North Carolina

Lew C. Schon, MD, FACS
Director of Foot and Ankle Fellowship and Orthobiologic
Laboratory
Chief of Foot and Ankle Division
Department of Orthopaedic Surgery
MedStar Union Memorial Hospital
Baltimore Maryland
Associate Professor
Department of Orthopaedics
Georgetown School of Medicine
Washington DC
Associate Professor
Departments of Orthopaedics and Biomedical Engineering
Johns Hopkins University
Baltimore Maryland
Fischell Literati Faculty
University of Maryland Fischell Department of Bioengineering
College Park, Maryland

R. Schuh, MD, PD
Department of Pediatric Orthopaedics and Adult Foot and
Ankle
Orthopaedic Hospital Speising
Vienna, Austria

Yoshiharu Shimozono, MD
Hospital for Special Surgery
New York, New York

Mary Kate Thayer, MD
Resident Physician
Department of Orthopaedics
University of Washington
Seattle, Washington

Matthew Stewart, MD
Orthopedic Surgeon
Hughston Clinic
Columbus, Georgia

Guglielmo Torre, MD
Department of Orthopedic and Trauma Surgery
Campus Biomedico University of Rome
Rome, Italy

H.J. Trnka, MD
Foot and Ankle Center, Vienna
Vienna, Austria

Francesca Vannini, MD, PhD
Bologna University
Clinical Orthopaedic and Traumatology
Rizzoli Orthopaedic Institute
Bologna, Italy

Chuanshun Wang, MD
Attending Physician, Orthopedic Surgeon
Shanghai General Hospital
Shanghai Jiao Tong University School of Medicine
Shanghai, China

Steven B. Weinfeld, MD
Associate Professor
Department of Orthopaedic Surgery
Chief; Foot and Ankle Surgery
Icahn School of Medicine at Mount Sinai
New York, New York

Brian S. Winters, MD
Orthopaedic Surgeon
Rothman Institute
Egg Harbor Township, New Jersey

Dane K. Wukich, MD
Chair
Department of Orthopaedic Surgery
University of Texas Southwestern Medical Center
Dallas, Texas

Youichi Yasui, MD
Department of Orthopaedic Surgery
Teikyo University School of Medicine
Tokyo, Japan

Nicholas E.M. Yeo, MD
Fellow
Foot and Ankle Program
University of British Columbia
Vancouver, British Columbia, Canada

Alastair Younger, MB ChB, MSc, ChM, FRCSC
Orthopaedic Foot and Ankle Surgeon
Professor
Head Division of Distal Extremities
Department of Orthopaedics
University of British Columbia.
Director of Foot and Ankle Research
St. Paul's Hospital
Vancouver, British Columbia, Canada

Jacob R. Zide, MD
Assistant Professor
Department of Orthopaedic Surgery
University of Texas Southwestern Medical School
Assistant Professor
Department of Orthopaedic Surgery
Texas A&M Health Science Center College of Medicine
Dallas, Texas

1   Hammertoe Correction (Proximal Interphalangeal Resection)

Richard M. Marks

Abstract

Symptomatic hammertoe deformity that is not amenable to shoe modifications and/or stabilization or protective devices requires surgical resection of the proximal interphalangeal (PIP) joint with K-wire stabilization. Associated soft-tissue contractures are addressed with capsular and/or tendon releases to balance the PIP and metatarsophalangeal (MTP) joints. PIP fusion may be performed for more advanced deformity or revision procedures, and may be stabilized with either a K-wire or intramedullary implant.

Keywords: *hammertoe, claw toe, proximal interphalangeal joint, lesser toes, lesser toe deformity*

1.1   Indications and Pathology

- Plantarflexion deformity of the proximal interphalangeal (PIP) joint due to imbalance between the intrinsic and extrinsic musculature.
- The deformity may be fixed or flexible.
- Frequently associated with dorsiflexion of the metatarsophalangeal (MTP) joint secondary to contracture of the extensor tendons.
- Medial or lateral deviation at the MTP joint may be present as a result of collateral ligament attenuation.
- Attenuation of the plantar MTP structures (plantar plate) with instability of the MTP joint is seen with more advanced deformities.
- Resultant deformity creates a painful bony prominence at PIP joint, frequently with associated callosity. Plantar pain at MTP joint results from protective soft tissues translated off weight-bearing surface.

1.1.1   Nonoperative Options

- Shoes with a soft leather and high toe box.
- Elasticized stabilization toe splint for flexible hammertoe.
- Gel protective sleeve over PIP joint.
- If metatarsalgia, accommodative orthotic with padding behind metatarsal head.

1.1.2   Clinical Evaluation of Pathology

- Observe patient in a standing (functional) position.
- Determine flexibility of PIP joint.
- Determine degree of contracture of the extensor tendons:
  ○ Does deformity correct with plantarflexion of foot? (Tight flexors.)
  ○ Does deformity correct with dorsiflexion of foot? (Tight extensors.)
- Is metatarsalgia present?
- Is the MTP joint unstable?

1.1.3   Radiology Studies

- Weight-bearing foot radiographs (anteroposterior, oblique, lateral).
- Advanced imaging studies not typically indicated.

1.1.4   Contraindications for Surgery

- Poor circulation to toe.
- Open/infected ulceration over PIP joint.

1.2   Goals of Surgical Procedure

- Correct bony deformity and soft-tissue inflammation at PIP joint.
- Correct dorsiflexion and medial/lateral deviation deformity of MTP joint.
- Alleviate associated metatarsalgia.

1.3   Advantages of Surgical Procedure

- Correction of painful deformity.
- Eliminates need for protective/supportive devices.
- Surgery associated with low recurrence and complication rate.

1.4   Key Principles

- Adequate bone resection to correct deformity; shorten as necessary.
- Avoid over-resection with excessive shortening of toe.
- Balance and release contracted soft tissues as necessary to obtain soft-tissue correction.
- Tendon transfers performed as indicated.
- Shortening metatarsal osteotomy for intractable metatarsalgia and excessive metatarsal length.
- Protect soft tissues during bony resection.
- Protect vasculature during dissection and bone resection.

1.5   Preoperative Preparation and Patient Positioning

- Ensure adequate peripheral digit perfusion.
- Ankle-brachial indexes (ABIs) if poor pulses.
- Ensure adequate soft tissues.
- Counsel patients about postoperative stiffness of the PIP joint and risk of compromised circulation in advanced, fixed deformities with MTP instability.

- Surgery typically performed under regional anesthesia (ankle block) with sedation.
- Patient positioned supine on operating room table.
- Limb typically prepped/draped to above ankle.
- Esmarch or ankle tourniquet may be used to ensure a bloodless field.

1.6 Operative Technique

1.6.1 Surgical Procedure

- Incision (**Fig. 1.1**) should be made in either of the following ways:
  - Longitudinal, centered over PIP joint: allows for proximal/distal extension.
  - Elliptical, centered over PIP joint: cosmetically more pleasing, not extensile.
- Flex PIP joint during incision (**Fig. 1.2**).
- Incise straight through extensor hood (**Fig. 1.3**).
- Centralize extensor hood with forceps, and excise (**Fig. 1.4**).
- Release collateral ligaments to fully expose head and neck of proximal phalanx (**Fig. 1.5**).
- Protect soft tissues with Hohmann retractors; secure proximal phalanx with small towel clip.
- Resect at level of head–neck juncture with a microsagittal saw (**Fig. 1.6**).
- Assess adequacy of resection (**Fig. 1.7**).
- Perform additional soft-tissue balancing as indicated (separate dorsal incision):
  - Dorsiflexion at MTP joint:
    - ❖ Perform MTP capsulotomy; if incomplete correction, then lengthen the extensor longus and brevis tendon medial or lateral deviation in frontal plane (crossover deformity).
    - ❖ Capsular release biased toward direction of deviation; if incomplete, collateral ligament release on contracted side, tendon lengthening/release as indicated.
  - Plantarflexion at distal interphalangeal joint:
    - ❖ Secondary to tight long flexor (claw toe, or neuromuscular disorder).
    - ❖ Isolate long flexor through dorsal PIP incision, and transect or percutaneous release from plantar aspect foot.
  - Sagittal instability:
    - ❖ Dorsal capsulotomy, extensor tendon release.
    - ❖ Plantar plate repair at surgeon's discretion.
    - ❖ Flexor-to-extensor transfer at surgeon's discretion.
  - Metatarsalgia:
    - ❖ Perform shortening metatarsal osteotomy.
  - Flexion deformity with clawing:
    - ❖ Flexor tendon release.
- Fixation of PIP resection:
  - Stabilize with K-wire (0.045, 0.054, 0.062); size determined by canal width.
  - K-wire placed antegrade from base of middle phalanx, exiting distal tip of toe (**Fig. 1.8**).
  - Align with canal of proximal phalanx and advance retrograde.
  - K-wire may be advanced across MTP joint if additional stability required.
  - Fusion of the PIP joint may be performed for instability of the PIP joint or revision hammertoe surgery, or if additional shortening of the toe is required. Fusion may be performed with a K-wire or intramedullary implant.
- Closure performed with simple 4–0 nylon sutures:
  - If separate incision for soft-tissue balancing, close in two layers: 3–0 or 4–0 absorbable suture for subcutaneous layer; 4–0 nylon for skin.
- Soft forefoot dressing applied.

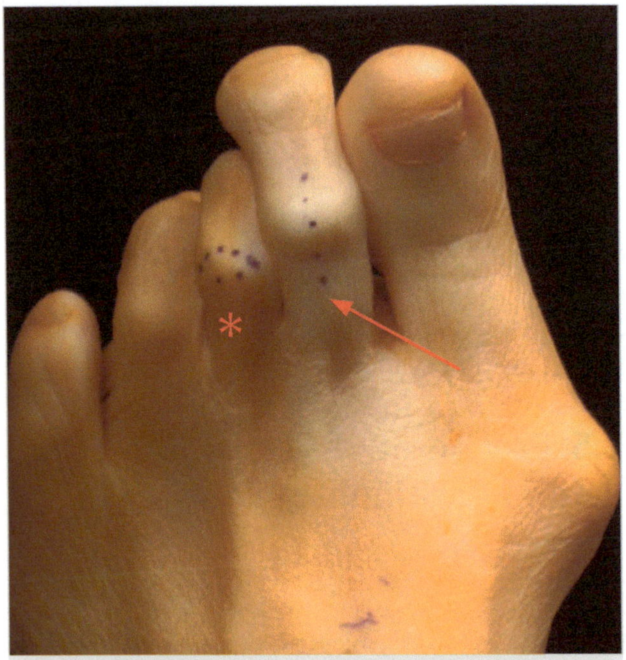

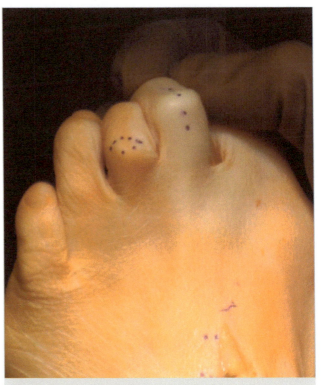

Fig. 1.1 A longitudinal (arrow) or elliptical (asterisk) incision may be utilized.

Fig. 1.2 The toe is flexed to perform incision.

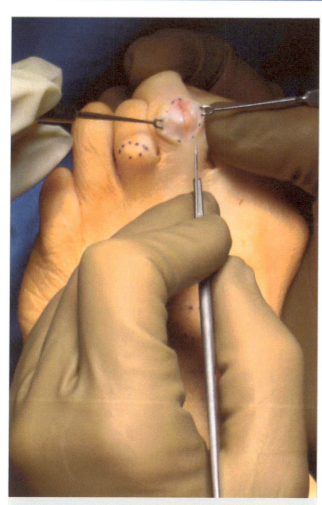

Fig. 1.3 Incision is completed through extensor hood.

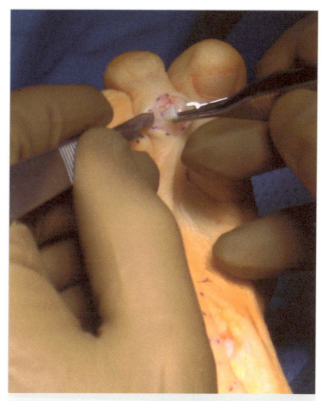

Fig. 1.4 Extensor hood is centralized and resected.

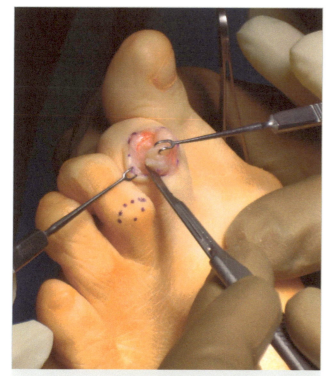

Fig. 1.5 Collateral ligaments are excised.

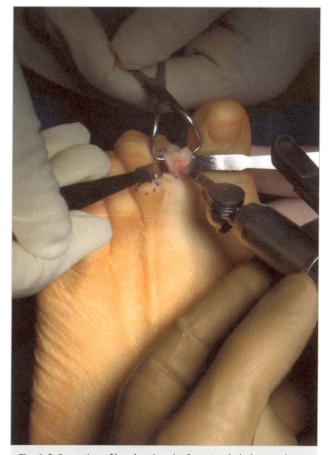

Fig. 1.6 Resection of head and neck of proximal phalanx with microsagittal saw.

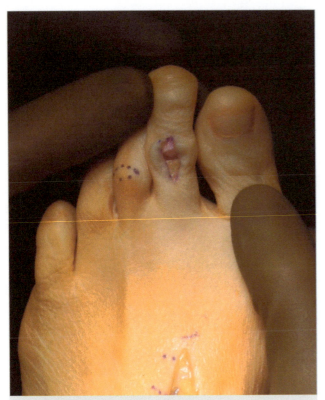

Fig. 1.7 Adequacy of resection evaluated.

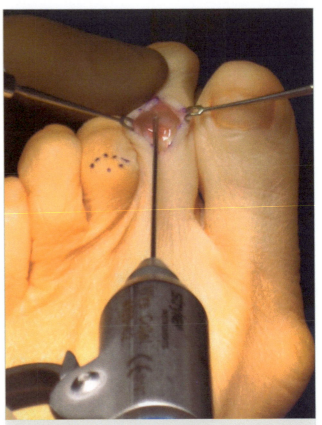

Fig. 1.8 Stabilization of resection performed with a K-wire placed antegrade (shown), then retrograde.

1.7 Tips and Pearls

- Evaluate digit perfusion and soft tissues preoperatively.
- Counsel patients that digit will be stiff postoperatively, but will not affect function.
- Assess need for soft-tissue balancing *prior* to Esmarch exsanguination (if tourniquet used).
- Evaluate adequacy of correction after bone resection; digit should extend without impingement.
- If additional shortening required after adequate resection, consider resection at base of middle phalanx (PIP fusion).
- Use a separate proximal incision when performing soft-tissue balancing; this creates more stability at base of proximal phalanx.
- When performing concomitant shortening metatarsal osteotomy, perform PIP resection *after* osteotomy.
- Sagittal instability may be adequately addressed with soft-tissue balancing and retrograde K-wire fixation across MTP joint.
- Slight plantarflexion of stabilization at MTP will assist with scarring of plantar soft tissues.
- Soft-tissue balancing can be evaluated with Esmarch released, prior to K-wire stabilization.
- Release tourniquet prior closure/dressing application to ensure perfusion of the digit:
  ○ If poor perfusion, back pin out of MTP joint, reposition.
  ○ May also distract or compress PIP joint.
  ○ If continued poor perfusion, reverse Trendelenburg position on table, use warm saline irrigation, consider Nitro-Dur paste.

1.8 Hazards and Pitfalls

- Avoid surgery on a poorly perfused digit.
- Avoid soft-tissue injury form microsagittal saw.
- Avoid under- or over-resection of proximal phalanx bone.
- Correct soft-tissue contracture/imbalance as completely as possible.
- Avoid incision extending proximal to MTP joint if possible; utilize a separate proximal incision.

1.9 Complications/Bailout/ Salvage

- Intraoperative poor toe perfusion:
  ○ Bailout: Reposition correction, reposition pin to avoid MTP joint, adjust length of correction of toe, pin removal completely.
- Bent pin postoperatively:
  ○ Bailout: Determine if pin is jeopardizing the soft tissues; if not, may remain. If yes, then remove and tape toe in corrected position.
- Pin track infection:
  ○ Bailout: Oral antibiotics, possible wound care.
  ○ Salvage: Remove pin, tape in corrected position.
- Loss of correction:
  ○ Bailout: Corrective taping, support devices.
  ○ Salvage: Revision correction, consider PIP fusion.

1.10 Postoperative Care

- Soft dressing, postoperative shoe or boot.
- Heel weight-bearing as necessary.
- Elevate when not ambulating.
- Suture removal between 10 and 14 days.
- Postoperative wraps determined by degree of swelling, additional procedures.
- Pin removal typically at 6 weeks (surgeon's discretion).
- Full weight-bearing in post-op shoe/boot allowed after pin removal.
- Wean from immobilization device after an additional 10 to 14 days.
- Physical therapy prescribed at surgeon's discretion; gait retraining, strengthening, edema control, modalities.
- Additional postoperative visits at
  - 10 weeks if concern for soft-tissue balance, swelling.
  - 3 months.
  - 6 months (surgeon's discretion).

1.11 Outcomes

Surgery is designed to correct deformity of the toe, relieve pain, and improve function. Patients should be counseled preoperatively to expect stiffness of the PIP joint. Swelling may persist for 3 to 4 months. A recent review of hammertoe correction with K-wire fixation in 2,698 procedures revealed maintenance of correction in 94.4%, with 3.5% of patients requiring revision for recurrent deformity. Complications associated with this procedure were quite low, including pin migration (3.5%), pin tract infection (0.3%), pin breakage (0.1%), recurrence (5.6%), and subsequent amputation (0.4%).[1]

Reference

1. Kramer WC, Parman M, Marks RM. Hammertoe correction with k-wire fixation. Foot Ankle Int 2015;36(5):494–502

2 Distal Oblique Metatarsal Osteotomy (Weil)

H.J. Trnka and R. Schuh

Abstract

Metatarsalgia secondary to mismatch within the metatarsal cascade due to a relatively long metatarsal can lead to deformities, such as claw toes, and pain particularly during the toe-off stage of gait. The distal oblique metatarsal osteotomy is a utilitarian procedure used to shorten the metatarsal, thereby elevating the metatarsal head and allowing relocation of the subluxed metatarsophalangeal joint and deformity correction. This can be achieved through a classical intra-articular osteotomy with screw fixation or through a minimally invasive extra-articular osteotomy at the metatarsal neck. Each of these options will be addressed and explained in this chapter.

Keywords: *distal metatarsal, osteotomy, oblique, metatarsalgia, Weil*

2.1 Introduction

Metatarsalgia is a widely used term for tenderness and pain in the forefoot. The many causes of metatarsalgia can be categorized in primary, secondary, and iatrogenic metatarsalgia.[1] Primary metatarsalgia refers to symptoms arising from innate abnormalities in the patient's anatomy, leading to overload of the affected metatarsal. These anomalies may include insufficiency of the first ray or a disproportionately long or plantarflexed metatarsal relative to the remaining rays of the forefoot. Secondary metatarsalgia includes metabolic disorders, gout, systemic disorders, rheumatoid arthritis, arthritides of metacarpophalangeal (MP) joints, trauma, neurological disorders, Morton's neuroma, tarsal tunnel syndrome, and Freiberg's disease. Iatrogenic metatarsalgia is caused by failed hallux valgus surgery, failed MP-I fusion, or failed corrective metatarsal osteotomies.

2.2 Pathobiomechanics

The basic knowledge of the gait cycle is mandatory in order to understand pathobiomechanic mechanisms causing metatarsalgia.[1] The stance (60% of the normal gait cycle) and the swing phase (40% of the normal cycle) form the normal gait cycle. The forefoot is in permanent contact with the ground throughout approximately half the gait cycle. In normal stance, the metatarsal heads all should rest evenly on the floor. The first, fourth, and fifth metatarsals are mobile in the sagittal plane. The second and third metatarsals are relatively fixed in position by rigid articulations with their corresponding cuneiforms. During walking, the foot functions as a three-rocker mechanism, providing physiologic balance between forward movement of the body and stability of the foot and leg during the stance phase.

The heel represents the first rocker, beginning with heel strike during the first 10% of the gait cycle. Metatarsalgia that is present in this particular phase of gait is usually caused by congenital deformities, for example, cavus foot or tight gastroc-soleus complex. A cavus foot has an abnormal increase in

longitudinal arch, which places all the weight-bearing on the heel and metatarsal heads, with little or no support from the lateral plantar midfoot. The toes commonly remain in extension in the metatarsophalangeal (MTP) joint with the greater flexion angles of the corresponding metatarsals. Weight-bearing pressure is concentrated under the metatarsal heads as a result of the abnormal foot position. Forefoot varus increases the amount of weight-bearing on the lateral aspect of the foot and leads to increased pressures under the fifth metatarsal head. In similar manner, forefoot valgus increases pressure under first metatarsal head.

The ankle is the second rocker during the next 20% of gait. In this phase (flat foot), the entire foot contacts the ground. Forefoot overloading occurs in this phase if ankle range of motion is restricted and if the plantarflexion of the metatarsals is increased. The pressure transfers rapidly toward the forefoot after heel strike. During toe-off, pressure moves rapidly toward the digits, primarily to the great toe. The first ray (first metatarsal or great toe) participates in 50% of weight-bearing and the lesser rays contribute the other 50%.

During the third rocker (toe-off), only the forefoot is in contact with the ground and the MTP joints are dorsiflexed. Therefore, deformities of the MTP joints can produce metatarsalgia. Additionally, pathologic conditions on one metatarsal can cause overload of the adjacent metatarsal. Hallux valgus alters first ray mechanics interrupting the windlass mechanism and weakening great toe flexion, which causes metatarsalgia. Hallux rigidus, first ray hypermobility, and iatrogenic weakening of the first MTP joint are common causes of metatarsalgia.

2.3 Indications

- Crossover toe deformity.
- Claw toe deformity.
- Dislocated or subluxed MTP joint.

2.3.1 Clinical Evaluation

- Clinical examination and a careful history and physical examination are the key to find the diagnosis. Patient's anamnesis is focused on pain localization, onset, and alleviating or aggravating factors. It is important to note skin changes and deformities such as claw toe, hammer toes, and hallux valgus because they increase pressure under the metatarsal heads.
- The patient's foot is evaluated in weight-bearing and non-weight-bearing position. Hindfoot pathologies are identified and ankle range of motion is evaluated.
- Second rocker keratosis is strictly plantar under the MT head located. The foot should be evaluated for abnormal plantarflexion of the lesser metatarsals. An elevated first metatarsal transfers the whole load to the second metatarsal. Gastroc-soleus contracture and pes cavus lead also to central keratoses under the lesser metatarsal heads.
- Third rocker keratosis is found more distal from the affected head.

- After inspection, the foot is palpated and functional evaluation is performed. Palpation begins systematically, from the front to the rear. The goals of palpation are the assessment of topographic anatomy and recognition of any deviations. All bony prominences, anatomic regions, and metatarsals should be palpated. The plantar aspect of the foot along with each digit must be examined for the development of callosities and MTP alignment. Each intermetatarsal web space is palpated to assess for tenderness of the intermetatarsal nerves.
- Stability of the MTP joints in the sagittal and transversal plane must be tested. The examiner stabilizes the metatarsal neck in one hand and attempts to displace the base of the proximal phalanx with the other hand while holding the joint in the neutral position (Lachman's test).
- Hypermobility of the first ray and limited dorsiflexion at the hallux-first MTP joint should be noted, as well as hallux rigidus. Also, inversion and eversion range of motion of the hindfoot as well as medial columns stability should be evaluated.[2]
- All muscles should be checked to assess strength and function. The Silfverskiöd method is used to evaluate for contracture of the gastroc-soleus complex.
- Ankle dorsiflexion is tested with the knee in full extension and in 90 degrees of flexion; the foot is maintained in an inverted position to avoid dorsiflexion movements at the midtarsal joints. Increased ankle dorsiflexion with the knee flexed indicates contracture of the gastrocnemius muscle.

2.3.2 Radiographic Evaluation

- Standard dorsoplantar and lateral weight-bearing radiographic views are obtained to evaluate the whole foot. The dorsoplantar view will help identify MTP joint congruency, arthritis, and metatarsal length, as well as the degree of hindfoot deformity accompanying the forefoot deformity. If metatarsus primus varus is present, hallux valgus angle and intermetatarsal angle can be assessed as well on dorsoplantar views.
- In a radiographic study, Maestro et al[3] introduced measures in order to assess forefoot geometry in detail on the dorsoplantar view.
- The lateral view can show collapse of the medial longitudinal arch and depict the magnitude of MTP joint dislocation.
- Plantarflexed metatarsals, bony and cutaneous prominences, and the sesamoids can be assessed upon axial radiograph. Bone scan and magnetic resonance imaging can be helpful adjuncts in the inspection of neoplasm and infection, whereas computed tomography scans can depict complex traumatic injuries. Ultimately, imaging should support the clinical examinations and the decision for operative intervention.[4]

2.3.3 Nonoperative Options

- For all causes, the first-line treatment of choice is nonsurgical therapy. This includes shoe modification (stiff sole, retro-capital metatarsal bar), custom foot orthoses with a metatarsal pad, and gastroc-soleus stretching exercises.
- Additionally, corticosteroid injections as well as shaving of callosities can be carried out.
- If nonoperative treatment fails, surgical options are considered.

2.3.4 Contraindications

- Impaired vascular blood supply.
- Chronic metatarsalgia without MTP joint involvement.
- Acute infection.

2.4 Goals of the Surgical Procedure

- Elevation of the metatarsal head.
- Decompression of the joint.
- Shortening of the metatarsal.
- Relocation of the joint.

2.5 Advantages of the Surgical Procedure

- Minimal surgical exposure.
- Ability to accurately realign the metatarsal cascade.
- Can be performed on multiple metatarsals.

2.6 Key Principles

- Dorsal incision centered over MTP joint.
- Z extensor tenotomy when needed.
- Dorsal capsular arthrotomy.
- Expose metatarsal head with McGlamry elevator.
- Osteotomy starts at the dorsal aspect of the articular cartilage of the metatarsal head and is directed parallel to the plantar aspect of the foot so as to exit within the distal plantar diaphysis of the metatarsal.
- Metatarsal head is shifted proximally (but not plantarly) so as to rebalance the metatarsal cascade.
- Fixation is undertaken with a headless "twist-off"-type screw.

2.7 Preoperative Preparation and Patient Positioning

All operations can be performed under a regional ankle block usually without Esmarch bandage as a tourniquet.

2.8 Operative Technique

2.8.1 Distal Oblique Metatarsal Osteotomy (Weil's Osteotomy)

The Weil osteotomy was first described by L.S. Weil in 1985 for the treatment of central metatarsalgia. In 1992, it was introduced in France by Barouk.[5] The goal of Weil's osteotomy is to achieve adequate proximal translation of the MT head in relation to the callus and to more evenly distribute pressure underneath the forefoot with adequate MT–ground contact during third rocker. It is an intra-articular osteotomy that achieves longitudinal decompression through shortening.[6]

A dorsal, longitudinal incision is made over the metatarsal for a single osteotomy and over the web space for a double osteotomy (**Fig. 2.1a, b**). The extensor tendons are usually lengthened (**Fig. 2.2**) and the metatarsal head and neck are identified. After incising the joint capsule, the toe is plantarflexed to expose the metatarsal head (**Fig. 2.3**). If needed, the collateral ligaments of the MTP joint are cut.

The plane of the osteotomy is parallel to the ground as if the foot was bearing weight Two osteotomies are performed (**Fig. 2.4**) and a slice of bone is removed (**Fig. 2.5**) to gain greater elevation of the metatarsal head. A pointed clamp is then used to grasp the mobile plantar fragment and shift it proximally to achieve the desired shortening. After the positioning is checked with the image intensifier, a screw is used to secure the two fragments (**Fig. 2.6**). The resulting dorsal protuberance on the metatarsal head is resected. We recommend the twist-off screw rather than K-wires for fixation of the Weil osteotomy. Most of the available minifragment screws need predrilling, which may dislocate the plantar fragment. The twist-off screw is used without predrilling. The resulting dorsal protuberance on the metatarsal head was resected.

Weight-bearing in a post-operative shoe is allowed immediately after surgery. A postoperative shoe is worn for 4 weeks and the patient is reviewed again at 4 weeks post surgery with standing anteroposterior (AP) and lateral radiographs to ensure position has been maintained. (**Fig. 2.7a-c**)

Postoperative complications include MTP joint stiffness, floating-toe deformity (**Fig. 2.8**, local second rocker metatarsalgia resulting from plantar shift of the lesser MT head, transfer metatarsalgia caused by extensive shortening, superficial wound healing problems and complex regional pain syndrome.[7]

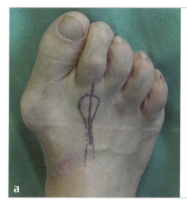
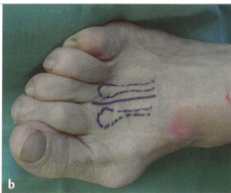

Fig. 2.1 (a) Longitudinal incision for a single Weil osteotomy centered over the shaft of the metatarsal. (b) Dorsal incision over the intermetatarsal space for two Weil's osteotomies.

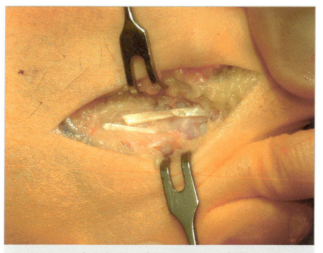

Fig. 2.2 Z-type lengthening of the extensor tendon.

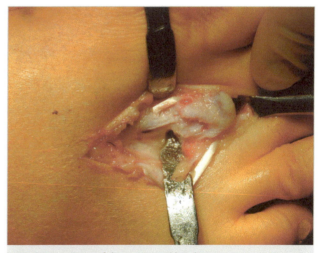

Fig. 2.3 Exposure of the metatarsal head.

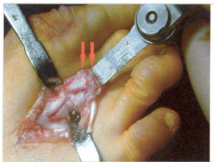
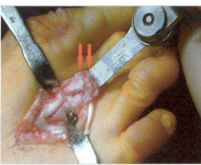

Fig. 2.4 Two osteotomies are performed in 2-mm distance parallel to the ground plane (*arrows*).

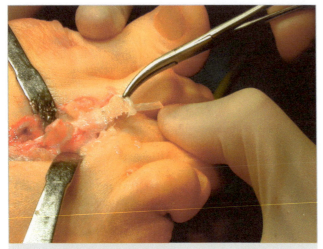

Fig. 2.5 A slice of bone is removed.

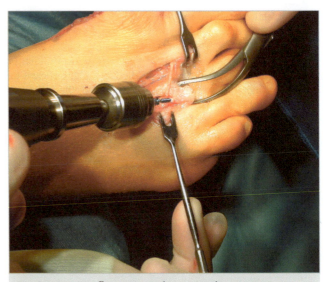

Fig. 2.6 A twist-off screw is used to secure the osteotomy.

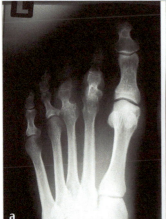
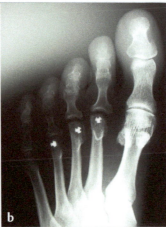
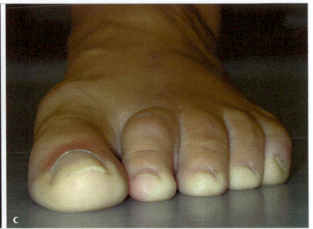

Fig. 2.7 (a) Preoperative radiograph with dislocation of the second and third MTP joint. (b) Two-year follow-up after Weil's osteotomies. (c) A clinically good result with ground contact of the toes.

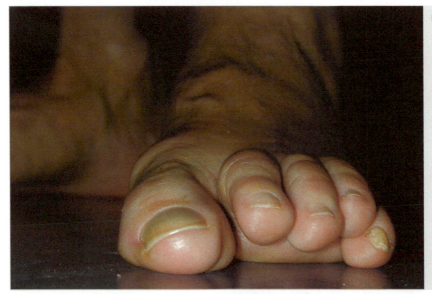

Fig. 2.8 Floating toes.

2.8.2 Minimally Invasive Weil's Osteotomy

Since its appearance, the Weil osteotomy has been the main surgical technique for the treatment of lesser metatarsal pathologies. However, from the early reports, postoperative stiffness and floating toes have been a serious issue. As already

mentioned, the resection of a slice of bone has been an approach to reduce the risk of floating toes. However, scarring and tendon shortening still contributed to prolonged stiffness and nonfavorable results.

The distal metatarsal mini-invasive Weil osteotomy is performed under fluoroscopic control. After marking the level of the metatarsal head, a stab incision is performed with a no. 11 scalpel. The stab incision is skin-deep only. Deepening of the incision or periosteal elevation is not required and might risk damaging the blood supply to the metatarsal head.

A rasp is used to create a working space around the metatarsal neck by elevating the soft tissue on either side of the osteotomy at the metatarsal neck.

A 12-mm Shannon burr is then inserted through this portal. The burr is then firmly rasped along the neck at an angle (45 degrees) relative to the metatarsal shaft at the level of the epiphysis–metaphysis junction to ensure the burr is on the bone (**Fig. 2.9**). The burr is then run on low speed and high torque. Once the burr has engaged the bone, the surgeon supinates the wrist in a smooth action until the burr lies flat on the foot at 90 degrees to the metatarsal axis in the AP plane (**Fig. 2.10**)

Once complete, the osteotomy should be mobile in the sagittal plane but should also telescope proximal–distal. If both these planes of motion are not present, then the osteotomy is not complete and the surgeon must replace the burr in the osteotomy to find where the intact bone remains, which must then be cut. No internal fixation is carried out. The incision is closed with nonresorbable suture.[6]

Since no internal fixation is used, the postoperative bandages are very important. The toes are strapped plantar side to ensure that with the plantarflexion of the toes the osteotomies are compressed. A postoperative shoe is worn for 4 weeks and the patient is reviewed again at 4 weeks postsurgical with standing AP and lateral radiographs to ensure position has been maintained.

The patient is allowed to return to his or her own footwear but can expect some limitation of choice of footwear for several months because of swelling.

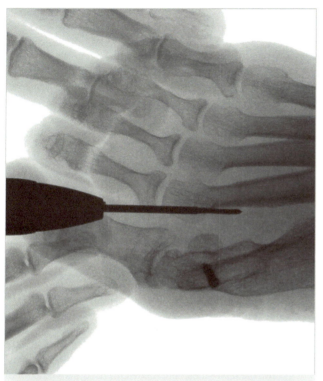

Fig. 2.9 Under fluoroscopic control, a 12-mm Shannon burr is placed at an angle of 45 degrees relative to the metatarsal shaft at the level of the epiphysis–metaphysis junction.

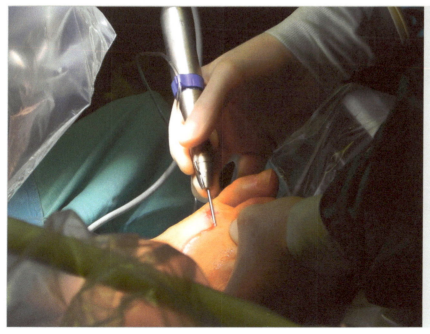

Fig. 2.10 Once the burr has engaged the bone, the surgeon supinates the wrist in a smooth action until the burr lies flat on the foot at 90 degrees to the metatarsal axis in the AP plane.

2.9 Tips and Pearls

2.9.1 Classic Weil

- In most cases, extensor tendon lengthening is necessary.
- The wedge resection is standard in our hands.

2.9.2 Minimally Invasive Weil

- Taping of the toes in slight plantarflexion.

2.10 Complications/Bailout/Salvage

Stiffness and floating toes are the major complications following the open Weil osteotomy. Extensor tendon lengthening and capsular release has shown to improve the ground contact of the toes. In the case of an additional hammertoe deformity, a proximal interphalangeal (PIP) fusion reveals better functional results than a PIP resection arthroplasty. If intraoperatively a hyperextension of the toe is already present, a temporary K-wire fixation of the toe into the metatarsal may reduce the extension.[8]

After minimally invasive Weil's osteotomy, prolonged swelling and even delayed bone healing may be seen. Usually, the bone heals without further intervention.

2.11 Postoperative Care

- Dressings and a tight bandage are used to protect the suture and to prevent swelling.
- Patient's toes are taped in a slight plantar flexion.
- Weight-bearing with a postoperative shoe is allowed immediately postoperatively.
- From time of surgery, patients will need the postoperative shoe for 4 weeks. Postoperative imaging includes dorsoplantar and lateral radiographs.
- Passive motion (starting on the fifth postoperative week) of the MTP joint is indicated and necessary to prevent postoperative extension contracture.
- If swelling occurs, foot elevation, cryotherapy, and wearing elastic stockings may keep the swelling under control.

2.12 Outcomes

The classic Weil osteotomy reveals excellent results in the correction of dislocated and subluxed lesser MTP joints.

Hofstaetter et al[9] showed in a previously published article with a follow-up of 7 years good clinical results and significant reduction of pain. Patients rated the outcome as excellent in 60% of the feet at 1 year and in 76% at 7 years postoperatively, respectively. Hart et al[4] reported 83% excellent results at 31 months after Weil's osteotomy. O'Kane and Kilmartin[10] reported about 85% completely satisfied patients 18 months postoperatively in 20 feet. At an average follow-up of 30 months, Vandeputte et al[11] reported excellent or good results for 32 of 37 feet (86%) in his series. Henry et al[12] performed a retrospective study on 39 patients operated by minimally invasive Weil's osteotomy and 33 patients operated by the standard Weil osteotomy technique. Sixty-seven patients were seen again with an average follow-up of 14.8 months (range, 12–24 months). The postoperative AOFAS score and the joint range of motion were comparable in both groups. After 3 months, edema and metatarsalgia were significantly greater in group 1. At the last follow-up, all the osteotomy sites had achieved union.

Our own preliminary study on the first 30 patients with minimally invasive Weil's osteotomies revealed a learning curve but the patient's satisfaction rate was high and the incidence of floating toes was less.

References

1. Espinosa N, Maceira E, Myerson MS. Current concept review: metatarsalgia. Foot Ankle Int 2008;29(8):871–879
2. Espinosa N, Brodsky JW, Maceira E. Metatarsalgia. J Am Acad Orthop Surg 2010;18(8):474–485
3. Maestro M, Besse JL, Ragusa,M, Berthonnaud E. Forefoot morphotype study and planning method for forefoot osteotomy. Foot Ankle Clin 2003 Dec;8(4):695–710
4. Hart R, Janecek M, Bucek P. The Weil osteotomy in metatarsalgia [in German]. Z Orthop Ihre Grenzgeb 2003;141(5):590–594
5. Barouk LS. Weil's metatarsal osteotomy in the treatment of metatarsalgia [in German]. Orthopade 1996;25(4):338–344
6. Redfern DJ, Vernois J. Percutaneous surgery for metatarsalgia and the lesser toes. Foot Ankle Clin 2016;21(3):527–550
7. Hofstaetter SG, Trnka HJ. Weil lesser metatarsal shortening osteotomyIn: Easley M, ed.Operative Techniques in Foot and Ankle Surgery. Philadelphia, PA: Lippincott Williams &Wilkins;2011:227–233
8. Highlander P, VonHerbulis E, Gonzalez A, Britt J, Buchman J. Complications of the Weil osteotomy. Foot Ankle Spec 2011;4(3):165–170
9. Hofstaetter SG, Hofstaetter JG, Petroutsas JA, Gruber F, Ritschl P, Trnka HJ. The Weil osteotomy: a seven-year follow-up. J Bone Joint Surg Br 2005;87(11):1507–1511
10. O'Kane C, Kilmartin TE. The surgical management of central metatarsalgia. Foot Ankle Int 2002;23(5):415–419
11. Vandeputte G, Dereymaeker G, Steenwerckx A, Peeraer L. The Weil osteotomy of the lesser metatarsals: a clinical and pedobarographic follow-up study. Foot Ankle Int 2000;21(5):370–374
12. Henry J, Besse JL, Fessy MH; AFCP. Distal osteotomy of the lateral metatarsals: a series of 72 cases comparing the Weil osteotomy and the DMMO percutaneous osteotomy. Orthop Traumatol Surg Res 2011 Oct;97(6 Suppl):S57–374

3 Treatment of Plantar Plate Tears of the Lesser Metatarsophalangeal Joints

Michael J. Coughlin, Wesley W. Flint, and Elizabeth H. Coughlin

Abstract

Instability of the lesser metatarsophalangeal joints has been appreciated since the original description of a crossover toe deformity in the 1980s. Only in the recent past has the actual pathology been described, which includes disruption or discontinuity of the plantar plate, with and without collateral ligament tears. By defining the actual pathologic issues, it has become possible to develop instrumentation and a surgical technique to perform a direct repair of plantar plate tears. A description of the pathology and the technique of surgical repair is provided in this chapter, as well as the postoperative regimen to assist in the rehabilitation process.

Keywords: *crossover second toe, plantar plate tear, instability lesser MTP joints, hammer toe deformity*

3.1 Indications

- Instability at the metatarsophalangeal (MTP) joint is due to ligamentous attenuation or rupture involving the supporting collateral ligaments along with the plantar plate.[1] Indication for surgery includes intractable pain and deformity due to an unstable lesser MTP joint.

3.1.1 Clinical Evaluation

- Plantar plate tears are diagnosed clinically using the drawer examination.[2] The drawer examination is graded 1 to 4 by the amount of subluxation achieved through dorsal translation of the proximal phalanx base at the MTP joint (**Fig. 3.1**).
- Grade 1 is less than 50% subluxation; grade 2 is between 50 and 100% subluxation; grade 3 is the ability to dislocate the MTP joint; grade 4 is a dislocated MTP joint.
- On intraoperative examination, tears of the plantar plate are graded into four types (**Fig. 3.2 a–d**):
- A grade 1 is a partial tear, with less than 50% of the distal plantar plate detached. A grade 2 tear is a distal plantar plate detachment between 50 and 100%. A grade 3 tear may have a distal transverse tear component, but also is characterized by a longitudinal plate tear. A grade 4 tear is an irreparable tear with little or no plantar plate available to reconstruct. (For these, a flexor tendon transfer is often performed.)

3.1.2 Radiographic Evaluation

- Weight-bearing plain radiographs are used to document the level of angular deformity at the lesser MTP joint and to rule out other bony causes of MTP joint pain.
- Magnetic resonance imaging (MRI) is not necessary to diagnose MTP instability; however, it may be helpful if confirming a suspicion.

- We find images from a 3-tesla MRI are most helpful to visualize the plantar plate when reformatted with fine sagittal slices.

3.1.3 Nonoperative Options

- Taping.
- Bracing.
- Orthotic inserts including metatarsal pads.
- Shoe modifications.

3.1.4 Contraindications

- Active infection.
- Vascular insufficiency.
- Severe deformity for which a soft-tissue repair would not be effective.
- Concomitant MTP joint arthrosis.
- Freiberg's infraction.
- Metatarsal head avascular necrosis.

3.2 Goals of Surgical Procedure

The goal of conservative treatment is to stabilize the deformity, reduce pain and swelling, and prevent the digit from further deformity. When pain and misalignment becomes more severe, the goals of surgical treatment are to stabilize the involved MTP joint, realign deformity, reduce pain, and return the patient to a higher level of function.[3]

3.3 Advantages of Surgical Procedure

Prior surgical treatment (1987–2011) involved indirect repairs of the misaligned digit including metatarsal and phalangeal osteotomies, soft-tissue releases and reefing, various tendon transfers, and even toe disarticulation.[4] Only with the definition of the true pathology of the plantar plate and collateral ligament dysfunction did a direct repair of the pathology become possible.[1]

3.4 Key Principles

- Dorsal approach with capsulotomy and collateral ligament release.
- Weil's osteotomy parallel to plantar aspect of the foot.
- Complete detachment of plantar plate distally.
- Plantar plate repair with horizontal mattress sutures.
- Proper collateral ligament tensioning as necessary.

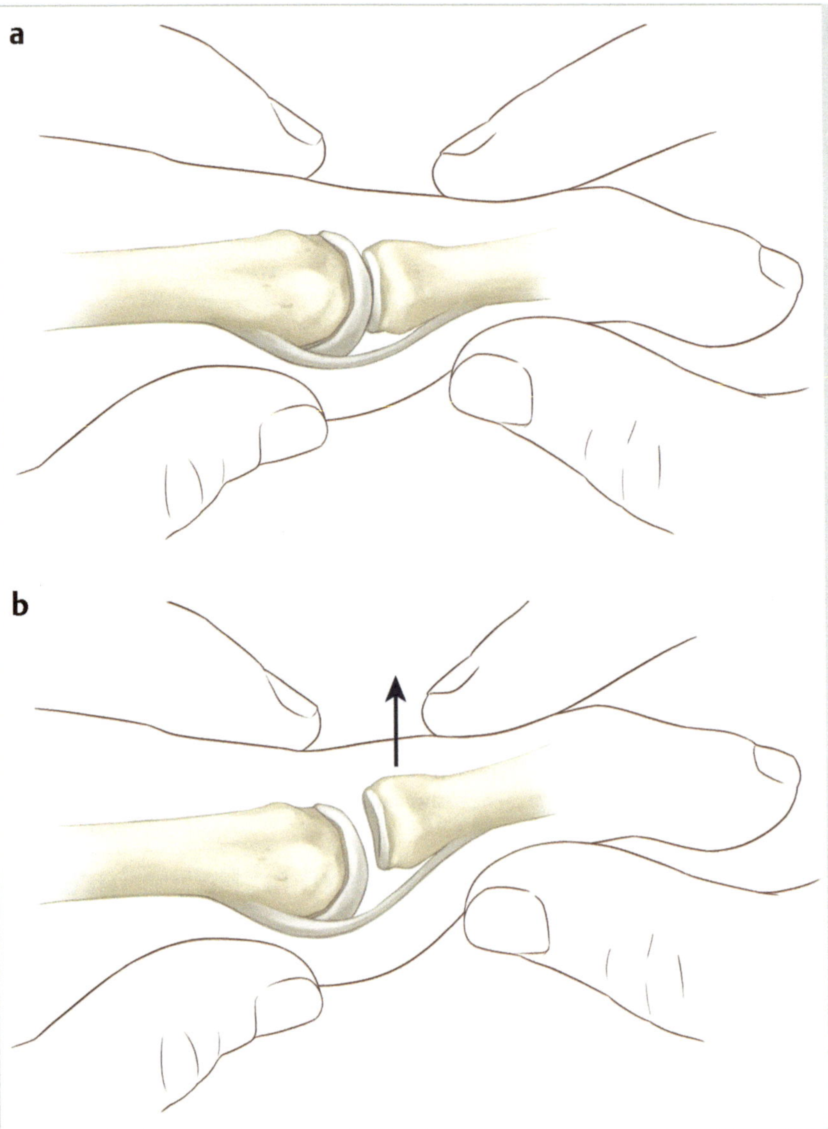

Fig. 3.1 (a,b) Drawer test. With the toe held between the examiners thumb and index finger, a dorsal force is placed on the digit. With instability, the proximal phalanx can be subluxated dorsally eliciting pain.

3.5 Preoperative Preparation and Patient Positioning

The patient is placed in a supine position on the operating room table with a bump beneath the ipsilateral hip. An Esmark bandage is used to exsanguinate the foot, and when properly applied, it may be used as a tourniquet as well.

3.6 Operative Technique

3.6.1 Anatomy

The lesser MTP joints are supported by the collateral ligaments on the medial and lateral aspect of the joint. There are both an accessory and proper collateral ligament; the accessory collateral ligament attaches to the plantar plate and supports the joint in a slinglike fashion. The proper collateral ligaments

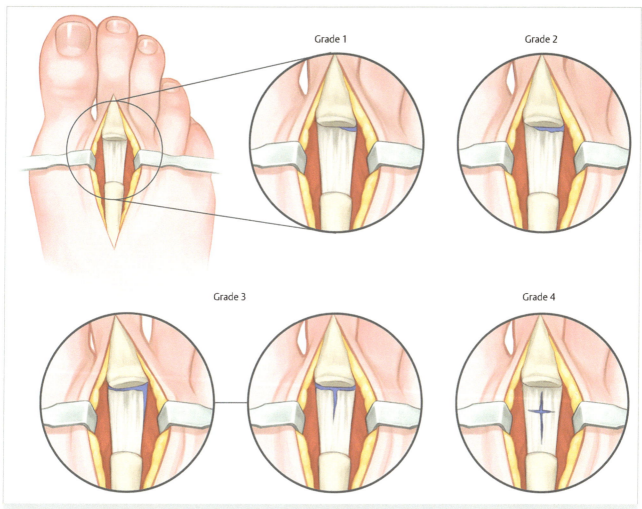

Fig. 3.2 Grading of plantar plate tears. Grading of types of plantar plate tears. (The metatarsal head has been removed and we are looking down on the plantar plate from dorsal approach). A grade 1 tear has a tear < 50% off of the base of the proximal phalanx, a grade 2 tear has a detachment greater that 50%, a grade 3 tear may have a transverse distal tear but also has a longitudinal component, and a grade 4 tear has an irreparable tear of the plantar plate.

span the MTP joint from a tubercle at the approximate center of rotation on the metatarsal head laterally and medially to the proximal phalanx base and control the varus/valgus orientation of the joint (**Fig. 3.3 a, b**). The area is further stabilized by the distal extension of the plantar fascia and the transverse intermetatarsal ligaments. On the dorsal aspect, the extensor expansion (**Fig. 3.3 c**) (including the long and short extensor tendons) and, on the plantar aspect, the plantar plate complete the soft-tissue envelope of the lesser MTP joint.

3.6.2 Description of the Procedure

A dorsal longitudinal incision may be centered either over the involved joint or along the adjacent interspace depending on other surgical procedures to be performed.

The approach is then deepened through the dorsal subcutaneous tissue to the dorsal joint capsule of the lesser MTP joint. A capsulotomy and synovectomy are performed exposing the joint. The collateral ligaments are released from the base of the proximal phalanx. A McGlamry elevator is used to release the

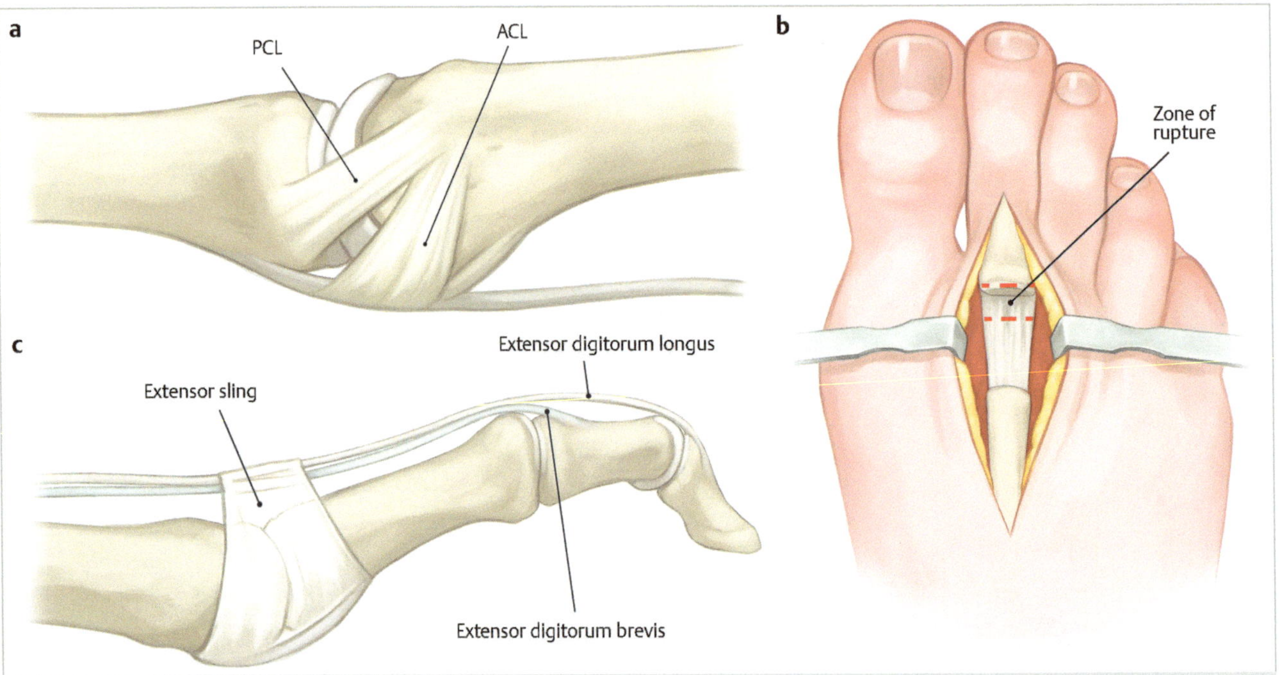

Fig. 3.3 Anatomy of the lesser MTP joint. (**a**) Lateral view demonstrating the proper (posterior cruciate ligament) and accessory (anterior cruciate ligament) collateral ligaments. (**b**) Dorsal view demonstrating the plantar plate. (**c**) Lateral view demonstrating the dorsal structures.

capsular attachment at the plantar proximal aspect of the metatarsal head; then, typically a Weil osteotomy is performed to increase exposure[5] (**Fig. 3.4**).

The metatarsal head is temporarily pushed proximally and then fixed with a vertical 0.62 Kirschner wire placed dorsal to plantar. The distal 2 mm of the metatarsal is removed with a rongeur. A second vertical Kirschner wire is placed in the proximal phalanx and a pin-to-pin distractor is applied and spread, distracting the joint space (**Fig. 3.5**). The plantar plate is then visualized and inspected with a freer. For a grade 1 to 3 tear, the plantar plate is released sharply from the insertion on the base of the proximal phalanx base with caution not to injure the flexor digitorum longus tendon just deep to the plantar plate.

Once the plantar plate is freed from the flexor tendon sheath, two no. 0 polyethylene braided sutures are placed in a horizontal mattress fashion using either a Mini Scorpion DX (Arthrex, Naples, FL) (**Fig. 3.6**) or a Micro SutureLasso (Arthrex, Naples, FL). A suture passer is used to pull the tails of these sutures from plantar to dorsal through two oblique tunnels drilled in the base of the proximal phalanx. The tunnels are drilled with a 0.62 smooth Kirschner wire from dorsal to plantar, staying proximal from the cartilaginous base (**Fig. 3.7**). The Weil osteotomy is then repaired in a slightly shortened position (2 mm) with two twist-off titanium screws. The joint is then reduced and held in approximately 20 degrees of plantar flexion as the sutures are sequentially pulled taut and tied over the dorsal cortex of the proximal phalanx.

The collateral ligaments are then assessed and reefed in the presence of residual transverse plane malalignment with a 2–0 braided polyglactin suture loaded on a UR-6 needle.

3.7 Tips and Pearls

• When performing the Weil osteotomy, the saw blade should parallel the plantar aspect of the foot. This technique prevents plantar translation of the capital fragment with proximal translation.[6]

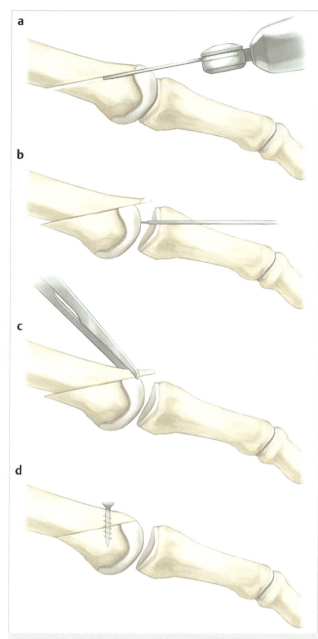

Fig. 3.4 Weil's osteotomy: view from lateral aspect. **(a)** Saw cut parallel to plantar aspect of foot. **(b)** Capital fragment translated proximally. **(c)** Removal of dorsal edge of bone. **(d)** Internal fixation with dorsal spin screw.

- When detaching the plantar plate from the base of the proximal phalanx, we find a sweeping motion with the scalpel blade from distal to proximal is helpful in freeing the plantar plate from plantar structures such as the tendon of the flexor digitorum longus.
- At times, a Weil osteotomy is not necessary, and the plantar plate can be visualized just with simple distraction. In this case, a Viper (Arthrex, Naples, FL) (**Fig. 3.8**) linear suture passer is used to place the securing suture in the prepared plantar plate. The rest of the reconstructive technique is identical.[7]

3.8 Hazards and Pitfalls

In the presence of longstanding lesser MTP joint subluxation, degenerative arthritis may develop. Cases with MTP joint osteoarthritis are contraindicated and tend to have restricted, painful postoperative motion. Dislocation of the joint often is associated with severe plantar plate degeneration, and resection arthroplasty or flexor tendon transfer may be a better surgical alternative. Plantar plate can be associated with longstanding inflammatory arthritis; however, in many of these cases, capsular and collateral ligament deterioration may preclude plantar plate repair.

3.9 Complications/Bailout/Salvage

3.9.1 Complications

In our current review of our cases, the more common complications are stiffness, ongoing pain, and recurrent varus or valgus deviation of the joint. This is attributed to arthrofibrosis, excessive tissue degeneration, or inadequate repair. In cases of more severe degeneration, a flexor tendon transfer (for grade 4 tears) may be considered.[8] Occasionally, loss of fixation of the Weil osteotomy or osteonecrosis of the metatarsal head may occur. The osteotomy should be avoided in osteopenic bone for which secure fixation is questioned. Excessive periosteal elevation should be avoided at the metatarsal head and the proximal phalanx. We believe early range-of-motion exercises should be initiated at 7 to 10 days following surgery to prevent postoperative stiffness.

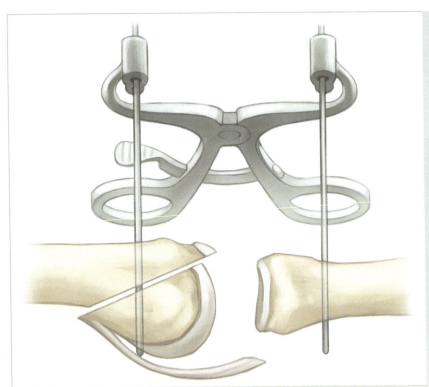

Fig. 3.5 Distraction of the joint. Two parallel Kirschner wires are placed in the phalanx and metatarsal to allow distraction.

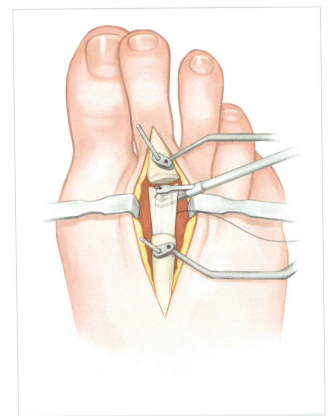

Fig. 3.6 Placement of horizontal mattress sutures in the plantar plate. Placement of sutures with Scorpion suture passer.

3.9.2 Bailout/Salvage

In our experience, failure is uncommon. However, with either severe arthrofibrosis or restricted motion, reoperation may be indicated. Initially, a soft-tissue arthroplasty and release of contracted tissue may be considered. With more severe changes, a resection of this joint and/or adjacent joints with a DuVries condylectomy or metatarsal head resection arthroplasty may be used as a salvage procedure.[9]

3.10 Postoperative Care

The foot is wrapped in a gauze and tape compression dressing and changed weekly. Toes are supported in slight plantar flexion with tape. At 7 to 10 days following surgery, a removable dressing is used and active and passive plantar flexion exercises are commenced. Toes are supported with tape in a plantar direction or placed in a dynamic splint (Darco TAS-Toe Alignment Splint, Darco International Inc., Huntington, WV) until 3 weeks following surgery. Then active and passive dorsiflexion exercises are started. Weight-bearing is initially allowed just on the heel, but at 3 to 6 weeks postoperatively, plantigrade weight-bearing is allowed at the forefoot.

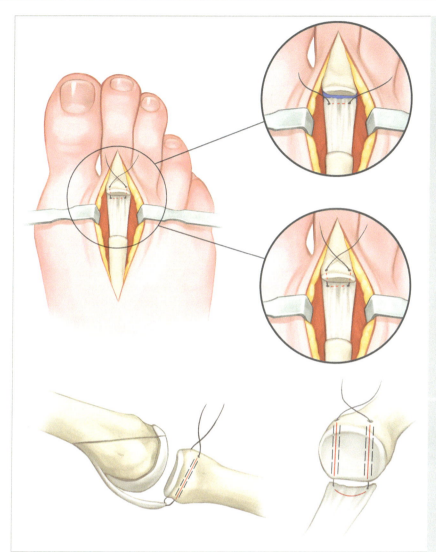

Fig. 3.7 Surgical technique. Placement of suture and passage through drill holes in base of proximal phalanx.

3.11 Outcomes

Nery et al[10] examined 22 patients following 40 plantar plate repairs. Their mean AOFAS (American Orthopedic Foot and Ankle Society) score at final follow-up was 92. Mean VAS scores dropped from 8 preoperatively to 1 at final evaluation. Of the 40, 32 had toe contact with the floor and 25 out of 40 toes had excellent toe purchase with the floor measured with the paper pullout test.

Our group prospectively followed over 138 plantar plate repairs for 12 months. Only 15 plantar plate repairs were completed without concomitant procedures. Subjectively, 80% of patients were satisfied with results of the procedure, including all patients in the cohort, and 100% were satisfied in those performed in isolation. Mean AOFAS scores at 1 year was 81 for all patients and 85 for those with isolated plantar plate repairs. Total active range of motion preoperatively was 43 degrees and postoperatively was 31 degrees at final follow-up.

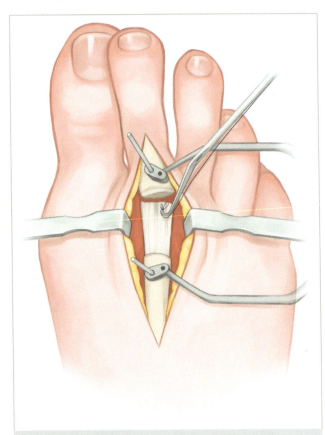

Fig. 3.8 Use of Viper suture passer. When a Weil osteotomy is not performed, a smaller suture passer can be used to place sutures in the plantar plate.

References

1. Coughlin MJ, Schutt SA, Hirose CB, et al. Metatarsophalangeal joint pathology in crossover second toe deformity: a cadaveric study. Foot Ankle Int 2012;33(2):133–140
2. Klein EE, Weil L Jr, Weil LS Sr, Coughlin MJ, Knight J. Clinical examination of plantar plate abnormality: a diagnostic perspective. Foot Ankle Int 2013;34(6):800–804
3. Coughlin M.J. Lesser Toe Deformities.Vol 1. 9th ed. Philadelphia, PA: Elsevier;2014
4. Coughlin MJ. Lesser-toe abnormalities. J Bone Joint Surg Am 2002;84(8):1446–1469
5. Cooper MT, Coughlin MJ. Sequential dissection for exposure of the second metatarsophalangeal joint. Foot Ankle Int 2011;32(3):294–299
6. Grimes J, Coughlin M. Geometric analysis of the Weil osteotomy. Foot Ankle Int 2006;27(11):985–992
7. Jastifer JR, Coughlin MJ. Exposure via sequential release of the metatarsophalangeal joint for plantar plate repair through a dorsal approach without an intraarticular osteotomy. Foot Ankle Int 2015;36(3):335–338
8. Coughlin MJ. Subluxation and dislocation of the second metatarsophalangeal joint. Orthop Clin North Am 1989;20(4):535–551
9. Kaz AJ, Mann RAKeratotic Disorders of the Plantar Skin.Vol 1. 9th ed. Philadelphia, PA: Elsevier;2014
10. Nery C, Coughlin MJ, Baumfeld D, Mann TS. Lesser metatarsophalangeal joint instability: prospective evaluation and repair of plantar plate and capsular insufficiency. Foot Ankle Int 2012;33(4):301–311

4 Extensor Digitorum Brevis Transfer for Crossover Toes

Elizabeth A. Cody and Scott J. Ellis

Abstract

The tendon transfer described in this chapter may be used to correct varus or valgus lesser toe deformity and dorsal elevation, seen typically as a second "crossover toe" associated with hallux valgus. The deformity arises from chronic attenuation of the collateral ligament and plantar plate on at least one side of the joint, allowing the toe to deviate in the opposite direction. This tendon transfer effectively reconstructs the collateral ligament on the attenuated side of the joint. Following a soft-tissue release of the metatarsophalangeal (MTP) joint, the extensor digitorum brevis tendon is released proximally and the distal segment, which remains attached distally, is used for the reconstruction. The tendon end is passed through bone tunnels created in the proximal phalanx and the metatarsal neck; it is tensioned and then anchored to a screw in the metatarsal shaft. This procedure provides a more anatomic reconstruction of the lateral collateral ligament compared to previously described tendon transfers. Surgeons and patients can expect good deformity correction and preserved MTP joint range of motion.

Keywords: *tendon transfer, extensor digitorum brevis, crossover toe, lesser toe deformity, varus lesser toe*

4.1 Indications

- Indicated for treatment of severe varus or valgus lesser toe deformity at the metatarsophalangeal (MTP) joint, with or without associated severe dorsiflexion of the MTP joint.[1]
  - Deformity is most commonly seen at the second toe in association with hallux valgus, in which the second toe deviates dorsomedially over the great toe ("crossover toe").
  - The procedure may be modified to treat other multiplanar lesser toe deformities.

4.1.1 Pathology

- The deformity arises from failure of the collateral ligament, which causes the toe to deviate in the opposite direction, as well as from failure of the plantar plate, which causes the toe to angulate dorsally.[2]
- As with hammertoes, this deformity is commonly seen in the setting of hallux valgus and may be due to relative muscle/tendon imbalance across the toe.
- It may result from MTP joint overload, poor shoe-wear, trauma, or connective tissue disorders.

4.1.2 Nonoperative Options

- Nonoperative management should be attempted prior to surgery.
- May include shoe-wear modification, taping, Budin splints, hammertoe crest pads, or orthotics.

4.1.3 Clinical Evaluation

- A thorough examination should be performed to identify any concomitant pathology.
  - Associated hallux valgus should be corrected at the same time as the lesser toe deformity.
  - Metatarsalgia will not improve with correction of the crossover toe and may require metatarsal-shortening osteotomy. This is especially true when a long metatarsal is present or a severe subluxation or dislocation has occurred in the setting of dorsiflexion.

4.1.4 Radiographic Evaluation

- Weight-bearing anteroposterior and lateral views of the foot are performed to assess the deformity in both planes.
- The MTP joint should be assessed for congruency, dislocation, and degenerative changes.
- Newer weight-bearing computed tomography (CT) scans may be helpful, but are not required.

4.1.5 Contraindications

- Pure vertical instability at the MTP joint: without varus or valgus deformity, this would be better treated with other options including a plantar plate repair and/or metatarsal-shortening osteotomy.
- Severe MTP arthritis: this may be exacerbated by relocating the toe in its anatomic position.
- History of previous surgery involving the extensor digitorum brevis (EDB) tendon.
- Current infection.

4.2 Goals of Surgical Procedure

- To provide a lasting correction of the multiplanar severe varus/valgus or crossover toe deformity while preserving MTP joint mobility and function.

4.3 Advantages of Surgical Procedure

- Allows for customized correction of deformity.
- Can assess and adjust tension intraoperatively prior to final fixation.
- MTP joint mobility is retained.
- Potentially less pain and stiffness relative to flexor digitorum longus transfer.[3]

4.4 Key Principles

- EDB transfer should be performed only if sufficient correction is not achieved after initial steps, namely, MTP joint release followed by release of up to one-third of the contracted plantar plate.
- Concomitant deformity, such as hallux valgus, should be addressed at the same time.

4.5 Preoperative Preparation and Patient Positioning

The figures shown in this chapter demonstrate correction of a classic second crossover toe, with varus deformity and dorsal angulation, in a cadaveric specimen. However, the procedure may be used to correct varus or valgus deformity in any of the lesser toes.

The patient is positioned supine and the limb is prepped in sterile fashion. A thigh tourniquet is applied prior to prepping and draping. We prefer a thigh tourniquet to an ankle tourniquet, which alters the tension in the extrinsic tendons around the ankle. For this reason, we use spinal anesthesia in addition to a long-acting popliteal block. A dorsal longitudinal incision is marked out over the affected MTP joint, extending from approximately 5 cm proximal to the joint to the proximal interphalangeal (PIP) joint. In the case of a bunion with second MTP deformity, the same skin incision may be used for both the lateral release of the bunion deformity and the second ray tendon transfer. The limb is then exsanguinated with an Esmarch bandage and the tourniquet inflated.

4.6 Operative Technique

The EDB and extensor digitorum longus (EDL) tendons are identified. The EDB tendon is smaller and located laterally to the EDL tendon, and can be further identified by its more distal muscle belly. The EDB tendon is then dissected out and transected as proximally as possible to ensure maximum length for the tendon transfer. The distal tendon end is tagged with a 2–0 fiberwire running suture, which will later be used to secure the tendon following transfer (**Fig. 4.1**). The EDL tendon should be released using a Z-lengthening technique and set aside for repair at the end of the procedure using absorbable suture at the correct tension.

With the extensor tendons out of the way, the dorsal capsule and contracted collateral ligament are released with a number 15 blade scalpel (**Fig. 4.2**). Care should be taken to preserve the extensor tendons' attachments to the extensor hood. If PIP joint resection is required, release of the extensor hood should be minimized. The MTP joint is then reduced. If the joint cannot be reduced to within 5 degrees of neutral, then the plantar plate is released on the contracted side by small amounts until reduction is maintained; care must be taken to avoid injury to the flexor tendons below. No more than one-third of the plantar plate should be released to avoid overcorrection. In some patients, the above-mentioned steps may be sufficient to correct the deformity. If this is the case, the EDB tendon transfer should not be performed, given it may cause overcorrection. If not needed, the remaining EDB can simply be excised. Intraoperative fluoroscopy can be used to verify adequate reduction.

If release of the contracted plantar plate does not fully correct the deformity, then EDB transfer is indicated. Briefly, starting from its distal insertion, the tendon is passed through a drill hole in the proximal phalanx going from dorsal-medial to plantar-lateral in the case of a varus deformity (dorsal-lateral to plantar-medial in the case of valgus). If there is significant dorsal angulation, the tunnel should be more vertical (exiting more plantarly) to enable plantar translation of the proximal phalanx, which to some degree reinforces the plantar plate. The tendon exits on the plantar-lateral side of the proximal phalanx and then enters a drill hole in the metatarsal neck going from plantar-lateral to dorsal-medial in the varus toe (plantar-medial to dorsal-lateral in the valgus toe), after which it is tensioned and secured to the metatarsal. The drill holes are always made from the dorsal side over a wire as described in the following. This reconstruction effectively recreates a collateral ligament situated plantarly on the attenuated side of the joint. In the case of a valgus deformity, the direction of the drill holes is reversed as noted earlier.

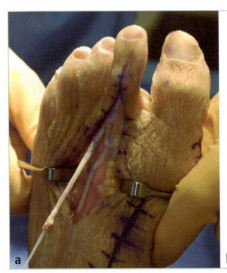 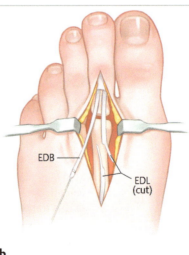

Fig. 4.1 (a,b) The EDB (extensor digitorum brevis) tendon is released proximally and tagged with fiberwire suture. EDL, extensor digitorum longus.

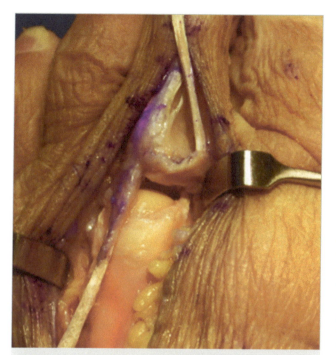

Fig. 4.2 The MTP (metatarsophalangeal) joint is well exposed following dorsal capsular release and release of the tight collateral ligament (medial collateral ligament in this case).

The proximal phalanx tunnel is drilled first. A 0.045 Kirschner wire (K-wire) is inserted in the desired trajectory (**Fig. 4.3**). The K-wire trajectory is inspected visually and adjusted if necessary. A 2.7-mm cannulated drill is then used to drill over the K-wire, taking care to avoid fracture. The metatarsal neck drill hole is then made in the same fashion (**Fig. 4.4**). A free Keith needle and Vicryl suture loops are used to facilitate passage of the tendon through the drill holes to create the construct described earlier (**Fig. 4.5**).

The tendon is then tensioned appropriately until the MTP is reduced and in neutral alignment with respect to the metatarsal shaft and the other toes. The sutures on the tendon end can be tied to a screw post (either a 2.0- or 2.4-mm screw) or a small suture anchor placed in the metatarsal shaft (**Fig. 4.6**). The screw or suture anchor should not be placed until correct tension has been confirmed. If there is residual extension at the MTP joint, a plantar dermodesis may be performed at this point. The completed reconstruction after EDL repair is shown in (**Fig. 4.7**). Final alignment should be checked on intraoperative fluoroscopy (**Fig. 4.8**). In some cases, a K-wire can be placed across the MTP joint to hold the toe in position for several weeks to take tension off the reconstruction. This is most often done when a concomitant PIP resection is performed, which already requires a more distal K-wire. This wire, however, should only be placed after final tensioning and positioning of the graft.

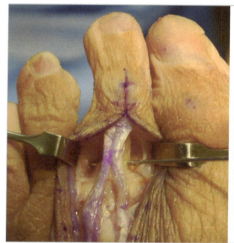
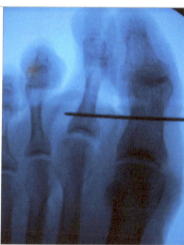

Fig. 4.3 A K-wire is inserted in the proximal phalanx in the planned trajectory of the proximal phalanx bone tunnel (left) with fluoroscopy confirming placement (right).

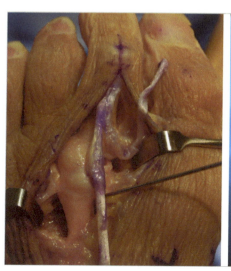
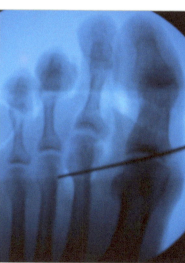

Fig. 4.4 A K-wire is also used to establish the trajectory of the drill hole in the metatarsal neck.

4.7 Tips and Pearls

- Do not perform the EDB transfer if MTP release and plantar plate release alone lead to adequate correction; performing the transfer in this setting is unnecessary and will lead to overcorrection.
- If hallux valgus is corrected concomitantly, we recommend performing the hallux valgus procedure first so that the lateral deviation of the great toe does not interfere with reduction and positioning of the second toe.

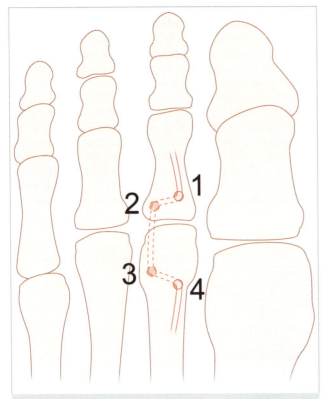

Fig. 4.5 The path of the tendon graft is shown schematically.

- The decision to perform a proximal phalangeal osteotomy of the great toe (i.e., Akin) is made after the second toe is in its final position.

4.8 Hazards and Pitfalls

- Do not release more than one-third of the plantar plate, given this can cause instability or overcorrection.
- Take care when releasing the EDB tendon proximally in order to ensure a distal segment that is long enough to perform the reconstruction.

4.9 Complications/Bailout/ Salvage

- Overcorrection can occur when EDB transfer is performed unnecessarily, as discussed earlier.
- Recurrence may occur if the graft is not placed in the correct location and orientation.
- Patients may have pain in the MTP joint especially if there was evidence of MTP arthritis before surgery.

4.10 Postoperative Care

- Postoperative care is usually dictated by any concomitant procedures, such as bunionectomy.
- Early weight-bearing (at 2 weeks postoperatively) may be allowed in the absence of other procedures that require non-weight-bearing status postoperatively.
- A protected boot should be worn until at least 6 weeks postoperatively.

4.11 Outcomes

- There are only two published case series in the literature describing outcomes.

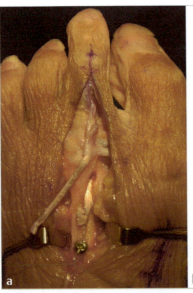
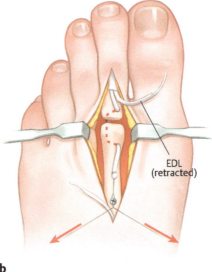

Fig. 4.6 After passage through the bone tunnels, the graft is tensioned to a screw placed in the metatarsal shaft. Note correction of the crossover toe deformity.

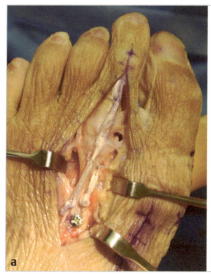 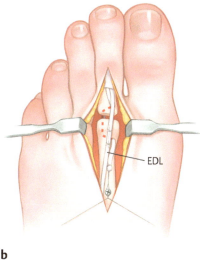

Fig. 4.7 (a,b) The complete reconstruction prior to closure is shown. The EDL tendon has been repaired side to side. The EDB graft sits in line with the metatarsal shaft after it exits its bone tunnel.

EDL

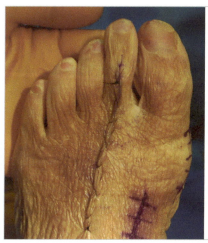 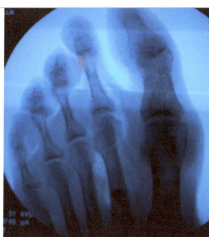

Fig. 4.8 Postoperative photograph (left) and final fluoroscopy (right) show excellent correction of the deformity, with the second toe now matching the alignment of the other lesser toes.

- The first case series reports 1-year outcomes in 11 patients with a second crossover toe and hallux valgus[4]:
  - Radiographic parameters significantly improved, in terms of both MTP varus and dorsal angulation; overcorrection was seen in some cases.
  - MTP joint range of motion was well maintained, with an average MTP dorsiflexion of 61 degrees and plantarflexion of 11 degrees.
  - Three patients had residual elevation of the affected toe from the plantar surface.
  - Subjectively, 9 of 11 patients were highly or moderately satisfied; no patients were dissatisfied.
  - A total of 10 of 11 patients reported the toe felt better postoperatively, although 3 of 11 remained mildly painful and 1 of 11 was moderately painful.
- Another more recent case series reported outcomes in six patients, all of whom had adequate deformity correction and were satisfied with their outcomes; however, the average follow-up was only 4 months.[5]
- In summary, this procedure provides a powerful means of deformity correction and has good reported outcomes.
- Patients cannot necessarily expect complete improvement in pain or deformity (especially dorsal angulation).

References

1. Mani SB, Ellis SJ, Deland JT. Correction of multiplanar lesser metatarsophalangeal joint deformity using an extensor digitorum brevis reconstruction. Tech Foot Ankle Surg 2014;13(1):59–63
2. Coughlin MJ, Schutt SA, Hirose CB, et al. Metatarsophalangeal joint pathology in crossover second toe deformity: a cadaveric study. Foot Ankle Int 2012;33(2):133–140
3. Haddad SL, Sabbagh RC, Resch S, Myerson B, Myerson MS. Results of flexor-to-extensor and extensor brevis tendon transfer for correction of the crossover second toe deformity. Foot Ankle Int 1999;20(12):781–788
4. Ellis SJ, Young E, Endo Y, Do H, Deland JT. Correction of multiplanar deformity of the second toe with metatarsophalangeal release and extensor brevis reconstruction. Foot Ankle Int 2013;34(6):792–799
5. Hobizal KB, Wukich DK, Manway J. Extensor digitorum brevis transfer technique to correct multiplanar deformity of the lesser digits. Foot Ankle Spec 2016;9(3):252–257

5 Fifth Metatarsal Osteotomy for Bunionette Deformities

Sandro Giannini, Cesare Faldini, and Francesca Vannini

Abstract:
A tailor's bunion or bunionette deformity is a combination of an osseous and soft-tissue bursitis located on the lateral aspect of the fifth metatarsal (MT) head, and is a condition caused by splaying of the fifth MT.

Many different techniques exist for bunionette correction, while the ideal treatment is still debatable.

Developed for hallux valgus correction, the SERI technique exhibits a high versatility and efficacy and can easily be applied to the treatment of bunionette with minimal morbidity for the patient and with easy and durable results.

A good correction is easily provided through a minimal incision and with the use of a single K wire, to be removed after 4 weeks, for osteotomy stabilization. The procedure is able to correct even major deformities by medially shifting the MT head, and a contact of less than 1 mm is needed between the MT head and the MT bone to obtain a safe consolidation.

After a learning curve, no technical problems are to be expected during surgery, as well as a very limited number of minor complications following surgery.

Keywords: *bunionette, Tailor's bunion, fifth metatarsal osteotomy, mini-invasive, linear distal osteotomy*

5.1 Overview

A tailor's bunion or bunionette deformity is a combination of an osseous and soft-tissue bursitis located on the lateral aspect of the fifth metatarsal (MT) head, and is a condition caused by splaying of the fifth MT.[1] The condition often presents with hallux valgus deformity and is characterized by a flexible splayfoot.

Several prospective studies indicate that the condition is 3 to 10 times more common in women than in men, but the incidence and prevalence remains unknown.[2]

Many different techniques exist for bunionette correction. Weil's osteotomy, scarfette, and lateral cheilectomy in cases with minimal deformity have been advocated, while the ideal treatment is still debatable.[3]

Surgical treatment for bunionette should be simple, effective, rapid, and inexpensive (SERI).

Developed for hallux valgus correction, the SERI technique is not a new technique because it uses an osteotomy and a stabilization method already described.[4,5] The osteotomy, in fact, is a linear distal osteotomy performed immediately before the MT head, as described by Hohmann, Wilson, and Magerl, through a minimal incision and stabilized by a single K-wire, as suggested by Kramer and by Bösch. Nevertheless, it exhibits a high versatility and efficacy given that it is a combination of the strength of these previously described procedures, resulting in a technique with unique characteristic of mini-invasivity, simplicity, versatility, and good stability of the construct.

This technique can easily be applied to the treatment of bunionette with minimal morbidity for the patient and with easy and durable result.[4]

5.2 Indications

- The main indication for bunionette correction is for pain relief, if painful callosities and reactive overlying bursa persist despite shoe modifications.
- Any bunionette, despite the degree of severity, may be corrected by SERI. This technique is particularly useful for the treatment of type 2 and 3 bunionettes where isolated shaving of the lateral eminence would remove a substantial portion of the head resulting in metatarsophalangeal (MTP) joint instability.
- Even if mild arthritis is evident, SERI may be performed, taking care to slightly incline the osteotomy in distal-proximal way, shortening the MT, and decompressing the metatarsophalangeal joint.

5.2.1 Pathology

- A tailor's bunion or bunionette deformity is a combination of an osseous and soft-tissue bursitis located on the lateral aspect of the fifth MT head.
- The fifth MTP and fourth and fifth inter-MT angles significantly increase as a result of rotational movement of the fifth ray at its articulation with the cuboid. The fifth ray excessively pronates, leading to a progressive deformity that is accompanied by the fifth toe developing an adductovarus position.[3,6]

5.2.2 Clinical Evaluation

- Pain is generally located over the lateral forefoot, corresponding to the lateral condylar process of the head of the fifth MT which protrudes laterally. This is often associated with a bursitis, which can also be painful as it rubs against the side of a shoe. The forefoot is generally splayed. Fifth toe range of motion in plantar-dorsiflexion should be assessed, as well as the presence of pain during this maneuver.
- Coughlin distinguished three types of bunionette:
  ○ Type 1, which has an enlarged fifth MT head and prominent lateral condyle (16–33%).
  ○ Type 2, which has a laterally bowed deformity of the fifth MT inducing symptomatic prominence of the lateral condyle (10%).
  ○ Type 3, which is characterized by an increased fourth and fifth intermetatarsal angle (IMA) (normal angle, < 12 degrees) with no particular distal fifth MT deformity (57–74%). There may be associated, usually congenital, fifth toe varus overlap, in infraductus or supraductus.[7]
- Because the condition is often present with hallux valgus deformity, the presence of hallux valgus should be also considered.

5.2.3 Radiographic Evaluation

- An anteroposterior (AP) and lateral weight-bearing radiographs of the standing patient are generally enough for a

bunionette deformity and permit to effectively plan the surgery.
- Computed tomography (CT) or magnetic resonance imaging (MRI) is needed only in cases in which the diagnosis is uncertain.

5.2.4 Nonoperative Options

- Footwear modifications.

5.2.5 Contraindications

- The presence of stiffness and/or arthritis of the fifth MTP joint of high degree.
- Skin ulceration or infection.
- Peripheral vascular disease.

5.3 Goals of Surgical Procedure

- The goal of distal osteotomies is to correct all the altered parameters typical of the bunionette, such as fifth MTP angle and the IMA and, furthermore, to derotate the MT head in order to address the supination of the toe or to reduce concomitant stiffness by shortening the MT bone.

5.4 Advantages of Surgical Procedure

- A good correction is easily provided through a minimal incision. The procedure is able to correct even major deformities

by medially shifting the MT head, and a contact of less than 1 mm is needed between the MT head and the MT bone to obtain a safe consolidation.
- Minimally invasive: no soft-tissue procedures, no opening of the capsule, or bursa removal. The whole procedure is made through a less than 1-cm access, under direct visual control. (Intraoperative X-rays are only needed during the learning curve).
- Straightforward: the entire procedure takes a very limited surgical time.
- Inexpensive: the stabilization of the osteotomy is obtained by a single K-wire, easy to remove after 1 month, during medication.

5.5 Key Principles

- Up to 1-cm incision just proximal to the MT head.
- Do not open the joint or the capsule.
- Make the osteotomy immediately proximally to the MT head.
- Incline the osteotomy in a dorsal to plantar direction of about 15 degrees to control the dorsal translation of the MT head with weight-bearing.
- Take care to make the osteotomy in the lateral to medial direction perpendicular to the fourth ray if the length of fifth MT bone was to be maintained (**Fig. 5.1**).
- Incline the osteotomy in a distal-proximal direction up to 25 degrees if a shortening of the fifth MT is needed (a lengthening is usually not required).
- Stabilize with a 1.6-mm K-wire, inserted from proximal to distal.

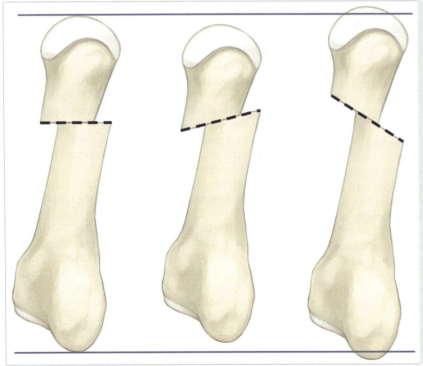

Fig. 5.1 The osteotomy should be inclined in the lateral to medial direction perpendicular to the fourth ray if the length of the fifth metatarsal bone was to be maintained; otherwise, by changing this inclination, the metatarsal may be shortened, as in the case of arthritis, or elongated, more rarely.

5.6 Preoperative Preparation and Patient Positioning

The patient is positioned on a radiolucent operating table in the supine position. A small lateral hip bump will improve ease of access to the fifth MT. Intraoperative imaging in two projections should be possible, in particular, during the learning curve; if performed by an experienced surgeon, the use of the C-arm is unnecessary.

5.7 Operative Technique

- The operation is usually performed under local or block anesthesia using ropivacaine hydrochloride monohydrate 7.5 mg/mL (Naropina; AstraZeneca Södertälje, Sweden).
- An Esmarch bandage or tourniquet may be optionally used at the ankle level.
- A 1-cm lateral incision is made just proximal to the lateral eminence through the skin, subcutaneous tissue, and down to the bone (**Fig. 5.2**).
- The soft tissues are separated dorsally and plantarly and held retracted with two small retractors 5 mm in width (**Fig. 5.3**).
- The lateral wall of MT neck is now well evident and the complete osteotomy is performed using a standard pneumatic saw with a 9.5 × 25 × 0.4 mm blade (**Fig. 5.4**).
- With a small osteotome, the head is mobilized.
- A 1.6-mm K-wire is inserted, using a normal drill passing through the incision, into the soft tissue adjacent to the bone in a proximal-distal direction along the longitudinal axis of the toe (**Fig. 5.5**).
- The K-wire exits at the lateral area of the tip of the toe; about 3 to 4 mm from the lateral border of to the nail, it is retaken by the drill (**Fig. 5.6**) and retracted up to the proximal end reaching the osteotomy line (**Fig. 5.7**).

- Using a small grooved lever to prize the osteotomy, the correction is obtained by moving, under visual control, the MT head depending on the pathoanatomy of the deformity (**Fig. 5.7**, **Fig. 5.8**).
- If the supination of the fifth MT bone is present, the correction is obtained also with a derotation of the toe up to the neutral position.
- The stabilization of the correction is obtained inserting the K-wire into the diaphyseal medullary canal of the fifth MT in a distal-proximal direction until its proximal end reaches the MT base (**Fig. 5.9**).
- The adjustment of the plantar dislocation of the MT head, more rarely of the dorsal dislocation, is obtained introducing the K-wire in the upper, or more rarely in the lower, site with regard to the long axis of the MT head (**Fig. 5.10a**, **b**).
- If the proximal stump of the osteotomy is medially prominent, a small wedge of bone is removed (**Fig. 5.11**).

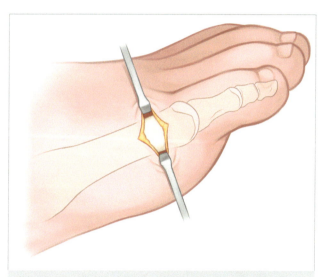

Fig. 5.3 The soft tissues are separated dorsalward and plantarward and divaricated by two small retractors 5 mm in width.

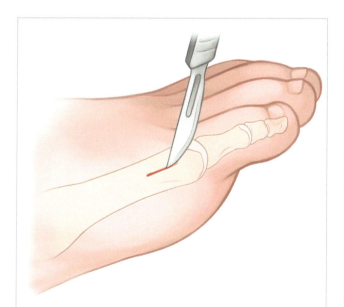

Fig. 5.2 A 1-cm lateral incision is made just proximal to the lateral eminence through the skin, subcutaneous tissue, down to the bone.

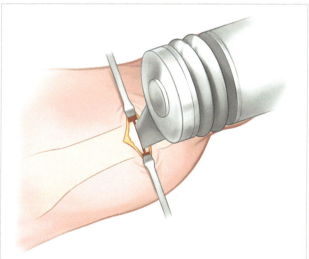

Fig. 5.4 The lateral wall of metatarsal neck is now well evident and the complete osteotomy is performed using a standard pneumatic saw with a 9.5 × 25 × 0.4 mm blade.

- The skin is sutured with only one 3–0 reabsorbable suture. The distal end of the K-wire is bent and cut distal to the tip of the toe.
- This technique can be performed bilaterally or combined with the correction of any other associated deformity of the forefoot or hindfoot, in the same surgical session.

5.8 Tips and Pearls

- Selecting the correct site for osteotomy is extremely simple, since the 1-cm incision should be performed immediately before the prominence of the MT head and the osteotomy should be performed just before the insertion of the capsule (**Fig. 5.2**).
- A key point of the stability of SERI technique is the 15-degree inclination to be given in a dorsoplantar direction, from distal to proximal. This helps in avoiding a possible dorsal dislocation of the MT head under weight-bearing.
- An adjustment of the mediolateral dislocation of the MT head is performed introducing the K-wire more or less adherent

to the medial eminence. (If the K-wire is inserted inside the eminence itself, the lateral displacement of the head will be reduced.)
- If additional shortening of the MT bone is needed, normally it is necessary to plantarly dislocate the MT head by many millimeters according to the extent of the shortening performed.
- A too proximal level of the osteotomy produces a higher risk of nonunion of the MT.
- A too distal osteotomy predisposes to osteonecrosis of the MT head.
- An osteotomy with excessive medial displacement of the head, without residual contact with the MT bone, is usually still capable to consolidate, but nevertheless produces a residual shortening of the MT bone (quite well tolerated in the fifth MT, anyway).
- An insufficient displacement of the MT head may produce a higher recurrence rate.
- The use of a K-wire of an incorrect size results in a strong decrease of the load applied to the osteotomy.

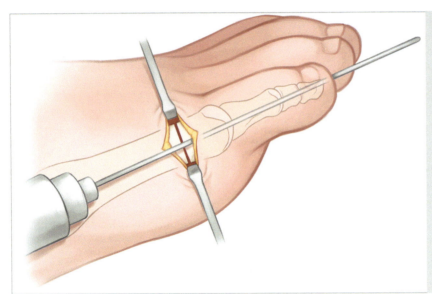

Fig. 5.5 A 1.6-mm K-wire is inserted, using a normal drill passing through the incision, into the soft tissue adjacent to the bone in a proximal-distal direction along the longitudinal axis of the toe.

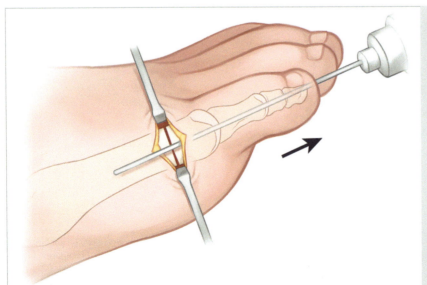

Fig. 5.6 The K-wire exits at the lateral area of the tip of the toe; about 3 to 4 mm from the lateral border of to the nail, it is retaken by the drill.

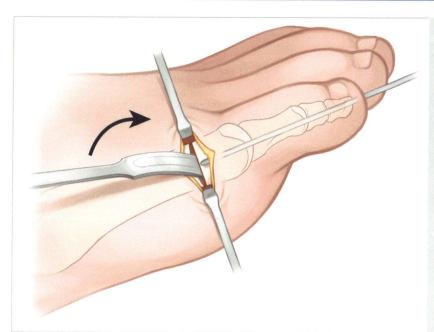

Fig. 5.7 Once the K-wire is retaken by the drill, it should be retracted up to the proximal end reaching the osteotomy line.

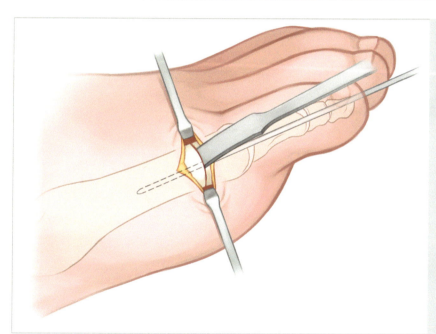

Fig. 5.8 Using a small grooved lever to prize the osteotomy, the correction is obtained by moving, under visual control, the metatarsal head depending on the pathoanatomy of the deformity.

5.9 Hazards and Pitfalls

- Do not open the capsule and take care to perform the whole procedure through the minimally invasive incision, otherwise the stability of the construct is compromised.
- Do not open the medication, unless abnormal pain or any clue of complications occurs, and maintain the same medication up to the 1-month control to ensure the stability of the construct.

5.10 Complications/Bailout/Salvage

- A very limited number of complications may occur intraoperatively during this surgery if attention is paid to the correct position and alignment of the osteotomy and of the K-wire insertion.
- A mild inflammatory reaction around the outlet of the K-wire at the tip of the toe may be experienced at medication removal, usually resolving in a few days. A gauze should be placed between the skin and the curved eminence of the K-wire itself.
- Nonunion is a very rare complication experienced by the authors in a negligible percentage of cases, and it may occur in cases of technical error, when the osteotomy is performed too proximally or the K-wire used is of an incorrect size.
- Another possible cause of residual pain is the prominence of the corner of MT bone, if it has not been adequately resected intraoperatively.

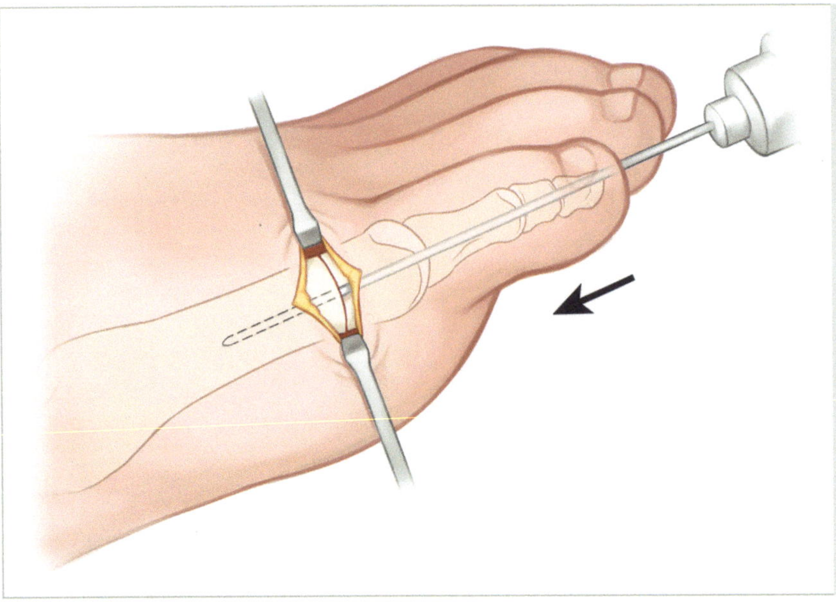

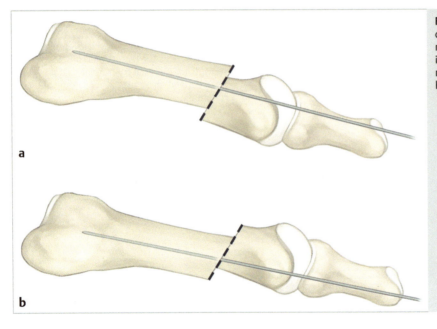

Fig. 5.9 The stabilization of the correction is obtained inserting the K-wire into the diaphyseal medullary canal of the fifth MT in a distal-proximal direction until its proximal end reaches the metatarsal base. If the supination of the fifth metatarsal bone is present, the correction is obtained also with a derotation of the toe up to the neutral position.

Fig. 5.10 (a,b) The adjustment of the plantar dislocation of the metatarsal head, more rarely of the dorsal dislocation, is obtained introducing the K-wire in the upper, or more rarely in the lower, site, with regard to the long axis of the metatarsal head.

a

b

5.11 Postoperative Care

After surgery, a gauze compression dressing is applied and radiographic control in AP and oblique views is performed to confirm the placement of the osteotomy and the correction of any characteristics of the deformity.

Ambulation is allowed immediately, for limited distances, using postoperative shoes, and foot elevation is advised when the patient is at rest. K-wire fixation due to wire bending upon insertion produces a viable stabilization, maintaining the same position obtained during surgery and favoring early healing of the osteotomy combined with early weight-bearing. Medication is not to be removed until 1 month, requiring no intermediate controls. This has the double advantage of protecting the osteotomy by the imbricate gauzes, which provide a mechanical containment.

After 1 month, the dressing, suture, and K-wire are removed. Passive and active toe mobilization, cycling, and swimming are advised, and comfortable normal shoes are recommended, gradually returning to former footwear.

5.12 Outcomes

In the paper published by Giannini et al,[4] using this technique for bunionette correction, the SERI minimally invasive distal osteotomy was found to be a reliable and adequate surgery for bunionette treatment (**Fig. 5.12a–c**). It does not need a capsulotomy or a permanent internal fixation device, but it achieved good clinical results with minimal morbidity. All but two of the patients in a series of 50 feet were satisfied with the procedure, with the clinical improvement reflected by an increase in the AOFAS score of 31.2 ± 13.2 ($p < 0.0005$).

No technical problems were observed in the series. In all the cases, the fifth MT head was translated according to the parameters of the deformity and stabilized with an optimal rate of bone healing. A correction of all the radiographic parameters was obtained, such as a correction of 5.3 ± 1.9 degrees ($p < 0.0005$) of the fourth and fifth inter-MT angle, and a correction of 8.9 ± 3.9 degrees ($p < 0.0005$) of the fifth

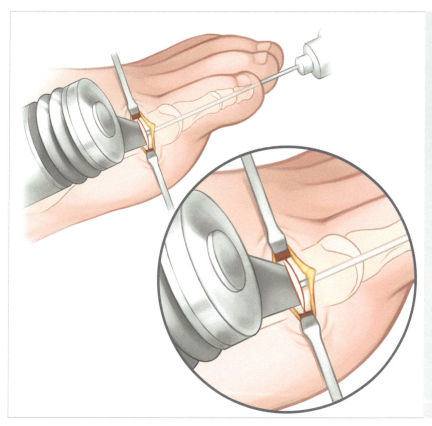

Fig. 5.11 If the proximal stump of the osteotomy is medially prominent, a small wedge of bone is removed.

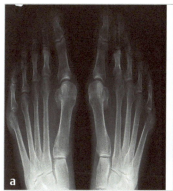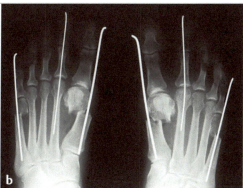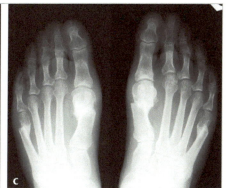

Fig. 5.12 **(a)** Preoperative X-rays of a 38-year-old woman affected by hallux valgus, second toe deformity, and bunionette. **(b)** Postoperative X-rays control after SERI procedures for hallux valgus, bunionette, and second toe correction. **(c)** Twelve-month X-rays control.

MTP angle. No severe complications, such as avascular necrosis of the MT head or nonunion of the osteotomy, occurred. The two feet rated as nonsatisfactory reported the persistence of callosity due to insufficient correction.

References

1. Deveci A, Yilmaz S, Firat A, et al. An overlooked deformity in patients with hallux valgus tailor 's bunion. J Am Podiatr Med Assoc 2015;105(3):233–237
2. Roukis TS. The tailor's bunionette deformity: a field guide to surgical correction. Clin Podiatr Med Surg 2005;22(2):223–245, vi
3. Weil L Jr, Consul D. Fifth metatarsal osteotomies. Clin Podiatr Med Surg 2015;32(3): 333–353
4. Giannini S, Faldini C, Vannini F, Digennaro V, Bevoni R, Luciani D. The minimally invasive osteotomy "S.E.R.I." (simple, effective, rapid, inexpensive) for correction of bunionette deformity. Foot Ankle Int 2008;29(3):282–286
5. Giannini S, Faldini C, Nanni M, Di Martino A, Luciani D, Vannini F. A minimally invasive technique for surgical treatment of hallux valgus: simple, effective, rapid, inexpensive (SERI). Int Orthop 2013;37(9):1805–1813
6. Laffenêtre O, Millet-Barbé B, Darcel V, Lucas Y Hernandez J, Chauveaux D. Percutaneous bunionette correction: results of a 49-case retrospective study at a mean 34 months' follow-up. Orthop Traumatol Surg Res 2015;101(2):179–184
7. Coughlin MJ. Treatment of bunionette deformity with longitudinal diaphyseal osteotomy with distal soft tissue repair. Foot Ankle 1991;11(4):195–203

6 Hoffman, Clayton Metatarsal Head Resection for Rheumatoid Forefoot

Graham McCollum

Abstract

Untreated or resistant rheumatoid arthritis can lead to significant forefoot deformities and morbidity. Typically, the hallux deforms into valgus and the lesser metatarsophalangeal joints dislocate dorsally with varying degrees of joint destruction and bone erosion. Surgical reconstruction entails creating a stable hallux with arthrodesis of the metatarsophalangeal joint and resection of the lesser metatarsal heads if the joints are not reducible or destroyed by the disease process. The hallux is generally fixed with a combination locking compression plate and the lesser toes held reduced with K-wire fixation. The results are generally good with high patient satisfaction long term if there are no complications. The most common complications are wound-healing problems, inadequate resection of the metatarsals, overgrowth of the resected bone, and hallux nonunion/malunion.

Keywords: *rheumatoid forefoot, hallux arthrodesis, Hoffman's procedure, Clayton's procedure, forefoot reconstruction*

6.1 Introduction

Rheumatoid arthritis (RA) is a systemic inflammatory disease that affects the forefoot, requiring surgical intervention in about 15% of cases. Between 85 and 92% of patients with RA will have some form of foot involvement, and it presents in the foot for the first time in around 20% of cases.[1]

With the introduction of disease-modifying drugs and biologics, the incidence of gross forefoot deformity and joint destruction has decreased. Deterioration after surgery in stable, well-controlled disease may also not be as prevalent.[2]

The timing of surgery is important to consider. Other joints are frequently affected and might need surgical intervention themselves. This might limit postoperative ambulation and affect the recovery of the foot surgery. The cervical spine, particularly the subaxial spine, can be unstable in uncontrolled disease, and stability should be confirmed prior to elective surgery.

The most common procedure performed for the management of these cases when advanced is the Hoffman or Clayton procedure.[3,4] This involves creating a stable hallux metatarsophalangeal joint (MTPJ) with an arthrodesis, resection of the lesser metatarsal heads, and correction of the lesser toes with osteoclasis of the proximal interphalangeal joints (PIPJs) or condylectomy of the proximal phalangeal heads. For patients who have endured longstanding suffering from walking on exposed metatarsal heads, often with gross deformity, the operation is life-changing, and it is rewarding for the surgeon too. With symptomatic lesser deformities and better management with disease-modifying drugs, joint-preserving procedures can be considered, such as shortening, elevating osteotomies of the lesser metatarsals, and correction of hallux valgus with conventional soft-tissue and bony work. This chapter focuses on the technique of hallux MTPJ arthrodesis and resection arthroplasty of the lesser metatarsal heads, the Clayton or Hoffman procedure.

6.1.1 Indications

- Advanced symptomatic disease with deformities not managed by conservative intervention.
- Subluxing or dislocated lesser MTPJs with joint destruction and erosion, plantar callus formation, and fat pad advancement. If the lesser MTPJs are passively reducible and the joints preserved on radiographs, shortening, elevating osteotomies can be considered.
- Hallux valgus or varus with joint destruction, instability, and subluxation. If the disease is well controlled and the joints preserved on radiographs with mild deformities, consider a joint-preserving procedure. If the interphalangeal joint is arthritic and symptomatic, consider a resection arthroplasty rather than an arthrodesis.
- Skin erosion or threatening of the skin from the bony prominences.

6.1.2 Clinical Evaluation

- Poorly treated or uncontrolled RA leads to deregulation of the cellular and humoral immune systems, resulting in synovial proliferation, pannus formation, capsuloligamentous destruction, and cartilage erosion.
- Initially, this presents as painful swelling of the MTPJs. If poorly treated or resistant, it proceeds to subluxation and dislocation of the joints with symptomatic plantar callus formation, metatarsalgia, fat pad migration, and dorsal callus formation over the lesser toes, which develop fixed flexion deformities.
- Typically, the hallux, together with erosive cartilage destruction, develops a valgus deformity of the MTPJ and sometimes subluxation. Hallux varus is a less common deformity (**Fig. 6.1**).[1]
- Patients typically experience pain under the exposed metatarsal heads, over the medial eminence of the hallux valgus and the dorsum of the lesser toes. Their skin is often thin from the systemic disease and prone to ulceration and skin breaches.

6.1.3 Radiographic Evaluation

- Global evaluation of the foot and the ankle is necessary for adequate surgical planning. Standing X-rays, three views, and anteroposterior (AP), lateral, and an oblique view are mandatory. Standing ankle views are also necessary if there is hindfoot malalignment, an acquired flatfoot, or rheumatoid ankle.
- Typically, the hallux is in valgus alignment, but sometimes it is in varus with varying degrees of bone erosion and loss. The proximal phalanx of the hallux can be very short if there is longstanding disease with erosion, which can make fixation for fusion difficult.

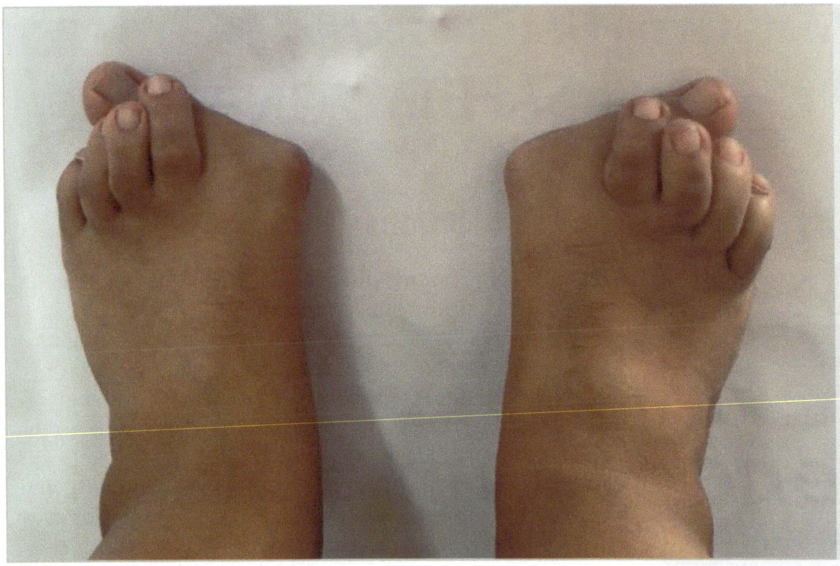

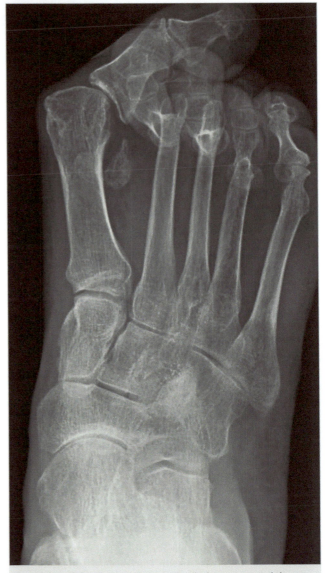

Fig. 6.1 Typical forefoot deformities. Photograph showing hallux valgus and dislocated lesser metatarsophalangeal joints.

- It is important to evaluate the interphalangeal joint (IPJ) of the hallux—this might sway you from fusion of the metacarpophalangeal (MP) joint. The lesser toes often have dislocated or subluxed MP joints and fixed flexion deformities of the PIP joints.
- Osteoporosis is common in these patients; they often are on longstanding corticosteroid treatment and have low activity levels; this might affect implant choice and fixation, and hence should be evaluated. If there is a concern with previous ulceration and osteomyelitis, a magnetic resonance imaging (MRI) scan is useful for detecting collections and bone involvement—otherwise, the role of further imaging is limited (**Fig. 6.2**).

6.1.4 Nonoperative Options

- The conservative treatments include.
  - ○ Shoes with a high and wide toe box.
  - ○ Metatarsal pads.
  - ○ Rocker bottom soled shoes.
  - ○ Metatarsal bars.
  - ○ Accommodating medium density orthotics.
- The goal is to offload the prominences and allows the callus formation to recede. These patients often suffer tremendous pain from their multijoint disease and cope with extreme deformity for a long time.

6.1.5 Contraindications

- Proven deep infection.
- Extreme skin fragility or soft-tissue infection.
- Vascular insufficiency.
- Other medical reasons and patient fragility, cervical spine instability and myelopathy, poor mobilization potential, etc.

6.2 Goals of Surgical Procedure

A successful procedure culminates in a stable united hallux in a good position, with resolution of the plantar calluses and correction of the deformities both in the hallux and the lesser

Fig. 6.2 Standing foot X-ray. Radiograph showing typical rheumatoid deformities, hallux valgus, and dislocated lesser metatarsophalangeal joints.

toes. These patients have tremendous pain from the disease and can be extremely grateful with improvement in their pain and function.

6.3 Advantages of Surgical Procedure

The fusion of the first MTPJ creates a stable medial column against which the lesser toes remain balanced. Prior techniques of resection arthroplasty (Keller's procedure) of the first MTPJ had no medial stability and recurrent valgus deformity of all the toes frequently occurred.

The resection of the lesser metatarsal heads alleviates the necessity of osteotomies of the metatarsals to heal in these patients with poor quality bone. Additionally, loss of plantar padding is no longer an issue given there is no metatarsal head to be prominent in this area after resection. Although the lesser MTPJs are unstable, this rarely causes any difficulty in low-demand rheumatoid patients.

6.4 Key Principles

• Perform an arthrodesis of the hallux in a good position for the patient's function.
• Remove the metatarsal heads at the appropriate level to form a cascade of decreasing lengths from medial to lateral.
• Hold the PIPJs and the distal interphalangeal joints in a reduced position after either an osteoclasis or proximal phalanx condylectomy and reduce the base of proximal phalanx onto the resected metatarsal with the extensor tendons acting as an interposition graft.

6.5 Preoperative Preparation and Patient Positioning

A thorough history and physical examination must be performed, looking for features of myelopathy including cervical spine instability, skin integrity, and ability to ambulate. Ankle, hindfoot, and midfoot involvement, including tendon function and involvement, must be examined and documented. In the forefoot, the hallux IPJ must be assessed for range of motion and pain and the lesser MTPJ dislocations/subluxations checked to see if they are reducible or not. Most patients have thin skin from the systemic disease and from prolonged steroid use, but extreme cases may be a contraindication to the surgery. Vascular competence, both venous and arterial, must be documented and areas of callus and threatened skin identified.

Consultation with their rheumatologist prior to the operation is mandatory. Most are on drugs to modulate their immune systems and theoretically could lead to an increased infection rate. This has not been proven in large retrospective studies.[5] The biologic drugs, tumor necrosis factor, should perhaps be discontinued for a month around the surgery but there is little high-level evidence to guide us.[6]

"Pre-hab" is essential to protect the surgery postoperatively. These patients often have upper limb involvement and are generally weak. Assisting devices and offloading shoes are required for safe ambulation postoperatively. We find that if the patient is introduced to the physical therapist and the rehab team before the surgery, the transition to independence is smoother and faster.

In cases of bilateral disease, staging the surgery is the safest option with the most symptomatic side operated on first (not necessarily the worst radiologically). The contralateral side should be treated surgically once the fusion of the hallux is proven and they can ambulate unassisted on the operated foot and have had time to appreciate the benefit of the surgery. Generally, this time frame is around 6 months but can be shorter if they recover fast. In certain circumstances, either for socioeconomic reasons or if there is equal bilateral threatened skin, they can be done at the same time, but this renders them extremely dependent and increases the complication rate.

Standing radiographs of both feet, AP, lateral, and an oblique view are necessary. The deformity of the hallux MTPJ, IPJ, and the lesser toes can be assessed, as well as the bone density, joint destruction, and bone stock. We like to take preoperative standing **photographs** of all patients given the deformity correction can be very dramatic and the patients seem to appreciate the operation even more when they see where they have come from.

The patients must be informed of the potential risks and complications. The most common of these are wound-healing problems, infection, nonunion of the hallux, IPJ degeneration, recurrent deformity of the lesser toes, and bony overgrowth of the metatarsal resection. Less commonly, in severe deformity, ischemia and digit loss of the hallux or the lesser toes is a possibility.

The patient is positioned supine with a sandbag or a bump under the ipsilateral buttock to position the foot facing the roof. We prefer to use a formal tourniquet and exsanguinate the limb with an Esmarch bandage prior to incision. The procedure can be time consuming, and duration of inflation must be monitored.

Meticulous handling of the skin and soft tissue, avoiding excessive retraction, exposing properly as opposed to forced retraction, will reduce the soft-tissue complications.

6.6 Operative Technique

6.6.1 Exposure

A three-incision technique should be used: one for the hallux MP fusion, one for the second and third metatarsal heads, and one for the fourth and fifth metatarsal heads. If the lesser toe flexion deformities are severe, then dorsal elliptical transverse incisions allow adequate exposure of the PIPJs. After reducing the joints, this skin incision removes the excessive skin on the dorsum of the toes and heals well.

The most common deformity of the hallux is valgus. By using a medial incision to approach the MTPJ, the skin bridge can be kept as wide as possible and in our experience the skin heals better. If there is a wound dehiscence, then the plate is covered with a decent flap and metal is not generally exposed. The medial skin is also less fragile. To correct gross hallux deformity, the joint must be circumferentially released and, in particular, the adductor tendon, medial capsule, and suspensory ligament of the sesamoids for adequate exposure of the joint for preparation.

The lesser metatarsals are approached through two dorsal incisions in the second and the fourth web spaces. We have found that if the incisions are gently curved, there is a better flap and there is less tension on the skin during the resection. It is helpful then to mark the incisions with crossed lines for the appropriate suturing of the skin. Other incisions include transverse plantar and dorsal plantar incisions, but we prefer the less invasive three-incision technique and have not had trouble with the wound if careful with the soft tissue.

6.6.2 Hallux Arthrodesis

Once the joint is exposed, there are several ways to prepare the surfaces for a successful arthrodesis. These include the cup and cone reamer technique, described first by McKeever,[7] burring the remaining cartilage and subchondral bone and making square cuts. If there is a prominent medial eminence, a sliver bunionectomy can be performed with an osteotome or oscillating saw, given that it is easier to appreciate the center of the metatarsal head after this is done. The cup and cone reaming technique allows the angle of the fusion to be adjusted and manipulated. It does not compromise stability and contact. This is the preferred method but can be dangerous in soft osteoporotic bone because the reamers can plunge into the metaphysis after penetrating the subchondral bone or can fracture the phalanx or metatarsal. Make sure the reamers are sharp and you do not have to apply too much pressure to ream. Great care must be taken not to plunge and destroy the bone necessary for fusion. If there is doubt, rather use a rongeur or burr to prepare the surfaces.

- Exposure for reaming is best done with the phalanx in plantarflexion, so the reamer clears the opposite bone. Place the appropriate guidewire in the center of the metatarsal head and make sure it follows the canal of the metatarsal. Trial the reamer sizes at this point as if the joint will be "resurfaced" and not excessive bone removed on the plantar or the dorsal sides. Sometimes, the wire has to be repositioned at this point if too plantar or dorsal.
- It is important to predetermine the amount of bone resection necessary. In extreme cases of hallux valgus, the metatarsal needs to be well shortened to limit the chance of ischemia. Once the metatarsal has been prepared, remove the loose bone and debris and use a rongeur to help fashion a smooth cone.
- The same guidewire (if not bent) can then be removed and placed into the middle of the proximal phalanx. Take care to seat the wire deep as it tends to back out, causing the reamer to slip off the bone and create an eccentric defect. Gently ream the phalanx. The subchondral bone can be quite resistant, and when more pressure is applied, it can literally explode. Ream just through the subchondral bone to good bleeding soft bone.
- If, after the reaming or resection during a trial reduction, the joint is still very tight and you cannot hold it in position easily, rather resect or ream more bone carefully until the reduced joint is decompressed. The reamed surfaces of the two bones should be gently drilled with a 2-mm drill bit to encourage bone bleeding. If the metatarsal is extremely soft, then abandon this because it may compromise fixation.
- The hallux should be set with the MTPJ in 8 to 15 degrees of valgus and with the distal phalanx just clearing the ground,

at a 10-degree dorsiflexed angle relative to the floor. Perform the "plate" test by placing a plate under the entire foot and loading it: the hallux should be sitting just off the plate by about 5 mm so that the distal hallux touches the plate in midflexion of the IPJ. This allows clearance during toe-off, but the distal phalanx can still engage the ground.

- The position can be altered and then held in the best position with K-wires. Intraoperative fluoroscopy is useful at this point to assess the coronal alignment but is difficult to assess the sagittal alignment because of the overlapping toes.
- A 2.5- to 3-mm cannulated transarticular screw is passed from plantar medial to dorsolateral at this point. It allows for immediate compression and stability. The position of the hallux should be rechecked, especially rotation, given that this can be overlooked. Sometimes, there is a ridge on the proximal phalanx that causes the plate to seesaw. It is a good time to use a rongeur or burr to make a flat surface on the dorsum of the hallux. The plate should be "fitted" to the bone, not the bone fitted to the plate. In other words, the position of the hallux should take priority intraoperatively. The low-profile plate should sit perfectly on the bone and not seesaw or be lifted up on one side, as, when the screws are placed, the bone will be pulled to the plate and the position possibly lost. In most cases, the plate has to be bent slightly to fit well.
- Given that these patients frequently have soft osteoporotic bone, a hybrid technique using a combination of nonlocking screws, to help hold the plate to the bone and achieve some compression, and locking screws, to resist pullout and achieve fixation, should be used. The sequence should be to place the two (preferably three) locking screws into the phalanx and then place a compression screw into the compression slot on the metatarsal. The rest of the holes should be filled with locking screws. In most cases, this provides good fixation, allowing the rest of the forefoot reconstruction to continue without compromising the position and fixation of the hallux.

6.6.3 Lesser Metatarsal Resection

This is the more destructive part of the operation but important to get right. In longstanding gross deformity, this can be difficult as the proximal phalanx dislocates dorsal of the metatarsal head and, with the extrinsic tendons, shortens significantly. The metatarsal head becomes adherent to what is left of the plantar plate and the diseased ligament structures. The skin over the dorsum is very fragile, and excessive retraction must be avoided. Rather, use longer incisions or try the slightly curved incision as the flap generated puts less tension on the skin.

- Make two incisions on the foot, as far apart as you can, one over the second web space and one over the fourth web space. Begin with the second metatarsal and move laterally. It can become confusing to find where you are when the toes are dislocated, but the long extensor tendon is usually tight and will be your guide to the proximal phalanx where you will find the metatarsal. Use harp to dissect down to the metatarsal neck and shaft and expose the joint and release as much of the capsule and the adherent joint as you can. At this point, cut the extensor tendons as proximal as you can so they can be used for an interposition graft.

- If possible, deliver the metatarsal head into the wound by reducing the released joint and plantar flexing the digit. This is not always possible, and if the skin is under extreme tension, then abandon and perform an in situ bone section. Check again where the level of the MTPJ fusion is. The level of resection of the metatarsal should be at or slightly longer than the first metatarsal.
- The resection should be done with an oscillating saw with the appropriate saw blade and angled retrograde to create a flattish surface for weight-bearing. Place two retractors around the metatarsal neck to protect the surrounding tissue and saw through. Once complete, remove the head and the neck. This can be difficult to do in one piece because the metatarsal head is very adherent to the plantar plate and the capsule. It has to be teased out and perform a "crocodile" role to get it out. If it breaks up, remove it piecemeal and put your finger in the defect, feeling for retained parts of head and remove them with a rongeur.
- Through the same incision, identify the extensors for the second toe and follow them to the joint. Once the metatarsal head and neck is visible, check the length of the second metatarsal and section the third about 3 to 5 mm shorter to achieve a cascade of lengths of the lesser metatarsals. If, after head resection, there is still a very tight space between the metatarsal and the phalanx, then remove some more metatarsal until there is a comfortable gap.
- Perform the same resection of the fourth metatarsal through the fourth web space incision noting the length of the third metatarsal. When it comes to the fifth metatarsal, we prefer to make an oblique cut in the metatarsal with the head resection so that there is a smooth lateral border to the forefoot. The same applies to judging length of resection (**Fig. 6.3**).
- An alternative approach is the plantar "fish-mouth" incision. This is a good alternative if there is gross advancement of the plantar fat pad, if there are severe plantar nodules and intractable callus that must be excised, and if the MTPJs are grossly dislocated and digits dorsally subluxed.
- Make two incisions on the sole of the foot, creating an ellipse over the plantar forefoot proximal and distal to the MTPJs including any plantar callosities. Remove the skin flap and dissect sharply down to the MTPJs. Take care to avoid plunging into the intermetatarsal spaces, given the neurovascular bundles are prone to injury.
- Open the MTPJ capsules longitudinally and expose the metatarsal heads. Resect them obliquely with a saw—creating a cascade from the second to the fifth metatarsal. Closure of the flap will help bring the lesser toes down and reduce the

clawing, but an extensor tenotomy will often be necessary to facilitate this. Interposition of the extensor tendons is not possible with this approach.
- Carefully close the plantar skin, making sure there are no overlaps and the skin edges marry up well. Wound complications with this approach are common. Close with nylon sutures, as they will have to remain in for at least 3 weeks to avoid the wound splitting open before healing (**Fig. 6.4**).

6.6.4 Lesser Toe Fixation

- The next part of the operation depends on the severity of the fixed flexion deformity of the lesser toe PIPJs. If they are fixed at 70 to 90 degrees, we prefer to do a P1 condyle removal through a transverse elliptical incision removing a piece of skin.
- The base of the middle phalanx is also prepared with a saw or the cartilage is removed with a rongeur. In these very fixed joints, forced osteoclasis sometimes causes the plantar skin to split open and there is an increased risk of vascular compromise. By removing the condyles, the PIPJs are open and K-wire fixation, first prograde and then retrograde, is easier than after the closed osteoclasis where the prograde wire can miss one of the phalanges. However, if the PIPJs are easily reducible with little force and the deformity is not severe, we

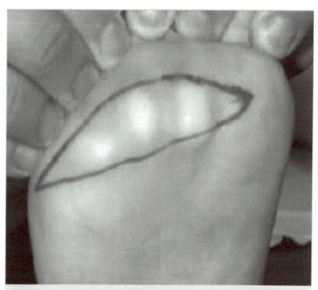

Fig. 6.4 Plantar approach. Photo showing the incision for the plantar approach.

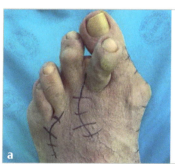
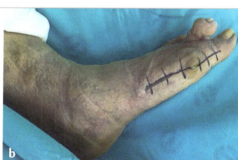

Fig. 6.3 (a,b) Incisions. Medial for the hallux and curved dorsal incisions. Photograph showing the placement of the incisions we typically use for the procedure.

perform a reduction of the joint closed and pass a 1.2- to 1.4-mm wire through the base of the proximal phalanx prograde to exit the toe just below the nail, trying to kebab the three phalanges. By holding the toe with two fingers and advancing the wire, you can almost feel it through the bones.

- Once out the digit, the wire is then pulled prograde so the other side is at the base of the proximal phalanx and visualized. At this point, gather the extensor tendon, which has been cut long, and use the wire to spear it once or twice so it is captured on the end of the wire exiting the P1 base. It will act as an interposition graft. The wire should then be placed in the canal of the resected metatarsal and advanced retrograde to the base of the bone just short of the tarsometatarsal joint.

- The interposed tendon should create a space between the end of the metatarsal and the base of the proximal phalanx. It is a good idea to use intraoperative fluoroscopy to confirm wire placement and metatarsal length.

- The wires exiting the toes should be bent and cut in a way that they are out of the way, will not catch on things, or put pressure on adjacent toes. Wire caps or beads are also a good idea and will limit the chance of being pulled out.

The tourniquet should be let down now and perfusion of the digits confirmed. If one of the toes is white, try hanging the leg over the bed or pour some warm water over the foot. If perfusion is still a problem, try and bend the wire in situ into more flexion, and if still nothing happens, then remove the wire and shorten the toe further through either the metatarsal neck or the PIPJ. These maneuvers will get the vast majority of dusky toes back.

The capsule of the MTPJ should be closed and then the three incisions with no tension. A bulky absorptive dressing with a postoperative wedge-type shoe should be applied in the operating room for protection (**Fig. 6.5, Fig 6.6**).

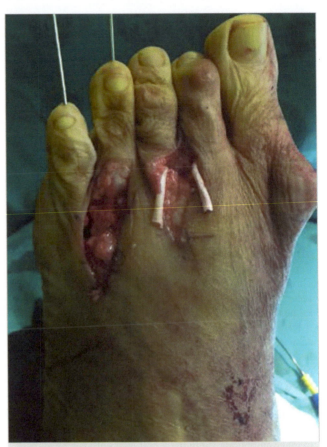

Fig. 6.5 Extensor tendons delivered and used as interposition graft. Photo showing the extensor tendons delivered through the dorsal incisions.

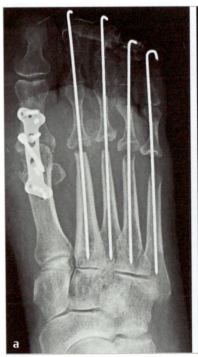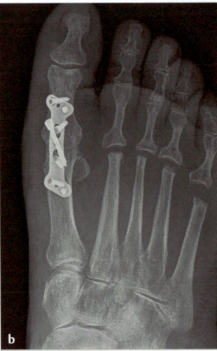

Fig. 6.6 (a) Postoperative X-rays and (b) X-rays at 2 years showing good spaces between the resected metatarsals and the phalanges.

6.7 Tips and Pearls

- Be gentle with the bone and the skin. They are fragile.
- With the MTPJ fusion, remove as little bone as you can, but with very extreme deformity (varus or valgus) with contracted tissue and neurovascular structures, shorten the metatarsal to a point where the reduction is easy. This will avoid an ischemic complication. Be wary of the cup and cone reamers—they can be dangerous.
- Fix the hallux accurately in about 8 to 15 degrees of valgus and enough dorsiflexion for the toe to clear the ground by 5 mm on standing.
- With the lesser metatarsal resection, create a cascade so there is no metatarsal that is more prominent than the other. Make sure you remove all the bone from the head if it comes out piecemeal. The fifth metatarsal should be resected at an angle. Use the extensors as an interposition graft—this keeps the phalanges from painful articulation with the excised metatarsal.

6.8 Hazards and Pitfalls

Intraoperatively, the most common hazard is too much resection of the metatarsal head or phalanx from an "explosion" or fracture. One may have to use a graft, either allograft or iliac crest, and a revision plate for fixation if it is a serious incident. In certain cases, the bone is so soft, it just cannot be held with a plate and screws. A good bailout is to pass multiple K-wires or Steinman pins across both the IPJ and the MTPJ and use a plaster slipper postoperatively. The pins need to remain in place for up to 8 weeks. Digital ischemia and its management were mentioned earlier.

6.9 Complications/Bailout/Salvage

- **Infection**: It is common for one of the dorsal incisions to dehisce slightly, requiring dressings for a couple of weeks or a small skin graft. The skin is fragile and healing can be a problem. Deep infection is uncommon but must be treated aggressively with appropriate antibiotics and possibly debridement and repeat surgery.
- **Nonunion of the hallux:** The risk is difficult to manage because it is often multifactorial and may include corticosteroid treatment, vitamin D deficiency, malnourished, etc. Meticulous surgery and obtaining good compression and fixation can limit this. If the nonunion is stable, it can be asymptomatic, in which case it can be observed, but if it becomes unstable and/or symptomatic, revision surgery will be required with bone grafting and better fixation. Always exclude an infection in a nonunion before revising.
- **Overgrowth:** Overgrowth of the resected metatarsal heads and insufficient metatarsal head resection with painful articulation is probably the most common reason for revision surgery. If painful, this must be managed surgically with further resection of the metatarsal making sure there

is a good space between the phalanx and the metatarsal. Since we began using the interposition technique, it seems to be less of a problem.

6.10 Postoperative Care

Patients are placed into a postoperative wedge shoe and instructed to maintain strict elevation for 2 weeks. They are permitted to ambulate around the house with two crutches, applying some weight on the heel. At 12 to 14 days postoperatively, the wounds are checked and re-dressed. The K-wires are left in for 6 weeks if there are no septic complications or problems. They have a postoperative X-ray at 6 weeks, and if the fusion looks good, they can transition into an open shoe with good support. Swelling is usual for up to 6 months or longer (**Fig. 6.7**).

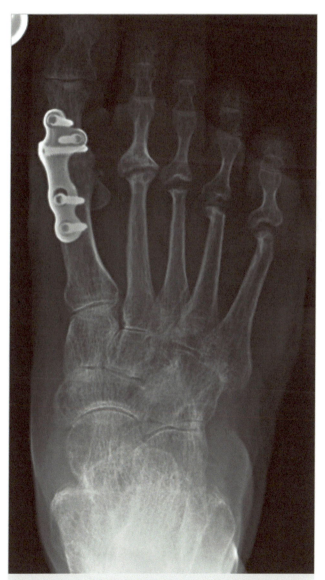

Fig. 6.7 Overgrowth and insufficient resection of the second and third metatarsals, requiring revision surgery. X-ray showing second metatarsal overgrowth impinging on the second proximal phalanx.

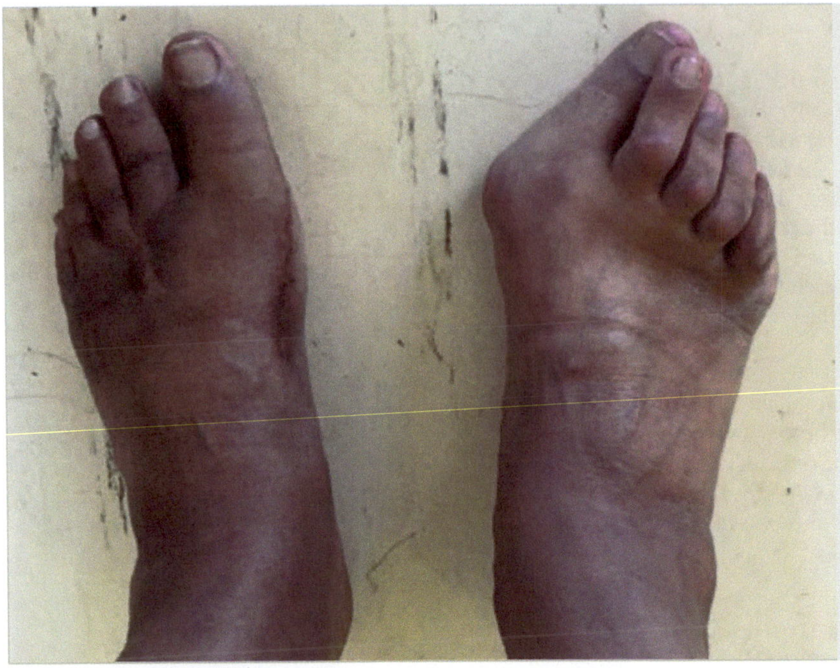

Fig. 6.8 Six months postsurgery on the left, and pending surgery on the right. Clinical photo showing a reconstruction of the left foot and typical forefoot surgery on the right.

6.11 Outcomes

Visually, when there is a large deformity and it is corrected surgically, the result can be quite dramatic. Generally, if there are no complications, the functional results are good. Coughlin[8] reported on his long-term results of the procedure in 43 patients and 58 feet at a mean follow-up of 6 years. The mean AOFAS forefoot score was 69 and subjectively rated as excellent or good in 45 of 47 feet and fair in 2, showing a high level (> 95%) of satisfaction. Thirty percent needed a secondary procedure to remove metal or to re-resect a metatarsal for pain. In contrast, Hulse and Thomas[9] noted significantly poorer results if a resection arthroplasty was done as opposed to an arthrodesis of the hallux.

Achieving a stable hallux is the key. This allows weight-bearing along the medial column, protecting the resected lesser toes from dorsal subluxation and lateral deviation. Poorer outcomes and subjective results have been reported when the hallux has been treated with a Keller-type resection arthroplasty.[10]

With low-profile plates and hybrid-type fixation, the need to remove the plate is reduced, and we have found that with appropriate resection of the metatarsal lengths and the interposition there is seldom overgrowth that requires reoperation. The majority of patients with bilateral disease choose to have the other side done as soon as they can. Some patients still have some symptoms and occasional pain, but when compared with the presurgery function, it is very rewarding for the patient and the treating surgeon (**Fig. 6.8**).

References

1. Jaakkola JI, Mann RA. A review of rheumatoid arthritis affecting the foot and ankle. Foot Ankle Int 2004;25(12):866–874
2. Niki H, Hirano T, Okada H, Beppu M. Combination joint-preserving surgery for forefoot deformity in patients with rheumatoid arthritis. J Bone Joint Surg Br 2010;92(3):380–386
3. Clayton ML. Surgery of the forefoot in rheumatoid arthritis. Clin Orthop 1960;16(1):136–140
4. Hoffman P. An operation for severe grades of contracted or claw toes. Am J Orthop Surg (Phila Pa) 1912;9:441–449
5. den Broeder AA, Creemers MC, Fransen J, et al. Risk factors for surgical site infections and other complications in elective surgery in patients with rheumatoid arthritis with special attention for anti-tumor necrosis factor: a large retrospective study. J Rheumatol 2007;34(4):689–695
6. Bibbo C, Goldberg JW. Infectious and healing complications after elective orthopaedic foot and ankle surgery during tumor necrosis factor-alpha inhibition therapy. Foot Ankle Int 2004;25(4):331–335
7. McKeever DC. Arthrodesis of the first metatarsophalangeal joint for hallux valgus, hallux rigidus, and metatarsus primus varus. J Bone Joint Surg Am 1952;34-A(1):129–134
8. Coughlin MJ. Rheumatoid forefoot reconstruction. A long-term follow-up study. J Bone Joint Surg Am 2000;82(3):322–341
9. Hulse N, Thomas AM. Metatarsal head resection in the rheumatoid foot: 5-year follow-up with and without resection of the first metatarsal head. J Foot Ankle Surg 2006;45(2):107–112
10. McGarvey SR, Johnson KA. Keller arthroplasty in combination with resection arthroplasty of the lesser metatarsophalangeal joints in rheumatoid arthritis. Foot Ankle 1988;9(2):75–80

7 Modified McBride's Bunionectomy

John Campbell

Abstract

Modified McBride's bunionectomy is a useful procedure for the correction of hallux valgus (bunion). Although it was originally described as an isolated technique, it is much more commonly performed in conjunction with proximal metatarsal osteotomy or tarsometatarsal arthrodesis in contemporary practice. A key goal of the procedure remains correction of the abnormal anatomy and mechanics while sparing the metatarsophalangeal joint and maintaining motion. Principles of the procedure include distal soft-tissue correction and balancing of the hallux metatarsophalangeal joint along with resection of the medial eminence. This requires release of the contracted lateral tissues, including the adductor hallucis tendon, intermetatarsal ligament, and lateral joint capsule. The medial eminence is removed, and a medial capsular imbrication removes redundant tissue and helps align the joint. Meticulous surgical technique is necessary to ensure good outcomes. This includes careful balancing of the soft tissues, avoidance of excessive removal of the medial eminence to prevent iatrogenic hallux varus, and minimizing capsular stripping to prevent osteonecrosis. Good clinical results can be expected in cases of flexible hallux valgus with mild to moderate deformity.

Keywords: *bunion, hallux valgus, bunionectomy, McBride's procedure, distal soft-tissue correction*

7.1 Indications

- A refinement of Silver's original bunionectomy procedure from 1923,[1] later modified by McBride.[2-4]
- Contemporary technique traces back to Mann and Coughlin,[5] who modernized McBride's and DuVries' method including two incisions.
- Relies on correction of abnormal anatomy and mechanics without joint destruction/ablation.[1-3]

- Can be used in isolation for mild to moderate hallux valgus and flexible deformity.
- Can be used for moderate to severe hallux valgus with flexible deformity in conjunction with proximal first metatarsal osteotomy or first tarsometatarsal (TMT) arthrodesis[5-7] (Chapters 9, 11, and 20).

7.1.1 Clinical Evaluation

- Determine location of tenderness.
- Assess range of motion of hallux metatarsophalangeal (MTP) joint.
- Determine flexibility/reducibility of hallux MTP joint.[4]
- Identify hypermobility of the first TMT joint.
- Assess lesser toe deformities.
- Confirm intact pulses and sensory function of the foot.

7.1.2 Radiographic Evaluation

- Weight-bearing radiographs of the affected foot, including anteroposterior, oblique, and lateral views.
- Identify degree of hallux valgus deformity, including
  ○ Congruent versus incongruent (subluxed) deformity (**Fig. 7.1**).
  ○ Measurement of hallux valgus angle (HVA), first/second intermetatarsal angle (IMA), and distal metatarsal articular angle (DMAA).
  ○ Presence of hallux MTP arthritis.
  ○ Assess lesser toe deformities.

7.1.3 Nonoperative Options

- Low-heeled, wide toe-box shoes.
- Foam or silicone gel spacers or pads.

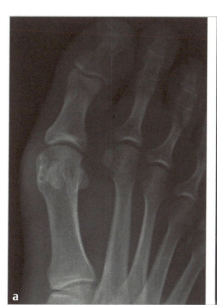 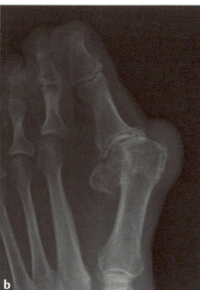

Fig. 7.1 (**a**) Congruent hallux valgus and (**b**) incongruent hallux valgus, with subluxation of the joint.

- Custom-molded orthotic insoles.
- Nonsteroidal anti-inflammatory medications.
- Avoidance of activities or shoes that exacerbate symptoms.

7.1.4 Contraindications

- Active infection of the foot.
- Severe peripheral vascular disease.
- Psychiatric disease, noncompliant patient.
- Congruent hallux valgus deformity (would cause subluxation or incongruence of joint).
- Severe hallux valgus deformity: IMA > 14 to 15 degrees; HVA > 30 to 40 degrees.[5-7]
- Rigid deformity or end-stage arthritis of MTP joint (better treated with arthrodesis).[2]
- Underlying inflammatory arthritides or neurologic disorders with high chance for recurrent deformity, e.g., rheumatoid arthritis, gout, cerebral palsy, spasticity (better treated with arthrodesis).

7.2 Goals of Surgical Procedure

- Release of contracted lateral structures—adductor hallucis tendon, transverse metatarsal ligament, and lateral capsule (**Fig. 7.2**).
- Removal of medial eminence.

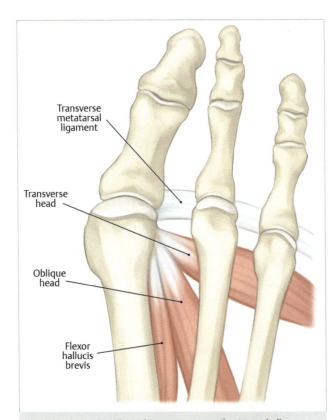

Fig. 7.2 Contracted lateral structures contributing to hallux valgus deformity; lateral slip of the flexor hallucis brevis inserting on the fibular (lateral) sesamoid; transverse metatarsal ligament between first and second MTP capsules; oblique and transverse slips of the adductor hallucis muscle inserting onto fibular sesamoid and lateral MTP capsule.

Image labels: Transverse metatarsal ligament; Transverse head; Oblique head; Flexor hallucis brevis

- Imbrication of medial soft tissues.
- Reduction of HVA and IMA.
- Improved congruence of MTP joint.

7.3 Advantages of Surgical Procedure

- Important technique in the foot surgeon's armamentarium.
- Technically facile and easily learned.
- Can be performed alone or in combination with proximal bony procedures based on the severity of deformity.[5,7]

7.4 Key Principles

7.4.1 Dorsal First Web Space Incision

- Release of adductor hallucis (conjoined) tendon.[1-7]
- Release intermetatarsal ligament.
- Incise suspensory (metatarsosesamoid) ligament.
- Stab incisions lateral capsule.[4]
- Suture adductor tendon stump into lateral capsule/periosteum on metatarsal head,[2-7] can also place sutures between first and second MTP capsules to close down IMA.[5,7]
- McBride's original technique of fibular sesamoidectomy and aggressive release of the lateral slip of the flexor hallucis brevis tendon[2-4] is no longer performed to avoid iatrogenic hallux varus.[8]

7.4.2 Medial Midline Incision[5,7]

- Medial bursectomy and capsulotomy.[1-5,7]
- Medial eminence resection.[1-5,7]
- Reduction and capsular repair.[1-5,7]

7.5 Preoperative Preparation and Patient Positioning

- Use of general anesthesia or regional block with intravenous sedation. Prophylactic antibiotics are administered.
- The patient is positioned supine on the operating room table with use of a thigh, calf, or ankle tourniquet. The operative limb should be freely movable to allow access to the dorsal and medial aspects of the foot.

7.6 Operative Technique (Author's Preferred Method)

- The dorsal web space between the first and second metatarsals is approached initially. The skin incision is created centrally in the web space and is followed by spreading of the subcutaneous tissues with scissors. Care should be exercised to avoid injury to the terminal branches of the deep peroneal nerve to the hallux and second toe. Thick bursal tissue may be encountered between the first and second metatarsal heads and should be dissected bluntly. A laminar spreader is useful to distract the first and second metatarsals to ensure good visualization of the deep structures of the web space.

- The adductor hallucis tendon is visualized inserting on the lateral aspect of the first MTP joint capsule and fibular sesamoid. The tendon has an oblique slip in addition to a transverse component. A pointed #11 scalpel blade is useful to meticulously release the tendon insertion on the capsule without excessive damage to the deeper structures (**Fig. 7.3**). Once the tendon insertion is released, scissors can be used in a proximal direction to ensure complete release of the tubular tendon. At the completion of the procedure, the stump of the released adductor hallucis tendon is sutured to the lateral capsule and periosteum of the metatarsal head with one or two 2–0 absorbable sutures to assist in correcting varus of the first metatarsal.
- Next, scissors are used to free both above and deep to the transverse metatarsal ligament between the first and second metatarsal heads. Care is taken to avoid injury to the deeper neurovascular structures. The ligament is then incised in a longitudinal direction with scissors, ensuring complete release (**Fig. 7.3**). The #11 scalpel blade can be used to create

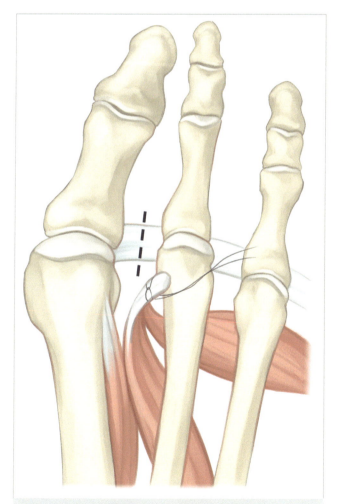

Fig. 7.3 Adductor hallucis tendon is released off fibular sesamoid and lateral capsule through dorsal web space incision. The tendon is reflected and the underlying transverse metatarsal ligament is incised (*dotted line*).

a longitudinal incision through the suspensory ligament, connecting the MTP capsule to the fibular sesamoid. Care is taken to avoid injury to the chondral surface of the sesamoid. Use of a Freer elevator to gently pry open the sesamoid articulation can allow exposure and facilitate complete release with the scalpel both proximally and distally.

- Release of the contracted lateral capsule is then carried out with the scalpel. In the majority of cases, multiple vertical stab cut incisions can be created in a "pie crust" manner to release the capsule. Gentle manipulation of the toe into varus can stretch the lateral capsular fibers. It is helpful to try to obtain at least 10 to 15 degrees of varus of the toe to ensure good release. In cases with severe lateral contracture, a more formal vertical lateral capsular incision may be necessary in order to minimize the risk of recurrence.
- A medial midline longitudinal incision is fashioned over the hallux MTP joint. The dorsal and plantar flaps are carefully elevated to allow full access and exposure to the capsule, with care taken to avoid injury to the dorsal cutaneous nerve to the hallux. Removal of the medial bursa is performed with scissors. Several different capsulotomy incisions have been described (**Fig. 7.4**). The author prefers an **L**-shaped capsulotomy with the vertical limb at the level of the joint line and the horizontal limb along the dorsal edge of the metatarsal head (**Fig. 7.4a**). This leaves the proximal capsular fibers attached near the first metatarsal neck and shaft. This flap is carefully elevated off the medial eminence in a full-thickness manner. It is important to extend the vertical limb plantarly to the tibial sesamoid to ensure adequate release and subsequent correction, while avoiding injury to the plantar nerve to the hallux in the plantar flap.
  - One alternative capsular incision involves a medial longitudinal capsulotomy in the midline (**Fig. 7.4b**). The dorsal and plantar flaps are carefully elevated off the medial eminence; at the completion of the procedure, a small wedge or **V**-shaped portion of capsule can be removed from the plantar flap, allowing side-to-side closure. Another alternative involves a **V**-, **Y**-, or chevron-shaped capsular incision (**Fig. 7.4c**), which allows advancement and imbrication at the time of closure to correct position of the toe.
- The medial eminence resection can be performed with either a power saw or a chisel at the surgeon's preference. This is typically performed after any proximal metatarsal osteotomy or first TMT arthrodesis is performed. The medial eminence resection is aligned parallel with the medial border of the foot. In order to avoid excessive bone resection and a potential for iatrogenic hallux varus, the author prefers to start the saw or chisel cut 1 mm medial to the sagittal groove on the metatarsal head with the exit point on the metatarsal neck flush with the diaphyseal bone (**Fig. 7.5**). The bony surface can be smoothed of any sharp edges using a synovial rongeur or small bone rasp.
- The hallux can be reduced to a congruent position on the metatarsal head and checked under fluoroscopy. Redundant medial capsular tissue can be sharply excised with a scalpel blade. The capsulotomy is then closed in side-to-side fashion with multiple figure-of-eight stitches using 2–0 absorbable suture to balance the soft tissues and maintain reduction of the joint (**Fig. 7.6**).

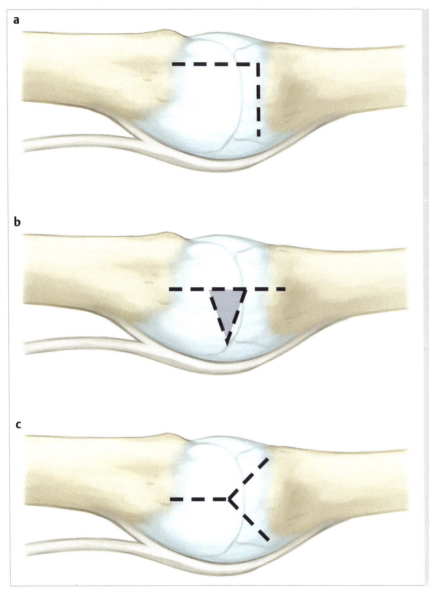

Fig. 7.4 Medial view of hallux MTP joint demonstrating various medial capsulotomy configurations. (**a**) Proximally attached **L**-shaped capsulotomy (author's preferred); (**b**) medial midline capsulotomy, with plantar wedge of tissue indicated for resection to reduce valgus of toe (cross-hatched section); (**c**) **Y**-shaped capsulotomy.

7.7 Tips and Pearls

- Use of a laminar spreader to distract between the first and second metatarsals drastically improves visualization of the contracted web space structures.
- More aggressive release of lateral structures is necessary for more severe deformity.
- Meticulous dissection of the capsule off the medial eminence provides better tissue for subsequent repair.
- Redundant medial capsule can be trimmed to allow better tensioning of the repair.

7.8 Hazards and Pitfalls

- Avoid excessive removal of the medial eminence to avoid creating iatrogenic hallux varus. It is recommended to make the medial eminence saw cut approximately 1 mm medial to the sagittal groove.
- Avoid excessive stripping of the lateral capsule off the metatarsal head to maintain vascularity to the head.

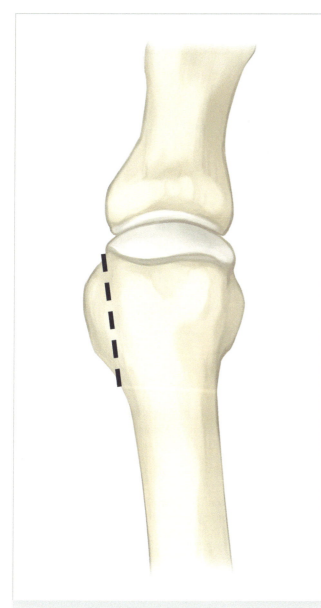

Fig. 7.5 Resection of medial eminence.

7.9 Complications/Bailout/ Salvage

7.9.1 Complications

- Recurrence.
- Contracture, stiffness.
- Wound complications.
- Infection.
- Neurapraxia, neuroma.
- Hallux varus.

7.9.2 Bailout/Salvage

In cases where the medial capsular tissue is not sturdy enough to perform adequate repair and balancing, the capsular sutures can be passed through bone for more reliable repair. This can be accomplished with use of a firm, tightly curved needle to push through the bone or even a drill hole created with a Kirschner wire through the edge of the metatarsal head or phalangeal base.

7.10 Postoperative Care

- The foot is bandaged with loose gauze fluffs between the lesser toes and gauze strips in a spica fashion around the hallux to maintain alignment and protect the repair. Gauze strapping around the metatarsals assists in reducing the IMA deformity. Soft cotton padding followed by a compressive bandage completes the bandaging.
- The operative foot is placed in a removable stiff-soled post-operative shoe or short fracture boot. In isolated McBride's bunionectomy, the patient can weight-bear on the heel for 4 weeks and then progress to flat-footed walking; if the distal soft-tissue correction is combined with a proximal meta-tarsal osteotomy or TMT arthrodesis, then weight-bearing restriction is dictated by the proximal bony procedure (as covered in Chapters 9, 11, and 20).
- The author straps or tapes the hallux in a reduced position every 10 to 14 days for roughly 4 to 6 weeks to allow soft-tissue healing. Following this, the taping is discontinued and the patient commences range-of-motion exercises of the toe.

7.11 Outcomes

- Numerous retrospective series demonstrate good clinical outcomes for mild to moderate hallux valgus.[5–8]
- All series showed improvements in HVA and IMA close to normal values (HVA, 14–18 degrees; IMA, 9–10 degrees).
- All authors noted improved outcomes when preoperative deformity was limited to mild to moderate deformities, with HVA < 30 to 40 degrees and IMA < 15 degrees[5–8]; for more severe deformities, proximal osteotomy in conjunction with distal soft-tissue correction is recommended.[5–8]
- Satisfaction averaged 90 to 92%.[7,8] In one series, 100% re-sumed jogging.[6]
- Iatrogenic hallux varus is described in 11 to 12% of cases.[5,7]
- When reported, 18 to 38% of patients demonstrated postop-erative stiffness of the MTP joint.[6,8]
- One series noted 14% incidence of nerve injury.[8]

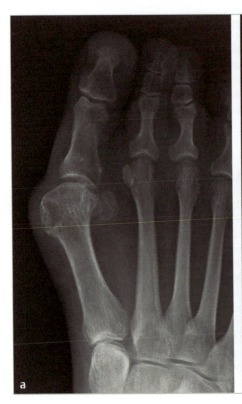 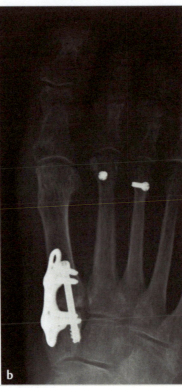

Fig. 7.6 (**a**) Preoperative and (**b**) postoperative views of MTP following modified McBride's procedure.

References

1. Silver D. The operative treatment of hallux valgus. J Bone Joint Surg 1923;5:225–232
2. McBride ED. A conservative operation for bunions.1928. J Bone Joint Surg Am 2002;84-A(11):2101
3. McBride ED. The conservative operation for "bunions". JAMA 1935;105:1164–1168
4. McBride ED. The McBride bunion hallux valgus operation. J Bone Joint Surg Am 1967;49(8):1675–1683
5. Mann RA, Coughlin MJ. Hallux valgus--etiology, anatomy, treatment and surgical considerations. Clin Orthop Relat Res 1981(157):31–41
6. Meyer JM, Hoffmeyer P, Borst F. The treatment of hallux valgus in runners using a modified McBride procedure. Int Orthop 1987;11(3):197–200
7. Mann RA, Pfeffinger L. Hallux valgus repair. DuVries modified McBride procedure. Clin Orthop Relat Res 1991(272):213–218
8. Johnson JE, Clanton TO, Baxter DE, Gottlieb MS. Comparison of Chevron osteotomy and modified McBride bunionectomy for correction of mild to moderate hallux valgus deformity. Foot Ankle 1991;12(2):61–68

8 Chevron Osteotomy for Hallux Valgus Correction

David I. Pedowitz and Walter J. Pedowitz

Abstract

The Chevron osteotomy is a reliable procedure for correction of mild to moderate hallux valgus. As with all hallux valgus correction, the Chevron osteotomy with or without distal soft-tissue realignment remains challenging, even for the most experienced foot surgeons. With careful clinical and radiographic evaluation, however, the Chevron osteotomy maintains its role as a dependable tool for correcting these deformities.

Keywords: *hallux valgus, bunion, metatarsus primus varus*

8.1 Indications

- Mild, moderate, or severe hallux valgus that have failed conservative care. Note: while absolute measurements of hallux valgus angles remain important in preventing recurrence and choosing the proper procedure for correction, it is a combination of these numbers with the clinical scenario that drives decision making.
- Intermetatarsal angle (IMA) < 14 degrees.

8.1.1 Clinical Evaluation

- Tenderness over the medial eminence of the first metatarsophalangeal (MTP) joint.
- Deformity should be passively correctable.
- Patients should have pain with weight-bearing activity and/or shoe wear.
- May present with or without significant ankle, midfoot, or hindfoot deformity.
- May have some decreased sagittal arc of motion at MTP joint.

8.1.2 Radiographic Evaluation

- Plain standing, weight-bearing X-rays of the foot looking for
  - MTP joint congruence.
  - Measurement of IMA between first and second metatarsal (MT) shafts; Mann's classification is as follows:
    - ✦ Mild: IMA < 13 degrees, HVA < 30 degrees.
    - ✦ Moderate: IMA > 13 degrees, HVA < 40 degrees.
    - ✦ Severe: IMA > 20 degrees, HVA > 40 degrees.
  - Presence of hallux valgus interphalangeus.
  - Increased distal metatarsal articular angle (DMAA).
  - Lateral sesamoid subluxation.
  - Arthritic change at the MTP joint.
  - Prior bony procedures or fractures which may affect corrective planning.
- Magnetic resonance imaging (MRI):
  - Generally not indicated in this setting.
  - Can be used if concerned about arthritic changes or an osteochondral defect in the MT head not seen on radiographs.
  - Indicated when pain in joint with range of motion or axial grinding is worse than would be suggested on radiographs.

- Computed tomography (CT) scan:
  - Rarely used.
  - Allows one to assess bone stock when cysts or osteochondral lesions can be seen with plain radiography.

8.1.3 Nonoperative Options

- Wide toe-box shoes with minimal stitching over region of medial eminence.
- Bunion spacers or silicone pads.
- Cutting hole in shoe over area of medial eminence.

8.2 Contraindications

- Impaired vascular status.
- Short first MT may predispose to transfer metatarsalgia postoperatively in the presence of a long second MT.
- Skeletal immaturity.
- Arthrosis at the MTP joint.
- An incongruent MTP joint with an IMA of >14 degrees is thought to be a relative contraindication.

8.3 Goals of the Surgical Procedure

- Translation of the first MT head laterally to correct the IMA to ≤ 9 degrees.
- Stable osteotomy with reduction of the MT head over the sesamoids.
- Stable, pain-free MTP joint correction with adequate great toe mobility for shoe wear.

8.4 Advantages of Surgical Procedure

- Modest surgical time.
- Stable osteotomy requires limited internal fixation.
- Less surgical dissection than other techniques.
- Allows one to assess and address intra-articular pathology and soft-tissue releases as well as bony correction through single incision.

8.5 Key Principles

- Adequate bony translation of the first MTP head fragment should correct the deformity (**Fig. 8.1**, **Fig. 8.2**).
- Careful soft-tissue balancing may fine-tune a bony correction and ensure a stable joint.

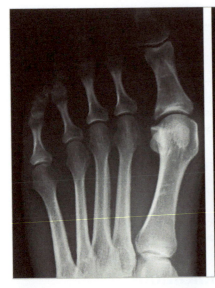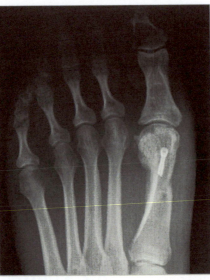

Fig. 8.1 A Radiographic example of a pre-operative deformity and status post surgical correction.

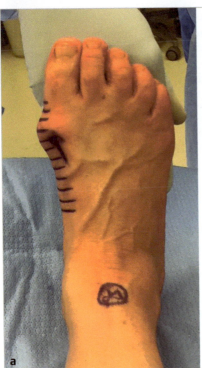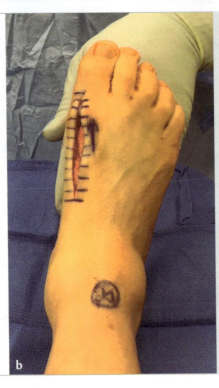

a   b

Fig. 8.2 (a,b) A clinical example of a preoperative deformity and status post surgical correction.

8.6 Preoperative Preparation and Patient Positioning

- Supine.
- General anesthesia with a regional ankle block for postoperative pain relief.
- Calf tourniquet or supramalleolar Esmarch tourniquet may be used.
- Prophylactic antibiotics.

8.7 Operative Technique

- Medial incision over first MTP joint for approximately 7 to 8 cm.
- Retract both dorsal and plantar medial cutaneous nerves to the great toe.

- A vertical capsulectomy at the level of the joint allows one to remove capsule so as to ensure that there is no redundant capsule once repaired.
- Capsule is then dissected off the medial eminences, leaving it attached to the plantar MT sesamoid complex.
- With axial traction on the MTP joint, a 15-blade is used to vertically incise and release the lateral capsule with care not to pivot with the blade too plantar as this could injure the flexor hallucis longus tendon.
- With a retractor pulling plantar on the capsule adjacent to the tibial sesamoid, the knife is then placed between the fibular sesamoid and the MT head, releasing the metatarsosesamoid ligament. This completes the distal soft-tissue release.
- The medial eminence is then resected in line with the sagittal sulcus and in a plane aligned with either the medial shaft of the first MT or the medial border of the foot. Note: lining up the medial eminence resection with the shaft of the first

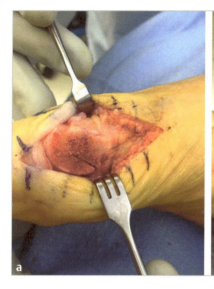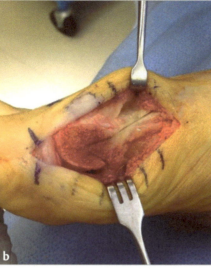

Fig. 8.3 (a,b) Plantar and dorsal limbs of osteotomy. A long dorsal limb provides ample room for screw placement. Ensure plantar limb exits proximal to sesamoid articulation.

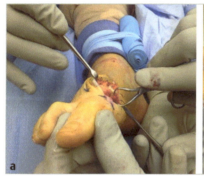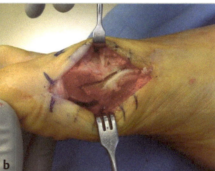

Fig. 8.4 (a,b) Once the osteotomy is completed, distraction on the great toe frees up the head fragment. Controlled with a small towel clamp, the proximal fragment is pulled medially while the head fragment is translated medially approximately 50% of the width of the shaft.

MT can, relatively speaking, make the head fragment more narrow, leaving one with less bone to work with for fixation and translation.

- Standard osteotomy is made with an apex distal 55- to 60-degree-angled Chevron-shaped bone cut within the MT head.
- We prefer an osteotomy made with a long dorsal limb. This provides a large surface for bony union as well as room for hardware placement (**Fig. 8.3**).
- The dorsal limb should exit on the dorsal cortex at about the midshaft.
- The plantar limb should exit proximal to plantar articular surface so as to avoid the metatarsosesamoid articulation.
- Once complete, the osteotomy may be freed up with a small osteotome or elevator.
- A small towel clamp is then used to pull medially on the MT shaft, while lateral pressure is used to translate the head fragment (**Fig. 8.4**).
- The MT head should be shifted adequately to correct the IMA to less than 9 degrees and reduce the MT head over the sesamoids. This should be checked with simulated weight-bearing intraoperative fluoroscopy.
- In males, the head can usually be shifted 6 mm, while in females only 5-mm translation is usually possible, while maintaining adequate bone contact and stability of the osteotomy.[1]
- A dorsal to plantar 3.0-mm headless compression screw may be used to fix the osteotomy (**Fig. 8.5**).
- The leading edge of remaining bone from the MT shaft is resected with a sagittal saw in line with the MT shaft.

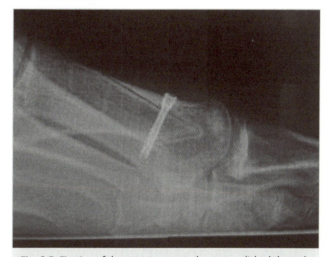

Fig. 8.5 Fixation of the osteotomy may be accomplished through a myriad of techniques. Shown here is a headless compression screw exiting proximal to the plantar limb of the osteotomy and metatarsosesamoid articulation.

- At this point, the toe should be in a nearly neutral position. If not, a medial-based closing wedge osteotomy of the proximal phalanx should be considered.
- If the correction is satisfactory, the capsule is then repaired using a 2–0 absorbable suture holding the toe in neutral to slight varus (**Fig. 8.6**, **Fig. 8.7**).
- Skin closure is with nylon running suture.
- A toe strapping dressing is applied and changed at 1 week.

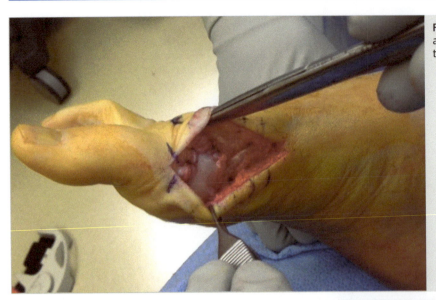

Fig. 8.6 The capsulotomy is closed with absorbable interrupted sutures holding the toe in neutral to slight varus.

8.8 Tips and Pearls

- Avoid aggressive periosteal stripping to minimize damage to MT head blood supply.
- Medial dissection and capsulotomy is unavoidable but leave dorsal and plantar soft-tissue attachments.
- If a distal soft-tissue procedure is necessary, this should be accomplished through MTP and metatarsosesamoid joints—not through a separate incision, which may increase the risk of vascular compromise.
- The osteotomy should be made perpendicular to the long axis of the foot (usually in line with the second MT) to prevent shortening of the first MT during translation of the MT head.
- A long dorsal limb increases bony contact and room for hardware placement.
- Inferior limb should exit proximal to the plantar extent of the articular surface of the MT head.
- If one displaces MT head greater than 50% of the width of the MT, the osteotomy may become unstable and require additional fixation and modifications to postoperative weight-bearing protocols.
- When one encounters a very high DMAA, a biplanar medial closing wedge Chevron osteotomy should be employed.
- This is accomplished by taking a medial-based wedge out of the residual MT once the osteotomy has been completed to allow the head fragment to be angulated into some additional varus.

8.9 Hazards and Pitfalls

- Metatarsus adductus must be appreciated preoperatively and may require additional extra-articular osteotomies.
- Hypermobility at the tarsometatarsal joint/generalized ligamentous laxity may predispose to recurrence.
- Excessive soft-tissue release may devascularize the MT head leading to osteonecrosis.
- Arthritis within the MTP joint (including the sesamoid MT articulation) may result in persistent pain despite deformity correction.
- If the osteotomy is angled proximally, the first MT will shorten during translation, which can result in transfer metatarsalgia to the second MT.

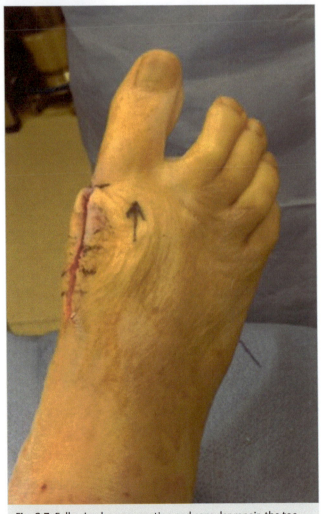

Fig. 8.7 Following bony correction and capsular repair, the toe should remain in the desired position on its own.

8.10 Complications/Bailout/ Salvage

- Excessive translation of the MT head can result in limited bone contact and an unstable osteotomy leading to nonunion or malunion at the osteotomy site. An aggressive medial eminence resection in line with the first MT shaft can also contribute to this technical complication.
- Transfer metatarsalgia (usually to the second MT) is managed by unloading orthotic inserts or surgical shortening of the second MT to rebalance the MT cascade. This should be assessed at the time of the initial bunionectomy surgery and can be performed as part of the initial procedure when necessary.
- Nonunion of Chevron osteotomy is rare, but can be managed with bone grafting and additional internal stabilization.
- Osteonecrosis is rare and may be associated with excess soft-tissue stripping. This will require a fusion of the MTP joint for salvage.

8.11 Postoperative Care

- Patients are made non-weight-bearing for 2 weeks to protect the incision and ensure that edema is kept to a minimum.
- Sutures are removed at 2 weeks.
- At 2 weeks, patients are made weight-bearing as tolerated in a stiff-soled postoperative shoe with a foam toe spacer between the first and second toes.
- Patients with right-sided surgery may drive at 6 weeks.
- At 8 weeks, patients may discontinue the postoperative shoe.
- Running and aggressive impact activities are resumed at 12 weeks postoperatively.
- Stiffness is common and often amenable to physical therapy.

8.12 Outcomes

- The Chevron has proved to be a stable, reproducible osteotomy with high patient satisfaction rates, to treat mild to moderate hallux valgus deformity for generations of surgeons.[2,3,4]
- While the historical risk of avascular necrosis of the head of the MT in combination with a lateral soft-tissue release has been reported to be as high as 40%, this has not been supported in more recent series.[5,6]

References

1. Badwey TM, Dutkowsky JP, Graves SC, Richardson EG. An anatomical basis for the degree of displacement of the distal Chevron osteotomy in the treatment of hallux valgus. Foot Ankle Int 1997 Apr;18(4): 213-5
2. Hattrup SJ, Johnson KA. Chevron osteotomy: analysis of factors in patients' dissatisfaction. Foot Ankle 1985;5(6): 327–332
3. Lewis RJ, Feffer HL. Modified chevron osteotomy of the first metatarsal. Clin Orthop Relat Res 1981;(157):105–109
4. Mann RA, Donatto KC. The chevron osteotomy: a clinical and radiographic analysis. Foot Ankle Int 1997;18(5):255–261
5. Mann RA. Complications associated with the Chevron osteotomy. Foot Ankle 1982;3(3):125–129
6. Trnka HJ, Zembsch A, Easley ME, Salzer M, Ritschl P, Myerson MS. The chevron osteotomy for correction of hallux valgus. Comparison of findings after two and five years of follow-up. J Bone Joint Surg Am 2000;82-A(10):1373–1378

9 Ludloff Proximal First Metatarsal Osteotomy for Hallux Valgus Correction

Steven B. Weinfeld

Abstract

The Ludloff osteotomy was initially described in 1918 for correction of deformities of the first metatarsal. Ludloff performed this procedure without internal fixation. With the addition of rigid fixation, it has gained popularity for correction of hallux valgus deformities because of its inherent stability and reproducible results. It is combined with soft-tissue realignment to correct moderate and severe hallux valgus deformities.

Keywords: *Ludloff, proximal osteotomy, hallux valgus, rotational osteotomy*

9.1   Indications

- Pathology of hallux valgus includes lateral deviation of the great toe, an increased intermetatarsal angle (IMA) between the first and second metatarsals, contracture of the lateral soft tissues, and displacement of the sesamoid complex. Pronation of the hallux may also be present along with a prominent medial eminence.[1]
- A proximal osteotomy, combined with soft-tissue realignment, is indicated for moderate to severe deformities including a hallux valgus angle (HVA) > 35 degrees and an IMA > 14 degrees.

9.1.1   Clinical Evaluation

- Patients should be assessed standing to evaluate true degree of deformity.
- Clinical evaluation of range of motion and pain with motion at the metatarsophalangeal (MTP) joint is essential to rule out arthritis within the joint.
- In most cases, there is no pain with motion at the MTP joint. Presence of pain may suggest arthritis or an osteochondral defect within the metatarsal head.
- Careful evaluation for associated lesser toe deformities and MTP instability must be performed
- Assess stability of first tarsometatarsal (TMT) joint for hypermobility or presence of arthritis.

9.1.2   Radiographic Evaluation

- Weight-bearing anteroposterior and lateral radiographs are used to assess the HVA and IMA along with any other associated pathology.
- Carefully assess first TMT for evidence of arthritis or hypermobility.
- Sesamoid view can be useful if sesamoid metatarsal arthritis is suspected.
- Associated planovalgus should be evaluated clinically and radiographically.
- Tertiary studies (computed tomography/magnetic resonance imaging [CT/MRI]) are not usually indicated, unless there is concern for intra-articular pathology not seen on plane radiographs.

9.1.3   Nonoperative Options

- Wide toe-box shoe.
- Padding.
- Orthotic inserts.
- Bunion spacers.

9.1.4   Contraindications

- This procedure should not be used in patients with significant degenerative changes of the first MTP joint. Consider first MTP arthrodesis in these patients.
- Hypermobility of the first ray also is a relative contraindication for the Ludloff osteotomy. A Lapidus fusion may be better suited for this population to address the first ray hypermobility.
- Severe osteopenia may prevent adequate fixation of the Ludloff osteotomy.
- A very narrow first metatarsal shaft may also be a contraindication to this procedure.
- Patients with an abnormal distal metatarsal articular angle may be better treated with a closing wedge chevron osteotomy.
- Patients with a small IMA but a large HVA may be better treated with a distal metatarsal osteotomy with the addition of an Akin osteotomy of the proximal phalanx.
- Mild deformities (IMA < 14 degrees or HVA < 35 degrees) may be better treated with a distal first metatarsal osteotomy.

9.2   Goals of Surgical Procedure

- The goals of the Ludloff osteotomy are to correct the IMA along with the hallux valgus deformity. This osteotomy is combined with a modified McBride soft-tissue realignment to achieve these goals.
- The Ludloff osteotomy allows for excellent correction of the IMA while providing stable fixation, which permits the patient early weight-bearing.[2]
- The Ludloff osteotomy can be performed to plantarflex or dorsiflex the first ray if desired. Stable fixation and reliable healing prevent malunion and nonunion of this osteotomy.

9.3   Advantages of Surgical Procedure

- Metaphyseal osteotomy allows excellent healing rates.
- Rotational osteotomy allows for unlimited angular correction.
- Initial rotational screw prevents any metatarsal shortening of the first ray, thereby avoiding stress transfer to the second metatarsal.

- Second fixation screw prevents loss of correction and creates rigid fixation.
- Due to the inherent stability of this procedure, patients can be weight-bearing as tolerated almost immediately.

9.4 Key Principles

- Medial first metatarsal approach from the MTP to TMT joint level.
- Always performed with associated distal soft-tissue release.
- Osteotomy extends from dorsal proximal first metatarsal in 20-degree plantar oblique angle to exit the plantar aspect of the first metatarsal neck just proximal to the capsular insertion.
- Do not complete the osteotomy cut plantarly until an initial rotational screw is inserted.
- Once initial length fixation has been achieved (but not tightened), the plantar osteotomy is completed.
- The metatarsal is rotated around the first screw until required IMA (< 9 degrees) is obtained.
- A second parallel fixation screw is then placed perpendicular to the osteotomy to maintain correction, and both screws are tightened to rigidly fix the osteotomy.
- The medial capsule is then repaired. The joint should be congruently aligned before repair so that the repair holds the joint in position and is not used to correct the joint alignment.

9.4.1 Operative Technique

- Patient placed supine on operating table.
- Regional anesthesia (popliteal block or ankle block) with sedation.
- I prefer to not use tourniquet.
- Sterile prep and draping to midcalf level.
- One medial incision from 2 cm distal to first MTP joint to first TMT joint proximally.
- Identify and protect the medial hallucal nerve.
- Inverted L-shaped capsulotomy to expose medial eminence.

- Resect medial eminence with sagittal saw parallel to medial aspect of first metatarsal.
- Make a 4- to 5-cm incision in first web space for lateral release.
- Perform release of intermetatarsal ligament, adductor hallucis tendon, lateral capsule, and sesamoid complex.
- Expose medial aspect of first metatarsal proximally to level of first TMT joint.
- Perform osteotomy from dorsal proximal aspect of first metatarsal to plantar distal aspect of metatarsal.
- Begin osteotomy 2 to 3 mm distal to the first TMT joint and complete the osteotomy 2 cm proximal to the sesamoids (**Fig. 9.1**).
- Osteotomy proceeds from proximal to distal at approximately 20-degree angle.
- Prior to completion of the osteotomy distally, a 3.5- or 2.7- mm cortical screw is placed across the proximal portion of the osteotomy using lag technique to engage both fragments. The screw is tightened and then loosened slightly to allow rotation of the distal fragment upon completion of the osteotomy (**Fig. 9.2**).
- The osteotomy is completed distally with the sagittal saw, and the distal aspect of the metatarsal is rotated laterally on the proximal screw to reduce the IMA (**Fig. 9.3**).
- Once the proper position is obtained, the proximal screw is tightened, being careful not to crack the dorsal bone. Countersinking of the screws is helpful to avoid fracture.
- A pointed bone reduction clamp is used to secure the distal part of the osteotomy.
- A second 3.5- or 2.7-mm cortical screw is then placed in the distal part of the osteotomy. This can be placed from either the dorsal-to-plantar or plantar-to-dorsal direction.
- It is critical to place the second screw carefully as the medial bone shelf that was produced from rotation of the metatarsal will be removed following secure fixation.
- Carefully remove medial bone shelf (**Fig. 9.4**) with sagittal saw, power burr, or rongeur.
- Assess correction and screw placement with image intensifier. Obtaining lateral image is the best way to check the first ray is not plantar or dorsally displaced and that proximal screw does not violate first TMT joint.

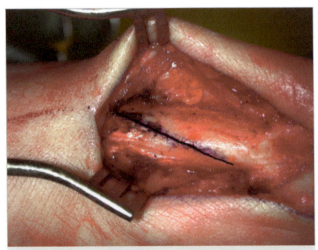

Fig. 9.1 Long oblique dorsal-proximal to distal-plantar osteotomy is initially left incomplete plantarly until the first screw is placed to prevent shortening.

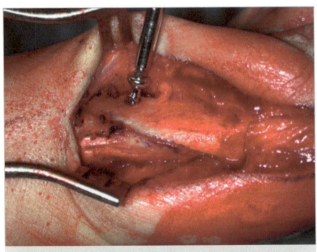

Fig. 9.2 The first screw is placed perpendicular to the osteotomy around which the deformity will be derotated to correct the IM angle.

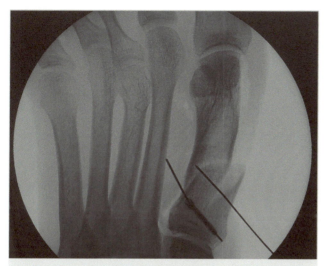

Fig. 9.3 Fluoroscopy view demonstrating appropriate IM correction and shaft derotation prior to inserting the second fixation screw.

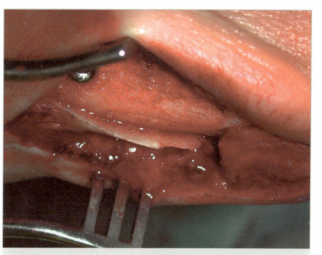

Fig. 9.4 After derotation of the osteotomy and fixation with the second screw, a medial shelf will be present which needs to be resected.

- The medial capsule is then closed using 2–0 absorbable sutures. The proximal soft tissues are closed first and then the L-shaped capsulotomy is repaired. The apex of the L capsular segment is closed by transferring this tissue slightly proximal and dorsal. This provides a stable repair while correcting the pronation of the hallux that often accompanies a hallux valgus deformity.
- Medial capsule is repaired, being careful not to overtighten and produce a hallux varus.

9.5 Tips and Pearls

- Do not remove too much of the medial eminence, as this can contribute to hallux varus. I like to begin medial eminence resection 2 mm medial to the sagittal sulcus in line with the medial shaft of the first metatarsal.
- The saw blade should be angled perpendicular to the shaft of the first metatarsal to avoid plantar or dorsiflexion of the metatarsal as it is rotated laterally.
- Slight angulation of the saw from medial dorsal to lateral plantar is used to prevent first metatarsal head elevation when the osteotomy is rotated.[3]
- The fixation screws should be placed in lag mode and countersunk to avoid splitting the metatarsal.
- In softer bone, cancellous screws may provide better fixation than cortical screws. Consider plate fixation in this situation.
- A longer osteotomy provides improved correction and more stable fixation.

9.6 Hazards and Pitfalls

- It is critical to avoid dorsiflexion or plantarflexion of the first metatarsal. This can cause overload of the first metatarsal head or transfer of stress to the second metatarsal. This problem is avoided by orienting the sagittal saw blade perpendicular to the shaft of the metatarsal.
- The Ludloff osteotomy provides a very powerful correction of the IMA. Care should be taken not to produce a negative IMA causing a subsequent hallux varus deformity.

- It is also important to make the first metatarsal osteotomy as long as possible given the patient's anatomy. If the osteotomy is too short, there may not be adequate room for two screws for fixation. In this situation, a contoured, flexible plate can be used for fixation of the osteotomy.[4]

9.7 Complications/Bailout/ Salvage

- One of the most frequent intraoperative complications with the Ludloff osteotomy is fracture of the first metatarsal. If this occurs, screw fixation alone is not possible, and a contoured, flexible plate can be used to secure the osteotomy.[4] If an appropriate plate is not available, multiple K-wires can be placed into the intramedullary canal of the first metatarsal to provide fixation.[5]
- If, upon completion of the osteotomy and repair of the medial capsule, there is a varus alignment of the hallux, first remove the sutures from the capsule and reevaluate the alignment of the toe. If varus of the toe persists, the first metatarsal osteotomy can be taken down and rotated to decrease the amount of IMA correction. Fixation then can be achieved with a flexible plate or multiple K-wires.
- If, upon completion of the Ludloff osteotomy, the hallux remains in valgus, the addition of an Akin osteotomy of the proximal phalanx can provide further correction.
- If the surgeon determines that the screw fixation is not completely stable, multiple K-wires can be used to augment fixation.[5]

9.8 Postoperative Care

- Patients are placed into a surgical shoe and are allowed flat foot weight-bearing at 3 to 5 days.
- Postoperative dressing change performed at 10 days with suture removal.
- Taping of the hallux in desired position is performed at first postoperative visit and every 2 weeks until 6 weeks postoperatively.

- Surgical shoe is used for 6 weeks.
- X-rays at 6 weeks are used to assess healing of the osteotomy (**Fig. 9.5**).
- Patients are placed into tennis shoe at 6 weeks and allowed low-impact activity.
- Full-impact sports including running and jumping are permitted at 3 months postoperatively.
- Patients should be informed that swelling may persist for 9 to 12 months postsurgery and can limit shoe wear options.

9.9 Outcomes

- The Ludloff osteotomy provides excellent correction of the first and second IMA associated with hallux valgus deformities (**Fig. 9.6a, b**). This osteotomy has been shown to be more stable than the proximal crescentic and other proximal first metatarsal osteotomies.[2,6] The surgeon can expect a powerful, reproducible correction of moderate to severe hallux valgus deformities when combined with soft-tissue realign-

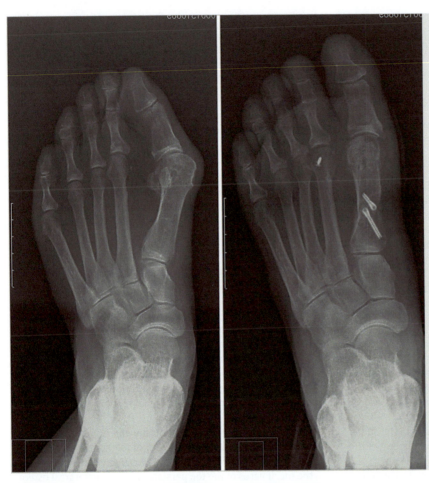

Fig. 9.5 Pre- and postoperative anteroposterior radiographs demonstrating deformity and correction with a Ludloff osteotomy.

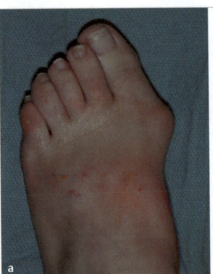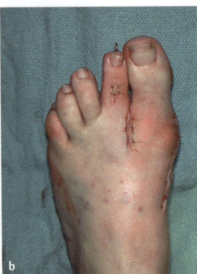

Fig. 9.6 Preoperative (a) and postoperative (b) clinical pictures of the hallux valgus deformity corrected with a Ludloff osteotomy.

ment. Chiodo et al reported correction of the HVA from 31 degrees preoperatively to 11 degrees postoperatively, with correction of the IMA from 16 to 7 degrees in 70 patients.[7] This author presented our results on 31 patients with moderated to severe hallux valgus treated with a Ludloff osteotomy and soft-tissue realignment.[8] The HVA improved from 36.7 degrees preoperatively to 10.8 degrees postoperatively, while the IMA improved from 14.8 degrees preoperatively to 3.9 degrees postoperatively. Complications included loss of fixation in one patient, along with three intraoperative fractures of the first metatarsal. These all occurred in older females with osteopenic bone. No hallux varus or transfer metatarsalgia was seen in this population. For patients with osteoporotic bone, the surgeon may consider using a contoured compression plate for fixation to avoid fracturing the first metatarsal. Neufeld and coworkers have reported good results with this technique.[4] The addition of multiple intramedullary K-wires has also been shown to be an effective augment to screw fixation for the Ludloff osteotomy.[5] Trnka et al reported on 111 feet with hallux valgus treated with the Ludloff osteotomy and soft-tissue realignment.[9] The HVA improved from 35 to 9 degrees, while the IMA improved from 17 to 8 degrees. This series found all osteotomies healed without dorsiflexion malunion but did have 2.2-mm shortening.

References

1. Ludloff K. Die beseitgung des hallux valgus durch die schrage planta-dorsale osteotomie des metatarsus I. Arch Klin Chir 1918;110:364–387
2. Trnka H-J, Parks BG, Ivanic G, et al. Six first metatarsal shaft osteotomies: mechanical and immobilization comparisons. Clin Orthop Relat Res 2000;(381):256–265
3. Beischer AD, Ammon P, Corniou A, Myerson M. Three-dimensional computer analysis of the modified Ludloff osteotomy. Foot Ankle Int 2005;26(8):627–632
4. Castaneda DA, Myerson MS, Neufeld SK. The Ludloff osteotomy: a review of current concepts. Int Orthop 2013;37(9):1661–1668
5. Schon LC, Dom KJ, Jung HG. Clinical tip: stabilization of the proximal Ludloff osteotomy. Foot Ankle Int 2005;26(7):579–581
6. Acevedo JI, Sammarco VJ, Boucher HR, Parks BG, Schon LC, Myerson MS. Mechanical comparison of cyclic loading in five different first metatarsal shaft osteotomies. Foot Ankle Int 2002;23(8):711–716
7. Chiodo CP, Schon LC, Myerson MS. Clinical results with the Ludloff osteotomy for correction of adult hallux valgus. Foot Ankle Int 2004;25(8):532–536
8. Weinfeld SB. The Ludloff osteotomy for correction of hallux valgus: results of 31 cases by one surgeon. Paper presented at: the 31stAnnual Meeting of the American Orthopaedic Foot and Ankle Society; March 3, 2001; San Francisco, CA/ conf
9. Trnka HJ, Hofstaetter SG, Hofstaetter JG, Gruber F, Adams SB Jr, Easley ME. Intermediate-term results of the Ludloff osteotomy in one hundred and eleven feet. J Bone Joint Surg Am 2008;90(3):531–539

10 Scarf Osteotomy

Andy Molloy and Lyndon Mason

Abstract

Burutaran first described the Z first metatarsal diaphyseal osteotomy for correction of metatarsus primus varus in hallux valgus deformities in four cases in 1976. Since then, the procedure has been refined and subsequently popularized internationally through the work of Barouk in France and Weil in the United States. The sagittal Z cut is based on a carpentry technique to longitudinally join two pieces of lumber called a scarf junction. In hallux valgus correction, this technique allows for accurate lateral translation of the first metatarsal to correct the deformity utilizing an inherently stable osteotomy. The diaphyseal location allows for rigid two-screw fixation, allowing for early weight-bearing ambulation. This chapter reviews the surgical technique of performing this procedure, giving tricks to optimize outcome and avoid complications.

Keywords: *scarf, metatarsal osteotomy, sagittal Z cut, hallux valgus*

10.1 Indications

- Hallux valgus without significant first tarsometatarsal instability.
- Hallux valgus deformity with or without a high distal metatarsal articular angle.
- Hallux valgus without arthritic changes.

10.1.1 Clinical Evaluation

- Although the scarf osteotomy is a highly versatile procedure for hallux valgus correction, it is important to have a number of other procedures in your arsenal to treat the myriad of hallux valgus deformities that can present.
- It is important to assess the stability of the tarsometatarsal joint (TMTJ), as a corrective distal or shaft osteotomy may struggle to correct or prevent recurrence in an unstable TMTJ.
- Arthritis in the first metatarsal phalangeal joint should be assessed. A positive midrange grind test should make you consider fusion surgery rather than an osteotomy.
- Consider the alignment of the entire limb. A pes planus deformity and supinated forefoot will exacerbate the deformity.
- Assess any lesser toe deformities. Firstly, these may require concurrent corrections. Secondly, a metatarsus adductus deformity with lateral deviated lesser toes can prove to be a significant challenge when correcting the hallux valgus deformity.

10.1.2 Radiographic Evaluation

- Weight-bearing anteroposterior, oblique, and lateral radiographs should be obtained.

10.1.3 Nonoperative Options

- The nonoperative options for a hallux valgus deformity aim to reduce the symptoms rather than the deformity itself.

- Modification of shoes by stretching constricting areas or relieving pressure areas may relieve symptoms. This can be achieved with commercially available ring shoe stretchers or by inserting additional material. Wider footwear with a roomy toe box may afford significant reduction in discomfort related to static forefoot abnormalities. However, the forefoot/hindfoot mismatch can be difficult to manage with off-the-shelf footwear, and custom-made shoe wear can resolve this.
- The use of pads, arch supports, and various insoles may assist in reducing a hallux valgus deformity if associated with a supinated forefoot.
- There is no evidence to support the use of any type of splint or brace and even very little for the long-term success of orthotics. Physiotherapy to stretch the lateral tissues will not reverse the problem but may help ease the pain and stiffness that is felt.

10.1.4 Contraindications

- Osteoarthritis.
- TMTJ instability.
- A narrow first metatarsal, meaning that maximum translation will be insufficient to correct the deformity.
- Severe hallux valgus deformity.

10.2 Goals of Surgical Procedure

- Our overall goal is to improve symptoms and decrease deformity. To be more specific, we aim to achieve a bony correction in order to balance the soft tissues to allow normal function to the hallucal metatarsal articulation.

10.3 Advantages of Surgical Procedure

- The scarf osteotomy is the "workhorse" procedure for the majority of hallux valgus reconstruction. It has great versatility given that it can be used to not only provide lateral shift of the first metatarsal, but also lower or elevate the metatarsal head, lengthen or shorten the first metatarsal, and even provide axial rotation.
- A survey of Australian orthopaedic surgeons found that greater than 50% would perform a scarf osteotomy for moderate to severe hallux valgus deformities.[1]
- A scarf osteotomy preserves the blood supply to the metatarsal head due to its long plantar limb.

10.4 Key Principles

- Lateral release.
- Lateral translation of metatarsal head to allow sesamoid coverage.
- Distal soft-tissue realignment.

10.5 Preoperative Preparation and Patient Positioning

- When assessing for appropriateness for scarf osteotomy, it is imperative to measure the width of the metatarsal head. A scarf osteotomy can only reliably translate the distal metatarsal 50% of the width of the metatarsal head, and therefore, if the intended correction is greater than this, another option should be considered (**Fig. 10.1**).

- Measure the medial and lateral walls of the proximal phalanx. If the length of the medial wall is more than 5 mm than that of the lateral wall, consider an Akin osteotomy (**Fig. 10.2**).

- Plan the transverse limbs of the osteotomy by drawing on the anteroposterior radiograph the proposed osteotomy 90 degrees to the second metatarsal. This is to ensure that minimal shortening occurs when translation is performed (**Fig. 10.2**). This can be used to choose an anatomical landmark to aim for the distal transverse cut. This is usually at the fourth metatarsophalangeal joint (MTPJ).

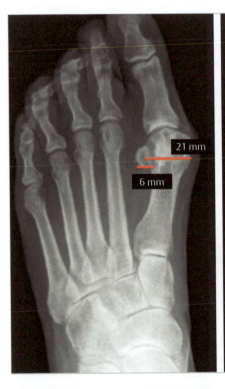
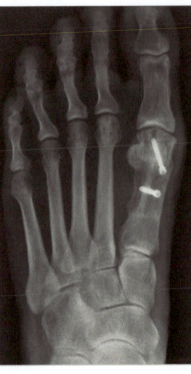

Fig. 10.1 Preoperative and 6-month postoperative radiographs of a hallux valgus correction showing a metatarsal head width measurement and intended correction measurement. Because it is only consistently possible to translate the metatarsal head by 50%, another option for correction should be considered if the intended correction measurement is greater than 50% of the metatarsal head width. In this example, the intended correction measurement is ideal for a scarf.

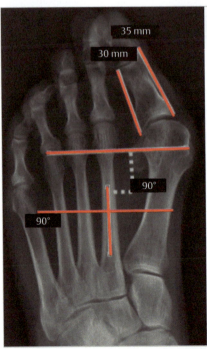
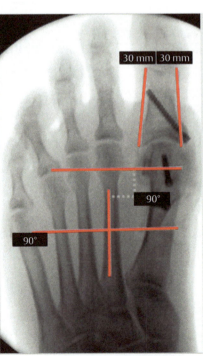

Fig. 10.2 Preoperative radiograph of templating a hallux valgus correction showing hallux interphalangeus (with the medial border of the proximal phalanx being longer than the lateral wall) and the templating for transverse osteotomy limbs so as not to produce shortening or lengthening. There is a 6-month postoperative radiograph showing that the correction has been achieved.

- The patient is positioned supine. Ensure the feet are on the end of the bed to allow easy access to the medial aspect of the first ray.

10.6 Operative Technique

- A midmedial approach is made to the first ray, from just distal to the MTPJ extending proximal, to where the metatarsal inferior flare starts descending to the TMTJ. Ensure the dorsal cutaneous nerve is taken superior to prevent damage.
- Open the capsule of the MTPJ with a midmedial longitudinal incision and elevate the capsule off the medial eminence and the dorsal aspect of the metatarsal head. Ensure that the inferior capsule is left unharmed, to maintain the vascular supply to the metatarsal head.
- A lateral release can be performed through the joint or over the dorsal aspect of the first metatarsal with division of the sesamoid suspensory ligament and the lateral collateral ligament plus, if necessary, adductor hallucis (**Fig. 10.3**). A successful lateral release will allow a varus position of 45 degrees of the hallux to be obtained on stressing.
- Excise the medial eminence if prominent, or at least provide a flat surface for ease of performing the osteotomy (**Fig. 10.4**).

Examining the site of the sesamoid ridges will indicate what is true metatarsal head and what is medial eminence. It is important to maintain metatarsal head anatomy where possible.

- A Z osteotomy is performed (**Fig. 10.5**). The longitudinal axial cut is performed by first ridging the medial cortex, starting 5 mm from the dorsal surface of the metatarsal head and moving proximally to the inferior flare of the metatarsal shaft. Angle the cut with a 10-degree declination angle to prevent dorsal malunions and subsequent transfer metatarsalgia.
- The two sagittal cuts are performed using the templated radiograph, 90 degrees to the second metatarsal shaft. They should be angled 80 degrees to the longitudinal cut. These need to be parallel, one distal dorsal and one proximal inferior. If an altered distal metatarsal articular angle has to be corrected (**Fig. 10.6**), a medial wedge of bone can be excised from the proximal dorsal limb, to allow easy rotation of the metatarsal head.
- The distal limb of the osteotomized metatarsal is translated laterally the required amount to improve the intermetatarsal angle (IMA). The bone is then held either manually or by a clamp (**Fig. 10.7**), allowing two 1-mm Kirschner wires

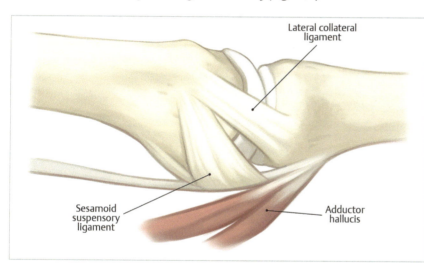

Fig. 10.3 Illustration showing the structure to be transected when performing a lateral release.

Lateral collateral ligament

Sesamoid suspensory ligament

Adductor hallucis

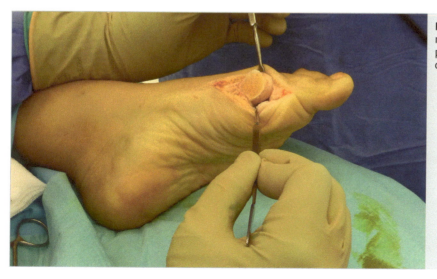

Fig. 10.4 Intraoperative photograph showing minimal resection of the medial eminence to provide a flat surface on which to perform the osteotomy.

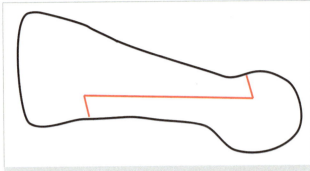

Fig. 10.5 Diagram of the Z osteotomy for the scarf procedure.

to be placed. Direct one wire from the middle of the dorsal proximal limb of the metatarsal toward the central aspect of the head. The second is placed from central aspect of the proximal limb to the central aspect of the distal limb of the metatarsal shaft.

- The metatarsal osteotomy is then secured using two self-drilling, self-tapping, 3.4-mm screws (**Fig. 10.8**).
- The medial remnant is then excised to give a smooth medial border of the metatarsal shaft. Any sharp edges should be paired down with the saw blade.
- A medial capsulorrhaphy is performed to reposition the sesamoids under the metatarsal head. This is performed using a 1 Vicryl suture, passing it from inside to out, starting just medial to the medial sesamoid and then through the dorsal

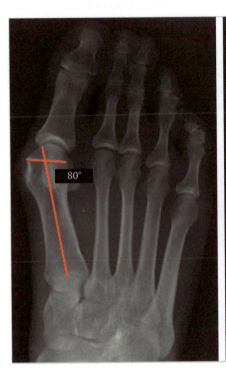
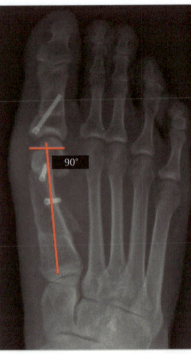

Fig. 10.6 Preoperative and 6-month postoperative radiographs of a hallux valgus correction showing an initial abnormal distal metatarsal articular angle and its subsequent correction.

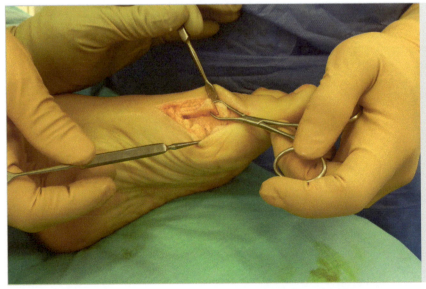

Fig. 10.7 Intraoperative photograph showing the translated osteotomy being held manually with a clamp to allow insertion of K-wires.

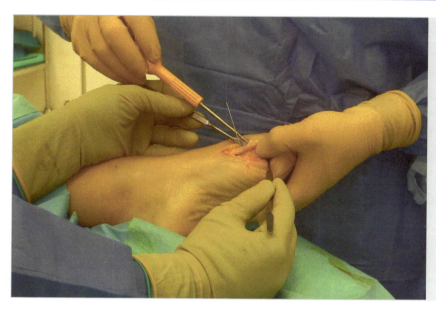

Fig. 10.8 Intraoperative photograph showing the insertion of a headless compression screw over the K-wires which are provisionally holding the osteotomy on the corrected position.

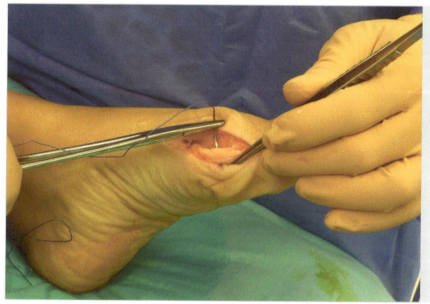

Fig. 10.9 Intraoperative photograph showing the initial suture pass of the capsulorrhaphy. The first pass of the suture is from inside to out going from adjacent to the medial border of the medial sesamoid.

capsule 5 mm more distal to the plantar suture (**Fig. 10.9**). This is then repeated again more distal. With the toe held in plantarflexion and varus, this suture is tightened.

- An Akin osteotomy should be considered in patients where the proximal phalanx medial cortex is longer than lateral cortex. It is also considered when the extensor hallucis longus is bowing medially, as it works to position the insertion point so that it lies on the mechanical axis of the first metatarsal.

10.7 Tips and Pearls

- Template the radiograph preoperatively as described earlier. It is useful to measure the distance from the lateral sesamoid to the expected normal sesamoidal position on the metatarsal head to give an estimate of the distance of correction that is required.

- The two sagittal cuts need to be parallel to allow easy translation. If the cuts are convergent, the bone will become wedged on translation. If this does occur, take a small slither of bone from the proximal aspect of the plantar distal bone fragment.
- If any soft tissue remains on the lateral aspect of the dorsal proximal limb, it will not allow you to translate the one limb on the other. Take special care in removing this soft tissue from the most distal lateral aspect of the proximal limb.
- To ensure that the lateral release has been successfully completed, pass a Freer retractor through medial side to the lateral side. If the lateral sesamoid suspensory ligament remains, the sesamoid relocation will not occur on medial capsulorrhaphy.
- Place the distal screw into the center of the metatarsal head in as vertical position as possible. If the screw is placed obliquely from medial to lateral, the screw will reduce your correction on compression by pulling the distal limb medially.

10.8 Hazards and Pitfalls

- Using a clamp to hold osteotomy reduction in osteoporotic bone will lead to troughing, which will ultimately lead to inadvertent metatarsal head elevation.
- Due to the complex three-dimensional osteotomy of the scarf, it is technically challenging with a substantial learning curve. Its versatility, although very advantageous, increases the risk of malunion as axial, sagittal, and coronal plane corrections are possible.

10.9 Complications/Bailout/Salvage

- Coetzee[2] described complications in 47% of cases. Troughing was the major complication that was reported, occurring in 35%. Other studies report complications occurring in 4 to 19%.[3–7] If troughing occurs, the bone resected from the initial saw cut of the medial eminence can be morcelized and inserted into the troughed area.
- Murawski et al[8] portrayed a reduction in troughing if a rotational scarf was performed, and the proximal end of the dorsal and distal end of the plantar bone was left very thin in order to reduce the trough in comparison to a traditional scarf.
- The technical difficulty with a scarf osteotomy was illustrated by Davies and colleagues,[9] where they found the production of unintentional malunions in a geometric study on scarf osteotomies.
- Valentin[10] reported a 27% rate of hallux limitus following scarf osteotomy for hallux valgus correction. It is essential not to inadvertently lengthen or dorsiflex the osteotomy. This can be avoided by accurate templating and ensuring that the longitudinal osteotomy is declined plantarward by around 10 degrees.
- Care needs to be taken not to crosshatch the limbs of the osteotomy so as to avoid acute or delayed fractures. If this happens, then for acute fractures additional fixation can be used or, for significant crosshatching, limitation of weight-bearing status.
- Fusion of the first TMTJ or MTPJ is a potential bailout/salvage operation of failed scarf osteotomies.

10.10 Postoperative Care

- A soft compression dressing is applied at surgery, wrapping the foot from medial to lateral, then allowing the dressing to wrap the toe, thus holding the toe in appropriate alignment
- A hard-soled shoe is appropriate for the first 6 weeks.
- At 6 weeks, repeat radiographs are obtained and the patient is transitioned to a comfortable shoe able to accommodate the swelling of the foot.
- Range-of-motion exercises are started between 3 and 6 weeks.
- Use of a silicone toe spacer for the first 12 weeks helps ensure soft-tissue tension of the medial capsulorrhaphy.

10.11 Outcomes

- A meta-analysis of scarf osteotomy for hallux valgus correction found that a mean reduction of 6.21 degrees in the first and second IMA was achieved in 300 cases.[11]
- De Vil et al reported on the longest prospective study available in the literature for scarf osteotomies. In this study, there was a mean improvement of first and second IMA of 6 degrees and hallux valgus angle of 19 degrees.[12] The AOFAS score improved from 47 to 83 at 1 year. These results were maintained at 8 years with no recurrence. The results in this study are comparable to other previous smaller follow-up studies.[4,5,13]
- Ballas et al found that after surgical correction for hallux valgus, patients who underwent scarf osteotomy had a gait pattern similar to that of their nonoperated foot in terms of forefoot propulsive forces.[14]

References

1. Iselin LD, Munt J, Symeonidis PD, Klammer G, Chehade M, Stavrou P. Operative management of common forefoot deformities: a representative survey of Australian orthopaedic surgeons. Foot Ankle Spec 2012;5(3):188–194
2. Coetzee JC. Scarf osteotomy for hallux valgus repair: the dark side. Foot Ankle Int 2003;24(1):29–33
3. Kristen KH, Berger C, Stelzig S, Thalhammer E, Posch M, Engel A. The SCARF osteotomy for the correction of hallux valgus deformities. Foot Ankle Int 2002;23(3):221–229
4. Garrido IM, Rubio ER, Bosch MN, González MS, Paz GB, Llabrés AJ. Scarf and Akin osteotomies for moderate and severe hallux valgus: clinical and radiographic results. Foot Ankle Surg 2008;14(4):194–203
5. Lipscombe S, Molloy A, Sirikonda S, Hennessy MS. Scarf osteotomy for the correction of hallux valgus: midterm clinical outcome. J Foot Ankle Surg 2008;47(4):273–277
6. Crevoisier X, Mouhsine E, Ortolano V, Udin B, Dutoit M. The scarf osteotomy for the treatment of hallux valgus deformity: a review of 84 cases. Foot Ankle Int 2001;22(12):970–976
7. Weil LS. Scarf osteotomy for correction of hallux valgus. Historical perspective, surgical technique, and results. Foot Ankle Clin 2000;5(3):559–580
8. Murawski CD, Egan CJ, Kennedy JG. A rotational scarf osteotomy decreases troughing when treating hallux valgus. Clin Orthop Relat Res 2011;469(3):847–853
9. Davies MB, Blundell CM, Marquis CP, McCarthy AD. Interpretation of the scarf osteotomy by 10 surgeons. Foot Ankle Surg 2011;17(3):108–112
10. Valentin B. Changing concepts in the surgery of hallux valgus. In: Jakob RP, Fulford P, Horan F, eds. European Instructional Course Lectures. London: British Editorial Society of Bone and Joint Surgery;1999:119–127
11. Smith SE, Landorf KB, Butterworth PA, Menz HB. Scarf versus chevron osteotomy for the correction of 1-2 intermetatarsal angle in hallux valgus: a systematic review and meta-analysis. J Foot Ankle Surg 2012;51(4):437–444

12. De Vil JJ, Van Seymortier P, Bongaerts W, De Roo PJ, Boone B, Verdonk R. Scarf osteotomy for hallux valgus deformity: a prospective study with 8 years of clinical and radiologic follow-up. J Am Podiatr Med Assoc 2010;100(1):35–40

13. Galli M, Muratori F, Visci F, Pezzillo F, Aulisa AG. Middle term results of I metatarsal "Scarf" osteotomy [in Italian]. Clin Ter 2007;158(3):209–212

14. Ballas R, Edouard P, Philippot R, Farizon F, Delangle F, Peyrot N. Ground-reactive forces after hallux valgus surgery: comparison of Scarf osteotomy and arthrodesis of the first metatarsophalangeal joint. Bone Joint J 2016;98-B(5):641–646

11 Proximal Opening Wedge First Metatarsal Osteotomy for Hallux Valgus Correction

Joseph N. Daniel and Steven M. Raikin

Abstract

Proximal opening wedge osteotomy of the first metatarsal is a reasonable treatment option for patients with symptomatic hallux valgus. Patient demographics, degree of symptoms, and the severity of the deformity should all be used to determine whether a proximal opening wedge osteotomy best suits a certain patient. This chapter provides a brief overview of the indications and contraindications for performing a proximal opening wedge osteotomy. In addition, the chapter contains a detailed preoperative planning guide, step-by-step operative technique, and potential risks or hazards that one might face intraoperatively. Expert advice and techniques are divulged to help avoid these hazards and minimize the risk for common postoperative complications. Overall, high patient satisfaction scores and equal results have been shown between proximal first metatarsal opening wedge osteotomy and alternative surgical options for patients suffering from hallux valgus.

Keywords: *proximal metatarsal osteotomy, opening wedge osteotomy, hallux valgus*

11.1 Introduction

- Utilization of proximal opening wedge osteotomy with exostosis for correction of hallux valgus first described by Trethowan in 1923 and Trott in 1972.[1,2]
- Historically utilized in adolescent hallux valgus.[3]
- Subsequent abandonment of procedure occurred with concerns for stability, dorsal malunion, and transfer metatarsalgia.[4]

11.2 Indications

- Patients with moderate or severe hallux valgus, which is symptomatic (i.e., pain in and out of shoe wear or limitations in reasonable shoe wear)[5,6] (**Fig. 11.1**).
- Patients having previous osteotomy with subsequent shortening of the first metatarsal.[7]

11.2.1 Clinical Evaluation

- Perform a complete neurovascular examination of the foot.
- Assess the range of motion of the first metatarsal-medial cuneiform joint.
- Assess the range of motion of the first metatarsal phalangeal joint (hypermobility or severe limitation of motion contraindication for procedure).
- Assess the pronation component to the deformity—if no pronation component is involved, deformity cannot be corrected with a proximal metatarsal osteotomy.

11.2.2 Radiographic Evaluation

- Measurements must be evaluated from weight-bearing radiographs of the foot (**Fig. 11.2**).
- Hallux valgus angle (HVA) > 30 degrees.[6]
- Intermetatarsal angle (IMA) > 13 degrees.[6]
- Normal to slightly elevated distal metatarsal articular angle (DMAA), normal being < 10 degrees.

11.2.3 Nonoperative Options

- Accommodative shoe wear.
- Shoes with < 1-inch heel to avoid progression of deformity.
- Insertion of toe spacer.
- No role for custom orthotic management.
- No role for steroid injection therapy.
- No role for physical therapy.

11.2.4 Contraindications

- Hypermobility or instability of the first tarsometatarsal (TMT) joint may have independent causation of increased IMA, one that will not be corrected with proximal metatarsal osteotomy. These patients may be treated more appropriately

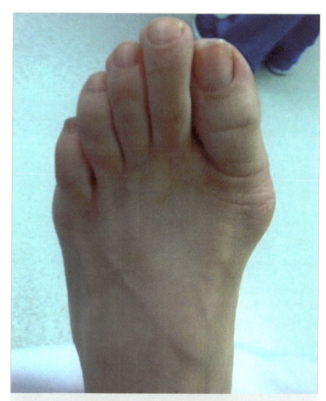

Fig. 11.1 Patient with symptomatic hallux valgus.

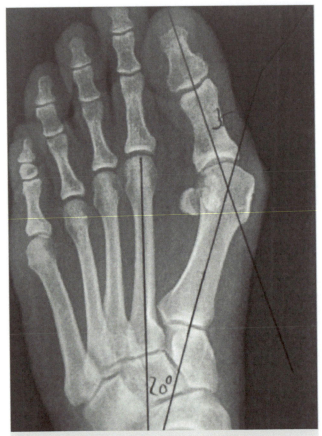

Fig. 11.2 Weight-bearing radiograph of patient demonstrating increased HVA and IMA angles.

with a first metatarsal-medial cuneiform arthrodesis (Lapidus' procedure).[5,6]
- Rotational deformities of the first metatarsal.[5]
- Anatomically narrow first metatarsal—due to the difficulty for obtaining stable fixation.[6]
- Severe arthritis of the metatarsophalangeal (MTP) joint.[3,6]
- Relative contraindication for severely osteoporotic patients.[6]
- Longer first metatarsal compared to the second metatarsal.[3]
- Large DMAA—due to further increase in DMAA with rotational component of osteotomy.[3]
- History of first metatarsal infection.
- Avascular necrosis of the first metatarsal.

11.3 Goals of Surgical Procedure

- Relieve pain and discomfort.
- Restore the physiologic function of the first ray and alignment of great toe.[5]
- Correction of hallux primus varus.
- Decrease IMA between first and second metatarsals.
- Preserve length of the first metatarsal.

11.4 Advantages of Surgical Procedure

- Ability to achieve a large correction of hallux primus varus without compromising length of first metatarsal.

- Less technically demanding and more straightforward of a procedure compared to proximal chevron osteotomy or biplanar osteotomy.[1]
- Low rates of nonunions.[5]
- Low rates of healing complications due to minimal periosteal stripping and intact lateral cortex.
- Rapid incorporation of selected bone graft supplement, if utilized.
- Decreased risk of hardware complications with new and improved fixation techniques.
- Less deviation against the mean absolute Meary's angle compared to proximal chevron osteotomy.[1]

11.5 Key Principles

- Step #1: perform distal soft-tissue procedure.[8]
- Step #2: excise the medial eminence of the first metatarsal.
- Step #3: perform proximal opening wedge osteotomy.
- Step #4: plication of medial MTP joint capsule.

11.6 Preoperative Preparation and Positioning

- Position patient supine and consider use of thigh or calf tourniquet.[6]
- Consider the use of a small hip bolster to provide neutralization of the lower extremity and minimize amount of external rotation.
- Consider the administration of regional anesthesia or nerve block for optimal postoperative pain control.[4,6]

11.7 Operative Technique

- Utilizing fluoroscopy and direct visualization, identify the location of the first TMT joint.
- Make a 2- to 3-cm medial longitudinal incision from the first metatarsal-medial cuneiform articulation, extending distally (**Fig. 11.3a,b**).
- Measure 1.5 cm distal to the first TMT joint, and mark site for correct osteotomy placement.
- Perform a transverse or oblique osteotomy.
- Maintain lateral cortex intact to serve as a hinge.[1]
- Open the osteotomy site.[1]
- Utilize fluoroscopy with different size wedges until achieving appropriate correction to the IMA (each 1 mm of wedge provides 3 degrees of correction).[1]
- Fixation of wedge plate onto the medial aspect of the metatarsal to maintain opening wedge.[1]
- Secure the plate with two distal and two proximal screws (paying close attention to not violate the TMT joint)[1] (**Fig. 11.4**).
- Insert the appropriate amount of bone graft into the osteotomy site from excised medial eminence or additional distal tibia harvest or autograft[1] (**Fig. 11.5**).
- Close tissue deeply over plate construct to decrease edema.
- Approximate skin edges of medial incision and recommend the use of interrupted simple sutures with nylon for closure (**Fig. 11.6**).

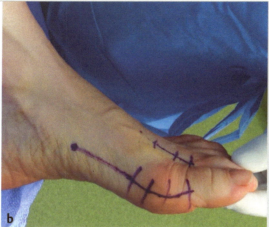

Fig. 11.3 (a) Photograph of modified McBride's dorsal first web space incision. (b) Medial incision from medial border proximal phalanx to first tarsal metatarsal joint.

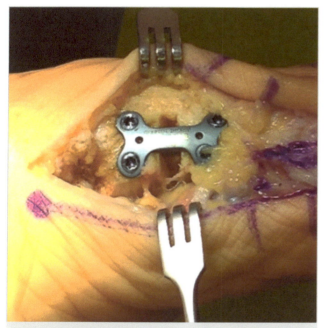

Fig. 11.4 Step-plate fixation with maintained opening at the site of proximal metatarsal osteotomy.

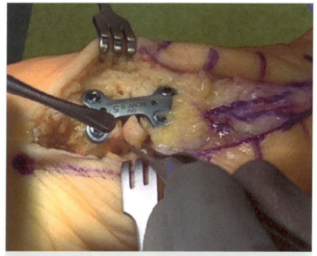

Fig. 11.5 Intraoperative photo demonstrating placement of harvested bone graft into osteotomy site.

- Recommend the application of a compressive bandage over the medial foot for the prevention of postoperative hematoma.
- Postoperative radiographs (**Fig. 11.7**).

11.8 Tips and Pearls

- May be necessary to address contributing conditions for improved results, including gastrocnemius tightness.[5]
- Oblique first metatarsal osteotomies yield better clinical and radiological outcomes—center of rotation of angulation (CORA) remains more proximal leading to decreased distance between first and second metatarsals.[8]
- Start with distal lateral soft-tissue release from first web space for better visualization.
- Transverse osteotomy safer 1.5 cm distal to TMT joint.

- Take care when opening osteotomy site—gentle use of flat osteotomes or distractor recommended.
- Location of the plate should be as plantar as possible on medial surface to counteract the tendency for the first metatarsal to plantarflex.
- Strongly recommend use of intraoperative fluoroscopy.
- Be sure not to overcorrect the first MTP joint.
- Always be conscious of rotational alignment of the hallux.
- Fifty percent of the success of the procedure deals with postoperative care, compliance, and patient education.
- Always utilize the correct-sized instrumentation (i.e., oscillating saw/blade, osteotome).

11.9 Hazards and Pitfalls

- Preserving the integrity of the lateral cortex remains paramount to achieving, maintaining, and stabilizing the correction.[6]
- Use of bone grafting can avoid the complication of nonunion at the osteotomy site.[6]

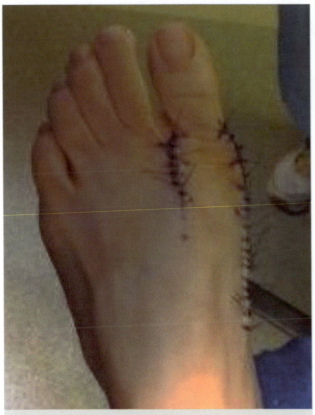

Fig. 11.6 Postoperative photo demonstrating approximated skin edges with simple interrupted nylon sutures.

- Although uncommon, be cognizant of a slight increase in first metatarsal length, which may lead to pressure on the MTP joint.[6]
- Be aware of possible donor-site complications if harvesting additional bone graft from separate location.[2]

11.10 Complication/Bailout/Salvage

11.10.1 Complications

- Occurrence of hallux varus with overcorrection:
  - Most common complication.[6]
  - Avoid this complication with the use of intraoperative fluoroscopy.[6]
- Overlengthening of the first metatarsal[6]:
  - No difference seen with lengthening between oblique and transverse osteotomies.[6]
  - Excessive length could lead to tightening of the soft-tissues correction and possible higher recurrence rate *and* decreased range of motion of the first metatarsal phalangeal joint.[6]
  - Overlengthening of the metatarsal may cause "jamming" of the MTP joint, with the possibility of subsequent symptomatic arthritis.[6]
  - Early identification of overlengthening with compensatory procedures (such as distal shortening chevron osteotomy) can negate these possible issues.[6]

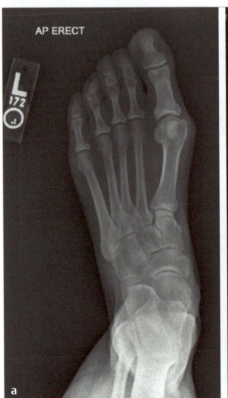
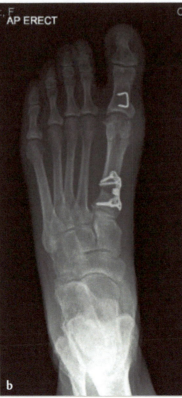

Fig. 11.7 (a) Preoperative and (b) postoperative anteroposterior radiographs.

- Recurrence of hallux valgus deformity[4]:
  - Occurs in approximately 3 to 11% of cases.[4]
  - Higher risk with greater preoperative HVA and higher DMAA.[4]
  - Supplementing with additional distal osteotomy may avoid recurrence in patients with higher preoperative DMAAs.[4]
  - Patients with hypermobility of the first ray may be at increased risk for recurrence.[4]
- Postoperative continuation of symptoms and pain at the first MTP joint[4]:
  - Higher likelihood of these patients developing symptomatic arthritis.[4]
- Development of irritation from prominent hardware:
  - Consider removal of hardware once bony healing is complete and correction stable.
- Postoperative infection:
  - Infection not responsive to local care and antibiotic treatment may require incision, drainage, and debridement with hardware removal and later revision surgery.

11.10.2 Salvage and Bailout

- If violation of the lateral cortex occurs while performing the osteotomy:
  - Consider insertion of a mini-fragment lag screw or K-wire across osteotomy site to hold the hinge intact while applying plate.[1]
  - Newer locking plate implant designs may be able to stabilize and hold fixation at the site of the osteotomy—even with disruption of the lateral cortex.
- If the proximal opening wedge osteotomy leads to excessive lengthening of the first metatarsal:
  - Consider additional distal chevron osteotomy to restore appropriate length.[7]
- If patients present with *significant* symptomatic or *prominent* hardware issues from the *plate placement*:
  - Consider *removal of hardware* and fixation of the osteotomy with two K-wires that can be removed 8 weeks postoperatively.[3]

11.11 Postoperative Care

- Dependent on patient factors, consider immobilization in *heel-bearing-only* wedge shoe, cam boot,[3] or strict non-weight-bearing for 4 to 6 weeks.[1,4]
- Recommend obtaining anteroposterior and lateral radiographs at 6 weeks postoperatively in order to verify alignment of the correction and bony healing.
- If radiographs reveal callus formation along the lateral cortex, this suggests disruption of the lateral cortex during procedure. Consider extended non-weight-bearing restrictions of these patients (2 weeks) to protect the correction. In addition, follow these patients closely to monitor for possible delayed union.[6]

- Infection not responsive to local care and antibiotic treatment may require incision, drainage, and debridement with hardware removal and later revision surgery.

11.12 Outcomes

- Patients have shown significant improvement in HVA, IMA, and AOFAS scores at midterm follow-up (approximately 5.2 years postoperatively).[5]
- Restoration of HVA and IMA improves the functional stability of the first ray with joint preservation by means of avoiding TMT joint arthrodesis.[5]
- Equivalent stability seen between proximal opening wedge osteotomy fixed with low profile plate and proximal chevron osteotomy.[4]
- Lateral cortex integrity and good bone density are important factors for achieving stable fixation with proximal opening wedge osteotomies.[6]
- High patient satisfaction rates—80 and 89% satisfaction rate.[6]

References

1. Glazebrook M, Copithorne P, Boyd G, et al. Proximal opening wedge osteotomy with wedge-plate fixation compared with proximal chevron osteotomy for the treatment of hallux valgus: a prospective, randomized study. J Bone Joint Surg Am 2014;96(19):1585–1592
2. Sammarco VJ. Management of soft tissue deficiency of the hallux: salvage in trauma, diabetes, and following surgical complications. Foot Ankle Clin 2005;10(1):55–74
3. Bagatur AE, Albayrak M, Akman YE, Yalcinkaya M, Ozer UE, Yalcin MB. A Simple Method for Fixation of Proximal Opening-Wedge Osteotomy of the First Metatarsal for Correction of Hallux Valgus. Orthopedics 2016;39(6):e1213–e1217
4. Iyer S, Demetracopoulos CA, Sofka CM, Ellis SJ. High rate of recurrence following proximal medial opening wedge osteotomy for correction of moderate hallux valgus. Foot Ankle Int 2015;36(7):756–763
5. Oravakangas R, Leppilahti J, Laine V, Niinimäki T. Proximal opening wedge osteotomy provides satisfactory midterm results with a low complication rate. J Foot Ankle Surg 2016;55(3):456–460
6. Ferrao PN, Saragas NP. Rotational and opening wedge basal osteotomies. Foot Ankle Clin 2014;19(2):203–221
7. Jeyaseelan L, Chandrashekar S, Mulligan A, Bosman HA, Watson AJS. Correction of moderate to severe hallux valgus with combined proximal opening wedge and distal chevron osteotomies: a reliable technique. Bone Joint J 2016;98-B(9):1202–1207
8. Han SH, Park EH, Jo J, et al. First metatarsal proximal opening wedge osteotomy for correction of hallux valgus deformity: comparison of straight versus oblique osteotomy. Yonsei Med J 2015;56(3):744–752

12   Akin's and Moberg's Osteotomies of the Hallux Phalanx

Adam G. Miller

Abstract
Proximal phalangeal osteotomies of the hallux serve to correct alignment when combined with hallux valgus corrective procedures or are used to alleviate hallux rigidus symptoms in combination with cheilectomy or in isolation. Multiple techniques have been described, and successful techniques are highlighted in this chapter. Careful correction avoids complication of tendon injury, overcorrection, or loss of fixation.

Keywords: *Akin, Moberg, proximal phalanx osteotomy, hallux rigidus, hallux valgus*

12.1   Akin's Osteotomy

12.1.1   Indications

- Hallux valgus interphalangeus.
- Congruent hallux valgus treated with double osteotomy (Akin's and metatarsal osteotomy).
- Residual hallux valgus after correction.

Pathology

Hallux valgus is a malalignment of the first ray with prominence over the medial eminence and resulting pain. The deformity also creates impingement in the first web space. Deformity can be congenital or acquired with age. While exact etiology is unclear, family history plays a role.

Clinical Evaluation

After diagnosing hallux valgus, one must rule out concurrent hallux rigidus. This diagnosis can require fusion of the great toe. Stability at the first tarsometatarsal (TMT) joint must be determined based on examination and radiographic studies. Instability requires a Lapidus fusion. Thereafter, the severity and congruence of the hallux valgus deformity must be determined. Akin's osteotomy can be used as part of a double osteotomy in congruent bunions or in conjunction with other hallux valgus corrections to augment the correction.

Radiographic Evaluation

A weight-bearing foot radiograph series including anteroposterior (AP), 30-degree oblique, and lateral views is indicated. One can evaluate arthritis of the metatarsophalangeal (MTP) joint, instability at the TMT joint, MTP congruency, hallux valgus angle, and hallux valgus interphalangeus angle (**Fig. 12.1**). Magnetic resonance imaging (MRI) and computed tomography (CT) are not indicated for treatment of isolated hallux valgus.

Nonoperative Options

Hallux valgus can be treated nonoperatively with attempts at relieving pressure in shoes or relieving pressure on the adjacent second toe. Wider shoes can be tried and stretching of the toe box with a shoe-tree may help. Protection of the great toe irritating the second toe with a silicone spacer may relieve pain. Lasting deformity correction without surgery is not possible.

Contraindications

- Performing an Akin osteotomy in isolation for incongruent hallux valgus.

12.1.2   Goals of Surgical Procedure

Akin's osteotomy is used for deformity correction and relieving impingement of the great toe in the first web space. Success can be defined by a congruent MTP joint with a healed proximal phalanx osteotomy and no symptomatic hardware.

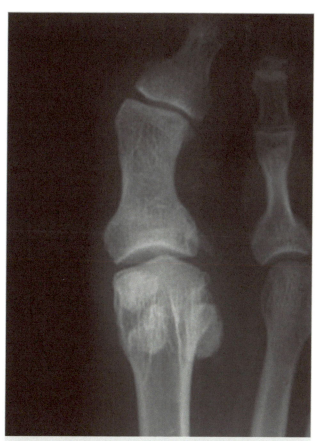

Fig. 12.1 Increased hallux valgus interphalangeus.

12.1.3 Advantages of Surgical Procedure

A proximal phalanx osteotomy is a useful adjunct to hallux valgus deformity correction. Instead of relying on a soft-tissue correction to maintain great toe position, one can dial in the correction with a bony correction of the proximal phalanx. This results in less long-term deformity recurrence and, after adequate bony consolidation, allows for more aggressive range of motion (ROM) in the great toe.

12.1.4 Key Principles

- Protect extensor and flexor tendons while limiting soft-tissue dissection.
- Take care not to overcorrect this powerful osteotomy by checking iterations of a unicortical osteotomy.
- Ensure secure fixation with no prominent hardware.

12.1.5 Preoperative Preparation and Patient Positioning

As most Akin's osteotomies are performed with a complete hallux valgus correction, position the patient at the edge of the operating table with slight external rotation. Calf tourniquet can be applied as needed.

12.1.6 Operative Technique

A longitudinal incision is made over the medial base of the proximal phalanx protecting the dorsomedial and plantarmedial nerve distributions. With concurrent bunion correction, continuation of the medial incision should be performed. Full-thickness dissection is made down to the medial aspect of the proximal phalanx. A Hohmann retractor is used to protect the extensor and flexor tendons. A guidewire is used to template the unicortical osteotomy. Transverse and oblique osteotomies have been described. An oblique osteotomy distal-medial to proximal-lateral will allow for normal compression with screw fixation. After satisfactory osteotomy position is determined under fluoroscopy, a microsagittal saw is used to perform the unicortical osteotomy, allowing compression of the medial cortex. Further correction can be obtained by compressing the medial osteotomy edges and using the kerf of the saw blade along the medial cortex. This ensures less overcorrection.

After satisfactory alignment and correction have been achieved, the correction can be maintained with hardware placement. Permanent suture,[1] staple, plate, and screw fixation have been described (**Fig. 12.2**). Transverse osteotomies may be better treated with plate or staple methods. Staple fixation has also been shown to be a viable option for fixation, with 5.9% of patients reporting tenderness over hardware.[2]

An oblique osteotomy, a solitary 2.4- or 3.0-mm screw perpendicularly to the osteotomy, provides enough stability and compression (**Fig. 12.3**).

For screw placement, template with guidewire starting at the medial base of the proximal phalanx. Some dissection of the capsule will need to be performed. The guidewire should be bicortical. The trajectory tends to be more dorsally driven

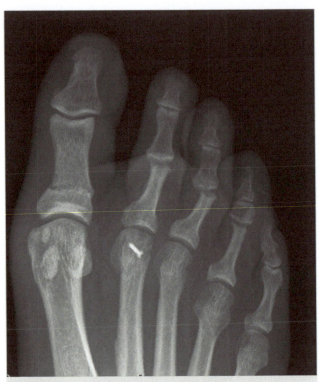

Fig. 12.2 Akin's osteotomy with suture fixation.

than expected. Check placement on AP and lateral fluoroscopic imaging. A headless screw or countersink should be used prior to screw placement. This limits hardware prominence. One should check for compression of the medial cortex after screw placement.

12.1.7 Tips and Pearls

- Do not overcorrect with an aggressive unicortical osteotomy. Use gradual correction to dial in alignment.
- Aim guidewire for screw fixation relatively dorsal to achieve appropriate positioning.
- Limit prominent hardware.

12.1.8 Hazards and Pitfalls

Protect the FHL and EHL with retractors during saw use. Iatrogenic injury to either tendon is possible and could lead to chronic deformity. Avoid overcorrection.

12.1.9 Complications/Bailout/Salvage

- *Too aggressive a resection*: Complete the osteotomy to allow for lateral cortex shortening. After alignment is reestablished, pinning the osteotomy while fixating helps maintain reduction and control.
- *Recurrence/wrong procedure for deformity*: If the prior procedure did not include an appropriate hallux valgus correction, one must determine if a complete revision is needed.[3]
- *Avascular necrosis soft-tissue stripping*: Limit dissection to the area of planned medial osteotomy only.

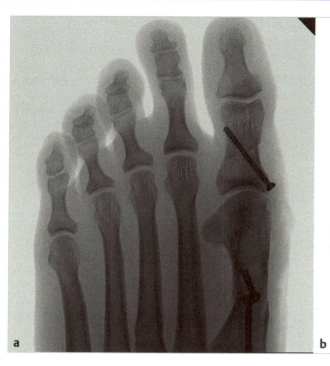

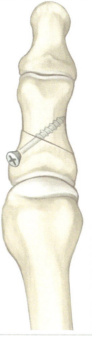

Fig. 12.3 (a,b) Solitary screw fixation of Akin's osteotomy.

- *EHL/FHL severed*: Typically, these complications may not be noticed until postoperatively. Often, stiffness complicates the postoperative presentation, and patients complain of transient stiffness or weakness initially that resolves afterward. If concerned for injury of either tendon, MRI or ultrasound can be used for diagnosis and repair is recommended. If found intraoperatively a tendon is severed, direct end-to-end repair of the tendon is recommended with permanent suture.
- *Poor cosmesis*: If an Akin osteotomy is planned, it is important to get a feel for where the toe must sit postoperatively. If all toes course laterally at the MTP joint and a correction of hallux valgus interphalangeus is performed, one must take into account the overall contour of the forefoot and not overcorrect. Overcorrection besides poor cosmesis may also lead to shoe impingement.

12.1.10 Postoperative Care

A protective bunion dressing reinforcing the correction should be applied with a surgical sandal. Limit forefoot weight-bearing until 6 weeks, but patients may weight-bear through heel or lateral foot depending on concomitant procedures. A first web space spacer is applied until normal shoe wear. At 4 to 6 weeks, begin passive ROM at the MTP joint based on the confidence in osteotomy healing. Walk in surgical sandal at 6 weeks until no pain and slowly transfer into normal shoe.

12.1.11 Outcomes

Outcomes and longevity of correction are reliable because the correction largely does not rely on soft tissue. The correction should not be done in isolation,[3] but in combination with hallux valgus correction. With a long oblique osteotomy, increased bony apposition affords better chance at bony union. The

patient can expect some stiffness in the great toe, and anecdotally the amount of stiffness relates to the amount of ROM exercises the patient does on his/her own. Outcomes reported are positive; hallux valgus interphalangeus improved in one study on average from 16 to 2 degrees with a distal Akin osteotomy.[4]

12.2 Moberg's Osteotomy

12.2.1 Indications

- Hallux rigidus in adolescent patient.
- Improve dorsiflexion of great toe in adult patient with concurrent cheilectomy treatment.

Pathology

Hallux rigidus is a progressive degeneration of the first MTP joint marked by loss of motion, osteophyte formation, pain, and potentially deformity. ROM is often limited in dorsiflexion. Focal joint changes in a younger population may be attributed to trauma and become an osteochondral lesion of the metatarsal head.

Clinical Evaluation

The overall alignment and any deformity should be noted with standing to rule out concurrent pathology. ROM should be tested paying particular attention to where in the arc of motion pain is elicited. Pain with end ROM early suggests less severe arthritis, whereas midrange of motion range signifies advanced arthritis in an adult or focal osteochondral lesion in a younger individual. Loss of dorsiflexion should be particularly evaluated when considering a Moberg osteotomy.

Radiographic Evaluation

A three-view standing radiograph series of the foot should be obtained paying particular attention to the MTP joint of the first ray. Classification of hallux rigidus has been previously described by Coughlin and Shurnas and is well accepted.[5] Cheilectomy has typically been indicated in less severe forms of hallux rigidus. In an adolescent, open physes should be noted when planning a Moberg osteotomy to ensure protection. Any metatarsal head cysts or signs of osteochondritis dissecans (OCD) should be noted. In a patient where pain is out of proportion to the imaging findings—particularly in a young patient—an MRI is of use to rule out OCD to the metatarsal head.

Nonoperative Options

A Morton's extension plate placed underneath the shoe insole limits ROM and stress to the MTP joint and therefore decreases pain in some individuals. Anti-inflammatories and activity modification are indicated. An intra-articular cortisone injection to the MTP joint may provide temporary relief.

Contraindications

• Maintained preoperative dorsiflexion ROM.

12.2.2 Goals of Surgical Procedure

A Moberg osteotomy attempts to take advantage of intact plantarflexion ROM in an effort to improve relative dorsiflexion ROM. While true improvement in ROM is often modest, pain improvement is often marked. The osteotomy should be performed in a manner sparing an open proximal phalanx physis and should be secure enough to attempt early ROM.

12.2.3 Advantages of Surgical Procedure

A Moberg osteotomy is a joint-sparing surgery for symptoms of hallux rigidus that can be applied in a younger population without significant spurring or MTP joint radiographic findings. It can also be combined with a cheilectomy in an older population.

12.2.4 Key Principles

• Protect an open proximal phalanx epiphysis and extensor tendon.
• Secure fixation to allow for early ROM.
• Medial approach for ease of dorsal wedge resection.

12.2.5 Preoperative Preparation and Patient Positioning

Position the patient at the edge of the operating table with slight external rotation or toes pointing upward. Exact position depends on concurrent procedures. Calf tourniquet can be applied as needed.

12.2.6 Operative Technique

A longitudinal incision is made over the medial aspect of the proximal phalanx. The dorsomedial cutaneous nerve is protected. The proximal phalanx base is identified and, if present, the open epiphysis protected. As an alternative, extension of a dorsal longitudinal incision can be made when concurrently performing a cheilectomy. A dorsomedial approach can also be employed; however, this risks the dorsomedial cutaneous nerve. If concurrent surgeries are planned such as OCD treatment to the metatarsal head or cheilectomy, these should be performed first.

A Hohmann retractor is placed dorsal to the phalanx near the planned osteotomy. A wedge osteotomy, apex plantar, is planned using a unicortical cut and maintaining the integrity of the plantar periosteum. This assists in hinging the osteotomy dorsally. Using the kerf of the blade, successive passes in the dorsal cortex can be made to achieve the desired amount of dorsal correction (**Fig. 12.4**). Appropriate amount of correction is 15 degrees in relation to the plantar aspect of the foot or 35 degrees dorsiflexion in relation to the first metatarsal on lateral imaging.

Once desired correction has been achieved, fixation can be performed with temporary Kirschner wire fixation, staple, permanent suture, or screws. Wire or screw fixation can be applied from a dorsal direction obliquely through the osteotomy.

12.2.7 Tips and Pearls

• Do not complete the osteotomy plantarly. This makes fixation more difficult.
• Kirschner wires in open growth plates protect against inadvertent physeal injury.
• Stable fixation allows for early motion.

12.2.8 Hazards and Pitfalls

Protect the FHL and EHL with retractors during saw use. Iatrogenic injury to either tendon is possible and could lead to chronic deformity. Avoid overcorrection.

12.2.9 Complications/Bailout/Salvage

• *EHL severed*: If found intraoperatively a tendon is severed, direct end-to-end repair of the tendon is recommended with permanent suture. Protect ROM for the first 4 weeks.
• *Fixation failure*: Screw or plate fixation capturing the proximal fragment of the osteotomy may be tenuous. Using Kirschner wire fixation as a bailout is useful.

12.2.10 Postoperative Care

A protective dressing reinforcing the correction should be applied with a surgical sandal. Limit forefoot weight-bearing until 4 to 6 weeks, patients may weight-bear through heel or lateral foot depending on concomitant procedures. (Weight-bearing acts to compress the osteotomy with inherent stability.) At 4 to 6 weeks, begin passive ROM at the MTP joint based on the confidence in osteotomy healing. Attempt earlier if combined with cheilectomy to

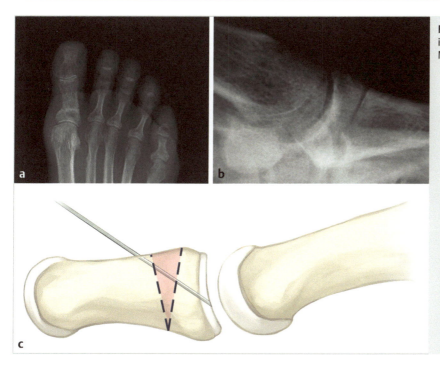

Fig. 12.4 **(a)** Anteroposterior and **(b)** Lateral images postoperatively and **(c)** illustration of Moberg's correction.

maintain ROM at the MTP joint. Walk in surgical sandal at 6 weeks until no pain and slowly transfer into normal shoe.

12.2.11 Outcomes

Symptomatic improvement is reliable; however, definitive ROM improvement is equivocal. When performing a cheilectomy, a Moberg osteotomy is most useful in advanced hallux rigidus cases. O'Malley et al reported 85% satisfaction with combined cheilectomy and proximal phalanx osteotomy with advanced hallux rigidus.[6] Only 5% of these patients underwent fusion. A review of outcome studies revealed a similar level of improvement (89%); however, most patients (72.3%) had a more moderate level (grade II) of hallux rigidus.[7] In another study, only 2 of 42 feet with moderate hallux rigidus required revision of isolated phalangeal osteotomy with screw irritation.[8] Hunt and Anderson described a combination of Moberg's and Akin's osteotomies as a biplanar osteotomy with all healing and 90% success.[9]

References

1. Roy SP, Tan KJ. A modified suture technique for fixation of the Akin osteotomy. J Foot Ankle Surg 2013;52(2):276–278
2. Neumann JA, Reay KD, Bradley KE, Parekh SG. Staple fixation for akin proximal phalangeal osteotomy in the treatment of hallux valgus interphalangeus. Foot Ankle Int 2015;36(4):457–464
3. Plattner PF, Van Manen JW. Results of Akin type proximal phalangeal osteotomy for correction of hallux valgus deformity. Orthopedics 1990;13(9):989–996
4. Vander Griend R. Correction of hallux valgus interphalangeus with an osteotomy of the distal end of the proximal phalanx (distal Akin osteotomy). Foot Ankle Int 2017;38(2):153–158
5. Coughlin MJ, Shurnas PS. Hallux rigidus. Grading and long-term results of operative treatment. J Bone Joint Surg Am 2003;85-A(11):2072–2088
6. O'Malley MJ, Basran HS, Gu Y, Sayres S, Deland JT. Treatment of advanced stages of hallux rigidus with cheilectomy and phalangeal osteotomy. J Bone Joint Surg Am 2013;95(7):606–610
7. Roukis TS. Outcomes after cheilectomy with phalangeal dorsiflexory osteotomy for hallux rigidus: a systematic review. J Foot Ankle Surg 2010;49(5):479–487
8. Perez-Aznar A, Lizaur-Utrilla A, Lopez-Prats FA, Gil-Guillen V. Dorsal wedge phalangeal osteotomy for grade II-III hallux rigidus in active adult patients. Foot Ankle Int 2015;36(2):188–196
9. Hunt KJ, Anderson RB. Biplanar proximal phalanx closing wedge osteotomy for hallux rigidus. Foot Ankle Int 2012;33(12):1043–1050

13 First Metatarsophalangeal Cheilectomy

Andrew D. Beischer

Abstract

Hallux rigidus is an arthritic condition affecting predominantly the dorsal aspect of the first metatarsal head with cartilage loss of dorsal spur formation. In early and moderate involvement (grade I–III) where the arthritis causes limited and painful dorsiflexion of the first metatarsophalangeal joint, a surgical debridement of the arthritic portion of the joint and spurs can be performed. The procedure, called cheilectomy after the Greek term *Cheilos* meaning "lip," removed the dorsal 30% of the metatarsal head and corrected the problem in about 90% of cases.

Keywords: *hallux rigidus, cheilectomy, dorsal cheilus*

13.1 Indications

- Primary osteoarthritis of the first metatarsophalangeal joint (MTPJ) often starts with a loss of cartilage over the dorsal aspect of the first metatarsal (MT) head.
- Frequently, a dorsal first MT osteophyte develops, and these two pathologies combined result in a painful restriction of dorsiflexion, particularly during the push-off phase of gait.
- The dorsal osteophyte, when large, may also cause the symptom of painful rubbing against the upper of a closed shoe.
- As the arthritis process progresses, the cartilage loss occurs in the more central and eventually plantar aspects of the joint.
- First MT head cheilectomy is appropriate when the loss of cartilage is confined to the dorsal third of the joint.

13.1.1 Clinical Evaluation

- Clinical evaluation is important to help select which patients suffering from osteoarthritis of the first MTPJ are appropriate candidates for this procedure.
- The ideal candidate reports painful dorsiflexion of the joint with walking. Rubbing of the dorsal osteophyte against the shoe may also be a presenting symptom.
- On examination, there should ideally be at least 40 to 50 degrees of total motion of the joint.
- The axial load grind test should be used to identify irritability of the joint in the midrange of motion; if present, this is indicative of central first MT head chondral loss, which is a relative contraindication for this procedure.
- An interesting common observation is that with passive range of motion of the joint, pain is induced particularly with plantar flexion of the great toe. This is likely caused by stretching of the inflamed capsule over the dorsal osteophyte.
- Digital compression under each sesamoid with passive motion of the toe can be used to illicit pain from an arthritic sesamoid—first MT articulation, which, if present, is a relative contraindication to this procedure.

13.1.2 Radiographic Evaluation

- In general, all that is required to assess the patient is a standard series (anteroposterior, lateral, and internal oblique view) of weight-bearing X-rays of the foot.
- The internal oblique view in particular is useful to assess how much of the plantar joint space is preserved.
- If clinical examination is suggestive of either central joint chondral loss or significant involvement of the sesamoid MT articulation and this is not apparent on standard X-rays, then a magnetic resonance imaging (MRI) can be useful to identify these pathologies given their presence is a relative contraindication to a cheilectomy (**Fig. 13.1**).

13.1.3 Nonoperative Options

- Activity modification.
- Shoe-wear modification:
  - Avoid heels.
  - Extra depth toe box.
  - Stiffened sole shoe with steel shank or carbon fiber plate.
- Nonsteroidal anti-inflammatory medications.

13.1.4 Contraindications

- Inflammatory arthritis.
- Chondral loss involving the lower half of the first MTPJ.
- Severe restriction of motion.
- Associated significant hallux valgus.

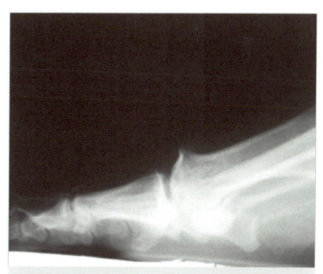

Fig. 13.1 Lateral radiograph demonstrating prominent dorsal osteophyte.

13.2 Goals of Surgical Procedure

• Reduce pain with motion of the great toe.
• Improve range of motion.
• Stop rubbing of the dorsal osteophyte against a shoe.

13.3 Advantages

• Simple procedure.
• Quick recovery.
• Reliable outcome in appropriately selected patients.

13.4 Key Principles

• Dorsal approach.
• Capsulotomy medial to extensor hallucis longus (EHL) tendon.
• Removal of dorsal 30% of first MT head plus osteophytes.
• Aim to get 90 degrees of dorsiflexion during the procedure.
• Consider a dorsal closing wedge osteotomy of the proximal phalanx base if unable to achieve 90 degrees of dorsiflexion.

13.5 Preoperative Preparation and Patient Positioning

• Day-case procedure.
• Supine positioning with bump under ipsilateral buttock so great toe points directly to the ceiling of the operating room.
• Easily done under intravenous sedation and local analgesia.
• Ankle tourniquet preferable but not essential.

13.6 Operative Technique

• A 4-cm longitudinal dorsal incision is made centered over the first MTPJ with care taken particularly to protect the dorsomedial hallucal nerve.

• The EHL tendon is retracted laterally and the capsule is incised longitudinally through its central aspect.
• The dorsal part of the joint is then exposed by sharp subperiosteal dissection and any loose bodies are removed.
• If present, the dorsolateral first MT head osteophyte is removed with 3-mm bone rongeur.
• The joint is then plantarflexed and the chondral surface of the central third first MT head is inspected to ensure it is intact. By gripping the hallux between thumb and index finger and applying an axial distraction force, the phalangeal articular surface can be examined.
• If the chondral loss is confined to the upper third of the first MT head, then proceed with the cheilectomy.
• If the chondral loss is more severe than what was anticipated based on clinical evaluation/imaging, then consideration of an alternative technique is warranted (provided that this had been discussed with the patient) (**Fig. 13.2**).
• The hallux is plantarflexed, which exposes the diseased portion of the first MT head. A 1-cm flexible chisel osteotome is used to remove the diseased portion (dorsal 30%) of the MT head (**Fig. 13.3**).
• The range of motion is then assessed. The aim should be to achieve 90 degrees of dorsiflexion of the first MTPJ. If this has not been achieved, then proceed to performing a dorsiflexion osteotomy of the proximal phalangeal base (Moberg's osteotomy) (**Fig. 13.4**, **Fig. 13.5**, **Fig. 13.6**).
• The wound is closed in layers. A #0 Vicryl for the capsule and #4/0 nylon for the skin.
• The foot is covered in a well-padded surgical dressing and the foot protected with a rigid-soled postoperative shoe.

13.7 Tips and Pearls

• When using the flexible chisel osteotome, it is critical that the beveled surface of the blade faces the plantar direction to ensure the blade will move in a dorsal/proximal direction when the chisel is struck with the mallet. The chisel is aimed to exit the dorsal aspect of the first MT neck approximately 1 cm proximal to the neck articular surface interface.

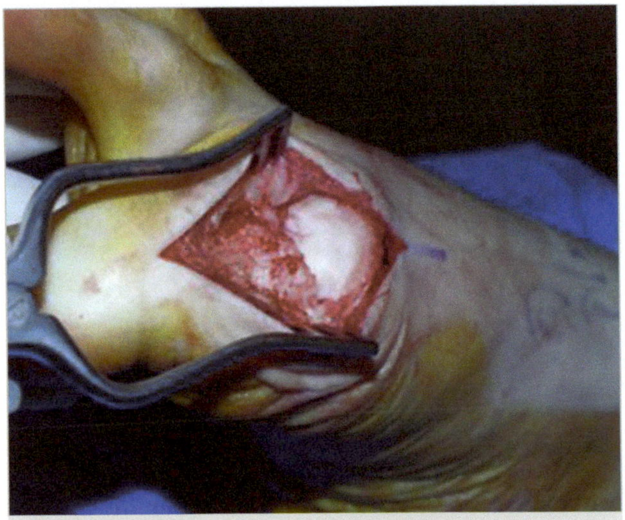

Fig. 13.2 Intraoperative photograph demonstrating dorsal osteophyte and diseased dorsal 30% of the first MT head.

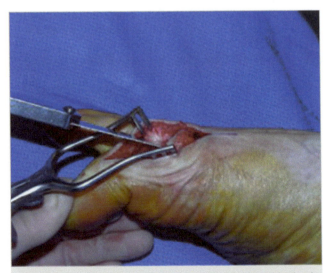

Fig. 13.3 Photograph demonstrating orientation of flexible chisel osteotome to perform the cheilectomy.

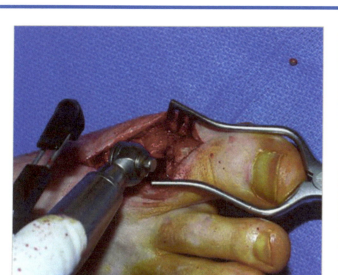

Fig. 13.4 Photograph demonstrating microsagittal saw being used to perform phalangeal dorsiflexion osteotomy.

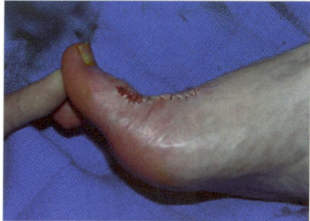

Fig. 13.6 Photograph demonstrating the 90 degrees of first MTPJ dorsiflexion that should be achieved at the end of the procedure.

13.9 Complications/Bailout/Salvage

- If inadequate motion is obtained through the cheilectomy, add a Moberg dorsal closing wedge osteotomy of the proximal phalanx, taking care not to penetrate the plantar cortex of the phalanx, which will lead to an unstable osteotomy.
- If plantar cortex is breached while performing phalangeal osteotomy, supplemental fixation (a 1.25-mm K-wire) is often needed to provide adequate stability.

13.10 Postoperative Care

- Full weight-bearing is allowed immediately after surgery.
- Suture removal at 2 weeks after surgery.
- If phalangeal osteotomy was not performed, the patient is allowed to wear accommodative shoe at 2 weeks after surgery. Active and passive dorsiflexion and plantar flexion of the first MTPJ is encouraged.
- If phalangeal osteotomy was performed, the patient uses postoperative shoe for 6 weeks while weight-bearing. Active and passive dorsiflexion of the first MTPJ is started at 2 weeks (compressive force to the phalangeal osteotomy). Active plantar flexion exercises commence 4 weeks from surgery. Passive plantar flexion exercises allowed once phalangeal osteotomy has united at 6 weeks following surgery.

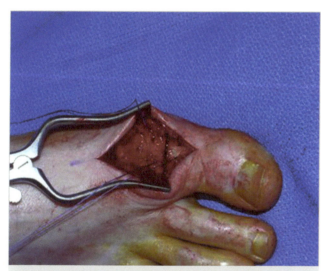

Fig. 13.5 Photograph demonstrating #0 PDS sutures that have been inserted through two pairs of converging holes made on opposing sides of the osteotomy using a 1.6-mm K-wire.

- A common error is to remove too little of the MT head. This may be because the dorsal osteophyte erroneously is being considered by the surgeon to be part of the head of the MT.
- If performing a phalangeal osteotomy, it is important to keep the plantar cortex intact as it protects the FHL tendon and maintains stability of the osteotomy.

13.8 Hazards and Pitfalls

- Removing too little of the true first MT head.
- Incorrect orientation of the chisel, which can result in excessive bone resection.

13.11 Outcomes

- In appropriately selected patients, the outcomes are good in a high proportion of patients for up to 10 years.[1,2]
- The addition of a phalangeal osteotomy may improve the outcome in those patients with restricted dorsiflexion after completion of the cheilectomy part of the procedure.[3,4]

References

1. Coughlin MJ, Shurnas PS. Hallux rigidus. Grading and long-term results of operative treatment. J Bone Joint Surg Am 2003;85-A(11):2072–2088

2. Nicolosi N, Hehemann C, Connors J, Boike A. Long-term follow-up of the cheilectomy for degenerative joint disease of the first metatarsophalangeal joint. J Foot Ankle Surg 2015;54(6):1010–1020

3. Thomas PJ, Smith RW. Proximal phalanx osteotomy for the surgical treatment of hallux rigidus. Foot Ankle Int 1999;20(1):3–12

4. Kim PH, Chen X, Hillstrom H, Ellis SJ, Baxter JR, Deland JT. Moberg osteotomy shifts contact pressure plantarly in the first metatarsophalangeal joint in a biomechanical model. Foot Ankle Int 2016;37(1):96–101

14 First Metatarsophalangeal Joint Fusion

Brian S. Winters

Abstract

Fusion continues to be the most successful and reproducible long-term option for reconstruction of the first metatarsophalangeal (MTP) joint in the setting of an unsalvageable joint or severe deformity, such as hallux rigidus, avascular necrosis, infection, rheumatoid/inflammatory arthropathy, and severe hallux valgus. A number of studies have described improved functional outcomes with this procedure that are associated with high success rates of union using various techniques of joint preparation and internal fixation, regardless of the etiology of degeneration. If you adhere to certain principles, you can expect your patients to achieve a good functional result and near-normal activity level. This chapter will help guide you to evaluate pathologies involving the first MTP joint and successfully perform a first MTP joint fusion when indicated.

Keywords: *first metatarsophalangeal joint, fusion, arthritis, degenerative joint disease, hallux rigidus*

14.1 Indications

14.1.1 Pathology

- Common etiologies of first metatarsophalangeal (MTP) joint pain include hallux rigidus, which can be caused by degenerative or posttraumatic arthritis; avascular necrosis; infection; rheumatoid/inflammatory arthropathy; and severe hallux valgus deformity.[1]
- The patient's major complaint is typically pain and stiffness.

14.1.2 Clinical Evaluation

- The initial step in assessing patients with first MTP joint pathology includes a thorough history to determine when they began to experience pain, its exact location, activities that exacerbate or relieve symptoms, and whether any constitutional symptoms are present.
- The physical examination should assess the overall alignment of the foot and ankle as deformity, such as an adult-acquired flatfoot or valgus ankle, can exacerbate symptoms by creating a pathologic pressure distribution and may also need to be addressed.
- If a prior surgery was conducted, scars and skin quality should be carefully evaluated.
- In the appropriate setting, infection needs to be ruled out as a cause of persistent pain.
- Palpate the distal pulses and obtain a vascular consultation if there is any concern for critical peripheral vascular disease.

14.1.3 Radiographic Evaluation

- Weight-bearing anteroposterior (AP), oblique, and lateral radiographs routinely provide sufficient information to make a definitive diagnosis and formulate a treatment plan.

- In some situations, advanced imaging modalities, such as magnetic resonance imaging (MRI) and computed tomography (CT), may be needed to further evaluate the underlying pathology, such as avascular necrosis.
- In cases where infection is suggested but not confirmed, a Ceretec bone scan or tagged white blood cell scan may be warranted.

14.1.4 Nonoperative Options

- Nonsteroidal anti-inflammatory medication.
- Custom-molded orthotics with a Morton extension.
- Steroid injections.
- Shoe-wear modification (i.e., rigid sole, deep/wide toe box).

14.1.5 Contraindications

- Active infection.
- Situations where approximately 1 cm or greater bone loss is anticipated.
- Severe peripheral vascular disease.
- Uncontrolled diabetes as determined by HbA1C.
- Active smoking.
- Poor soft-tissue envelope.

14.2 Goals of the Surgical Procedure

The ultimate goal is to decrease pain, correct forefoot alignment, and restore patient function.

14.3 Advantages of the Surgical Procedure

Several procedures have been described,[2] but fusion continues to be the most successful and reproducible long-term option for reconstruction in the setting of an unsalvageable joint or severe deformity, with rates of union being described ranging from 77 to 100%.[1,3,4]

14.4 Key Principles

Meticulous surgical technique must be adhered to throughout the entire procedure in order to decrease soft-tissue trauma and potential for wound complications.

- The length of the first ray must be maintained. Significant shortening can result in pain at the MTP joint region and subsequent transfer metatarsalgia.[5–7]
- Both sides of the joint must be thoroughly debrided to a healthy, bleeding bed of bone in order to maximize the chance of union.

- After the joint is debrided, the hallux needs to be appropriately aligned:
  - 10 to 15 degrees of valgus.
  - Neutral rotation.
  - 10 to 15 degrees of dorsiflexion relative to the floor.
- Rigid internal fixation is used to compress and stabilize the joint.

14.5 Preoperative Preparation and Patient Positioning

The patient should be placed in the supine position with the foot about a fist length from the end of the operating table. If significant external rotation of the operative extremity is present, a well-padded bump should be placed under the ipsilateral hip so that the foot is pointing toward the ceiling. It is recommended to use a tourniquet, either at the thigh or calf, in order to prevent excessive bleeding into the soft tissues and improve intraoperative visualization. Despite this, meticulous hemostasis still needs to be obtained throughout the procedure in order to prevent a postoperative hematoma and reduce the risk of wound complications/infection. The foot and ankle is then prepped and draped in the standard sterile fashion.

14.6 Operative Technique

14.6.1 Surgical Approach

The first MTP joint is best accessed through a dorsal midline approach (**Fig. 14.1**). This allows for an expansile incision, if necessary, to obtain adequate exposure. It also avoids the area of the dorsal medial cutaneous nerve. Before making your skin incision, it is imperative that any old scars are noted and incorporated into the new incision, if possible. Unfortunately, this is not always feasible, and in these situations, it is best to make your incision as dorsal as possible. The incision should start approximately 2 cm proximal and extend approximately 2 cm distal to the first MTP joint. The incision is then extended in both directions as needed in order to gain access to the joint while minimizing soft-tissue tension. Therefore, the length of the incision will vary from patient to patient. After the skin and subcutaneous tissue are retracted, the extensor hallucis longus (EHL) tendon will be encountered, which should be isolated and retracted laterally (**Fig. 14.2**).

The joint capsule should then be incised in line with your skin incision directly down to bone. The capsule and medial/lateral collateral ligaments are then released on both sides of the joint, full thickness, as a continuous envelope using sharp

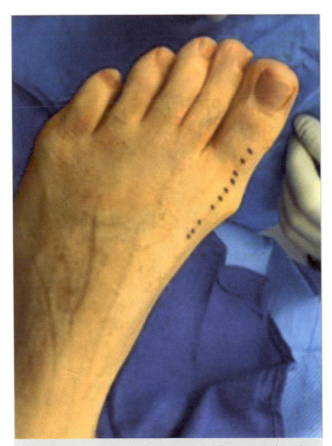

Fig. 14.1 Planned incision for the dorsal midline approach to the first MTP joint.

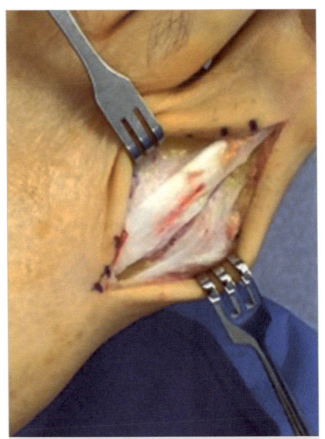

Fig. 14.2 Exposure of the extensor hallucis longus tendon. This should be retracted laterally.

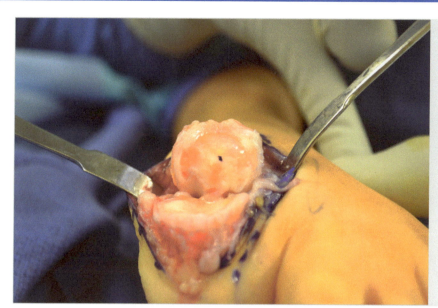

Fig 14.3 Exposure of the first MTP joint following full-thickness release of the capsule and collateral ligaments. The central marking on the metatarsal head is your planned entry point for the guidewire.

dissection (**Fig. 14.3**). This will ensure a sufficient release and provide adequate soft-tissue coverage during your closure, which is particularly important when a plate is used. The plantar aspect of the joint should be left intact in order to preserve the blood supply to the proximal phalanx and metatarsal head. Any osteophytes, remaining soft tissue/cartilage, and implants should then be removed.

14.6.2 Fusion Technique

At this point, the proximal phalanx base and metatarsal head are debrided to healthy, bleeding bone in a way to allow for complete bone-on-bone apposition in the desired alignment. My preferred technique involves using cup-and-cone reamers (**Fig. 14.4**), which have the advantages of minimizing bone resection and allowing one to place the hallux in multiple different positions. The diameter of the metatarsal head is first measured to determine what size reamers should be used. A guidewire (usually supplied with the specific reamers used) is then inserted into the center of the metatarsal head. Using fluoroscopic guidance, it is important that the wire is placed in the center of the head and shaft both on the AP and lateral views (**Fig. 14.5**, **Fig. 14.6**). Once appropriate placement of the guidewire is confirmed, the soft tissues should be protected with Hohmann's retractors and the toe hyperflexed prior to reaming (**Fig. 14.7**, **Fig. 14.8**). Care should be taken to debride just enough to cancellous bone. If significant sclerosis is present, a K-wire can be used to create bleeding "channels" that will optimize your fusion rate while avoiding additional bone loss. This same process is then repeated on the proximal phalanx base using the corresponding reamer (**Fig. 14.9**). Once the MTP joint has been prepared and all bony debris removed, the hallux is positioned for internal fixation.

My preferred construct is two cannulated, headless, partially threaded cross-screws. This technique is quick, allows for excellent rigid fixation and compression, and is low profile and relatively inexpensive. The most difficult part about this

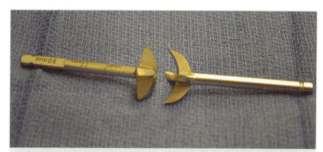

Fig. 14.4 Clinical picture of the proximal phalanx and metatarsal head cup-and-cone reamers, respectively.

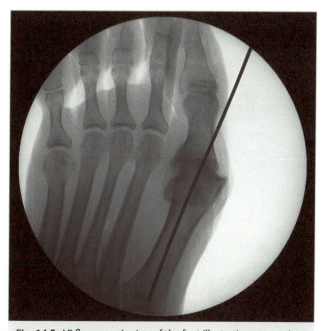

Fig. 14.5 AP fluoroscopic view of the foot illustrating appropriate guidewire placement in the center of the first metatarsal.

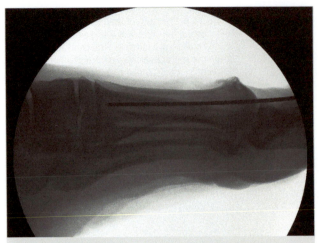

Fig. 14.6 Lateral fluoroscopic view of the foot illustrating appropriate guidewire placement in the center of the first metatarsal.

technique is placing the two screws in a fashion where they will not converge into each other. The best way to avoid this is to place both pins in the desired position from within the joint. This way you will know exactly where the screws will ultimately cross. Using a double-ended guidewire, start one wire at the dorsal, central to medial aspect of the proximal phalanx, aiming slightly dorsal to the long axis of the proximal phalanx and advance it out the medial aspect of the toe percutaneously. Then retract it until the tip is at the border of the proximal phalanx base. A second double-ended guidewire is then placed from the plantar, central to medial aspect of the metatarsal head aiming slightly plantar to the long axis of the metatarsal and advanced out the medial aspect of the foot percutaneously. Then retract it until the tip is at the border of the metatarsal head. Use fluoroscopy to confirm that once the wires are advanced, you will have enough screw purchase at both their proximal and distal ends (**Fig. 14.10**).

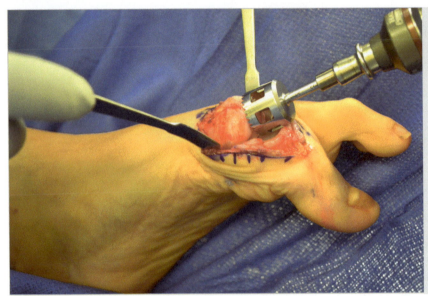

Fig. 14.7 Clinical picture of the initial barrel reamer used on the metatarsal head, which quickly removes any surrounding osteophytes.

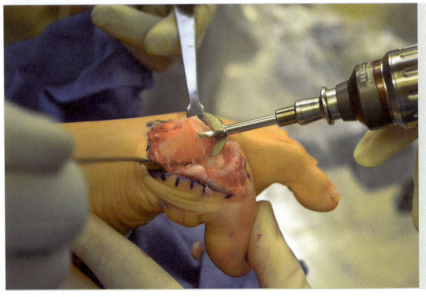

Fig. 14.8 Metatarsal head reamer.

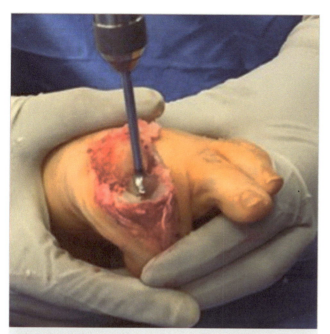

Fig. 14.9 Proximal phalanx reamer (retractors removed for picture clarity).

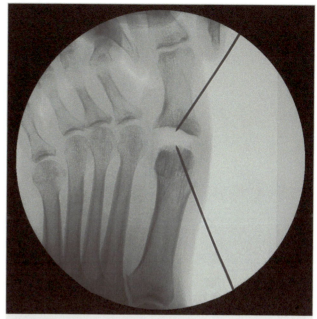

Fig. 14.10 Appropriate guidewire starting positions for cross-screw internal fixation.

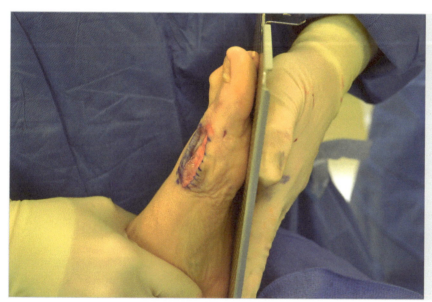

Fig. 14.11 Assessment of first MTP joint dorsiflexion using a flat plate. The pulp of the toe should be just touching the plate when simulating a standing position.

At this point in time, the toe is held in the desired position while maintaining compression (10–15 degrees of valgus, neutral rotation, and 10–15 degrees of dorsiflexion relative to the floor). Have your assistant or scrub nurse advance the two guidewires across the joint and past the far cortex. The toe should be stable at this point and can be released. Then confirm the appropriate alignment of the hallux. First, clinically assess the valgus from above the foot, as this is what the patient will see. This is done by simulating weight-bearing utilizing a solid flat plate (such as a lid of one of the surgical trays which one should save at the start of the case) and placing the foot flat down onto the plate. First, evaluate the rotation by looking at the toe nail/hallux axially from the foot of the bed. Next, assess its dorsiflexion of the hallux. Here, the pulp of the hallux should be just touching the lid (**Fig. 14.11**). You then want to make sure

that the hallux will have adequate clearance in order to avoid premature contact with the ground by lifting the hallux off the plate (**Fig. 14.12**). Once satisfied with the above, intraoperative fluoroscopy should be used to confirm appropriate guidewire placement and then use AO technique to measure, drill, and place two cross-screws under compression (**Fig. 14.13**, **Fig. 14.14**). I like to place the distal to proximal screw first in order to compress the hallux to the metatarsal. Final fluoroscopic views are then obtained and the wound copiously irrigated. The deep capsule is closed with 0 Vicryl, the dermis with 3–0 Monocryl, and skin with 3–0 nylon.

An alternate form of fixation can be performed utilizing a dorsal fusion plate. Most companies now have specific precontoured anatomic plates for this purpose which are either flat or dorsiflexed 8 to 10 degrees, and distally oriented in valgus for

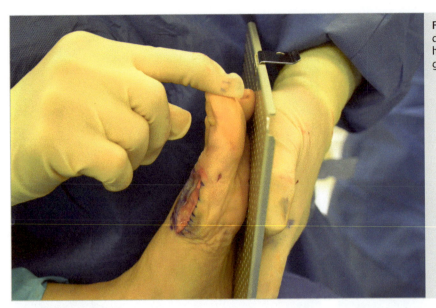

Fig. 14.12 Assessment of first MTP joint dorsiflexion using a flat plate. Ensure that the hallux will not prematurely impinge on the ground with walking.

accurate positioning. When utilizing plate fixation, one should always include an axial compression screw first to compress the joint. Plate fixation can be undertaken with locking or nonlocking screws, but rigid stability and compression must be obtained.

14.7 Tips and Pearls

- Proper patient placement allows for direct access to the joint and easy use of fluoroscopy.
- Respect the soft tissues from the initial incision until when the last stitch is placed. The tissues should always be "manipulated" and never "grabbed" to avoid tissue ischemia and subsequent necrosis.
- Ensure that the first MTP joint is adequately debrided to healthy, bleeding, cancellous bone prior to placement of your internal fixation. If there is any uncertainty, the tourniquet can briefly be let down to help determine whether this has been achieved. Minimize your bony resection in order to maintain the length of the first ray.
- Critique the position of the hallux both clinically and radiographically prior to placing your internal fixation. If adjustments need to be made, use a marking pen to make a transverse line at the joint line and a longitudinal line crossing the MTP joint. Use this as a guide when fine-tuning your hallux position. Guidewire adjustments should be made by only backing them out to the joint level so you do not lose your starting position.
- After joint debridement and prior to internal fixation, ensure that the joint will be compressed evenly, while maintaining the desired position of the hallux.

14.8 Hazards and Pitfalls

- The skin, capsule, EHL tendon, and dorsal medial cutaneous nerve are at risk of injury throughout the procedure and need to be protected accordingly.
- Inadvertent reaming of the opposite side of the joint can easily occur if the hallux is not sufficiently hyperflexed or retractors are improperly positioned.

- If the guidewire is not centrally placed, eccentric reaming will occur leading to unwanted bone loss and difficulty with positioning the hallux in the desired position.
- The cup-and-cone reamers are very aggressive and over-resection can easily occur, especially in soft bone. Debride the joint in a controlled fashion by performing a "tapping" technique instead of applying continuous pressure.
- Always check proper placement of the hallux prior to internal fixation by simulating weight-bearing with the flat plate. Assessing it in a resting position can be misleading. A varus position can make finding comfortable shoe wear difficult, while a valgus position can irritate the second toe. Excessive dorsiflexion of the toe can lead to overload of the sesamoids, symptomatic irritation of the hallux in a shoe, and poor cosmesis. On the contrary, excessive plantarflexion can lead to irritation of the distal phalanx during the push-off phase of gait and eventual interphalangeal joint arthrosis.

14.9 Complications/Bailout/ Salvage

- *EHL tendon laceration*: a repair should be performed in order to maintain extension of the interphalangeal joint.
- *Tenuous fixation with the cross-screw construct*: Either change the position of your screws or consider augmenting with a plate, which you should always have available.
- *Nonunion*: consider a bone stimulator at 3 months from surgery. Ensure no underlying metabolic conditions are present (i.e., low 25-hydroxy vitamin D level).
- *Malunion*: if symptomatic, attempt shoe wear modification and/or custom orthotics.
- *Infection*: Superficial infection can be treated with local wound care and oral antibiotics. Deep infection should be appropriately debrided and treated with intravenous antibiotics.
- *Excessive shortening of the first ray*: You want to anticipate this preoperatively and consider simultaneous lesser metatarsal shortening osteotomies to balance the cascade and avoid transfer metatarsalgia. This can occur with revision first MTP joint surgery in particular. In some revision set-

tings, especially after a failed arthroplasty, lesser metatarsal osteotomies might be not powerful enough to balance out the cascade. Here, a distraction, bone-block first MTP joint fusion should be considered instead of an in situ fusion.

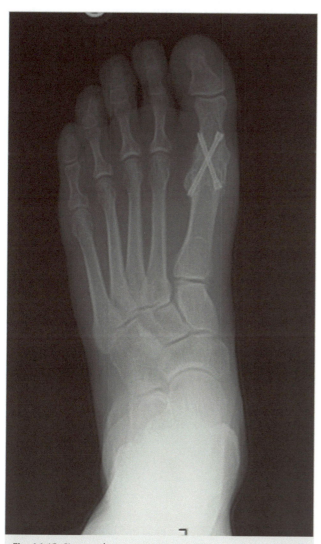

Fig. 14.13 Six-month postoperative AP X-ray.

14.10 Postoperative Care

At the conclusion of the procedure, a well-padded, sterile dressing should be applied to the foot and placed into a forefoot offloading postoperative shoe. It is recommended that the patient be heel-weight-bearing only in this shoe for transfers and bathroom privileges for 2 weeks in order to control pain/swelling and allow the wound to heal. The patient should keep the limb elevated well above the level of the heart during this time period. At 2 weeks, the incision should be evaluated, sutures removed if healed, and non-weight-bearing AP, lateral, and oblique X-rays obtained to ensure that the position of the reconstruction remains unchanged. The patient should then be placed back in the forefoot offloading postoperative shoe and allowed to heel weight-bear as tolerated for 4 more weeks. I recommend that the shoe be worn to sleep for protection but can be taken off daily for personal hygiene purposes. At 6 weeks, weight-bearing foot X-rays are obtained to assess for signs of progressive healing. If there is radiographic evidence of union, the patient can be progressed to full weight-bearing as tolerated in a regular postoperative shoe for another 6 weeks. At this point, the patient is allowed to also take off the postoperative shoe to sleep. At 3 months, weight-bearing foot X-rays are again obtained, and if union is achieved, the patient can wean from the postoperative shoe into a supportive sneaker.

14.11 Outcomes

Fusion is a well-recognized procedure that continues to be the most successful and reproducible long-term option for reconstruction of the first MTP joint in the setting of an unsalvageable joint or severe deformity.[8,9] A number of studies have described improved functional outcomes with this procedure that are associated with high success rates of union using various techniques of joint preparation and internal fixation, regardless of the etiology of degeneration.[8-18] As long as you adhere to the principles of respecting the soft-tissue envelope, meticulous joint preparation, appropriately positioning the hallux under compression, and using rigid internal fixation, you can expect your patients to achieve a good functional result and near-normal activity level.

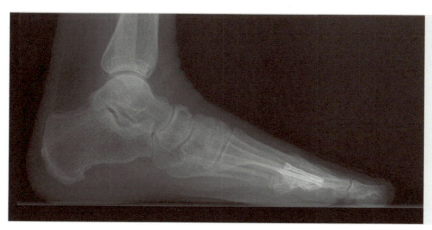

Fig. 14.14 Six-month postoperative lateral X-ray.

References

1. Bennett GL, Kay DB, Sabatta J. First metatarsophalangeal joint arthrodesis: an evaluation of hardware failure. Foot Ankle Int 2005;26(8):593–596

2. Kumar V, Clough T. Silastic arthroplasty of the first metatarsophalangeal joint as salvage for failed revisional fusion with interpositional structural bone graft. BMJ Case Rep 2013;2013:bcr2013008993

3. Hecht PJ, Gibbons MJ, Wapner KL, Cooke C, Hoisington SA. Arthrodesis of the first metatarsophalangeal joint to salvage failed silicone implant arthroplasty. Foot Ankle Int 1997;18(7):383–390

4. Whalen JL. Clinical tip: interpositional bone graft for first MP fusion. Foot Ankle Int 2009;30(2):160–162

5. Cole GK, Nigg BM, van Den Bogert AJ, Gerritsen KG. The clinical biomechanics award paper 1995 Lower extremity joint loading during impact in running. Clin Biomech (Bristol, Avon) 1996;11(4):181–193

6. Schuh R, Trnka HJ. First metatarsophalangeal arthrodesis for severe bone loss. Foot Ankle Clin 2011;16(1):13–20

7. Stokes IA, Hutton WC, Stott JR, Lowe LW. Forces under the hallux valgus foot before and after surgery. Clin Orthop Relat Res 1979;(142):64–72

8. Brodsky JW, Passmore RN, Pollo FE, Shabat S. Functional outcome of arthrodesis of the first metatarsophalangeal joint using parallel screw fixation. Foot Ankle Int 2005;26(2):140–146

9. Womack JW, Ishikawa SN. First metatarsophalangeal arthrodesis. Foot Ankle Clin 2009;14(1):43–50

10. Beertema W, Draijer WF, van Os JJ, Pilot P. A retrospective analysis of surgical treatment in patients with symptomatic hallux rigidus: long-term follow-up. J Foot Ankle Surg 2006;45(4):244–251

11. Bennett GL, Sabetta J. First metatarsalphalangeal joint arthrodesis: evaluation of plate and screw fixation. Foot Ankle Int 2009;30(8):752–757

12. Coughlin MJ, Shurnas PS. Hallux rigidus. Grading and long-term results of operative treatment. J Bone Joint Surg Am 2003;85-A(11):2072–2088

13. DeFrino PF, Brodsky JW, Pollo FE, Crenshaw SJ, Beischer AD. First metatarsophalangeal arthrodesis: a clinical, pedobarographic and gait analysis study. Foot Ankle Int 2002;23(6):496–502

14. Goucher NR, Coughlin MJ. Hallux metatarsophalangeal joint arthrodesis using dome-shaped reamers and dorsal plate fixation: a prospective study. Foot Ankle Int 2006;27(11):869–876

15. Kumar S, Pradhan R, Rosenfeld PF. First metatarsophalangeal arthrodesis using a dorsal plate and a compression screw. Foot Ankle Int 2010;31(9):797–801

16. Poggio D, de Retana PF, Borda D, Hortua P, Asunción J, Rios J. Analysis of the clinical score progressions during the first year after first MTPJ fusion. Foot Ankle Int 2010;31(7):578–583

17. Raikin SM, Ahmad J, Pour AE, Abidi N. Comparison of arthrodesis and metallic hemiarthroplasty of the hallux metatarsophalangeal joint. J Bone Joint Surg Am 2007;89(9):1979–1985

18. Roos EM, Brandsson S, Karlsson J. Validation of the foot and ankle outcome score for ankle ligament reconstruction. Foot Ankle Int 2001;22(10):788–794

15 Morton's Neurectomy

Christopher P. Chiodo

Abstract

The plantar interdigital neuroma or Morton's neuroma is caused by a thickening of the interdigital nerve as it crosses under the intermetatarsal ligament just distal to the division of the nerve traveling to the two adjacent toes. The third web space nerve is the most commonly affected due to its relative immobility as the junctional terminal nerve between the medial and lateral plantar nerves. Patients present with pain in the ball of the foot, often radiating to the third and fourth toes, and numbness. A cortisone injection can be used therapeutically and diagnostically to confirm the diagnosis. Failure of nonoperative modalities is treated with surgical neurectomy, usually through a dorsal third web space approach, as outlined in this chapter.

Keywords: *interdigital, Morton's neuroma, neurectomy*

15.1 Indications

- Mild intermittent nerve pain is not necessarily an indication for surgery and may respond to nonoperative measures or may be tolerable to the patient.
- Surgery is indicated in patients who have at least 3 months of daily or regular pain that is refractory to nonoperative measures and interferes with activities of normal living.
- It is recommended that all patients undergo a cortisone injection into the web space before surgery given this will help confirm the diagnosis (if the pain is temporarily relieved), and may resolve the swelling and cure the neuroma.
- Finally, patients may occasionally present with numbness but no pain. Neurectomy is contraindicated in these instances, as it will not improve sensation.

15.1.1 Pathology

- In 1876, Morton described painful thickening of the interdigital nerves at the level of the metatarsal heads. Such "in situ" neuromas are histologically characterized by concentric perineural fibrosis.
- The vast majority of these lesions occur between the third and fourth metatarsals. In those cases in which symptoms are attributed to a second interdigital neuroma, the alternative diagnosis of second metatarsophalangeal (MTP) synovitis and instability should be carefully considered.
- The exact etiology of a Morton neuroma is not entirely understood and may be multifactorial.
- Potential intrinsic factors include irritation of the nerve as it crosses under the intermetatarsal ligament, bursa formation, ischemia, tethering of the nerve, and the fact that the third interdigital nerve is thicker than the other interdigital nerves.[1]
- Potential extrinsic factors include high-heeled shoes, shoes with a narrow toe box, and proximal nerve compression.

15.1.2 Clinical Evaluation

- A Morton neuroma may occur in any of the lesser web spaces, with pain radiating to the two adjacent toes supplied by the nerve.
- As mentioned previously, the third web space is the most commonly affected, followed by the second and fourth web spaces, respectively.
- A small number of patients may have more than one neuroma, although the additional neuromas may not contribute to the patients' symptoms.
- Patients with interdigital nerve pain are typically tender with palpation of the soft tissues between the metatarsal heads and distal metatarsals. With a primary neuroma, there is often a painful "click" with palpation of the intermetatarsal space while simultaneously compressing the metatarsal heads (i.e., Mulder's sign).
- Additionally, pain is reproduced by squeezing the forefoot medially–laterally, rather than plantar-dorsal as is seen with MTP pathology. MTP synovitis and instability is characterized by pain and tenderness located more medial, at the base of the toe.
- The second MTP joint will also be unstable and painful with dorsal translation of the toe (a positive "drawer" test).

15.1.3 Radiographic Evaluation

- Preoperative diagnostic studies should include weight-bearing radiographs of the foot. These are important to rule out other potential sources of pathology, including pain from a long second metatarsal (e.g., second MTP synovitis and instability), stress fracture, or Freiberg's disease.
- Advanced imaging, specifically magnetic resonance imaging (MRI), is not routinely necessary, but may be helpful to confirm the presence of a neuroma or multiple neuromas in atypical presentations. It may also help to rule out other potential diagnoses such as MTP capsulitis, plantar plate injuries, stress fracture, or Freiberg's infraction.
- Ultrasound evaluation can give real-time imaging of the plantar foot structures and help identify a neuroma, the presence of multiple neuromas, or the presence of plantar plate MTP pathology or synovitis.
- Finally, the treating physician should have a low threshold to use diagnostic lidocaine injections. These injections are invaluable when it comes to confirming or ruling out the diagnosis of neurogenic pain.

15.1.4 Nonoperative Options

- Pain due to a Morton neuroma may often respond to accommodative orthotics and a cortisone injection, as well as nonsteroidal anti-inflammatory medications and oral nerve stabilizing agents (e.g., gabapentin or pregabalin).

- More than one cortisone injection should be used with caution, however, given that this can lead to plantar fat-pad atrophy or MTP instability.

15.1.5 Contraindications

- Active infection.
- Vascular insufficiency.
- Uncontrolled complex regional pain syndrome.
- Lack of a clear diagnosis.

15.2 Goals of Surgical Procedure

The primary goal of a neurectomy is pain relief. Neurogenic pain can be disabling, especially in the foot where cyclic loading can lead to thousands of painful stimuli each day. Neurectomy alleviates the majority of symptoms in most patients. Nevertheless, patients must be counseled about the fact that there will be permanent postoperative numbness in the foot. Additionally, they should be aware that any peripheral nerve transection can result in a recurrent stump neuroma, albeit one that is less painful or asymptomatic.

15.3 Advantages of Surgical Procedure

The main advantage of neurectomy is long-term pain relief. The interdigital nerves generally travel in the second plantar layer of the foot. The advantages of performing this procedure through a dorsal approach are that a plantar scar is avoided and that patients can bear weight in the immediate postoperative period. While a plantar approach has been described for the treatment of primary neurectomy,[2,3] it is more useful for a recurrent neuroma in which more proximal exposure is necessary.

15.4 Key Principles

- Adequate exposure is essential.
- An appropriate level of proximal transection is critical for success. Ideally, the distal aspect of the residual proximal nerve segment should be well proximal to the weight-bearing portion of the forefoot.
- All nerves must be handled with delicacy to avoid scarring and iatrogenic damage. This can theoretically lead to pain in the residual nerve ending.

15.5 Preoperative Preparation and Patient Positioning

The patient is positioned supine with the operative extremity elevated on blankets or a foam wedge. If necessary, a bump is placed under the ipsilateral hip so that the toes are oriented toward the ceiling. The use of a calf or ankle tourniquet facilitates visualization, as does the use of loupe magnification. Regional anesthesia with sedation is preferred, specifically either an ankle or popliteal fossa block.

15.6 Operative Technique

- A 3- to 4-cm longitudinal incision is made on the dorsal aspect of the foot centered between the metatarsal heads and extending to the distal web space (**Fig. 15.1**).
- The underlying subcutaneous adipose and dorsal fascia of the foot are sharply divided. The latter structure is thin and membranous and should not be confused with the more robust and plantar transverse intermetatarsal ligament.
- A smooth lamina spreader is then placed between the metatarsal necks and used to gently distract the metatarsals. This tensions the intermetatarsal ligament and thereby facilitates its identification and exposure (**Fig. 15.2**).
- The intermetatarsal ligament is then sharply divided after its proximal and distal edges are identified. Passing a Freer elevator deep to the ligament will minimize inadvertent damage to the nerve or artery.

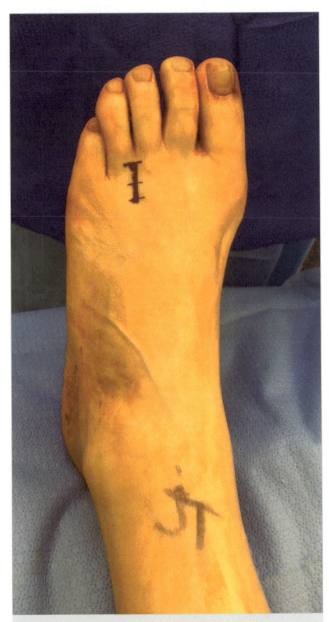

Fig. 15.1 Planned skin incision.

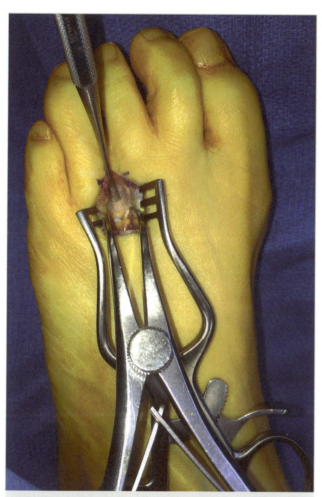

Fig. 15.2 With a lamina spreader placed between the metatarsal necks, a Freer elevator is passed deep to the distal edge of the intermetatarsal ligament.

- The interdigital nerve is then identified and isolated. The artery runs in close proximity and the use of vessel loops during this portion of the procedure helps with isolating the nerve. Often, a bursal-like structure is also present and should carefully be resected with Stevens scissors.
- The two distal branches of the nerve are then identified and transected distal to the bifurcation (**Fig. 15.3a,b**).
- Next, the cut ends of the nerve are grasped and reflected dorsally with a hemostat. Small plantar nerve branches are then visualized and divided.
- The nerve is then dissected proximally until robust intrinsic foot musculature is encountered. This is facilitated by using a small thyroid pole retractor in the proximal extent of the wound. The adjacent fascia of the intrinsic musculature of the foot is divided (**Fig. 15.4**).
- Gentle traction is then applied to the nerve, which is then transected as far proximally as possible (**Fig. 15.5**), and the resected nerve is removed (**Fig. 15.6**).
- Hyperdorsiflex the ankle to allow the nerve stump to retract into the deep submuscular area of the foot. This allows any traumatic neuroma formation to be proximal to the weight-bearing area of the foot, and not to be symptomatic.
- The tourniquet is let down and meticulous hemostasis obtained with cautery.
- The subcutaneous tissues are closed with a 4–0 absorbable suture and the skin closed with 4–0 nylon using a no-touch technique.
- A compression dressing is applied followed by a postoperative shoe.

15.7 Tips and Pearls

Especially when considering a neuroma of the second interdigital nerve, great care must be taken to confirm the diagnosis and

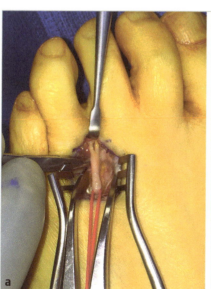
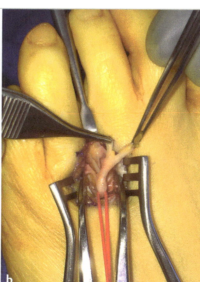

Fig. 15.3 The nerve is distally dissected (a) and then transected (b) beyond the bifurcation.

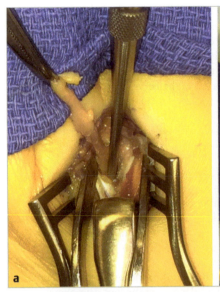
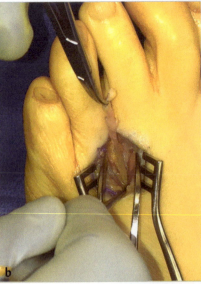

Fig. 15.4 The nerve is dissected as far proximally as possible. A Freer elevator is passed between the nerve and the adjacent fascia of the intrinsic musculature of the foot (a). The latter is then transected allowing an even more proximal transection (b).

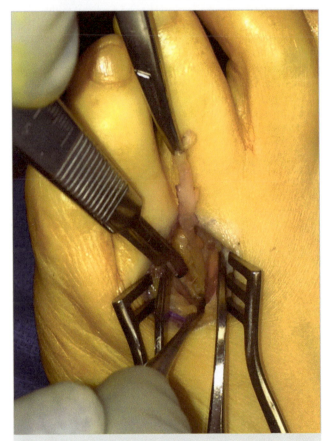

Fig 15.5 Proximal nerve transection.

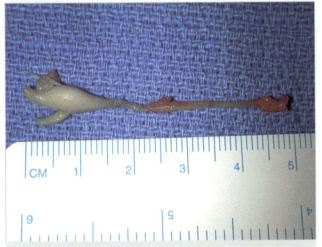

Fig. 15.6 The transected nerve removed from the foot demonstrating the neuroma in the one limb after the bifurcation. Additionally, note that a long segment of nerve is removed proximal to the transverse metatarsal ligament to prevent recurrence.

rule out second MTP synovitis and instability with advanced radiologic studies.

In some patients, there may actually be more than one neuroma present; however, the additional neuroma may not contribute to the patients' symptoms. In these instances, only the symptomatic neuroma should be removed. If the surgeon truly believes that there are symptomatic neuromas present in both the second and third web spaces, and if second MTP instability has been ruled out, then one strategy is to resect the third in-terdigital neuroma while performing a neurolysis of the second interdigital nerve.

Additionally, there are several pearls that facilitate a smooth and efficient surgery.

- The exposure and level of transection should be sufficiently proximal. Specifically, this should be 1 to 2 cm proximal to the metatarsal necks. With this, recurrent neuroma tissue will be proximal to the weight-bearing portion of the forefoot and also not crowded by the adjacent metatarsal heads.
- The use of a lamina spreader placed between the metatarsal necks greatly facilitates visualization and expands working space throughout the procedure.
- The use of loupe magnification also facilitates visualization and isolation of the nerve.
- Be careful to adequately cut and release the plantar branches of the interdigital nerve. Failure to do so will prevent the remaining nerve stump from retracting into the submuscular region of the foot, resulting in painful recurrent neuromas.
- Finally, an alcohol-based skin prep as well as meticulous

hemostasis and a layered closure will minimize wound complications. It is the author's belief that most postoperative foot infections are actually secondary to wound dehiscence.

15.8 Hazards and Pitfalls

- Multiple cortisone injections can result in irreversible loss of the plantar fat pad of the ball of the foot. This should be avoided to prevent ongoing metatarsalgia even after resolution of the neuroma.
- Mistaking second MTP synovitis and instability for neuroma pain can lead to poor results. Resection of the second interdigital nerve in this scenario will leave the patient with persistent joint pain as well as numbness and possible iatrogenic nerve pain.
- As noted, if the proximal nerve transection level is too distal, the outcome of surgery may be jeopardized by recurrent neuroma pain.
- Every attempt should be made to preserve the digital artery and thus minimize the chance of toe ischemia. This is especially important if there has been prior surgery and the possibility of occult vascular injury. As noted, the use of loupe magnification helps in this regard.

15.9 Complications/Bailout/ Salvage

- A postoperative infection can be extremely challenging for both the patient and surgeon. In these instances, early and aggressive wound care is critical, with appropriate antibiotic management. The use a subatmospheric wound dressing may also be necessary.
- Recurrent nerve pain must always be considered in patients with persistent or recurrent symptoms beyond 3 months postoperatively. As noted, some degree of neuroma tissue will form whenever a peripheral nerve is transected. If a recurrent neuroma is sufficiently symptomatic, then revision surgery should be considered. Traditionally, this is performed through a plantar approach, which allows improved proximal exposure. In some patients, however, revision surgery can be performed through a dorsal approach, especially if the primary incision is small and does not extend proximally past the metatarsal necks.

15.10 Postoperative Care

Immediate weight-bearing is allowed in a postoperative shoe. Sutures are removed at approximately 14 days and thereafter the patient may cautiously and responsibly progress activities and shoe wear as dictated by symptoms. Full recovery and maximal subjective improvement takes approximately 3 months.

15.11 Outcomes

Patient satisfaction with neurectomy as reported in the literature varies. Akermark and colleagues recently reported good clinical outcomes in 34 of 41 patients (83%) at an average follow-up of 34 months.[2] A significant reduction in pain with activities of daily living was noted in 96% of patients. In the longer term, Coughlin and Pinsonneault reported good or excellent overall satisfaction in 56 of 66 patients (85%) at an average of 5.8-year follow-up, while Keh et al reported a 93% satisfaction rate at an average of 4.8 years postoperatively.[4,5] Womack and colleagues, however, reported less encouraging results with only 51% of patients having good or excellent results noted at an average follow-up of 66.7 months.[1] These authors noted that surgery for second web space neuromas had significantly worse results when compared to third web space neuromas.[6] This may underscore the importance of establishing an accurate diagnosis and assessing for alternative pathology of the second MTP joint.

References

1. Womack JW, Richardson DR, Murphy GA, Richardson EG, Ishikawa SN. Long-term evaluation of interdigital neuroma treated by surgical excision. Foot Ankle Int 2008;29(6):574–577
2. Akermark C, Crone H, Skoog A, Weidenhielm L. A prospective randomized controlled trial of plantar versus dorsal incisions for operative treatment of primary Morton's neuroma. Foot Ankle Int 2013;34(9):1198–1204
3. Faraj AA, Hosur A. The outcome after using two different approaches for excision of Morton's neuroma. Chin Med J (Engl) 2010;123(16):2195–2198
4. Coughlin MJ, Pinsonneault T. Operative treatment of interdigital neuroma. A long-term follow-up study. J Bone Joint Surg Am 2001;83-A(9):1321–1328
5. Keh RA, Ballew KK, Higgins KR, Odom R, Harkless LB. Long-term follow-up of Morton's neuroma. J Foot Surg 1992;31(1):93–95
6. Singh KS, Ioli JP, Chiodo CP. The surgical treatment of Morton's neuroma. Curr Orthop 2005;19:379–384

16 Revision Intermetatarsal Neurectomy

David R. Richardson

Abstract

Interdigital neuromas are a common cause of forefoot pain. Recurrent or persistent symptoms are common after primary excision and may lead to significant impairment. Failure of initial excision may result from incorrect diagnosis, inadequate excision, or formation of a stump neuroma. Symptoms usually recur within the first 12 months. History and physical examination are the mainstays of diagnosis. Corticosteroid injection may be beneficial but should be limited. Conservative treatment is usually warranted but there is a high failure rate. Results of revision intermetatarsal neurectomy are satisfactory but less gratifying than those of primary excision.

Keywords: *interdigital neuroma, recurrent, metatarsalgia, Morton's neuroma, forefoot, surgical treatment, nerve transposition*

16.1 Indications

- Approach revision intermetatarsal neuroma surgery with circumspection.
- Presumed recurrence may be due to previous wrong diagnosis, inadequate resection, or inadequate preparation and placement of nerve trunk following resection.[1–4]
- Histologic changes in a primary interdigital neuroma occur distal to the transverse intermetatarsal ligament and represent an entrapment neuropathy resulting in perineural fibrosis.[5,6]
- Recurrence following interdigital neuroma resection represents a true histopathologic stump neuroma (haphazard proliferation of axions)[6] (**Fig. 16.1**).
- Stump (true) neuromas tend to form at the transected end of nerves, and proliferation is directed toward the skin or distal portion of the transected nerve.[7,8]
- Differential diagnosis includes
  - Distal resection of previous neuroma.
  - Failure to excise correct structure (e.g., lumbrical).
  - Adjacent web space neuroma.
  - Metatarsophalangeal (MTP) joint synovitis.
  - Freiberg osteochondrosis.
  - Stress fracture of the metatarsal neck.
  - Tarsal tunnel syndrome.
  - Peripheral neuropathy.
  - Lumbar radiculopathy.
  - Unrelated soft-tissue tumor (e.g., ganglion, synovial cyst, lipoma).

16.1.1 Clinical Evaluation of Pathology (History)

- Two-thirds of patients present with symptoms of "recurrent" neuroma within 12 months of index surgery.[2] This probably represents an original misdiagnosis or resection of the wrong structure or original inadequate resection.[9,10]

- An incisional neuroma of a branch of the superficial peroneal nerve may occur and will result in primarily dorsal pain.
- It is important to obtain a thorough, detailed history and physical examination in patients suspected of having a recurrent interdigital neuroma.[4,5,11–15]
- Those with a stump neuroma often complain of plantar pain (burning, aching, electrical) radiating proximally (unlike an original Morton neuroma in which the pain radiates distally).
- Patients often relate the sensation of "walking on a rock" and pain relieved by removing tight shoes and walking on soft surfaces.[2] However, unlike an original Morton neuroma in which the symptoms can be quite vague, a true stump neuroma usually results in very localized, reproducible pain.
- If the patient denies digital numbness, even in the immediate postoperative period following the index procedure, a true stump neuroma is doubtful. If this history is given, it is necessary to rule out other causes in the differential including original inadequate resection.

16.1.2 Clinical Evaluation of Pathology (Physical)

- Plantar tenderness in the web space is the most common physical examination finding.[5,6,11–13] Usually, more localized, reproducible, and intense than with an original Morton neuroma.
- Pain is aggravated by ambulation and shoe wear and relieved with rest.[2,3,12,14,15]
- Patients likely have a positive "Tinel sign," although the pain often radiates proximally.
- Plantar flexion of the corresponding MTP joint can help differentiate joint synovitis from a neuroma. This maneuver causes increased pain with a synovitic joint, but pain is uncommon in patients with a neuroma.
- The Mulder test often is useful.[5,6,11–14,16] This test is best performed with the patient positioned prone with the knees flexed 90 degrees. Pain often is more pronounced and the "click" less pronounced in patients with recurrent neuromas compared to those with primary Morton neuromas (**Fig. 16.2**).

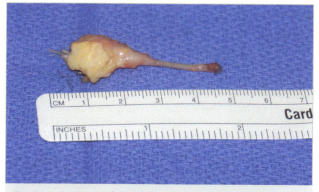

Fig. 16.1 Recurrence following previous interdigital neuroma resection represents a true histopathologic stump neuroma (haphazard proliferation of axions).

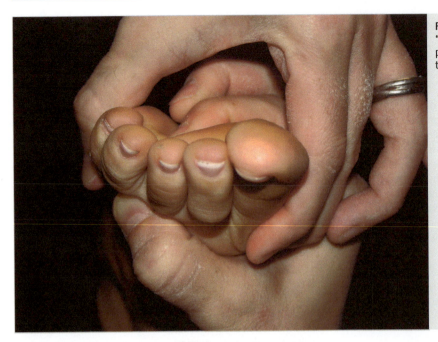

Fig. 16.2 Mulder test is useful; however, the "click" is less pronounced in patients with previous neuroma excision. Performing this test with the patient prone has proved useful.

- Metatarsal fat-pad atrophy may occur after primary neuroma excision (perhaps due to poor technique), but also may result from aging, trauma, medications, or other conditions. Fat-pad atrophy increases the risk of continued pain after surgery and must be discussed with the patient.

16.1.3 Radiographic Evaluation

- The diagnosis of recurrent intermetatarsal neuroma is primarily a clinical exercise, relying on history and physical examination.[2,5,12–14,16]
- Standing anteroposterior, lateral, and oblique radiographs are necessary to assess the MTP joint and osseous structures.
- Electromyographic nerve conduction studies are rarely useful in diagnosing a recurrent intermetatarsal neuroma, but may be beneficial in cases of suspected concomitant tarsal tunnel syndrome or lumbar radiculopathy.[3,10]
- In the case of an ambiguous clinical examination, a magnetic resonance imaging (MRI) or ultrasound (US) may help identify conditions such as a stress fracture or a space-occupying lesion causing neuritic pain. US appears more helpful than MRI in the diagnosis of a recurrent neuroma.
- However, both of these imaging modalities have a high false-negative rate (approximately 20%), especially for small neuromas.[17,18]

16.1.4 Nonoperative Options

- Nonoperative treatment results in varying degrees of relief, but only 20 to 30% get complete, lasting resolution of symptoms.[12]
- Approximately 40% of those treated conservatively experience enough symptomatic relief to avoid surgery. Therefore, nonoperative treatment is recommended before surgical intervention.
- Wide, soft inner–soled, stiff, laced shoes with a low heel are recommended.[12–14]

- An accommodative orthotic with a metatarsal support can be placed proximal to the point of maximal tenderness[11,12,14,19] (**Fig. 16.3**).
- A corticosteroid injection may provide symptomatic relief for up to 2 years in approximately 30% of patients[2,4,11,20] (**Fig. 16.4**).
  - This injection can be both diagnostic and therapeutic; however, caution is required to ensure the medication is placed around the neuroma (not intraneural) and the MTP joint is avoided.
  - US guidance may help direct the injection and document appropriate placement.
  - Injections should be attempted with caution given fat-pad atrophy, skin discoloration, or MTP joint instability may occur.
  - No more than two injections should be attempted.
  - We use a mixture of 40-mg Depo-Medrol:1-mL 0.25% Marcaine and a dorsal approach for the injection.

16.1.5 Contraindications

- Pain control after surgical intervention is less predictable in patients being treated for chronic pain, diagnosed with a mood disorder, taking preoperative narcotics, or using tobacco products. Obesity has not been associated with worse outcomes.[21–23]
- A lengthening procedure should be considered in those with a tight gastroc-soleus complex (Silfverskiöld's test).
- Absolute and relative surgical contraindications are the same as for any forefoot surgery, for example, peripheral vascular disease, poorly controlled diabetes mellitus (A1C > 8), and local infection.[23]

16.2 Goals of Surgical Procedure

The goal of revision intermetatarsal neurectomy is relief of pain and dysfunction. It must be made clear to the patient that intermetatarsal neurectomy is more unpredictable in terms of

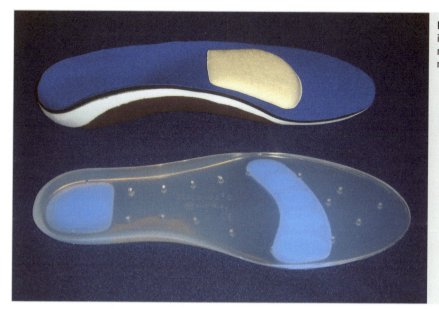

Fig. 16.3 Conservative treatment should include accommodative orthotics and a metatarsal pad placed proximal to point of maximal tenderness.

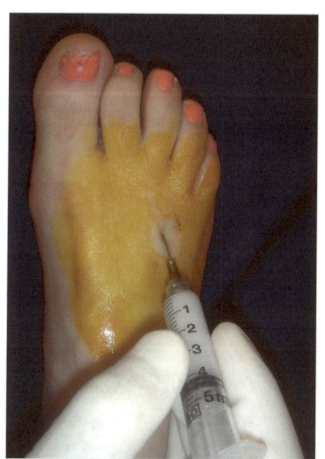

Fig. 16.4 A corticosteroid injection can provide temporary and even long-term relief.

permanent, complete symptomatic relief than many other surgeries of the foot and ankle. Revision surgery adds to the unpredictability, and results appear to be worse than after primary excision; however, the literature suggests reasonable results in patients in whom conservative treatment has failed.[16]

16.3 Advantages of Surgical Procedure

The advantages of revision neuroma excision include improved outcomes compared to conservative treatment.

16.4 Key Principles

- As far as is possible, the primary diagnosis must be ensured to be correct and secondary conditions must be treated as effectively as possible (neuropathy, radiculopathy, gastroc-soleus contracture).
- Patient education is critical to prevent unrealistic expectations and prepare for possible complications:
  ○ The patient should be aware that numbness is expected and "mild aching" pain often exists, especially after increased activity.[5, 11-14,16,19] The sharp, stabbing pain should be significantly improved.
  ○ If a plantar incision is planned, the patient should be aware that the scar often is sensitive for several months postoperatively.[2,19,24]

16.5 Preoperative Preparation and Patient Positioning

- An ankle or forefoot block is administered using a 50/50 mixture of a long- and short-acting anesthetic (e.g., lidocaine and Marcaine). Approximately 20 to 30 mL are used for an ankle block, while 10 to 20 mL is adequate for a forefoot block.
- An examination under anesthesia should be performed because a Mulder click may be present, especially in those with

an inadequate resection at index procedure, or an interspace mass may be more easily appreciated.[14]

- Instruments needed include a Freer elevator, Weitlaner or neuroma retractor, hemostats, small tenotomy retractor, and Senn retractor.
- A sterile ankle tourniquet is used with cast padding and an Esmarch wrap.
- With a plantar incision, care must be used to position the incision proximal to the metatarsal heads and centered on the neuroma.[2,19,24]

16.5.1 Patient Positioning

- After standard preparation and draping, a 3-inch bump is placed under the distal leg, proximal to the ankle, such that the heel is floating. This will allow the ankle to be flexed as needed for visualization.
- If the surgery is to be performed with the patient supine using a dorsal approach, the surgeon should sit or stand proximal to the foot with an assistant at the end of the bed to help with retraction. If the surgery is to be performed with the patient supine through a plantar approach (easier if only local anesthesia administered), in addition to the bump under the heel, the patient is placed in a mild Trendelenburg position (**Fig. 16.5**).
- If a plantar approach is used (preferable for visualization but patients often need general anesthesia), the patient is placed prone with a 3-inch bump under the distal leg just proximal to the ankle. The patient's feet must be at the distal end of the operative table to allow the surgeon to stand (or sit) at the foot of the bed.
- Surgical loupes are recommended.

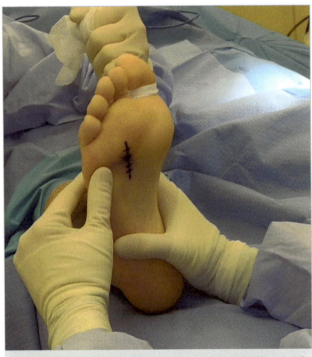

Fig. 16.5 For the plantar approach, the surgeon should be seated at the end of the operative table and a 4-cm incision is made centered over the point of maximal tenderness.

16.6 Operative Technique

16.6.1 Dorsal Approach

- Reserved for revision cases in which inadequate or incomplete resection is suspected. Due to the convergence of the metatarsals at their base, it is very difficult to identify a true stump neuroma and dissect the common digital nerve adequately proximal.
- A dorsal incision is made 4 cm proximal to the web, extending distally to the web space.
- The incision is slightly oblique from proximal-lateral to distal-medial but does not follow the extensor tendons (as this would be too laterally oriented in the proximal direction).
- The dorsal sensory nerves are retracted to the side of least resistance.
- The lumbrical tendon is to the lateral side of the dissection.
- The dorsal interosseous fascia and muscle belly are identified proximally and followed distally to the bursa overlying the transverse metatarsal ligament.
- A neuroma or Weitlander retractor is placed to distract the metatarsals and improve visualization.
- The bursa is incised to expose the transverse metatarsal ligament.
- The interspace is manually palpated to insure that the transverse metatarsal ligament has been released (it can reconstitute or scar after the index procedure).
- A Freer elevator is placed under the transverse ligament (or scar tissue) to protect the underlying structures and then the ligament is released with a no.15 blade knife.
- The lumbrical tendon is in the lateral aspect of the dissection just plantar to the intermetatarsal ligament.
- The neurovascular bundle is identified medial and plantar to the lumbrical.
- Despite the size of the nerve or obvious presence of a neuroma, the nerve should be resected as planned.
- Structures that may be mistaken for the nerve (and therefore may be resected from the previous index procedure) include the lumbrical tendon, which passes to the medial portion of the adjacent proximal phalanx (extension expansion) and therefore is lateral to the nerve or the common digital artery which usually crosses proximal-medial to distal-lateral lying dorsally over the nerve.[2,12,14]
- The nerve is identified proximally and followed distally to the stump (or Morton) neuroma.
- The transverse head of the adductor hallucis may need to be retracted dorsally to gain access to the plantar-directed common digital nerve.
- Any branches of the common digital nerve are divided to allow it to retract 1 to 2 cm.
- The common digital nerve itself is divided while both sides are gently held with an Adson forceps and the damaged portion of the nerve is removed.
- If the recurrence was due to incomplete resection at the index procedure, the distal remaining nerve is circumferentially dissected to the bifurcation and divided just distal to the bifurcation.
- The proximal portion of the nerve is transposed into the intrinsic musculature of the foot (usually the interosseous muscle).[25]
- If desired, a 6–0 nylon epineural stitch can be used to secure the distal aspect of the remaining nerve into muscle belly.

- The specimen is sent for pathologic examination if desired.
- The tourniquet is released, and hemostasis is obtained.
- The wound is irrigated with sterile saline and closed with an interrupted 4–0 nylon suture in an everted, nontensioned manner.
- A Xeroform gauze is placed on the wound, followed by a mildly compressive forefoot dressing.

16.6.2 Plantar Approach

- Preferred for recurrence due to true stump neuroma.
- If a longitudinal incision is preferred, a 4-cm longitudinal incision is made centered over the previously determined point of maximal tenderness. The incision usually begins 1 cm proximal to the first web space and extends 4 cm proximally. The incision is made between the metatarsal heads, which must be carefully located and marked before the incision is made (**Fig. 16.5**).
- If a transverse incision is preferred, a 4-cm transverse plantar incision is made over the point of maximal tenderness. This usually is 1 cm proximal to the weight-bearing pad and parallel to the natural crease.
- The metatarsal heads are repeatedly palpated to provide a reference point for dissection.
- A small Weitlaner retractor is placed to retract the fat overlying the plantar aponeurosis.
- Careful dissection using tenotomy scissors is needed to expose the septa of the plantar fascia.
- The interval between the longitudinal limbs of the plantar fascia septa is exposed.
- A no. 15 blade knife is used to incise the aponeurosis longitudinally.
- The bands of the plantar fascia are retracted medially and laterally with a Senn retractor, and the interspace is carefully explored to identify the common digital nerve and vessel.
- The common digital nerve will lie just dorsal (deep) to the plantar fascia and just plantar (superficial) to the flexor digitorum brevis muscle or tendon.

- Tenotomy scissors are used to bluntly spread until the common digital nerve is identified proximally.
- The dissection then proceeds distally to identify the stump neuroma and proximally to expose 2 cm of the common digital nerve.
- The intermetatarsal ligament is often scarred or reconstituted but does not need to be resected because the stump neuroma is well proximal and plantar.
- The transverse head of the adductor hallucis may need to be retracted dorsally to gain access to the plantar-directed common digital nerve.
- Any branches of the common digital nerve are divided to allow retraction of 1 to 2 cm.
- The stump neuroma itself is removed while both sections are gently held with an Adson forceps and the damaged portion of the nerve is removed (**Fig. 16.6**).
- The proximal portion of the nerve is transposed into the intrinsic musculature of the foot (usually the interosseous muscle).[25]
- If desired, a 6–0 nylon epineural stitch can be used to secure the distal aspect of the remaining nerve into muscle belly.
- The tourniquet is released, and hemostasis is obtained.
- The wound is irrigated with sterile saline and closed with an interrupted 4–0 nylon suture in an everted, nontensioned manner (**Fig. 16.7**).
- A Xeroform gauze is placed on the wound, followed by a mildly compressive forefoot dressing (**Fig. 16.8**).
- A short leg posterior splint is worn for 10 to 14 days.

16.7 Tips and Pearls

- History and physical examination are the primary basis for diagnosis and treatment.
- Attempt conservative treatment before surgery; 6 months is reasonable but depends on patient personality and symptom severity as well whether the index procedure resulted in symptom relief.

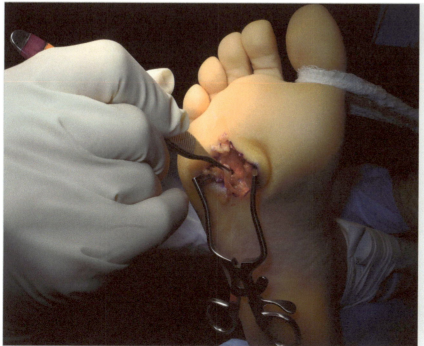

Fig. 16.6 Remove the stump neuroma while gently holding the proximal segment. Transpose the proximal segment into intrinsic musculature.

- Discuss possible complications, especially the relatively high risk of incomplete symptom relief and recurrence.[5,11,12,16,19]
- For a plantar incision, avoid placing the incision directly under the metatarsal heads.

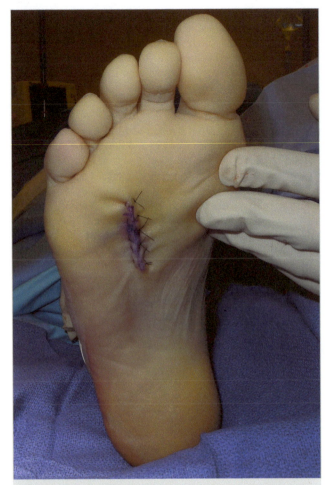

Fig. 16.7 Obtain strict hemostasis and create a nontensioned everted closure with 4–0 nylon suture.

- Transect the common digital nerve 2 cm proximal to the stump neuroma and transpose the nerve into the intrinsic musculature of the foot.[25]
- Obtain hemostasis prior to closure.
- Keep patients non-weight-bearing until the wound is healed.

16.8 Hazards and Pitfalls

- Good to excellent results may be less frequent than previous literature suggests.
- Avoid a plantar incision in those known to form keloid or with thick callosities. Hypersensitivity may occur.
- Avoid hematoma formation to lessen risk of wound problems and infection.

16.9 Complications/Bailout/ Salvage

- Complications include those associated with most surgeries: infection, wound complications, continued pain, and those particular to surgery of nerves and foot in particular, numbness, "shocking" pain, limited shoe wear, and activity limitations.
- Resect the nerve (whether intact due to prior incomplete resection or transected) proximally despite gross appearance. A "normal-appearing" nerve may still have cellular pathology.
- The salvage procedure is revision surgery as described earlier. Caution is advised if two previous resections have failed.
- Conservative treatment should be attempted prior to any revision and a full work-up for other etiologies should again be undertaken.

16.10 Postoperative Care

- After a mildly compressive dressing and short leg splint are placed, the operative limb should be elevated most of the time for 3 days.

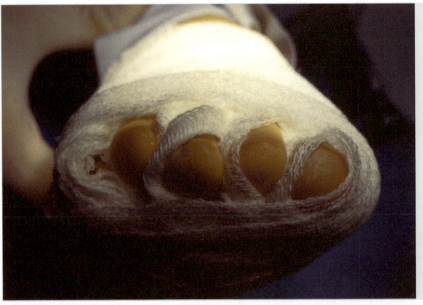

Fig. 16.8 Place a mildly compressive dressing.

- Sutures should remain until the wound is completely healed (2–3 weeks).
- A stiff-soled shoe is worn for 2 weeks after suture removal, and then the patient is transitioned into a wide toe-box shoe until asymptomatic.

16.11 Outcomes

- The patient should expect long-term numbness.
- Shoe wear restrictions are a common complaint after revision neuroma excision.[2,4,6,14]
- Recovery from revision surgery often takes longer than patients expect (often 4 months).
- Reported good to excellent outcomes of surgical treatment of interdigital neuromas are variable but range from 50 to 85%.[1,5,11–13,20,26,27]
- Our experience is on the less encouraging side with 50% good and excellent results at an average of 67-month follow-up.[13,14]
- Good to excellent results after revision surgery may be lower than those of primary excision.[4,6,16]
- In patients with significant preoperative symptoms, revision surgery offers a reasonable expectation of benefit.

References

1. Bradley N, Miller WA, Evans JP. Plantar neuroma: analysis of results following surgical excision in 145 patients. South Med J 1976;69(7):853–854
2. Beskin JL, Baxter DE. Recurrent pain following interdigital neurectomy—a plantar approach. Foot Ankle 1988;9(1):34–39
3. Benedetti RS, Baxter DE, Davis PF. Clinical results of simultaneous adjacent interdigital neurectomy in the foot. Foot Ankle Int 1996;17(5):264–268
4. Stamatis ED, Myerson MS. Treatment of recurrence of symptoms after excision of an interdigital neuroma. A retrospective review. J Bone Joint Surg Br 2004;86(1):48–53
5. Giannini S, Bacchini P, Ceccarelli F, Vannini F. Interdigital neuroma: clinical examination and histopathologic results in 63 cases treated with excision. Foot Ankle Int 2004;25(2):79–84
6. Johnson JE, Johnson KA, Unni KK. Persistent pain after excision of an interdigital neuroma. Results of reoperation. J Bone Joint Surg Am 1988;70(5):651–657
7. Colgrove RC, Huang EY, Barth AH, Greene MA. Interdigital neuroma: intermuscular neuroma transposition compared with resection. Foot Ankle Int 2000;21(3):206–211
8. Dellon AL. Treatment of recurrent metatarsalgia by neuroma resection and muscle implantation: case report and proposed algorithm of management for Morton's "neuroma". Microsurgery 1989;10(3):256–259
9. Amis JA, Siverhus SW, Liwnicz BH. An anatomic basis for recurrence after Morton's neuroma excision. Foot Ankle 1992;13(3):153–156
10. Wolfort SF, Dellon AL. Treatment of recurrent neuroma of the interdigital nerve by implantation of the proximal nerve into muscle in the arch of the foot. J Foot Ankle Surg 2001;40(6):404–410
11. Coughlin MJ, Pinsonneault T. Operative treatment of interdigital neuroma. A long-term follow-up study. J Bone Joint Surg Am 2001;83-A(9):1321–1328
12. Mann RA, Reynolds JC. Interdigital neuroma--a critical clinical analysis. Foot Ankle 1983;3(4):238–243
13. Womack JW, Richardson DR, Murphy GA, Richardson EG, Ishikawa SN. Long-term evaluation of interdigital neuroma treated by surgical excision. Foot Ankle Int 2008;29(6):574–577
14. Richardson DR, Dean EM. The recurrent Morton neuroma: what now? Foot Ankle Clin 2014;19(3):437–449
15. Bennett GL, Graham CE, Mauldin DM. Morton's interdigital neuroma: a comprehensive treatment protocol. Foot Ankle Int 1995;16(12):760–763
16. Bucknall V, Rutherford D, MacDonald D, Shalaby H, McKinley J, Breusch SJ. Outcomes following excision of Morton's interdigital neuroma: a prospective study. Bone Joint J 2016;98-B(10):1376–1381
17. Sharp RJ, Wade CM, Hennessy MS, Saxby TS. The role of MRI and ultrasound imaging in Morton's neuroma and the effect of size of lesion on symptoms. J Bone Joint Surg Br 2003;85(7):999–1005
18. Torres-Claramunt R, Ginés A, Pidemunt G, Puig L, de Zabala S. MRI and ultrasonography in Morton's neuroma: diagnostic accuracy and correlation. Indian J Orthop 2012;46(3):321–325
19. Richardson EG, Brotzman SB, Graves SC. The plantar incision for procedures involving the forefoot. An evaluation of one hundred and fifty incisions in one hundred and fifteen patients. J Bone Joint Surg Am 1993;75(5):726–731
20. Pace A, Scammell B, Dhar S. The outcome of Morton's neurectomy in the treatment of metatarsalgia. Int Orthop 2010;34(4):511–515
21. Bettin CC, Gower K, McCormick K, et al. Cigarette smoking increases complication rate in forefoot surgery. Foot Ankle Int 2015;36(5):488–493
22. Mulligan RP, McCarthy KJ, Grear BJ, Richardson DR, Ishikawa SN, Murphy GA. Psychosocial risk factors for postoperative pain in ankle and hindfoot reconstruction. Foot Ankle Int 2016;37(10):1065–1070
23. Stewart MS, Bettin CC, Ramsey MT, et al. Effect of obesity on outcomes of forefoot surgery. Foot Ankle Int 2016;37(5):483–487
24. Nery C, Raduan F, Del Buono A, Asaumi ID, Maffulli N. Plantar approach for excision of a Morton neuroma: a long-term follow-up study. J Bone Joint Surg Am 2012;94(7):654–658
25. Rungprai C, Cychosz CC, Phruetthiphat O, Femino JE, Amendola A, Phisitkul P. Simple neurectomy versus neurectomy with intramuscular implantation for interdigital neuroma: a comparative study. Foot Ankle Int 2015;36(12):1412–1424
26. Friscia DA, Strom DE, Parr JW, Saltzman CL, Johnson KA. Surgical treatment for primary interdigital neuroma. Orthopedics 1991;14(6):669–672
27. Lee KT, Kim JB, Young KW, Park YU, Kim JS, Jegal H. Long-term results of neurectomy in the treatment of Morton's neuroma: more than 10 years' follow-up. Foot Ankle Spec 2011;4(6):349–353

17 Tarsal Tunnel Release

Sheryl de Waard and Daniel Haverkamp

Abstract

Tarsal tunnel release is a surgical decompression by dividing the flexor retinaculum to relieve the symptoms of a tarsal tunnel syndrome. The tarsal tunnel syndrome is a compression neuropathy of the tibial nerve or its branches. The etiology is still not completely understood, which could explain the variable outcomes of release in the literature.

Keywords: *tarsal tunnel syndrome, neuropathy tibial nerve, release flexor retinaculum*

17.1 Introduction

17.1.1 History

- Tarsal tunnel syndrome was described in 1960 by Kopell and Thompson,[1] and it was named by Keck[2] and Lam[3] in 1962.
- Synonym: posterior tibial neuralgia.

17.1.2 Anatomy

The tarsal tunnel is a fibro-osseous space at the posteromedial side of the ankle. Its anatomical boundaries are the flexor retinaculum, the posteroinferior side of the medial malleolus, the medial wall of the talus, and calcaneus. The following structures pass through the tarsal tunnel: tibialis posterior tendon, flexor digitorum longus tendon, tibialis posterior artery, tibialis posterior vein, tibial nerve, and the flexor hallucis longus tendon (also known as "Tom, Dick, And Very Nervous Harry") (**Fig. 17.1**). The tibial nerve divides into the nerve to the calcaneus, medial plantar nerve, and the lateral plantar nerve within the tarsal tunnel. The first branch of the tibial nerve in the tarsal tunnel is the nerve to the calcaneus, which goes from the tarsal tunnel through the flexor retinaculum to the surface. More distal in the tarsal, the tibial nerve splits into the medial and lateral plantar nerve, with the lateral nerve giving off a branch to the adductor digiti quinti muscle just as it exits the tunnel and passes under the abductor hallucis muscle.

17.2 Indications

- If the patient has complaints of compression neuropathy of the tibial nerve and conservative therapy fails; *or*
- If there is a benign (bone) tumor, such as lipoma, ganglia, or exostosis.

17.2.1 Pathology

- The clinical presentation of tarsal tunnel syndrome is pain behind the medial malleolus, which radiates to the plantar side of the foot. The medial side of the ankle or toes can also be involved.
- The pain can be described as burning, tingling, or dysesthesia/paresthesia.
- Worsening of the symptoms can be provoked by prolonged walking, standing still, or lying in bed.
- The diagnosis is not always easy to make due to other lower limb conditions such as polyneuropathy with diabetes or radiculopathy of L5–S1. If patients have unexplained paresthesias in the foot, toes, or medial side of the calf, physicians must keep this disorder in mind.[4]

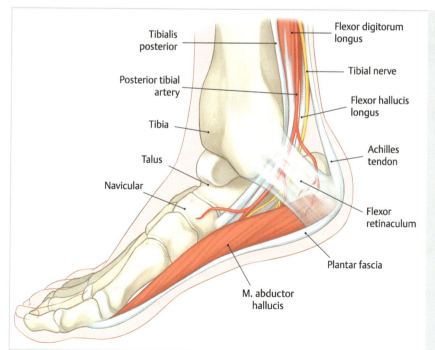

Fig. 17.1 The anatomy of the tarsal tunnel with the structures passing through.

Labels: Tibialis posterior; Posterior tibial artery; Tibia; Talus; Navicular; M. abductor hallucis; Flexor digitorum longus; Tibial nerve; Flexor hallucis longus; Achilles tendon; Flexor retinaculum; Plantar fascia

• Causes of tarsal tunnel syndrome can be divided into three groups:
  ○ Idiopathic.
  ○ Intrinsic (pressure within the tarsal tunnel), such as osteophytes, hypertrophic retinaculum, ganglia, lipoma, neuroma, or enlarged veins.
  ○ Extrinsic (pressure out of the tarsal tunnel), such as direct trauma, constrictive foot wear, hind foot varus or valgus, postsurgical scarring, diabetes, or generalized lower limb edema.[5]

17.2.2 Clinical Evaluation

• Begins with examination of the foot and ankle; look for deformation of the foot such as pes planovalgus or a varus position of the hind foot.
• Let the patient show where he or she experiences the pain. With palpation, the physician can check for soft-tissue tumors.
• Tinel's sign can be positive; but if it is negative, this does not exclude tarsal tunnel syndrome.
• Provocation maneuvers, such as the dorsiflexion-eversion test, can be useful.
• In chronic complaints, also intrinsic muscle weakness or contractures can be found.[5]

17.2.3 Radiographic Evaluation

• After clinical examination, an X-ray of the ankle is made for eventual deformities of the bone. If this shows nothing, compression due to soft tissue must be evaluated due to ultrasound or magnetic resonance imaging (MRI).
• Irritation in the tarsal tunnel can be seen on the MRI without direct soft-tissue compression, which can indicate tarsal tunnel syndrome. However, MRI findings must correlate with clinical findings. Pathophysiological findings can also be found in asymptomatic patients.[6]
• Another diagnostic tool described in the tarsal tunnel is an electromyogram (EMG). An EMG does not exclude tarsal tunnel syndrome if this is normal. Also, an abnormal EMG does not show any correlation with the final outcome of surgical decompression.

17.2.4 Nonoperative Options

• Nonsteroidal anti-inflammatory drugs.
• Corticosteroid injection.
• Physiotherapy.
• Walking cast/sleeping splint.

17.2.5 Contraindications

• Peripheral artery disease with insufficient blood flow to the ankle/foot.
• Idiopathic cause of tarsal tunnel syndrome has inferior outcomes compared to cases where the cause of compression is found.[7]

17.3 Goals of Surgical Procedure

• Release of the tibial nerve or its branches by splitting the flexor retinaculum and if needed excision of the benign (bone) tumor. Goal is to decompress the tibial nerve.

17.4 Advantages of Surgical Procedure

• Good exposure of structures.
• Direct identification and freeing of the tibial nerve and its branches.
• Ability to evaluate for and remove any space-occupying lesions/masses within the tarsal canal.

17.5 Key Principles

• Make an adequately long incision to allow full visualization and release of the tunnel and the tibial nerve.
• Perform an extraneural release only. Intraneural neurolysis should be avoided to prevent excess scar tissue formation within the nerve.
• Ensure full hemostasis has been obtained before incision closure. Bleeding around the nerve can result in excess scar tissue and recurrent compression.

17.6 Preoperative Preparation and Patient Positioning

Apply a tourniquet around the upper leg for good view during the operation. The patient should lie on his or her back with the operated leg in external rotation (**Fig. 17.2**). This can be aided by placing a hip bump under the contralateral hip. The foot is in 70-degree plantar flexion. Depending on the wishes of the patient and anesthesiologist, patient can get a distal nerve block in the popliteal fossa.

17.7 Operative Technique

17.7.1 Incision

The longitudinal incision is made on the medial side of the ankle at the height of the medial malleolus, in the soft spot between the tibia and Achilles tendon. The incision must almost form a straight line until the navicular tuberosity (**Fig. 17.3**). Coagulate any superficial veins which obstructs further incision. Use small dissecting scissors for splitting the subcutaneous fatty tissue and the fascia until the muscle tissue is visible (proximally the flexor digitorum longus and distally the abductor hallucis).

An alternate incision is more longitudinal placed midway between the posteromedial border of the tibia and the anteromedial border of the Achilles tendon, starting about 6 cm proximal to the medial malleolus. This lies directly over the path of

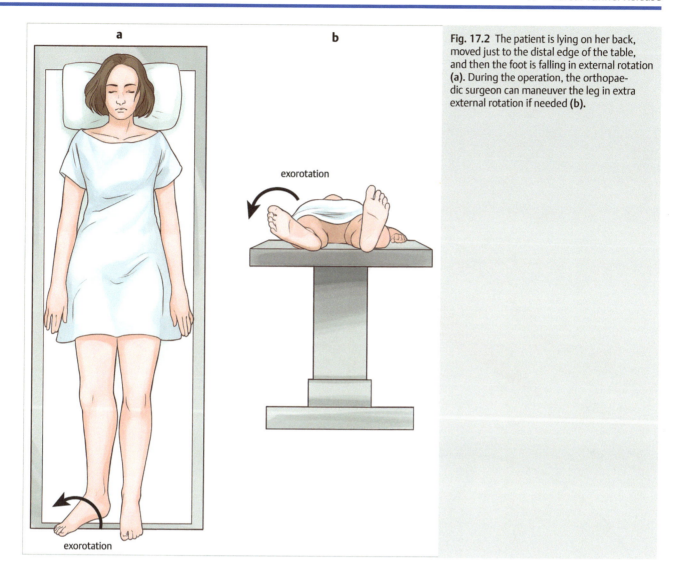

Fig. 17.2 The patient is lying on her back, moved just to the distal edge of the table, and then the foot is falling in external rotation **(a)**. During the operation, the orthopaedic surgeon can maneuver the leg in extra external rotation if needed **(b)**.

the tibial nerve. Distal to the malleolus, the incision is curved slightly anteriorly along the path of the nerve to cross the medial heel over the proximal aspect of the abductor hallucis muscle belly under which the first branch of the lateral plantar nerve (Baxter's nerve) runs and is often entrapped.

17.7.2 Release of the Tarsal Tunnel

After dissection, the neurovascular bundle can be seen before it dives into the tarsal tunnel. Release the flexor retinaculum from proximal to distal and stop until you see the muscle of the abductor hallucis longus. Watch out for the nerve to the calcaneus, which goes through the flexor retinaculum to the surface. After splitting the flexor retinaculum, cut off 5 mm extra of the retinaculum for optimal release (**Fig. 17.4**). Follow the tibial nerve and its branches, making sure there is no further entrapment found. Sometimes, it is necessary to release the abductor halluces from its origin. If any space-occupying masses, such as a ganglion cyst, are present, these should be removed to further decompress the nerve. Full hemostasis must be obtained before closure.

17.7.3 Closing the Incision

Close the subcutaneous layer and skin with whatever surgical thread the surgeon prefers. The subcutaneous layer is stitched with standard interrupted sutures. The skin, however, must be done with continuous suture for best skin contact exposure and thus healing.

17.8 Tips and Pearls

- Positioning of the patient, if the surgeon prefers, can also be done while the patient is lying on the side of the operated foot.
- Always make sure that a complete release is achieved, and make sure that the surgical exposure is adequate.

17.9 Hazard and Pitfalls

- The most important thing during surgery is the view, so make sure there is no underexposure of the structures to prevent inadequate release or damage.

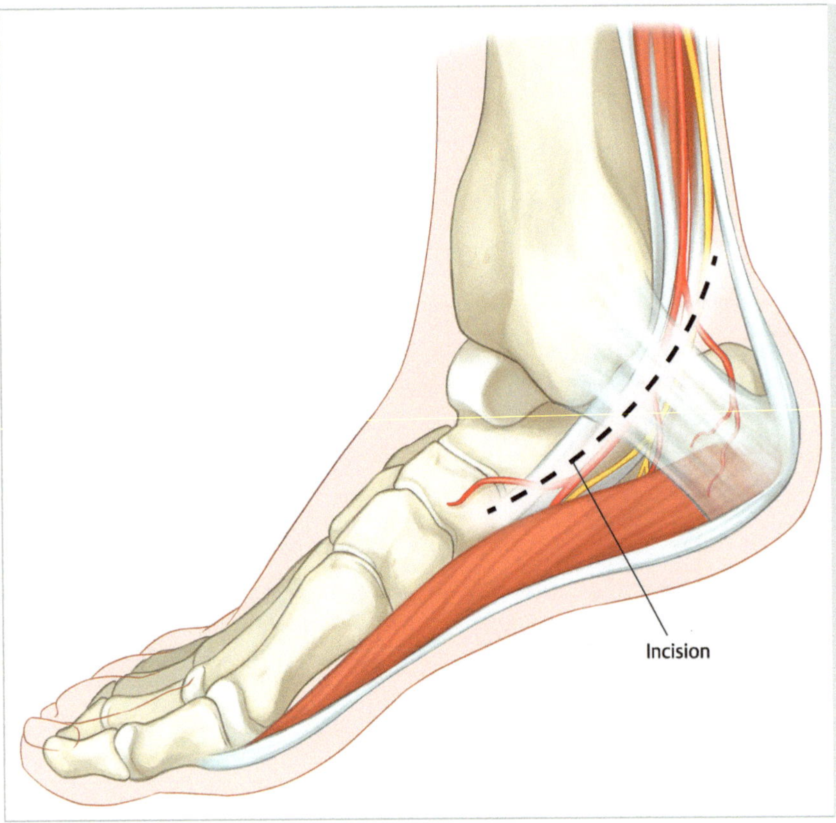

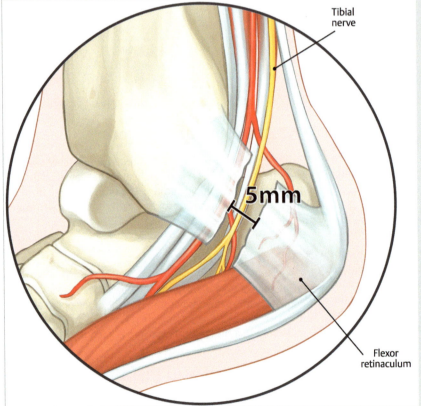

Incision

Fig. 17.3 The marking of the incision in the position of the foot in 70 degrees plantar-flexion.

Tibial nerve

5mm

Flexor retinaculum

Fig. 17.4 Cutting of 5 mm of the flexor retinaculum for adequate release.

- The nerves damage easily; use adequate tools during surgery.
- There is variability in where the branches split from the tibial nerve. In 5% of the cases, the splitting of the medial plantar and lateral plantar nerve occurs proximal in the tarsal tunnel.

17.10 Complications/Bailout/ Salvage

- *Wound dehiscence*: depending on the width and length, instructions for wound cleaning are given and if necessary and possible new sutures.
- *Wound infection*: instructions for wound cleaning are given and if necessary antibiotics. In the worst case, another operation is needed for debridement.
- *Neurovascular damage*: If there is a perforation of the artery during the operation, the vascular surgeon is to be consulted. If there is nerve damage during surgery, consult the neurosurgeon. If you find postoperative damage of the nerve, there is no indication for reoperation.
- *Deep venous thrombosis*: after confirmation, it must be treated with anticoagulants, so a direct consult and follow-up with an internal medicine specialist is in order.

17.11 Postoperative Care

After closing the wound, apply a compress for 5 days. Patients may walk on the foot, if pain allows this. After 5 days, the compress is removed and a normal bandage can be used. The sutures can be removed after 2 weeks. Patients are usually discharged the same day. Postoperative walking cast can be preferred in some type of patients.

17.12 Outcomes

The patient can have edema for the first 6 to 12 weeks, which gradually lessens. After activity, the ankle can get swollen again. This can continue up until 1 year postoperative. The prognosis after surgery depends on the pathology, duration of the compression, and decompression technique. Outcomes are better when caused by a space-occupying mass than when caused by a tight compressive retinaculum.

About 70 to 85% of patients will obtain complete objective correction of their symptoms,[7,8] but the patient's subjective improvement may not be as good.[8]

References

1. Kopell HP, Thompson WA. Peripheral entrapment neuropathies of the lower extremity. N Engl J Med 1960;262:56–60
2. Keck C. The tarsal tunnel syndrome. J Bone Joint Surg Am 1962;44:180–182
3. Lam SJ. A tarsal-tunnel syndrome. Lancet 1962;2(7270): 1354–1355
4. Lareau CR, Sawyer GA, Wang JH, DiGiovanni CW. Plantar and medial heel pain: diagnosis and management. J Am Acad Orthop Surg 2014;22(6):372–380
5. Ahmad M, Tsang K, Mackenney PJ, Adedapo AO. Tarsal tunnel syndrome: a literature review. Foot Ankle Surg 2012;18(3):149–152
6. Wong GNL, Tan TJ. MR imaging as a problem solving tool in posterior ankle pain: a review. Eur J Radiol 2016;85(12):2238–2256
7. Reichert P, Zimmer K, Wnukiewicz W, Kuliński S, Mazurek P, Gosk J. Results of surgical treatment of tarsal tunnel syndrome. Foot Ankle Surg 2015;21(1):26–29
8. Gondring WH, Shields B, Wenger S. An outcomes analysis of surgical treatment of tarsal tunnel syndrome. Foot Ankle Int 2003;24(7):545–550

18 Plantar Fasciectomy and First Branch Lateral Plantar Nerve Release

Omar F. Rahman, David J. Love, and Steven K. Neufeld

Abstract

Plantar fasciitis is one of the most common orthopaedic conditions affecting the hindfoot. Patients complain of excruciating heel pain, especially with the first step in the morning, that tends to resolve throughout the day with walking and tenderness to palpation of the plantar foot. This pain is related to repetitive tensile stresses on the plantar fascia. Many of these patients also complain of neuritic pain that is associated with impingement of the first branch of the lateral plantar nerve, or Baxter's nerve, as it traverses deep to the abductor hallucis. This combination of pathology has been described as distal tarsal tunnel syndrome in the literature. Nonsurgical, conservative therapy is the treatment of choice for plantar fasciitis and this condition. After conservative treatments fail, patients can elect for surgical intervention. In this chapter, we describe the benefits of a partial plantar fasciectomy and release of Baxter's nerve. Prior to surgical intervention, it is critical for the surgeon to obtain a detailed history and physical examination to determine the nature and origin of the heel pain. With the guidance of imaging modalities, the surgeon can more reliably identify potential sources of pain that can help guide surgical management. This surgical intervention provides definitive treatment of plantar fasciitis and nerve impingement and can provide pain relief and a gradual return to daily and recreational activities.

Keywords: *recalcitrant plantar fasciitis, plantar fasciectomy, Baxter's nerve release, first branch of lateral plantar nerve, distal tarsal tunnel syndrome*

18.1 Indications and Pathology

- Chronic degenerative condition at the origin of the plantar fascia on the medial calcaneal tuberosity.
- Repetitive microtrauma and injury-reparative processes lead to micro-tears, necrosis, and chondroid metaplasia.
- Traction irritation of the first branch of the lateral plantar nerve (Baxter's nerve) as it traverses under the deep fascia of the abductor hallucis and over the superficial fascia of the quadratus plantae.
- Neuropathic pain due to compression of Baxter's nerve is referred to as "distal tarsal tunnel syndrome."[1]
- Repetitive tensile forces on the plantar fascia with dorsiflexion of the ankle and metatarsophalangeal (MTP) joints during toe-off (windlass mechanism).
- Radiation of neuritic pain along lateral aspect of the plantar heel.
- Tight Achilles tendon complex and restricted ankle dorsiflexion.

18.1.1 Clinical Evaluation

- Severe morning heel pain, especially when taking the first step.
- Resolution of pain with stretching and walking, and throughout the day.
- Worsening pain when barefoot or with flat shoes due to decreased medial longitudinal arch support.
- Two primary sources of pain on physical examination:
  - Pain or point tenderness at the medial calcaneal tuberosity.
  - Medial hindfoot tenderness at the origin of the abductor hallucis due to compression of Baxter's nerve traversing underneath.
- Positive Tinel's sign with radiating pain in the distribution of the first branch of the lateral plantar nerve (lateral plantar foot, lateral fourth toe, and fifth toe).
- Pain on passive toe dorsiflexion (tension on the plantar fascia):
  - Also demonstrated in S1 radiculopathy, but patients will lack localized tenderness at the plantar heel.

18.1.2 Radiographic Evaluation

- X-ray: lateral weight-bearing views of the affected foot:
  - To rule out calcaneal stress fracture or hindfoot degenerative joint disease.
  - May demonstrate plantar spur at the calcaneal origin of the flexor digitorum brevis but is not considered a reproducible source of pain.[2,3]
- Electromyogram (EMG):
  - Abnormalities of abductor hallucis and/or abductor digiti minimi due to compression of Baxter's nerve.[4]
  - May also demonstrate S1 radiculopathy in the lateral plantar foot.
- Magnetic resonance imaging (MRI): sensitive for frank rupture of plantar fascia but not indicated in most cases:
  - Selective atrophy of abductor digiti minimi indicated by high-signal areas in T1-weighted and low-signal areas in T2-weighted images (**Fig. 18.1**).[5]
  - Focal thickening of plantar fascia with edema.[5]

18.1.3 Nonoperative Options

- Relative rest from exercise.
- Stretching of plantar fascia, Achilles tendon, and gastrocnemius/soleus complex.
- Semi-rigid, triple-layered orthotic devices for arch support and heel cup cushioning.
- Night splinting with dorsiflexion.
- Nonsteroidal anti-inflammatory drugs.

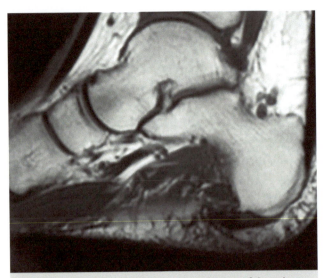

Fig. 18.1 Sagittal T1-weighted suppressed image of the right foot. The image demonstrates high signal demonstrating thickening of the plantar fascia and adjacent edema in the subcutaneous fat tissue.

- Extracorporeal shock wave lithotripsy therapy.
- Cortisone injection at medial calcaneal tuberosity if persistent pain.
- Cold therapy.

18.1.4 Contraindications

- Nonsurgical therapy is the treatment of choice for patients with less than 6 months of symptoms.
- Surgical intervention is considered only if patients are refractory to conservative measures or symptoms last more than 6 months.

18.2 Goals of Surgical Procedure

The purpose of surgical intervention for recalcitrant plantar fasciitis and nerve impingement is to relieve pain refractory to conservative options. Alleviation of or decreased heel pain can effectively improve functional limitations in daily and recreational activities.

18.3 Advantages of Surgical Procedure

The primary advantage of surgical resection of the plantar fascia and release of the first branch of the lateral plantar nerve is definitive treatment. Fasciectomy of at least one-third of the medial band of the plantar fascia has been demonstrated to yield the most patient satisfaction with heel pain relief.[6] The release of the nerve relieves pain and paresthesia associated with nerve compression. This procedure addresses the two primary sources of pathology related to plantar fasciitis and can provide definitive treatment of the disorder.

18.4 Key Principles

- Incision of one-third to one-half of the medial band of the plantar fascia.[6]
- Avoid overexcision of the medial or central band of the plantar fascia, given that complete resection is associated with dorsal foot pain.
- Baxter's nerve dissection between the deep fascia of the abductor hallucis and the superficial fascia of the quadratus plantae.
- Complete release of the deep fascia of the abductor hallucis to allow for gliding of Baxter's nerve.
- Avoid over-dissection of the calcaneal branches of the posterior tibial nerve.
- Excision of an existing calcaneal spur is not necessary.

18.5 Operative Technique

18.5.1 Preoperative Preparation and Patient Positioning

The patient is placed on the operating room table in the supine position with the affected lower extremity in extension and external rotation. A bump can also be placed under the contralateral hip to allow for full external rotation. Regional anesthesia via a popliteal nerve block is recommended, and an ipsilateral calf tourniquet can improve intraoperative visualization. Using a surgical marker, the medial malleolus is outlined and a straight line is drawn from the heel to the posterior malleolus. The midpoint is marked between the posterior border of the medial malleolus and the medial border of the Achilles. The medial edge of the heel is palpated posteriorly and distally to feel for the "soft spot" where the neurovascular bundle is located. This area is marked as well for orientation. These superficial landmarks help delineate the medial oblique incision to be made from the origin of the abductor hallucis to the plantar foot (**Fig. 18.2**).

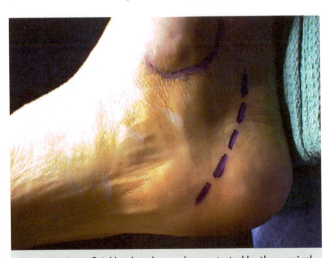

Fig. 18.2 Superficial landmarks are demonstrated by the surgical markings. The medial malleolus is outlined and the incision course is marked by the interrupted line. The oblique marking between the posterior border of the medial malleolus and the medial border of the Achilles tendon overlies the origin of the abductor hallucis.

18.5.2 Surgical Procedure

A 3-cm oblique incision is made over the medial calcaneal tubercle. The incision is located over the proximal aspect of the abductor hallucis muscle. The surgeon should proceed with sharp dissection until the superficial fascia of the abductor hallucis is identified. Superficial vessels may bleed and should be cauterized appropriately (**Fig. 18.3**).

A self-retaining retractor is inserted and blunt dissection is used to identify the interval between the superficial fascia of the abductor hallucis and the muscle body. Using a number 15 blade, the superficial fascia of the abductor hallucis is divided and the muscle belly is retracted superiorly to expose the deep fascia layer. Blunt dissection is used again to adequately expose the deep fascial layer. The deep fascia of the abductor hallucis comprises two layers and is located directly over Baxter's nerve and the superficial fascia of the quadratus plantae muscle. The deep fascia is then sharply divided. The muscle belly is then retracted inferiorly to expose the rest of the deep fascia. Once the deep fascia is divided again, the area in which Baxter's nerve traverses is adequately decompressed (**Fig. 18.4**).

Attention is then directed distally toward plantar fascia release. The medial band of the plantar fascia can be palpated at the inferior border of the deep fascia of the abductor hallucis. Using a number 15 blade, an incision is made into one-third to one-half of the medial band of the plantar fascia. Keep the windlass mechanism taught by dorsiflexing the MTP joints so as to cut the plantar fascia under tension. Resect a 1-cm segment of the plantar fascia 30 to 50% across to ensure adequate release of the tension in the fascia and to prevent re-scarring and recurrence.

After the plantar fasciectomy, attention is then redirected to Baxter's nerve. The course of the nerve is examined to ensure it is free of compression (**Fig. 18.5**). The wound is then irrigated and the tourniquet, if used, is deflated to examine hemostasis. For subcuticular closure, 3–0 Monocryl sutures are used, and for skin closure, 3–0 nylon interrupted vertical mattress sutures are used. A sterile, bulky dressing is then applied to the heel and ankle, and the foot is placed in a short-leg plaster splint with the ankle in neutral dorsiflexion.

18.6 Tips and Pearls

- By not exsanguinating the leg, it may be easier to differentiate the vascular structures from the nervous structures.
- A monopolar Bovie cautery is safer than a bipolar Bovie cautery for hemostasis. The monopolar cautery avoids the larger area of heat that can injure the small nerves.
- After release, we bathe the nerves in dexamethasone to help with postoperative neuritis.
- Though the inferior calcaneal "spur" does not need to be excised, it can be safely removed if neurovascular structures are carefully protected with retractors. It is done in line with the plantar cortex using an osteotome and smoothing the edges with a power rasp.
- The deep layer of the incision is not closed in order to avoid scarring and compression of the nerves postoperatively.
- It is important to not release more than 50% of the fascia so as to avoid postoperative lateral column and calcaneal-cuboid pain.

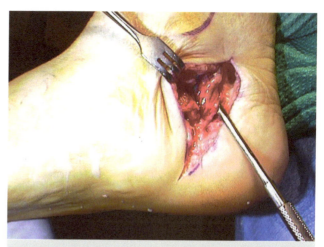

Fig. 18.3 The abductor hallucis origin is exposed after sharp dissection of the superficial layers.

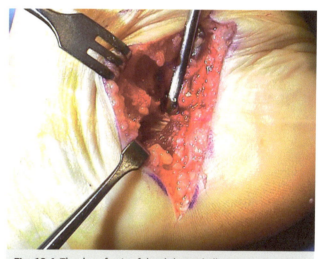

Fig. 18.4 The deep fascia of the abductor hallucis is retracted inferiorly to expose the course of Baxter's nerve.

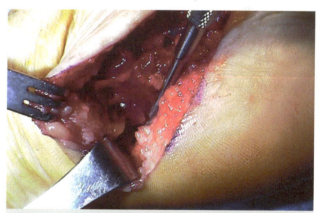

Fig. 18.5 The plantar fascia is divided at the inferior border of the deep fascia of the abductor hallucis.

- Endoscopic plantar fascia release remains a controversial procedure; furthermore, calcaneal spurs and decompression of the first branch of the lateral plantar nerve cannot be addressed endoscopically.

- Postoperatively, the patient remains non-weight-bearing in a splint for 10 to 14 days. Only after the incision is completely healed is range of motion and stretching initiated.

18.7 Hazards and Pitfalls

Once Baxter's nerve is identified under the deep fascia of the abductor hallucis, it is not necessary to dissect through the perineural fat. Excessive dissection around the nerve can cause perineural scarring and devascularization. The neurovascular bundle containing the tibial nerve and posterior tibial vessels is at risk if the medial oblique incision is created too anteriorly or proximally. By maintaining the incision over the medial calcaneal tuberosity, the neurovascular bundle is preserved under the flexor retinaculum. Terminal branches of the posterior tibial artery also traverse around the medial calcaneus and may be inadvertently divided. Once the plantar fascia is incised, if a tourniquet is used, it should be deflated to ensure adequate hemostasis of these branches. Resection of the calcaneal spur is not routinely performed, given there is no evidence demonstrating the spur as a reproducible source of pain. Aggressive excision of the spur requires excess muscle and fascia dissection, which increases postoperative pain and can also cause a calcaneal stress reaction.[7,8]

18.8 Complications/Bailout/ Salvage

There is a relatively low rate of complications during and after the surgical procedure. These complications include wound dehiscence, perineural injury, and direct nerve injury. Postoperatively, complications of surgical intervention revolve around residual heel pain. With complete release of the plantar fascia, the affected extremity is prone to longitudinal arch collapse due to abnormal foot biomechanics. Frank rupture of the plantar fascia will lead to lateral column overload and metatarsalgia due to increased stress transfer to the ligaments of the midfoot and the metatarsals. Patients can also develop heel cord contracture and dorsal midfoot paresthesia.

18.9 Postoperative Care

After the procedure, the patient is placed in a well-padded, compressive dressing and a posterior splint. The patient is kept on crutches/walker and non-weight-bearing for 10 to 14 days. Gentle range-of-motion exercises of the ankle are encouraged. Level I and II literature discusses the plantar fascia–specific stretch, which consists of maintaining ankle and toe dorsiflexion with gentle massage of tight plantar fascia bands upon active stretch.[9,10] The patient is then moved to partial weight-bearing as tolerated in a postoperative shoe with a custom medial longitudinal arch support orthotic. The orthotic should be used for at least 9 months before phasing out, given that arch strain at the dorsolateral foot border can develop with noncompliance. After 3 to 4 weeks, if the incision is healed, the patient is allowed full weight-bearing status as tolerated. After 8 weeks, the patient is encouraged to perform balance and proprioceptive exercises and is permitted for light endurance activities.

18.10 Outcomes

Postoperatively, the patient should expect minimal pain and a gradual return to daily and recreational activities. Patients who receive both a fasciectomy and nerve release should expect greater satisfaction, given that all potential sites of pathology are adequately addressed. In a retrospective study by DiGiovanni et al, 75% of the patients with open plantar fascia release and distal tarsal tunnel release had improved functional outcomes and 82% were satisfied with the procedure.[9] The study stressed the importance of the postoperative protocol, which involved 4 weeks of weight-bearing restrictions and 6 months of strict use of medial longitudinal arch support orthotic. Previous studies by DiGiovanni et al reported less than 50% of total satisfaction by patients who underwent limited plantar fascia release and Baxter nerve release or nerve release without plantar fascia release.[9,10] Moreover, Conflitti and Tarquinio reported that patients with partial fasciectomy and nerve release returned to work or daily activities at an average of 1.5 months and 96% of the 23 patients returned within 3 months.[4] These studies emphasize the point that a comprehensive surgical approach with dedicated postoperative rehabilitation is required to decrease residual pain and improve activity limitations.

References

1. Martin BD, McGuigan FXPlantar fasciitis. In: Wiesel BB, Sankar WN, Delahay JN, Wiesel SW, eds.Orthopaedic Surgery: Principles of Diagnosis and Treatment. Philadelphia, PA: Lippincott Williams & Wilkins; 2011:792–794
2. Cottom JM, Maker JM. Endoscopic debridement for treatment of chronic plantar fasciitis: an innovative surgical technique. J Foot Ankle Surg 2016;55(3):655–658
3. Cottom JM, Maker JM, Richardson P, Baker JS. Endoscopic debridement for treatment of chronic plantar fasciitis: an innovative technique and prospective study of 46 consecutive patients. J Foot Ankle Surg 2016;55(4):748–752
4. Conflitti JM, Tarquinio TA. Operative outcome of partial plantar fasciectomy and neurolysis to the nerve of the abductor digiti minimi muscle for recalcitrant plantar fasciitis. Foot Ankle Int 2004;25(7):482–487
5. Dirim B, Resnick D, Ozenler NK. Bilateral Baxter's neuropathy secondary to plantar fasciitis. Med Sci Monit 2010;16(4):CS50–CS53
6. DiGiovanni BF, Dawson LK, Baumhauer JF. Plantar heel pain. In: Coughlin MJ, Saltzman CL, Anderson RB, eds. Mann's Surgery of the Foot and Ankle. Philadelphia, PA: Saunders; 2014:685–701
7. Gould J, DiGiovanni BF. Plantar fascia release in combination with proximal and distal tarsal tunnel release. In: Wiesel SW, ed. Operative Techniques in Orthopaedic Surgery. Philadelphia, PA: Wolters Kluwer;2016:4620–4630
8. McGarvey WC. Chronic heel pain: surgical management. In: Wulker N, Stephens M, Cracchiolo A, eds. An Atlas of Foot and Ankle Surgery. New York, NY: Taylor & Francis; 2005:207–213
9. DiGiovanni BF, Abuzzahab FS, Gould JS. Plantar fascia release with proximal and distal tarsal tunnel release: surgical

approach to chronic, disabling plantar fasciitis with associated nerve pain. Tech Foot Ankle Surg 2003;2:254–261

10. Digiovanni BF, Nawoczenski DA, Malay DP, et al. Plantar fascia-specific stretching exercise improves outcomes in patients with chronic plantar fasciitis. A prospective clinical trial with two-year follow-up. J Bone Joint Surg Am 2006;88(8):1775–1781

19 Posterior Tibial Tendon Transfer (Including Bridle's Procedure) for Drop-Foot

Carroll P. Jones

Abstract

Drop-foot is a common problem that may result from anterior compartment syndrome, peroneal nerve palsy, incomplete sciatic nerve injuries, lumbar spinal disease, or other inherited or acquired neuromuscular diseases. If there is no potential for nerve recovery and bracing is unfeasible or poorly tolerated, then a posterior tibial tendon (PTT) transfer or Bridle's tendon transfer may be considered. The ideal candidate, to ensure a successful clinical outcome, has a mobile nonarthritic ankle with maintained passive range of motion, minimal deformity, and at least 4/5 PTT strength. The PTT transfer technique has been modified multiple times over the years. The current technique, described here, includes a harvest of the tendon at its insertion on the navicular, and transfer from posterior to anterior through the interosseous membrane (IM). The tendon is secured to the middle or lateral cuneiform with a biotenodesis interference screw. The Bridle procedure, which has also evolved over the last few decades, includes the PTT transfer through the IM. It is then passed through the anterior tibial tendon (ATT) before reattachment in the middle cuneiform bone. The peroneal longus is transected proximally and transferred from the cuboid level to the anterior lower leg, just above the ankle, and secured to the ATT and PTT, completing a tritendon anastomosis. Compared to the PTT transfer alone, the Bridle procedure provides better coronal plane balance and stability and potentially greater dorsiflexion strength. With either of these tendon transfer procedures, patients can expect a brace-free lifestyle and near-normal ambulation on even ground. Assuming careful attention to technique is followed, complications are very uncommon and satisfaction rates are very high.

Keywords: *drop-foot, foot drop, posterior tibial tendon transfer, Bridle's procedure, peroneal nerve palsy, anterior compartment syndrome*

19.1 Indications

19.1.1 Pathology

- Peroneal nerve palsy.
- Spinal cord injury (incomplete).
- Sciatic nerve injuries (partial).
- Anterior compartment deficiency.
- Upper motor neuron disease (i.e., cerebral palsy).
- Hereditary neurologic disorders (i.e., Charcot–Marie–Tooth).

19.1.2 Clinical Evaluation

- Gait consistent with drop-foot (i.e., steppage).
- Weak or absent active ankle dorsiflexion.

- Ideally at least 4/5 posterior tibial tendon (PTT) strength (anything less will result in a tenodesis).
- Intact peroneal longus (PL) tendon and anterior tibial tendon (ATT; for Bridle).
- Normal ankle joint and well-maintained passive range of motion (ROM).
- Gastroc-soleus motor strength of 4/5 or greater.

19.1.3 Radiographic Evaluation

- Standing ankle and foot radiographs.
- Consider electromyogram (EMG) if clinical exam unclear (rarely necessary).

19.1.4 Nonoperative Options

- Physiotherapy if motor strength recovery a possibility.
- Ankle-foot orthosis (AFO).

19.1.5 Contraindications

- Weak or absent PTT strength (less than 4/5).
- Absent anterior tibial or PL tendon (for Bridle).
- Severely arthritic, deformed, and/or contracted ankle joint.
- Incomplete nerve injury with likelihood of recovery.
- Vascular insufficiency.

19.2 Goals of Surgical Procedure

The primary goal of the Bridle and PTT transfer procedures is to obtain a balanced foot and ankle that will permit brace-free ambulation. A successful transfer will ideally result in a normal gait pattern on even ground and at least 5 degrees of active ankle dorsiflexion, with limited plantarflexion. Running, wearing high heels, and walking on uneven ground may not be possible, and the patient should be counseled in this regard.

19.3 Advantages of Surgical Procedure

These procedures have numerous advantages and relatively little downside. A brace-free lifestyle is almost universally well received given that bracing is expensive, cumbersome, and often uncomfortable. The patient is also afforded the maintenance of ankle and hindfoot motion, an obvious advantage over arthrodesis. The operation is relatively simple to perform for the experienced surgeon, and the results are very predictable. Complications are relatively rare and the recovery is straightforward.

19.4   Key Principles

- Transferring a functional tendon (PTT 4/5 strength or greater).
- "Powering" a mobile joint (preserved ankle joint with reasonable passive ROM).
- Ensuring soft-tissue balance around the ankle (i.e., Achilles lengthening if necessary).
- Correct any foot deformities at same time or in staged fashion (i.e., calcaneal osteotomy).
- Establishing the right amount of tension on the transfer.
- In-line tendon transfers with minimal soft-tissue friction (i.e., subcutaneous vs. below retinaculum).
- Stable fixation to allow quicker and safer rehabilitation.

19.5   Preoperative Preparation and Patient Positioning

The patient is positioned supine for the procedure, typically with a bump under the ipsilateral hip to ensure balanced access to the medial and lateral sides of the foot and ankle. Peripheral nerve blocks are usually avoided, particularly in the presence of an established neurologic deficit. General anesthesia and a thigh tourniquet are recommended.

19.6   Operative Technique

19.6.1   Isolated Posterior Tibial Tendon Transfer

For peroneal neuropathy or other conditions only affecting the anterior compartment musculature, without hindfoot deformity or imbalance, a PTT transfer alone can be considered. The tendon, in its entirety, is transferred through the interosseous membrane (IM) to the middle cuneiform or lateral, as first described by Mayer.[1]

The technique involves four incisions. The first incision, utilized to harvest the PTT, is made along the medial hindfoot at the level of its insertion on the navicular bone. The dissection is started proximally and the PTT sheath is opened to expose the tendon. The dissection extends distally to the tendon insertion. To maximize tendon length, the PTT is harvested with a periosteal flap to the most distal extent of the navicular. The end of the harvested tendon is tagged with a 0–0 absorbable suture.

The second incision, longitudinal, is made along the posteromedial border of the distal tibia, 4 to 5 cm proximal to the medial malleolus. The fascia is incised and the PTT is identified. A right-angled clamp is used to pull the distal part of the tendon out of the incision. The tendon is wrapped with a saline-soaked gauze to prevent desiccation.

A third incision, longitudinal, is made along the anterior lower leg, 5 to 6 cm above the level of the ankle joint, just lateral to the tibial spine. The fascia is incised and dissection extends deep and directly along the lateral border of the tibia, medial to the anterior tibial tendon. A hemostat is used to carefully penetrate the IM, which is then opened proximally and distally 10 cm or more, in line with the skin incision. A right-angled clamp is then carefully passed from the *medial* lower leg incision, subperiosteally, to the anterior incision. To pass the PTT

through the IM, it is easiest to first pass a looped suture with the right-angled clamp from medial to lateral between the incisions and through the IM. The looped suture can then be passed around the PTT and used to pull it through the IM out of the anterior incision.

Lastly, a fourth longitudinal incision is made directly over the middle cuneiform. Fluoroscopy is used to identify the bone before the incision is made. Blunt dissection then proceeds carefully down to the middle cuneiform and a Bovie is used to mark the center of the bone. A biotenodesis screw set is used for the next step. The diameter of the PTT is measured and a drill hole of similar, or slightly larger, size is made from dorsal to plantar over a guide pin. The entire depth of the bone is drilled so that the tendon transfer can be appropriately tensioned without "bottoming out" in an incomplete osseous tunnel.

The PTT is then passed subcutaneously with a long clamp from the incision over the IM to the distal wound over the middle cuneiform. The tendon is then passed through the middle cuneiform with a straight needle. The ankle is positioned in 5 degrees of dorsiflexion and the PTT is tensioned by pulling the attached suture from the bottom of the foot. If the Achilles is tight, a heel cord lengthening is performed before securing the tendon transfer. Finally, a biotenodesis screw (usually 5–6 mm in diameter) is placed from dorsal to plantar, securing the tendon in the osseous tunnel. The tendon can be oversewn to the surrounding periosteum for additional stability if necessary.

The wounds are closed in routine layered fashion, followed by application of a well-padded short-leg splint with the ankle in maximal dorsiflexion.

19.6.2   Bridle's Tendon Transfer

As reported by McCall et al, and later modified by Rodriguez, a Bridle procedure may also be considered to treat drop-foot, particularly if associated with hindfoot imbalance (i.e., cavovarus).[2,3] It provides a more robust tenodesis affect and stronger medial to lateral balancing than the PTT transfer alone. In fact, it was designed for cases in which a too-far medial or too-far lateral transfer of the PTT alone may result in a coronal plane deformity.

The Bridle procedure includes a slight modification of the PTT transfer (as described earlier) with the additional involvement of the PL tendon and ATT.

The PTT is harvested, tagged, and passed around the IM exactly as described earlier. The ATT is split longitudinally just distal to the level where the PTT traverses the IM. The PTT is passed from posterior to anterior through the ATT (**Fig. 19.1**). After identification under fluoroscopy, a short longitudinal incision is made just lateral to the middle cuneiform (may consider transferring to the lateral cuneiform if there is significant varus and/or supination deformity). As described earlier, the PTT is passed subcutaneously to the cuneiform. An osseous tunnel is drilled into the center of the cuneiform and the PTT is passed, tensioned, and secured with a biotenodesis screw.

A 4-cm longitudinal incision is made over the peroneal tendons, retrofibular, centered 8 cm proximal to the tip of the lateral malleolus (**Fig. 19.2**). The fascia is incised and the peroneal tendons are exposed. A side-to-side tenodesis between the longus and brevis tendons is performed with nonabsorbable suture. The PL tendon is transected just distal to the tenodesis and the tendon end is tagged.

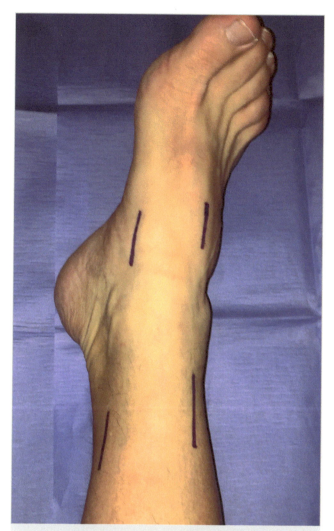

Fig. 19.1 Bridle's procedure: medial and anterior incisions.

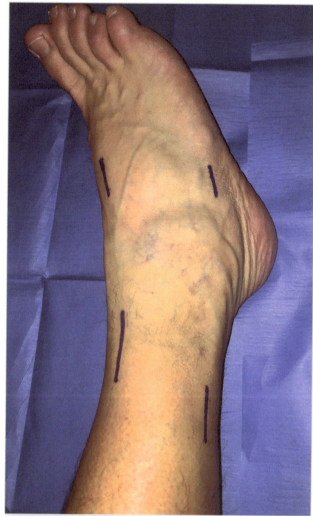

Fig. 19.2 Bridle procedure: lateral incisions.

A short longitudinal incision is then made along the distal aspect of the PL, at the level of the cuboid. The tendon is exposed and then the proximal aspect is pulled distally, out of the wound with a clamp. Using a large, curved clamp, the PL is then transferred subcutaneously, from distal to proximal, into the incision over the ATT. The PL is then woven, in Pulvertaft fashion, through the PTT and ATT. This tritendon anastomosis is then secured with several figure-of-eight nonabsorbable suture passes (**Fig. 19.3**). It is critical to ensure the tension is set with the ankle in 5 degrees of dorsiflexion. The PL and suture can be used to tighten the anastomosis accordingly.

The incisions are closed in typical layered fashion and a well-padded double short-leg splint is applied.

19.7 Tips and Pearls

• Whether to transfer the PTT to the middle or lateral cuneiform is surgeon's choice—for an isolated PTT transfer in the setting of a flexible varus deformity, I prefer the lateral cuneiform to assist with deformity correction.
• Maximizing the length of the PTT harvest is critical to ensure enough length to pass into the cuneiform and obtain good purchase with the interference screw.

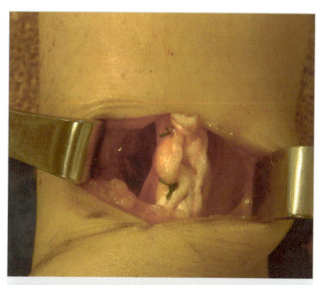

Fig. 19.3 Tritendon anastomosis.

• Before tagging the PTT, without compromising length, sharply trim the bulbous distal part of the tendon to facilitate passing it through the cuneiform bone.

- The PTT is typically the second deepest tendon visualized when approaching from the posteromedial distal tibia (flexor digitorum longus [FDL] is often the most medial at this location).
- After piercing the IM with a hemostat, it is critical to fully open this as far proximal and distal as possible (10–15 cm) to limit friction on the transferred PTT.
- When pulling either the PTT or the PL subcutaneously, first spread the clamp to create an open pocket for easier passage.
- Tension the PTT to 50 to 75% of its full passive excursion before securing.
- Before tensioning and securing the PTT in the cuneiform, harvest and pass the PL tendon to minimize ankle manipulation after the interference screw is placed.
- For the Bridle procedure, first passing the PTT only through the ATT and tensioning it in the cuneiform and *then* completing the tritendon anastomosis is easier than initially passing it through both tendons.

19.8 Hazards and Pitfalls

- If inadequate length of PTT is harvested, it is difficult to transfer it to the cuneiforms in a stable fashion.
- Passing the PTT through the IM can be a tedious step and consume tourniquet time—first pass a suture loop as described earlier and use large right-angled clamps.
- Drilling an osseous tunnel off-center on the cuneiform is a common mistake—a cannulated system ensures the guide pin is centered, using fluoroscopy.
- If a line-to-line interference screw results in a loose fit, upsize the screw by one size.
- Attempting to pass the PTT and/or PL beneath the extensor retinaculum can be difficult, and is not necessary.

19.9 Complications/Bailout/Salvage

Intraoperative complications are rare, and this is consistent with a recently published series by Johnson et al.[4] If, after harvesting the PTT, inadequate length is available for a stable transfer to the cuneiforms, a proximal "Z" lengthening of the tendon can be considered. Alternatively, the PTT can be transferred to the peroneus tertius for a soft-tissue repair alone.

As noted earlier, in cases of soft bone, upsizing the interference screw may be preferable. If the transfer is still unstable, an attempt to transfer to the adjacent (lateral, if medial failed, and vice versa) can be made. As a last result, the PTT can be secured to the peroneus tertius.

To avoid inadvertent pull-out of the PTT, the surgeon or an assistant should hold the foot in dorsiflexion until the procedure is complete and the splint is fully applied and stable.

Although uncommon, flatfoot deformity after transfer of the PTT alone has been reported.[5] Hansen has described performing an FDL transfer to the navicular concomitantly with PTT transfer through the IM for drop-foot to prevent this from occurring.[6] This may be considered for cases of preexisting pes planus or as a salvage procedure if it occurs.

19.10 Postoperative Care

A non-weight-bearing sugar-tong and posterior splint is applied intraoperatively. The patient returns 10 to 14 days later for suture removal and transition to a non-weight-bearing fiberglass cast with the ankle in neutral to 5 degrees of dorsiflexion. It is critical that the ankle is held in dorsiflexion during suture removal and cast application. Six weeks after surgery, the patient is placed into a walker boot and full weight-bearing is permitted. Physical therapy is initiated at this time, with an emphasis on active and passive dorsiflexion and gentle active plantarflexion. The boot can be removed in the evening, but a night-splint or AFO is required during sleep until 3 months after surgery. Eight to ten weeks after surgery, swelling permitting, the patient may transition to an AFO with an athletic-type shoe, which is worn until the 3-month mark. If an AFO is not feasible or available, the walker boot is utilized during this period of time. After 3 months, the patient may transition entirely out of the brace or boot.

19.11 Outcomes

In a series of 19 patients treated with the Bridle procedure with minimum 2-year follow-up, Johnson et al reported a 100% satisfaction rate. All subjects were brace-free for regular everyday activity and two patients utilized a brace for athletic endeavors. There were no significant radiographic changes in foot position compared to preoperative imaging at final follow-up.[4]

With modern techniques, particularly the use of the biotenodesis interference screws, short- and long-term complications are relatively rare. The vast majority of patients are able to resume brace-free ambulation in regular shoes and achieve 5 degrees of active dorsiflexion. Although not necessarily the primary goal of the procedure, the tendon transfer(s) at least provide a tenodesis effect and maintain the ankle in neutral position.

References

1. Mayer L. The physiological method of tendon transplantation in the treatment of paralytic drop-foot. J Bone Joint Surg Am 1937;19(2):389–394
2. McCall RE, Frederick HA, McCluskey GM, Riordan DC. The Bridle procedure: a new treatment for equinus and equinovarus deformities in children. J Pediatr Orthop 1991;11(1):83–89
3. Rodriguez RP. The Bridle procedure in the treatment of paralysis of the foot. Foot Ankle 1992;13(2):63–69
4. Johnson JE, Paxton ES, Lippe J, et al. Outcomes of the Bridle procedure for the treatment of foot drop. Foot Ankle Int 2015;36(11):1287–1296
5. Vertullo CJ, Nunley JA. Acquired flatfoot deformity following posterior tibial tendon transfer for peroneal nerve injury : a case report. J Bone Joint Surg Am 2002;84-A(7):1214–1217
6. Hansen ST. Transfer of the posterior tibial tendon to the dorsolateral midfoot. In: Functional Reconstruction of the Foot and Ankle. Philadelphia, PA: Lippincott, Williams, & Wilkins;2000:442–447/bok19 Posterior Tibial Tendon Transfer (Including Bridle's Procedure) for Drop-Foot

20 Tarsometatarsal Fusions

J. Chris Coetzee

Abstract

Tarsometatarsal (TMT) fusions have always been challenging due to several reasons. The anatomy is complicated: there are always branches of the saphenous, deep, and superficial peroneal nerves that will cross the surgical field. Surgical neuromas in any of these digital nerves could severely compromise an otherwise excellent arthrodesis result. The dorsalis pedis artery also traverses from dorsal to plantar at the base of the first and second interspace. Furthermore, the TMT joints are essentially "flat-on-flat" surfaces with no inherent stability, therefore completely reliant on ligamentous structures. With the joints perpendicular to the axial force across the joints during weight-bearing, the bending force across the joint during walking predisposes it to a higher risk for nonunion. Lastly, the real estate in the cuneiforms is small, and the angle of screw placement could be challenging. Over time, arthrodesis techniques changed a little, but the fixations options expanded significantly to accommodate the challenges posed by getting the TMT joints to fuse. There is fairly informed consensus that one should not fuse the fourth and fifth TMT joints, while the first, second, and third could be fused individually or in any combination depending on the pathology. Optimum treatment still includes adequate preparation of the joints, correction of deformity in all planes, and stable fixation, followed by appropriate postoperative management to allow the fusions to consolidate.

Keywords: *tarsometatarsal joints, arthrodesis, Lisfranc's injuries*

20.1 Indications

- Posttraumatic degenerative joint disease (DJD) after Lisfranc's injuries.
- Idiopathic/primary tarsometatarsal (TMT) DJD.
- First ray hypermobility.
- Rheumatoid arthritis.
- Stable/chronic Charcot's neuro-arthropathy or other complications of diabetes.
- Major ligamentous disruptions with multidirectional instability/dislocation of the Lisfranc joints.
- Comminuted intra-articular fractures at the base of the first or second metatarsal.
- Crush injuries of the midfoot with intra-articular fracture dislocation.

20.1.1 Pathology

- There is a wide variety of causes for midfoot arthritis.[1]
- In the acute injury situation, it is most often a dislocation of the TMT joints, with or without fractures:
  - The ones with intra-articular, comminuted fractures usually need a primary arthrodesis.
  - Complete ligamentous disruptions alone still create a little controversy whether they should be fused or not.
  - Minor ligamentous injuries should be temporarily stabilized with screws or plates, but do not need fusions.

- Secondary DJD of the TMT joints is very common and the deformity can vary from subtle to severe with a complete collapse into valgus and extension.
- Midfoot Charcot's neuro-arthroplasty can result in very severe deformities:
  - As a rule, midfoot Charcot is initially treated nonsurgically in the hope it will stabilize in a plantigrade, stable foot.
  - However, there are situations where one might have to do surgery early on to prevent ulcerations.[2] Late deformities can be difficult to correct.

20.1.2 Clinical Evaluation

- Evaluate with the patient if possible—it is most helpful to understand the severity of the deformity.
- Palpation and manipulation of the individual TMT joints will establish which joints are most affected, and also the potential for passive correction of the deformity.
- In posttraumatic cases, the soft-tissue envelope should be inspected to look for issues that could compromise healing and increase risk of infection.
- Look for second and third metatarsal overload. This is common in chronic cases and should be addressed during the correction.
- Always do a Silversköld test to see if there is an equinus contracture, which should be addressed with any midfoot arthrodesis procedure, given this will limit the torque placed across the midfoot joints and risk for nonunion.
- The hindfoot and ankle should also be examined to look for other pathology.

20.1.3 Radiographic Evaluation

- Weight-bearing anteroposterior (AP), lateral, and oblique weight-bearing views of the foot are routinely performed for evaluation of the midfoot[3]:
  - AP view: evaluation of the medial column:
    - ❖ Look for collapse into valgus at the TMT joint but also at the naviculocuneiform joint.
    - ❖ Look for relative shortening of the first ray compared to the second and third.
  - Oblique view: to evaluate the middle and lateral columns.
  - Lateral view: dorsal bossing, osteophytes, and early joint-space narrowing:
    - ❖ Look for collapse of the medial arch.
- Comparison to the uninvolved, contralateral foot can provide a valuable model for preoperative planning.
- For severe, complex deformities, a computed tomography (CT) scan can be very helpful in planning the correction.

20.1.4 Contraindications

- Skeletal immaturity—open physes.
- Simple, incomplete ligamentous injuries.
- Active infection.

20.2 Goals of Surgical Procedure

- To provide a stable, well-aligned midfoot which is plantigrade with normal weight distribution throughout the foot.

20.3 Advantages of Surgical Procedure

- Open debridement of arthritic changes of the midfoot.
- Allows anatomic alignment of the midfoot and reconstruction of the tripod effect of the foot.
- Improves stability of the midfoot and arch.
- Only sacrifices the "nonessential," low-mobility TMT and intercuneiform joints.
- Allows for rigid stabilization of the medial and central columns of the midfoot.

20.4 Key Principles

- Plan incisions well, and know the anatomy. Identify and protect the neurovascular structures.
- Have a very low threshold to do two incisions. It reduces the risk of injury to the soft tissue as well as wound complications. It also allows for much better visualization of the joints.
- Reduce the deformity in all planes prior to fixation. In situ arthrodesis of a deformity is not acceptable.
- Stable fixation is essential. It could be done with screws, staples, or plate constructs.

20.5 Preoperative Preparation and Patient Positioning

- Supine, usually with a bump under the ipsilateral hip to allow easier exposure to the lateral side.
- Thigh tourniquet.

20.6 Operative Technique

20.6.1 In Situ TMT Joint Arthrodesis

- Depending on the number of TMT joints involved in the injury or arthritic process, one or two dorsal, longitudinal incisions are made:
  - The first incision is made over the first metatarsal, just lateral to the extensor hallucis longus. This will allow access to the first and most of the second TMT joints. Pathology involving only the medial two TMT joints can be corrected with this single incision.
- If there is any concern about the accuracy of the reduction, it is advisable to do a second more lateral incision to facilitate exposure and visualization of the joint:
  - The second incision is centered over the fourth metatarsal; it is much further lateral than what is appreciated (**Fig. 20.1**).
  - The most common mistake is to make the incision too far medial; incision placement may be aided by fluoroscopic

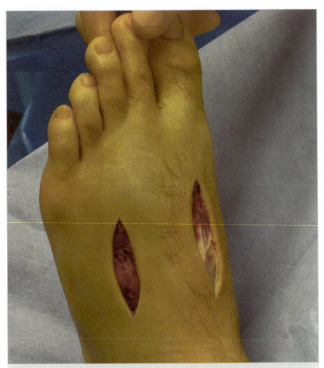

Fig. 20.1 For an arthrodesis in situ, one could use one or two incisions depending on how many joints are involved

guidance and identification of the intended bony targets.
  - The foot should be internally rotated to get an end-on view of the fourth metatarsal. If the X-ray is done with the foot in a neutral position, there is too much overlap between the third, fourth, and fifth metatarsals to accurately determine the position of the fourth ray.
- Adequately expose the joints and then remove all remaining cartilage with small osteotome and curette.
- Be very careful not to use a saw to create flat cuts. Once you start, it is difficult to get all the joint to be adequately apposed. I prefer to use an osteotome to correct minor alignment issues.
- Most critical is to remember the first TMT is about 30 mm deep. A mini-lamina spreader is invaluable to allow proper visualization down the depths of the joint:
  - All plantar cartilage and prominent spurs must be removed to prevent a dorsiflexion malunion.
- Meticulous bone preparation is critical to the success of the case, with a goal to expose a bleeding cancellous bone surface.
  - A small curved osteotome is used to microfracture the subchondral bone.
  - Could also use a 2-mm drill bit to perforate the surfaces.
- Bone graft is not typically required to achieve fusion:
  - If there is a localized defect, a cancellous graft could be harvested to fill the defect.
- Fixation is generally performed from medial to lateral and a reduction clamp is placed prior to fixation to achieve compression across the prepared joints.

20.6.2 Fixation: Screws versus Plates[4]

- Screws are indicated for "simple" fusions (**Fig. 20. 2a–c**):
  - No bone loss.

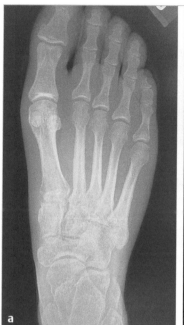
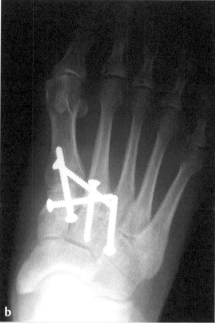
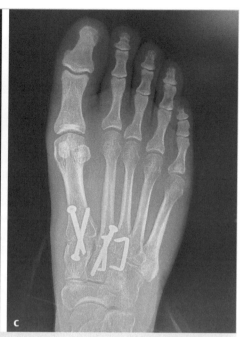

Fig. 20.2   (a) Shows a primary DJD of the TMT joints without collapse or deformity. (b) Simple screw fixation in this situation usually gives adequate stability. (c) In certain situations, staples could be used for the second and third TMT joints, and are generally easier to insert.

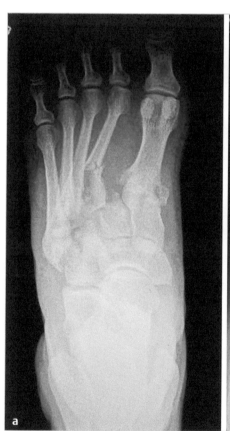
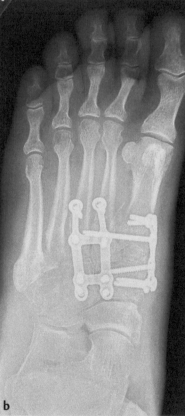

Fig. 20.3   (a) This is a case with a severely comminuted intra-articular fracture dislocation. (b) The most reliable way to secure the fractures and achieve an arthrodesis is with spanning plate fixation.

- ○ Minimal correction needed.
- ○ Good bone quality.
- ○ It might be easier to use staples for especially the second and third TMT joints due to the acute angle of screw placement.

- Plates are useful for "complicated" fusions:
  - ○ Where corrective osteotomies are required.
  - ○ Bone loss that requires grafting.
  - ○ Poor bone quality.
  - ○ Comminuted fractures (**Fig. 20.3**).
  - ○ Complex reconstructions where maximum stability is needed.

- In good quality bone, use 3.5- or 4.0-mm screws:
  - Solid or cannulated.
  - First TMT joint is stabilized with two crossed screws.
  - A Lisfranc screw is then placed from the medial cuneiform to the base of the second metatarsal:
    - ❖ Correct lateral translation of the second metatarsal base.
    - ❖ Help restore midfoot alignment.
  - The second and third TMT joints can be difficult to secure with a single screw due to the acute angle of the screw placement:
    - ❖ One could use a nitinol staple or a two-hole compression plate with a screw on both sides of the joint.
- Meticulous closure of incisions.
- Dressings and a well-padded splint with the ankle in neutral dorsiflexion are applied.

20.6.3 Realignment Arthrodesis

- Greater than 15 degrees of angular deformity or 3 mm of displacement in either the transverse or sagittal plane is noted; a wedge resection is indicated to restore plantigrade alignment of the foot.
- A large C-arm may be helpful to increase the field of view needed to appreciate the achieved degree of correction.
- The initial incision is along the medial border of the foot to allow access to the dorsal and plantar aspects of the first TMT joint (**Fig. 20.4**):
  - The tibialis anterior tendon will be in the way, and should be protected.
  - A biplanar medial and plantar-based wedge, including the medial and middle columns, is resected for the typical abduction and dorsiflexion midfoot deformity:

- ❖ It is often required to do a second dorsolateral incision to adequately visualize and complete the second and third TMT osteotomies.
- ❖ A Steinmann pin is placed through the metatarsals from medial to lateral, perpendicular to the axis of the metatarsals and placed at the proximal aspect of the metatarsals, marking the location of the osteotomy.
- ❖ A second guidewire is placed into the cuneiforms from medial to lateral, perpendicular to the axis of the talus and placed at the distal aspect of the cuneiforms.
- ❖ The wires should meet at an apex at the lateral border of the middle column. A wedge is created with an oscillating saw, progressing from medial to lateral along the guidewires.
- ❖ Angular correction in the sagittal plan is achieved by angling the oscillating saw during the osteotomy and resecting more plantar than dorsal bone.
- ❖ Remove any deep plantar fragments of bone, which may lead to malunion.
- ❖ Reduce the osteotomy in all planes and held with temporary K-wires.
  - Due to the nature of the medial/plantar wedge, the first ray is usually shortened more than the second and third:
    - ❖ This should be corrected with bone grafting of the first to lengthen or the preferred method of shortening the second and third metatarsals either midshaft or distal.
- Specialized plates designed for midfoot fusions are available and may provide additional stability to the final construct (**Fig. 20.5a,b**).
- Closure follow as for in situ arthrodesis.

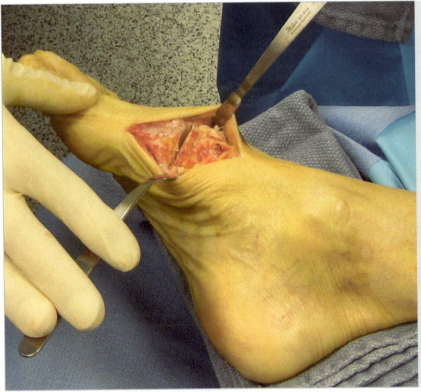

Fig. 20.4 In situations with a severe medial column collapse, it is advisable to make the first incision medial along the border of the foot, to allow access to the plantar and dorsal aspects of the first TMT joint.

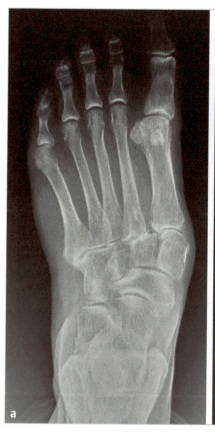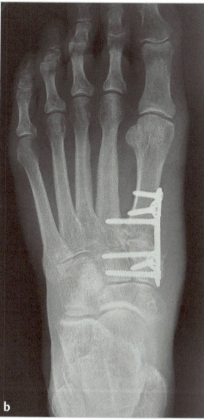

Fig. 20.5 (a) This represents a chronic, progressive collapse of the midfoot secondary to an old Lisfranc injury. (b) After correction in two planes and medial plate fixation.

20.7 Tips and Pearls

- Protect the neurovascular structures.
- Do an adequate exposure and soft-tissue release to allow reduction.
- Do not fuse a deformity in situ. Always correct in all planes!
- Bone graft as needed, especially if there are dorsal and lateral defects after reduction.
- Use adequate fixation. The forces over the TMT joints are large.

20.8 Hazards and Pitfalls

20.8.1 Preparation of the Plantar Joint Surface

- This cannot be overemphasized! The first TMT joint is 30 mm deep. Inadequate plantar preparation will lead to a fusion in dorsiflexion.
- Use a small lamina spreader to aid visualization, preparation, and reduction.

20.8.2 Shortening

- Chronic midfoot collapse can be very difficult to correct. Most common mistake is to remove a wedge from the first metatarsal and not the remainder of the TMT joint:
  - That invariably leads to a short first ray and lesser metatarsophalangeal joint overload.

20.8.3 The Use of Wedge Resections

- Wedge resections are powerful tools to correct severe deformities, but should be carefully planned.
- Best to start with small wedges and verify reduction under fluoroscopy.
- Almost always biplane osteotomies with medial and plantar wedges to correct out of abduction and extension.

20.9 Complications/Bailout/Salvage

Total complication rate could be as high as 30%.
- Skin/wound complications:
  - Wound dehiscence, neuropraxis, hardware pain or breakage, and tendon adhesions.
  - Infection in 3 to 11%.
- Mechanical complications:
  - About 25% complain of metatarsalgia, second metatarsal stress fractures, and neuromas.
  - Malunion of arthrodesis in 6% of cases.
  - Nonunion in 3 to 7%.

20.10 Postoperative Care

- Procedure is usually performed on an outpatient basis:
  - Cast or splint for 2 weeks.
  - Elevation is important for the first 2 weeks following surgery.
  - Non-weight-bearing for the first 2 weeks.

- At 2 weeks, the sutures are removed if the wounds look good.
  - CAM (controlled ankle motion) walking boot is used for the following 4 weeks. The patient may remove the boot for hygiene and application of ice, but must remain non-weight-bearing.
- At 6 weeks, X-rays are done and if there are adequate signs of healing:
  - Start gentle PT to allow range of motion and nonimpact activities. Biking/swimming.
  - Remain partial weight-bearing in the boot or shoe for another 2 to 6 weeks postoperatively, until clinical and radiographic signs of healing are noted.
- Once radiographically healed, start gait training and gentle, progressive strengthening of the leg.
- Takes 4 to 6 months to fully mature, so might have to wait that long before returning to high-impact activities.
- Might continue to swell for up to a year.

20.11 Outcomes

- Primary fusions without deformity correction generally have a very satisfactory result with a high return to previous level of activity.[5-7]
- Severe deformities are harder to correct, and good and excellent results are lower.[8-10]

References

1. Patel A, Rao S, Nawoczenski D, Flemister AS, DiGiovanni B, Baumhauer JF. Midfoot arthritis. J Am Acad Orthop Surg 2010;18(7):417–425

2. Simon SR, Tejwani SG, Wilson DL, Santner TJ, Denniston NL. Arthrodesis as an early alternative to nonoperative management of charcot arthropathy of the diabetic foot. J Bone Joint Surg Am 2000;82-A(7):939–950

3. Younger AS, Sawatzky B, Dryden P. Radiographic assessment of adult flatfoot. Foot Ankle Int 2005;26(10):820–825

4. Alberta FG, Aronow MS, Barrero M, Diaz-Doran V, Sullivan RJ, Adams DJ. Ligamentous Lisfranc joint injuries: a biomechanical comparison of dorsal plate and transarticular screw fixation. Foot Ankle Int 2005;26(6):462–473

5. Espinosa N, Wirth SH. Tarsometatarsal arthrodesis for management of unstable first ray and failed bunion surgery. Foot Ankle Clin 2011;16(1):21–34

6. Coetzee JC, Ly TV. Treatment of primarily ligamentous Lisfranc joint injuries: primary arthrodesis compared with open reduction and internal fixation. Surgical technique. J Bone Joint Surg Am 2007;89(Suppl 2 Pt.1):122–127

7. Rammelt S, Schneiders W, Schikore H, Holch M, Heineck J, Zwipp H. Primary open reduction and fixation compared with delayed corrective arthrodesis in the treatment of tarsometatarsal (Lisfranc) fracture dislocation. J Bone Joint Surg Br 2008;90(11):1499–1506

8. Komenda GA, Myerson MS, Biddinger KR. Results of arthrodesis of the tarsometatarsal joints after traumatic injury. J Bone Joint Surg Am 1996;78(11):1665–1676

9. Sangeorzan BJ, Veith RG, Hansen ST Jr. Salvage of Lisfranc's tarsometatarsal joint by arthrodesis. Foot Ankle 1990;10(4):193–200

10. Sammarco VJ, Sammarco GJ, Walker EW Jr, Guiao RP. Midtarsal arthrodesis in the treatment of Charcot midfoot arthropathy. J Bone Joint Surg Am 2009;91(1):80–91

21 Naviculocuneiform Fusion to Treat Midfoot Arthritis and Deformity

Alastair Younger and Nicholas E.M. Yeo

Abstract

Naviculocuneiform (NC) fusion is not a new concept and was first described in the literature in the early 20th century. However, over the years, it has played second fiddle to various other procedures as the workhorse for flatfoot deformity correction due to its perceived unreliability. In recent years, foot and ankle surgeons are reevaluating the role of NC fusions in the treatment of deformity correction and symptomatic arthritis. A better appreciation of NC collapse in a certain subgroup of patients with planovalgus feet where the apex of the deformity lies in the NC joint has highlighted the role of deformity correction through the NC fusion. Biomechanically, fusion of the NC joint is the most effective procedure to correct the forefoot varus in a planovalgus deformity. This medializes the joint reaction force in the ankle and restores more normal ankle joint mechanics while preserving motion at the ankle and Chopart's joints. Recent literature suggests that NC fusion is a safe and reliable procedure. Fusion rates have been shown to be upward of 95% when performed for the correct indication and with good surgical technique. Complication rates are similar to that of other joint fusions in the foot. Our experience is in keeping with that of the literature and we recommend NC fusion as an option for pes planovalgus deformity correction and symptomatic arthritis of the medial column. It may be performed in isolation or in conjunction with other soft-tissue and bony procedures.

Keywords: naviculocuneiform, fusion, planovalgus

21.1 Indications and Pathology

- **Flat foot deformity.** Naviculocuneiform (NC) fusion within our practice is most commonly used to derotate the forefoot in flatfoot correction. In symptomatic flatfoot deformity such as in posterior tibial tendon dysfunction, the joint reaction force in the ankle joint is laterally placed. This needs to be corrected. There are three components to the deformity that causes the lateral load. The hindfoot may be in valgus and this may occur through the subtalar joint, through the ankle, or be supramalleolar in origin. The larger mechanical component of the lateral load arises in the forefoot. This is because the forefoot makes for a larger lever arm at the ankle. There are two components to the forefoot malposition in flatfoot. The forefoot may be externally rotated on the hindfoot. This places a valgus load on the ankle. The second forefoot deformity, which may laterally load the ankle, is forefoot varus on the hindfoot.
  The hindfoot position can be corrected by a medializing calcaneal osteotomy, a subtalar fusion, or a lateral column lengthening. The lateral or externally rotated position of the forefoot can be corrected by a lateral column lengthening or a talonavicular (TN) fusion. Both procedures may leave the forefoot in varus, and the TN fusion may cause stiffness that can be avoided. The NC fusion is the most powerful and effective fusion to correct the forefoot varus in a flat foot deformity. It will medialize the joint reaction force in the ankle and restore more normal ankle joint mechanics.
  In addition, there is a group of patients with symptomatic flatfoot deformity where the apex of the deformity is centered at the NC joint. This is readily apparent on the lateral weight-bearing radiographs of the foot. In such cases, correction of the deformity at the NC joint is indicated.
- **Posttraumatic arthritis.** The midfoot can be involved in crush injuries and trauma. These include navicular crush or impaction injuries, navicular cuneiform dislocations, and variants of the Lisfranc fracture–dislocation pattern. Traumatic injuries resulting in medial column dissociation with significant osteochondral injuries and gross instability will benefit from primary in situ or corrective fusion.
- **Post–tumor resection.** Following excision of a tumor, the NC joint may need to be fused.
- **Inflammatory arthritis.** Patients with rheumatoid arthritis may have degenerative change at this level, with or without a flatfoot deformity.
- **Correction of forefoot deformity in ankle joint replacement.** In patients with forefoot varus who are undergoing an ankle joint replacement, an NC fusion may be required to correct the forefoot deformity to ensure that the medial side of the ankle (the medial malleolus and deltoid ligament) is not overloaded (**Fig. 21.1**).
- **Muller–Weiss disease.** Muller–Weiss disease is an avascular collapse of the navicular. Typically, the collapse can involve the TN and navicular cuneiform joints. The navicular cuneiform joint may need to be fused in conjunction with the TN and possible triple arthrodesis.

21.1.1 Clinical Evaluation

- The patient is observed walking and standing. The forefoot external rotation will be manifest by the "too many toes" sign when the patient is observed from behind. The forefoot varus will be visible when the patient sits and the hindfoot is corrected to a neutral position. The forefoot position is assessed by determining the degree of forefoot varus on the long axis of the tibia. This may reach 40 to 50 degrees.
- Assessment of the tibialis posterior tendon is important especially in the setting of medial-sided symptoms. Clinical tenderness and weakness on resisted eversion is suggestive of some element of inflammation or dysfunction. Clinical assessment of the TN, NC, and first tarsometatarsal (TMT) joints may point to degenerative or inflammatory arthritis as the underlying etiology.

21.1.2 Radiographic Evaluation

- Standing anteroposterior (AP) and lateral radiographs of the ankle and foot are required to assess the deformity.
- Lateral views will show if the apex of the collapse of the flat foot is at the NC joint or at the TMT joints.

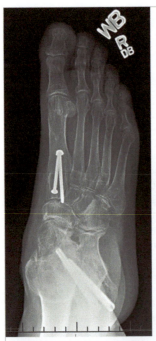
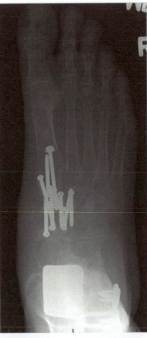
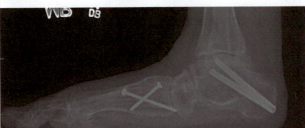
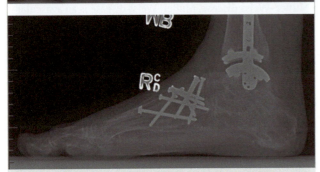

Fig. 21.1 Pre- and post-op radiographs of pes planus reconstruction through naviculocuneiform (NC) fusion in conjunction with total ankle replacement to correct the forefoot position and offload the NC joint.

- The AP view will show if the translation is at the TN joint.
- If needed, three-dimensional imaging may be required. This will almost certainly be required if arthritis is present. The imaging will allow the midfoot to be more clearly seen than on plain radiographs. AP and lateral views of the ankle will also be needed to rule out injury to the deltoid ligament (**Fig. 21.2**).

21.1.3 Nonoperative Options

- Custom rigid orthotic inserts.
- Rigid soled shoes (full-length carbon fiber or steel shank).

- Rocker-bottom soled shoes.
- Ankle foot orthosis.
- Combined orthotic and double upright brace.

21.1.4 Contraindications

- Inadequate circulation.
- Active infection at the surgical site.
- Poor local soft-tissue envelope.
- Severe osteoporosis preventing adequate fixation and healing of fusion.

21.2 Goals of Surgical Procedure

- Reconstruction of the medial longitudinal arch.
- Rigid stabilization of the navicular cuneiform joints.
- Rebalancing of the foot tripod creating a plantigrade foot.

21.3 Advantages of Surgical Procedure

- Ability to resect arthritis from the NC joint.
- Restabilization of the medial arch.
- Only sacrifices noncrucial anatomically stable joints.

21.4 Key Principles

- Exposure of the appropriate joint:
  - Anatomic deformity can make the NC joint easy to miss and cause inadvertent arthrotomy of the TN or TMT joints.
- Joint preparation:
  - Removal of any remaining arthritic cartilage.
  - Removal of sclerotic subchondral or necrotic bone to ensure adequate bleeding surfaces for fusion.
- Reduction and alignment of the joint to recreate normal foot anatomy and stable plantar grade foot for ambulation.
- Rigid compressive fixation of the joint to maximize fusion.

21.5 Operative Technique

21.5.1 Open Technique

Positioning

A popliteal block is administered. The patient is positioned on the table with the foot toward the bottom of the table. The ipsilateral hip is bumped up so that the foot points directly vertical. The concomitant lateral column lengthening in many of these patients will require the lateral foot to be exposed. A thigh tourniquet is preferable.

Exposure

The foot is approached through a dorsal incision centered over the NC joint. The tibialis anterior tendon is mobilized medially. The neurovascular bundle is typically mobilized laterally, but the lateral aspect of the NC joint may be accessed via a

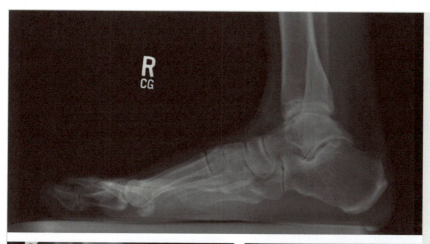
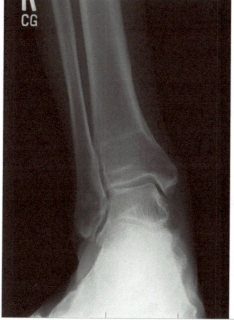
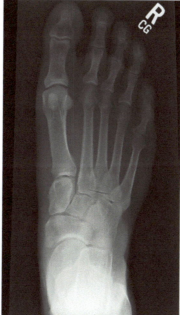

Fig. 21.2 Preoperative anteroposterior and lateral standing radiographs of a patient with a planovalgus foot.

soft-tissue window lateral to the neurovascular bundle if necessary. The NC joint is identified and exposed via sharp subperiosteal dissection (**Fig. 21.3**).

Care is taken to ensure that the correct joint is exposed. There is a possibility that the TN joint is exposed inadvertently. The TN joint can be identified by palpation because it will be proximal to the tuberosity of the navicular as opposed to distal. The plane of motion of both joints is different with the TN joint moving in a transverse plane and the NC joint, if any motion exists, will be in a dorsiflexion plantar flexion direction.

The intercuneiform joint between the medial and intermediate cuneiforms can also be inadvertently dissected. This should be avoided given that it may compromise the blood supply of the medial cuneiform, particularly if the NC joint and TMT joints are fused. Finally, the TMT joints should not be exposed inadvertently. The anatomy of these is quite different and the surgeon should be aware of the difference. If there is any doubt, then the C-arm can be used to confirm the level of the fusion.

The NC joint is then prepared using a combination of a curved osteotome and curettes to remove all cartilage till subchondral bone is visible. The subchondral plate is then perforated with a 1.6-mm K-wire (Kirschner wire). The cuneiform is then plantarflexed and compressed on the navicular to achieve correction of the deformity.

The plantar cartilage can be hard to remove with the open technique. The joint can be better visualized once all three joints have been exposed and released. A small curette (OOO) can be placed between the medial cuneiform and the navicular. This will open the joint and can be used to carefully release the plantar capsule. The curette can be used to keep the joint open, while a 5-mm curved osteotome is used to remove the cartilage (**Fig. 21.4**).

Care should also be taken to remove all cartilage from all three joints. The lateral side of the lateral joint can be challenging to reach. All cartilage is then removed using a pituitary rongeur. The cartilage fragments can release factors preventing neovascularization and migration of osteoblasts. Cartilage therefore works against the factors released by the bone graft or bone graft substitute.

Reduction of the Joint

Once debrided, the joint is held reduced. Correction of the NC joint is often required, and usually into plantar flexion. Temporary fixation is achieved with a 1.6-mm K-wire.

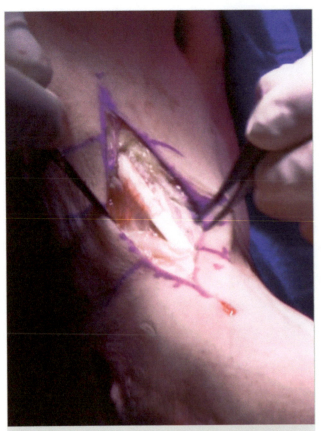

The forefoot is inspected and correction reviewed. The medial three metatarsals should all be correctly oriented to each other, with the first slightly more plantar than the second and third (**Fig. 21.5**).

If there is instability of the first ray and the reduction is compromised, then first TMT fusion should be considered at this point. First TMT fusion should be expected if there is a hallux valgus deformity and should be part of the consent.

The joint is correctly reduced if the forefoot is perpendicular to the tibial axis with the knee bent at 90 degrees and the ankle at neutral. The forefoot position is also checked for internal and external rotation. Some correction can be achieved at the NC joint. If it cannot be corrected, then a lateral column lengthening or TN joint release may be required. In severe deformities, this should be anticipated and be part of the consent.

Screw Position

Once reduction is achieved, the screws are placed. Two to three screws should be placed across each joint. The NC joint should be considered as three joints because any one joint can go on to nonunion in isolation. The medial cuneiform to navicular can be transfixed first. A lag screw technique can be used. The 3.5-mm drill is placed first, followed by a 2.5-mm drill. The drill hole starts on the dorsal medial side of the cuneiform and is placed down toward the plantar and tuberosity portion of the navicular. A second drill bit can be placed alongside using X-ray and the screws are placed. These are usually in the 30- to 45-mm range (**Fig. 21.6**).

Fig. 21.3 Dorsal exposure, naviculocuneiform joint accessed lateral to extensor hallucis longus tendon.

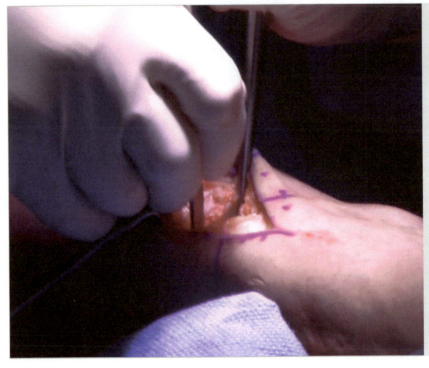

Fig. 21.4 Naviculocuneiform joint debridement.

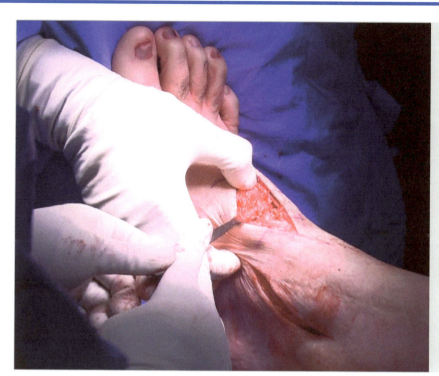

Fig. 21.5 Reduction maneuver.

A lag screw technique can also be used to fix the intermediate cuneiform. The screws are placed from the mid to distal dorsum of the intermediate cuneiform into the plantar midpoint of the navicular. The degree of correction of the alignment can also be increased slightly as the screws and drills are placed. These screws are usually in a 26- to 36-mm range. The lateral cuneiform to navicular screw may require dissection lateral to the neurovascular bundle. The nerve branch to the extensor digitorum brevis should not be damaged. The drill is placed from the midpoint of the cuneiform and needs to aim dorsal to hit the navicular. This screw is usually around 26-mm long.

Proximal to distal fixation can be achieved from the dorsal navicular and the navicular tuberosity. From the dorsal side, a 2.5-mm drill can be placed into the medial cuneiform around the distal to proximal screws. The screw will usually be around 40-mm long. The second screw starts just adjacent to the first on the dorsal navicular and goes into the intermediate cuneiform. This screw is usually 32 to 40 mm long. The final screw goes from the lateral navicular to the lateral cuneiform. This is usually 30 to 40 mm long. Some of the screws from the dorsal navicular can be doubled up in larger patients. From the tuberosity, a screw can be placed from proximal to distal and into the medial or intermediate cuneiform. The tuberosity can be exposed open or percutaneously (**Fig. 21.7**). Final C-arm views are obtained to ensure that all bones are immobilized and that no screws penetrate into the TN and TMT joints (**Fig. 21.8**).

Bone graft may be placed into the fusion site following fixation. This can be in the form of autogenous bone graft or bone graft substitutes.

21.5.2 Arthroscopic Technique

Positioning

The patient is positioned the same way as described in the open technique. The arthroscopy tower is placed toward the head of the bed on the opposite side to the surgical side. A thigh tourniquet is used because the compression of a calf tourniquet on the calf muscles will prevent the joint from being distracted open.

The arthroscopic fusion can be used for patients with either wound-healing issues or the potential to devascularize the navicular with an open fusion (**Fig. 21.9, Fig. 21.10**).

Instruments

A 2.4- or 2.9-mm arthroscope can be used. A 3.5-mm shaver will assist in visualization. The 4.5-mm burr with an auger can also be used. This will help remove debris. For a smaller patient, the smaller wrist instruments and shavers can be used.

Portals

To access the NC joint, the portals are placed each side of the joint on the dorsal medial and dorsal lateral side (**Fig. 21.11**). The joint is often quite mobile in the planovalgus foot so there is a reasonable amount of space on the dorsal side for access. The dorsalis pedis artery and deep branch of the peroneal nerve should be avoided in the dorsal midline. An accessory portal can be made from the plantar medial side. Because the TMT and NC

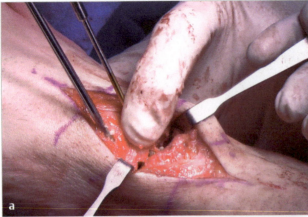

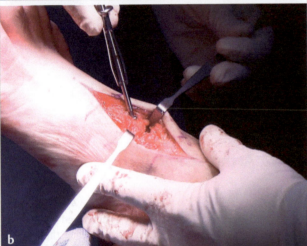

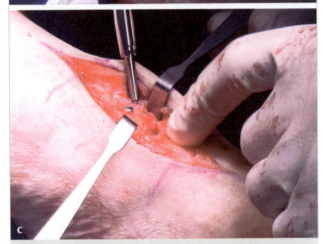

Fig. 21.6 (a) Fixation of the medial cuneiform to the navicular bone. (b) Fixation of the intermediate cuneiform to the navicular bone. (c) Fixation of the lateral cuneiform to the navicular bone.

joints are close, confirmation of access to the joint is advisable using imaging. The joint line is best palpated by identifying the TN joint via the tuberosity of the navicular. The NC joint is distal to this level (**Fig. 21.12**). The correct level can also be identified by the appearance of the joint. The two joint lines between the cuneiforms should be visible. Care should be taken not to drift

into these joints mistaking them for the NC joint. Equally, the NC joint should not be mistaken for the TN joint. Once the joint is correctly identified, more space can be created using a small curette (O, OO, or OOO) to release the capsule around the joint.

The burr is then used to sequentially remove the cartilage surface. Once the joint is debrided, it is held reduced. A percutaneous 1.6-mm K-wire can be placed and the forefoot position checked.

Screw Fixation

Screw fixation for an arthroscopic NC fusion is a little more challenging than an open fusion. Cannulated screws can be used, although they use up more space. For this reason, we prefer to use 3.5-mm solid screws placed percutaneously. Screw fixation should immobilize all three cuneiforms to the navicular. The joint should be considered as three joints, not one.

Two or three screws can be placed across the first cuneiform to navicular joint (**Fig. 21.13**). A dorsal stab wound is used and blunt dissection continued down onto the medial cuneiform lateral to the neurovascular bundle. A 2.5-mm drill is then placed distal to proximal from the medial cuneiform into the tuberosity zone of the navicular. This placement is then confirmed on C-arm views. From the C-arm, the space available next to the drill is assessed. A second drill bit is then placed parallel just medial, just lateral, just proximal, or just distal depending upon the access. If need be, a 3.5-mm drill hole is also used for compression of the first screw. The second drill bit, once positioned, is then used to measure length. A drill bit the same length can be placed on the bone and a depth gauge used to determine the difference, which is the same as the required screw length. The drill bit is removed and the screw is placed with the position indexed by the original drill bit being left in place.

On the medial side, a screw can also be placed from the tuberosity of the navicular down into the medial and intermediate cuneiforms. The tuberosity is palpated, and a percutaneous drill placed. The screw is placed in a similar manner as described earlier. Using a similar technique as used for the medial cuneiform, percutaneous wounds are made for the intermediate and lateral cuneiforms (**Fig. 21.14, Fig. 21.15**). The landmark for the intermediate is just lateral to the neurovascular bundle, and aiming from dorsal lateral to plantar medial. The lateral cuneiform is identified in a similar manner. Once the screws have been placed and the position confirmed (no placement into the TN joint or TMT joints), bone graft or bone graft substitute can be placed. Bone marrow aspirate may be easier to insert because cancellous graft will require an extended portal. Closure is with interrupted nylon and the patient placed in a below-the-knee walker boot.

21.6 Tips and Pearls

- Make sure that the cartilage is debrided to the plantar side of the medial cuneiform and over to the lateral side of the lateral cuneiform.
- Ensure that the cartilage and cartilage fragments are all removed to assist in fusion.

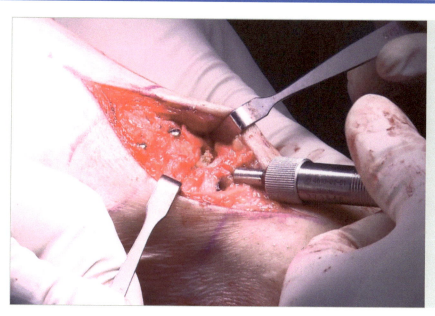

Fig. 21.7 Fixation from the navicular to the cuneiforms.

- If there is a dorsal gap, bone graft the defect.
- Ensure that the forefoot is correctly positioned before the placement of hardware.
- The correction can be improved by holding the navicular dorsal while holding the medial cuneiform plantar.
- Ensure that each of the three joints has at least two screws across the joint.

21.7 Hazards and Pitfalls

- Failure to achieve complete correction of the forefoot.
- Inadequate fixation resulting in failure of fusion.
- Penetration of the navicular cuneiform or TMT joints by the screws.

21.8 Complications/Bailout/Salvage

NC union rates in the literature range from 6 to 14%. More recently, Ajis and Geary in 2014 reported a union rate of 97% in a cohort of 33 NC fusions performed for symptomatic arthritis or deformity correction.[1] This is closer to the union rates of adjacent joints in the foot. It should be noted that the average time to union was 21.7 weeks, much longer than most joints in the foot.

Other complications related to open arthrodesis include delayed wound healing, infection, neurovascular injuries, complex regional pain syndrome, venous thromboembolic events, malunion, and adjacent joint arthritis. Most early complications can be avoided with careful patient selection, recognition of high-risk patients, careful dissection, and meticulous soft-tissue handling.

21.9 Postoperative Care

The patient is kept strictly non–weight-bearing for 6 weeks. A backslab is applied immediately after the surgery in the op-

erating room with care to ensure that the foot is in a planti-grade position. The wound is inspected and sutures removed at 2 weeks postsurgery. The patient is then placed in an air-cast boot but kept non–weight-bearing for another month. At 6 weeks, a weight-bearing radiograph is performed to assess alignment and interval fusion. A further 6 weeks in the aircast boot ensues, with progressive weight-bearing allowed under guidance of a physiotherapist. At 3 months, another set of interval radiographs is obtained. Provided it shows good interval union, the patient is weaned off the aircast boot and allowed full weight-bearing as tolerated (**Figs. 21.16, 21.17**).

21.10 Outcomes

Few publications exist on the NC fusion. A review of our billings show that we have performed 495 NC fusions. When we reviewed the revision rate for nonunion, we identified three revisions out of 265 fusions performed in a paper presented at the AOFAS meeting in 2013.[2] Ajis and Geary published a series of 33 NC fusions that were performed for deformity correction and symptomatic arthritis. Mean time to union was 21.7 ± 2 weeks. There was one case of nonunion requiring revision surgery, indicating a fairly high union rate of 97%. There were two superficial wound infections that were successfully treated with oral antibiotics. Time to union of approximately 5 months appears to be longer than other foot joints, but overall it appears to be a safe and reliable procedure.[1]

A case report exists using the NC fusion to successfully treat a fracture nonunion of the navicular bone using a locked plating system.[3] There is a report on the use of the NC fusion to treat acute NC dislocations. The authors report two cases of NC dislocations with damage to the medial facet of the distal navicular articular surface, separation of first and second cuneiforms, and an unstable first ray. NC fusion in conjunction with an intercuneiform fusion was performed with good results.[4] The fusion may be required to treat naviculo–first cuneiform coalition, a rare form of tarsal coalition.[2]

NC fusion can be combined with triple arthrodesis to treat Müller–Weiss disease that usually traverses both TN and NC

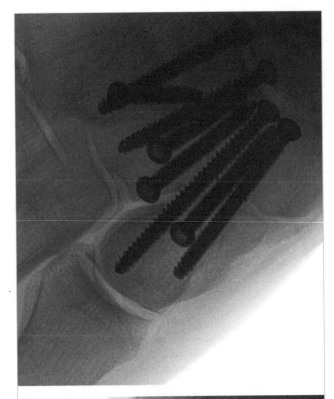

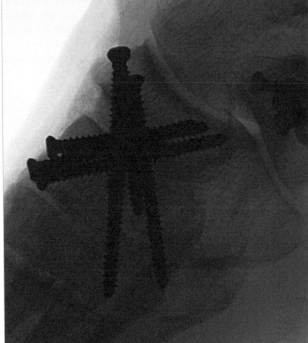

Fig. 21.8 Intra-op C-arm imaging (anteroposterior and lateral) following fixation of naviculocuneiform joint.

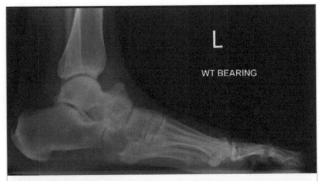

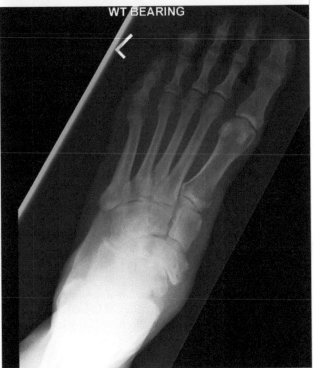

Fig. 21.9 X-rays of a patient undergoing a combined naviculocuneiform (NC) and triple arthrodesis for a fractured navicular with talonavicular and NC joint arthritis.

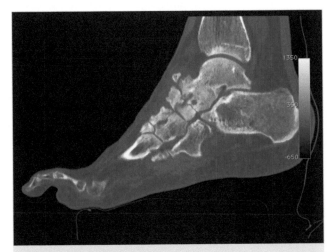

Fig. 21.10 Sagittal CT view of the same patient.

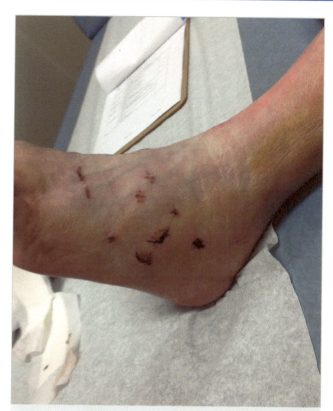

Fig. 21.11 Views of the portals used in an arthroscopic naviculo-cuneiform and triple fusion.

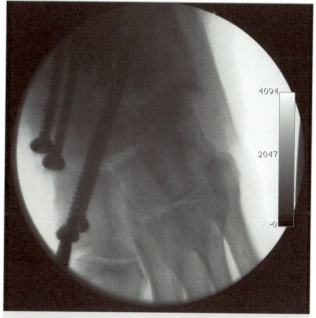

Fig. 21.13 Percutaneous placement of the medial cuneiform screws.

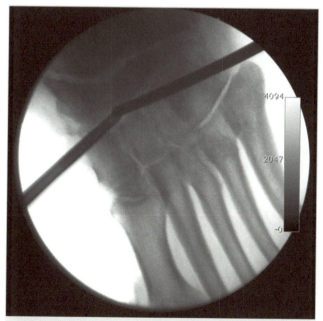

Fig. 21.12 Confirmation of placement of the scope and shaver into the navicular cuneiform joint.

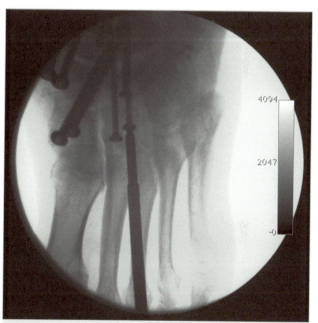

Fig. 21.14 Placement of the middle cuneiform screws.

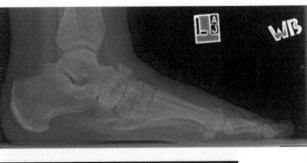

Fig. 21.15 Position of the percutaneous placement of the lateral cuneiform screws after insertion of the lateral cuneiform screws.

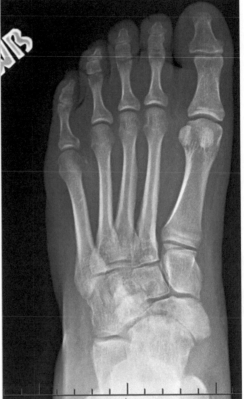

Fig. 21.16 Another case: a patient with diabetes and a Charcot fracture of the navicular.

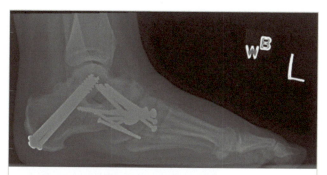

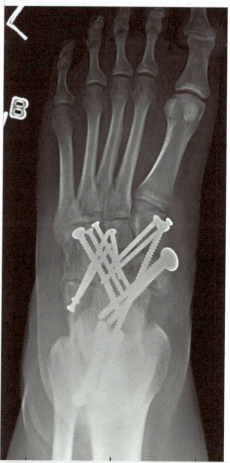

Fig. 21.17 Postoperative: with early healing of the triple and naviculocuneiform joints.

joints. A study by Chi et al[5] in 1999 outlined the use of NC fusion in combination with lateral column lengthening to correct flat foot deformity. Another author used an NC fusion after excision of a schwannoma and we have performed NC fusion after excision of plantar midfoot pigmented villonodular synovitis.

The very first reports in the literature on NC fusion was as early as 1927, when Miller[6] described this procedure for treatment of symptomatic flat feet in older children and adolescents. Subsequent reports in the late 1950s and 1960s reported on their outcomes.

References

1. Ajis A, Geary N. Surgical technique, fusion rates, and planovalgus foot deformity correction with naviculocuneiform fusion. Foot Ankle Int 2014;35(3):232–237
2. Younger AS, Steeves M, Wing K, Penner M. Revision Rates for Nonunions after Foot and Ankle Fusions Maybe Decreasing in time: Experience within a Canadian Teaching Hospital Foot and Ankle Program. San Diego, CA: American Orthopaedic Foot and Ankle Society; 2013
3. Fujioka H, Nishikawa T, Kashiwa K, et al. Localized naviculocuneiform arthrodesis combined with osteosynthesis of fracture nonunion of the tarsal navicular bone using a locked plating system. J Orthop 2014;11(4):188–191
4. Byun SE, Lee HS, Ahn JY, Seo DK, Seo JH. Treatment of naviculo-first cuneiform coalition of the foot. Foot Ankle Int 2014;35(5):489–495
5. Chi TD, Toolan BC, Sangeorzan BJ, Hansen ST Jr. The lateral column lengthening and medial column stabilization procedures. Chin Orthop Relat Res 1999;365:81–90
6. Miller OL. A plastic flat foot operation. J Bone Joint Surg 1927;9:84–91

22 Subtalar Joint Fusion

Ben Hickey and Anthony M.N.S. Perera

Abstract

Subtalar fusion is a successful operation for patients with symptomatic degeneration of the subtalar joint. Open and arthroscopic approaches provide good union rates, consistently above 90% and the majority of patients experience significant improvements in pain and functional outcomes. Careful surgical technique is important to minimize wound complications and maximize chances of union. Attention to patient selection, joint preparation, alignment, and adequate compression is vital.

Keywords: *subtalar, arthrodesis, fusion*

22.1 Indications and Pathology

- Primary osteoarthritis isolated to the subtalar joint.
- Posttraumatic arthritis.
- Inflammatory arthropathy.
- Subtalar tarsal coalitions in adults.
- Failed nonoperative management.

22.1.1 Clinical Evaluation

- Patients complain of symptoms of pain in the sinus tarsi and distal to the fibula, typically this is worse on walking on uneven surfaces. With more advanced disease, pain will be present while walking on flat ground and also at rest.

- Clinical examination will reveal painful, restricted movement in the subtalar joint. Typically the tenderness is most apparent in the sinus tarsi.
- It is important to evaluate the coronal plane alignment of the midfoot and the forefoot, and in particular their relationship with the hindfoot. With increasing valgus deformity, there will be supination of the foot. If this is marked or if it is not passively correctable, it will need to be addressed at the same time as the subtalar fusion.
- Similarly assess for a contracture of the gastrocnemius in severe deformity. These biomechanical risk factors need to be addressed to minimize the risk of recurrence of the deformity.

22.1.2 Radiographic Evaluation

- Weight bearing radiographs of the ankle will usually demonstrate subtalar joint posterior facet arthritis, particularly on the lateral radiograph. Confirmation can be obtained with preoperative computed tomography (CT) scan or magnetic resonance imaging (MRI; see **Figs. 22.1**, **22.2**). This also enables assessment of the talonavicular joints and calcaneocuboid joints.
- If adjacent joints are painful or appear to be degenerate, it may be helpful to perform preoperative steroid and local anesthetic injection under ultrasound scan (USS)/CT guidance to confirm that the subtalar joint is symptomatic. Contrast is helpful as joints can frequently communicate, especially in late stages of disease (**Fig. 22.3**).

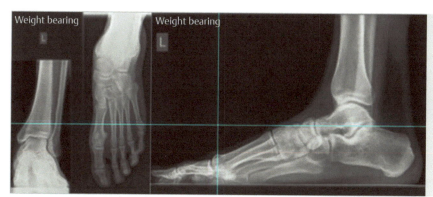

Fig. 22.1 Subtle radiographic signs of subtalar joint osteoarthritis. Note normal appearance of talonavicular and calcaneocuboid joints.

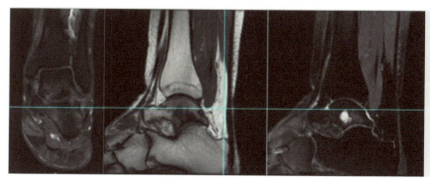

Fig. 22.2 MRI (magnetic resonance imaging) showing involvement of posterior and middle facets of subtalar joint.

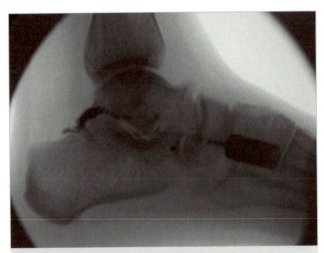

Fig. 22.3 Fluoroscopic guided injection of subtalar joint with local anesthetic and contrast.

22.1.3 Nonoperative Options

• UCBL (University of California at Berkeley Laboratory) inserts.
• Custom rigid ankle–foot orthosis (AFO) bracing (Arizona or molded ankle–foot orthosis [MAFO]).
• Intra-articular steroid injections.
• Anti-inflammatory medications.
• Activity modification.

22.1.4 Contraindications

• Infection: if there is a history of infection inflammatory markers, white cell scan and bone biopsies may be necessary.
• Forefoot supination: long-standing valgus can be associated with first ray elevation; if this is not correctable, then it may require middle column osteotomy or triple fusion instead.
• Smoking should be stopped; nonunion is more common than for some other fusions.

22.2 Goals of the Surgical Procedure

Our aim is to provide pain relief, by achieving a solid bony fusion, which we achieve in the majority of cases.

22.3 Advantages of the Surgical Procedure

22.3.1 Open Procedure

• Shorter learning curve than arthroscopic approach.
• Ability to correct defects or bone loss in the posterior facet with graft.
• Can be quicker.

22.3.2 Arthroscopic Fusion

• Smaller incision with less wound complications.
• Full visualization of the posterior facet.
• Visualization of the medial ST joint and middle facet.
• Easier deformity correction.

In the authors' opinion, the arthroscopic approach is preferable, particularly in the presence of severe deformity or where the lateral skin is poor/has had previous surgery.

22.4 Key Principles

• Remove all cartilage: use laminar spreaders to inch inward toward the medial side. You need to see the flexor hallucis longus (FHL) tendon moving to know that you have gotten to the medial extent.
• Avoid undercorrection of hindfoot deformity. Even in normal alignment, it is easy to take more bone off the lateral side than the medial side. It is very important to avoid this especially when there is a preoperative valgus deformity. In that case, it is necessary to take more of the medial side than the lateral and the middle facet can be a block to reduction.
• Feather the bone surfaces and achieve adequate compression with partially threaded screws, with entry point in calcaneus to try to avoid symptomatic hardware. Make sure all the threads cross the fusion site and in osteoporotic bone it may be helpful to not drill all the way in order to ensure the best hold possible in the talus.
• After correction and fixation, check the first ray and midfoot for supination and the gastrocnemius for contracture. These are risk factors for recurrence of deformity.

22.5 Operative Technique

22.5.1 Open Fusion

Setup and Positioning

The patient is supine in a semilateral position, achieved by placing a sandbag under the ipsilateral buttock. X-ray comes in from the same side.

Incision

A lateral sinus tarsi approach, from the tip of the fibula to the fourth tarsometatarsal joint (**Fig. 22.4**). Avoid fixed retraction of the skin with self-retainers; instead use assistant to retract intermittently with Langenbeck's retractors.

Surgical Procedure

Superficially identify extensor digitorum brevis and the sinus tarsi fat pad. It is important that some of the sinus tarsi fat pad is preserved. It may be easier visualization to re-

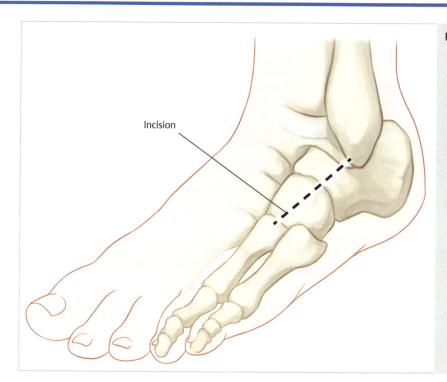

Fig. 22.4 Incision.

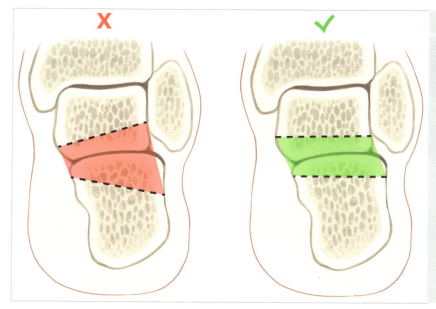

Fig. 22.5 Coronal sketch to show tendency to take too much bone laterally and create trapezoidal bone resection. Aim to create rectangular bony resection.

move it, but if it is completely removed it may result in skin devascularization and a dead space, which may compromise wound healing. Identify and protect the superficial peroneal nerve anteriorly.

The first landmark is to identify the lateral process of the talus; this is now removed using a sharp osteotome. Anteriorly the bifurcate and cervical ligaments can be cut; this will allow the joint to start to become mobile. These are tough structures that require release.

To expose the subtalar joint, place a Trethowan retractor under the peroneal tendons anteriorly and retract them posteriorly. Place a laminar spreader into the sinus tarsi and open this to expose the subtalar joint. Once this is identified, change the Trethowan retractor posteriorly for a second laminar spreader and place this at the level of the posterior facet. To prepare the

subtalar joint, it is important to use sharp osteotomes and remove the cartilage and hard subchondral bone.

It is critically important to realize that because you are starting to remove bone laterally and working medially, there is a tendency to remove more bone laterally, which will create a trapezoidal bone resection (Fig. 22.5). This should be avoided, in order to avoid placing the subtalar joint into excessive valgus. In order to achieve parallel bone removal, constantly adjust the position of the laminar spreaders, moving medially, and bear in mind the tendency to remove too much bone laterally in error.

The middle facet is a very deep structure that is never easy to see with an open approach. Beware of the FHL tendon, which is posterior to this and is a structure at risk of injury. A vision of this ensures a good clearance of medial bone and the medial extent of the joint has been reached. Prepare the bone surfaces using a fish-scale technique and a 2-mm drill. Then insert bone graft and ensure you pack this as far medial as possible. This sinus tarsi can also be grafted if required, but the bone will need to be prepared.

The next step is to reduce the joint prior to fixation with 2 × 6.5 mm partially threaded screws, which are inserted from the posterolateral aspect of the calcaneus, heading in a super-omedial direction in order to end in the central position of the talar body. The screws should diverge (**Fig. 22.6**). In order to achieve reduction of the subtalar joint, invert and supinate the foot while holding the ankle in dorsiflexion. Remember that the goal is to reduce the talus, which has subluxed medially, back onto the calcaneus. This requires significant force and may

seem an unusual position; however, we are yet to over-reduce one. Once the position is achieved, insert the screws.

It is important that the screw threads are engaged only in the talus in order to achieve compression and to not traverse the joint. In some situations, even after insertion of two screws, the talus may still try to rotate off the calcaneus if the bone is osteoporotic for instance. In this situation, one can pass a third (6.5 mm), extra-articular screw from the calcaneus, vertically/obliquely into the talar neck (**Fig. 22.7**). Caution must be taken when doing this due to risk of talar neck fracture, but we are yet to experience this.

Close the fat pad with Vicryl suture and skin with interrupted nylon 3.0. Take care to evert the skin edges to avoid wound complications.

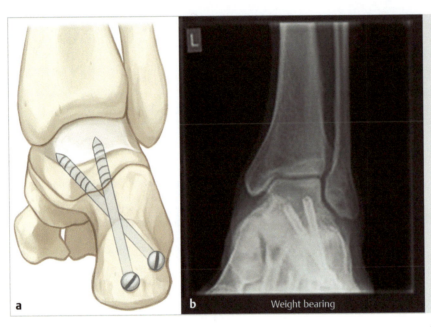

Fig. 22.6 (a) Illustration and **(b)** radiograph demonstrating divergence of partially threaded screws.

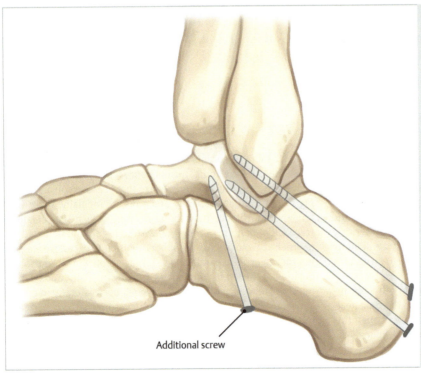

Additional screw

Fig. 22.7 Sketch to show additional screw that may be required if subtalar joint is still unstable after insertion of two screws.

22.5.2 Arthroscopic Subtalar Joint Fusion

Equipment

• 4.0-mm, 30-degree scope.
• Arthroscopic burrs.

Setup and Positioning

Semilateral position with sandbag under ipsilateral buttock as per open fusion.

Portals

Portal 1 is made via the peroneal sheath, 1.5 cm posterior and 1.5 cm proximal to the tip of the fibula. Portal 2 is made over the sinus tarsi.

Surgical Procedure

A 4.0-mm scope is inserted into the subtalar joint through portal 1 and the shaver is inserted into the sinus tarsi through portal 2. The fat is cleared, in order to visualize the lateral process. Next, switch the scope to portal 2 and the shaver to portal 1, which will give a full view of the lateral process of the talus. Debride the lateral process of the talus to gain access to the posterior facet and use a curette to remove cartilage. Work from lateral to medial. Identify FHL medially and follow this anteriorly onto the middle facet and the anterior facet. Pass a small osteotome to achieve fish-scaling preparation of the joint surfaces. Once the joints are prepared, reduce the subtalar joint and fix with 6.5-mm screws as per open fusion.

22.6 Tips and Pearls

• Screw starting point should be posterolateral, heading to a superomedial position in the talus.
• If the subtalar joint is still unstable with two screws, consider placing a third screw anteriorly, heading across the sinus tarsi vertically into the talar neck.

22.7 Hazards and Pitfalls

• Avoid removing the entire fat pad from the sinus tarsi; this will risk wound complications.
• Avoid making trapezoidal joint preparation with more bone removed from the lateral side than the medial side; this is an easy trap to fall into when starting out.
• Avoid malreduction; supinate and invert the foot with the ankle plantarflexed and then dorsiflex in order to lock this position.

22.8 Complications/Bailout/Salvage

• Infection.
• Neurovascular injury.
• Nonunion.
• Fibrous union; may be asymptomatic. May require revision.
• Progression of adjacent joint symptoms/disease.
• Prominent metalwork causing symptoms may require removal.
• Symptoms from bone graft harvest site (if necessary).

22.9 Postoperative Care

All patients should be non–weight-bearing for 2 weeks, and start weight-bearing in cast as comfort allows at between 2 and 6 weeks postoperative. At week 6, we remove the cast and apply a boot. CT scan is the only way to confirm successful union (**Figs. 22.8–22.10**).

22.10 Outcomes

In a recent systematic review of subtalar arthrodesis, nonunion occurred in 14% of 953 cases (range: 2–46%).[1] For open procedures, Dahm and Kitaoka reported fusion in 96% of 25 patients at a mean follow-up of 4 years.[2] Easley et al reported similar rates of union (92%), but found that smokers had a significantly higher rate of nonunion (27%).[3] Patients who have previously had ankle fusion have even higher rates of nonunion (39%).[4]

For patients who undergo arthroscopic subtalar fusion, union rates are consistently above 90%. In a series of 37 patients

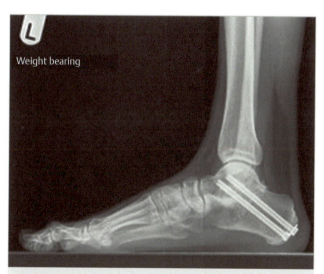

Fig. 22.8 Postoperative weight-bearing radiograph showing position of screws.

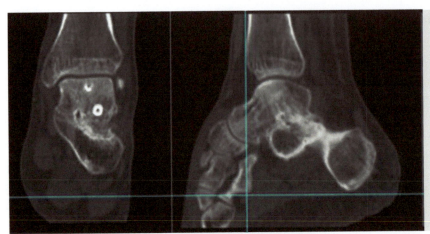

Fig. 22.9 CT scan confirming middle facet fusion.

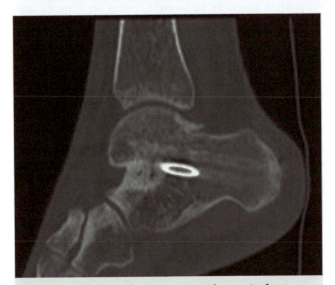

Fig. 22.10 CT scan confirming extra-articular anterior facet fusion.

In view that undercorrection of hindfoot deformity occurs in almost a quarter of patients,[1] intraoperative fluoroscopic imaging has been advocated to reduce the chance of malalignment. Hentges et al have suggested intraoperative fluoroscopic axial imaging, with the aim to achieve parallel tibial mid-diaphyseal and calcaneal bisector lines. In order to minimize malalignment of the ground reaction forced through the ankle joint, it is advocated that the calcaneus should be translated medially so the weight-bearing axis of the calcaneus and tibia are collinear.[8]

After surgery, it can be anticipated that there will be a reduction in transverse tarsal motion, dorsiflexion, and plantar flexion by 40, 30, and 9%, respectively.[9] Some patients will develop radiographic adjacent joint arthrosis of talonavicular and ankle joints, which may become symptomatic.[2]

with posttraumatic arthritis who underwent arthroscopic subtalar fusion, union rates of over 95% were reported.[5] Rungprai et al achieved union in 94.2% of patients at mean follow-up of 22.7 months (±22.4).[6]

Both arthroscopic and open subtalar fusion techniques result in significant improvements in pain and functional outcome.[6] After open subtalar fusion, over 80% of patients are very satisfied with the outcome.[7] Approximately 80% of patients report no pain or mild pain and over 70% report excellent or good American Orthopaedic Foot and Ankle Society (AOFAS) scores at fusion.[2] In a series of 184 feet at average, who underwent open subtalar fusion, AOFAS scores improved from 24 preoperatively to 70 at follow-up of 51 months (24–130).[3] For those who undergo arthroscopic subtalar fusion, results are similar. In a series of 64 patients who underwent arthroscopic subtalar fusion, mean improvement of visual analogue scale (VAS) for pain was 5.1 (±2.2).[6] AOFAS scores improve by an average of 27 points (±9.1).[5]

Worse outcomes are expected in those who develop nonunion or reflex sympathetic dystrophy.[2] In approximately 14% of patients (range 10–32%), screws will be symptomatic and require removal.[1,7] Approximately 10% will experience lateral impingement and 3% will experience an infection.[3]

References

1. Tuijthof GJ, Beimers L, Kerkhoffs GM, Dankelman J, Dijk CN. Overview of subtalar arthrodesis techniques: options, pitfalls and solutions. Foot Ankle Surg 2010;16(3):107–116
2. Dahm DL, Kitaoka HB. Subtalar arthrodesis with internal compression for post-traumatic arthritis. J Bone Joint Surg Br 1998;80(1):134–138
3. Easley ME, Trnka HJ, Schon LC, Myerson MS. Isolated subtalar arthrodesis. J Bone Joint Surg Am 2000;82(5):613–624
4. Zanolli DH, Nunley JA II, Easley ME. Subtalar fusion rate in patients with previous ipsilateral ankle arthrodesis. Foot Ankle Int 2015;36(9):1025–1028
5. Vilá y Rico J, Jiménez Díaz V, Bravo Giménez B, Mellado Romero MÁ, Ojeda Thies C. Results of arthroscopic subtalar arthrodesis for adult-acquired flatfoot deformity vs post-traumatic arthritis. Foot Ankle Int 2016;37(2):198–204
6. Rungprai C, Phisitkul P, Femino JE, Martin KD, Saltzman CL, Amendola A. Outcomes and complications after open versus posterior arthroscopic subtalar arthrodesis in 121 patients. J Bone Joint Surg Am 2016;98(8):636–646
7. Diezi C, Favre P, Vienne P. Primary isolated subtalar arthrodesis: outcome after 2 to 5 years followup. Foot Ankle Int 2008;29(12):1195–1202
8. Hentges MJ, Gesheff MG, Lamm BM. Realignment subtalar joint arthrodesis. J Foot Ankle Surg 2016;55(1):16–21
9. Mann RA, Beaman DN, Horton GA. Isolated subtalar arthrodesis. Foot Ankle Int 1998;19(8):511–519

23 Triple Arthrodesis

W. Hodges Davis

Abstract

The triple arthrodesis includes fusion of the subtalar, talonavicular, and calcaneocuboid joints to address hindfoot deformity and arthritis. It is crucial to fuse the joints in an anatomic alignment to rebalance the tripod effect of the foot and prevent deformity and pain at adjacent joints, particularly the ankle joint. In many cases, the calcaneocuboid joint can be spared from inclusion in the fusion (double arthrodesis) obtaining similar correctability of the deformity while maintaining more flexibility of the lateral column of the foot. This chapter outlines the indication, advantages, and the surgical technique focusing on the tricks to obtaining the most optimal outcome.

Keywords: *triple, double, pes planovalgus, hindfoot arthritis*

23.1 Indications

- Degenerative flatfoot (stage 3 adult acquired flatfoot).
- Posttraumatic hindfoot disease.
- Rheumatoid/autoimmune hindfoot disease.
- Charcot's hindfoot dislocation.
- Spastic hindfoot instability.

23.1.1 Clinical Evaluation

- Stiff hindfoot in gait and manual testing.
- Tender and painful in sinus tarsi, subfibular area, and transverse tarsal joints.
- Varus/valgus collapse on standing exam.
- Most often tight Achilles complex.

23.1.2 Radiographic Evaluation

- Flatfoot series (standing anteroposterior [AP]/lateral of both feet, standing AP/mortise of both ankles; **Fig. 23.1a,b**).
- Axial alignment view.

- Computed tomographic (CT) scan if concerned about the involvement of the calcaneal cuboid joint and bone stock for the fusion.
- Magnetic resonance imaging (MRI) if concerned with talar or navicular vascularity.
- MRI to confirm degenerative changes in flatfoot deformity unclear on radiographs.
- Fluoroscopically directed selective injections can be helpful to only fuse the joints that are causing the pain.

23.1.3 Nonoperative Options

- Brace (soft hindfoot ankle brace up to a rigid ankle–foot orthosis [AFO] or an Arizona brace).
- Repetitive injections.

23.1.4 Contraindications

- Active infection.
- Dysvascular limb.

23.2 Goals of Surgical Procedure

- Realignment of the hindfoot in relation to the rest of the lower extremity.
- Realign the forefoot to the hindfoot (correct residual forefoot varus and valgus).
- Fuse affected/painful joints.

23.3 Advantages of Surgical Procedure

- Creation of a stable plantar grade hindfoot.
- Realigns the foot under the ankle.
- Can address massive deformities.

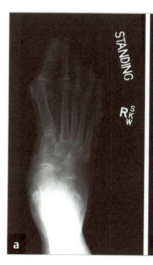 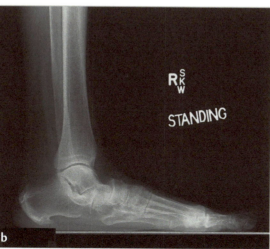

Fig. 23.1 **(a)** Standing anteroposterior view of the foot. Valgus collapse shows the lateral peritalar subluxation of the talonavicular (TN) joint. **(b)** Standing lateral view of the foot shows collapse at the TN joint.

- Reliable and reproducible results.
- Disadvantages:
  - The patient loses the ability for foot to accommodate uneven surfaces.
  - Stress on the joints adjacent to the fusion (ankle and navicular cuneiform most common) can result in degeneration in those joints.
  - Potential for nonunion.

23.3.1 Triple versus Double Arthrodesis

We have evolved to more double arthrodesis (subtalar [ST] and talonavicular [TN] joints) and then true triples (including the calcaneocuboid [CC] joint) in the last 10 years. The reasoning is that we are only fusing the joints that need to be fused. This ends up being less surgery for the patients. The troublesome healing of the lateral incision becomes less of an issue with large corrections from planovalgus deformities. In addition, the lateral column maintains more flexibility if the CC joint is left alone. If the CC joint is symptomatic preoperatively, it can be addressed without changing the approach. We have also trended away from the "medial double" (fusing TN and ST through and extensile medial approach). Concern with the deltoid release required with this approach resulting in some cases of talar AVN (avascular necrosis) and valgus collapse has tempered our enthusiasm for the all medial approach.

23.4 Key Principles

- Soft-tissue contracture releases.
- Exposure and removal of blocking bony prominences.
- Removal of chondral surfaces of joints to fuse.
- Preparation of those joints.
- Graft defects.
- Correct all deformities.
- Rigid compressive fixation.
- Radiographic confirmation.
- Layered closure.

23.5 Preoperative Preparation and Patient Positioning

- Place sandbag under operative hip. The tibial tubercle should point to the ceiling. This allows access to the lateral foot. If the limb is externally rotated, a larger bump or wedge may have to be used.
- Prep and expose the limb to the knee. This helps with alignment and gives access to the proximal tibia for bone graft.

23.6 Operative Technique

23.6.1 Soft-Tissue Contracture Release

The type of deformity determines the releases necessary. The Achilles tendon (AT) tends to be consistently tight in varus and valgus as well as neutral degenerative cases. In hindfoot fusions, we recommend an AT lengthening rather than a gastrocnemius recession. Make incisions over the center of the AT. Make the

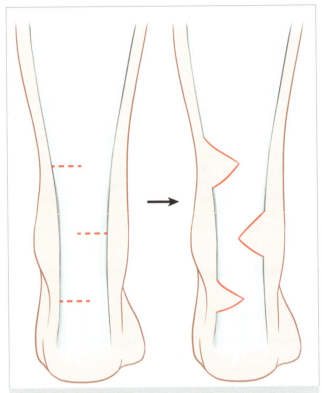

Fig. 23.2 Drawing showing the incisions and the Achilles hemisection using the Hoke technique.

three incisions: (1) distal just above the insertion, (2) proximal just distal to the musculotendinous junction of the muscle and the tendon, and (3) the middle equidistant from the distal and proximal (**Fig. 23.2**). Use a no. 15 blade. Cut through the AT in line with the fibers, turn the blade in the direction you want to cut, and finish the hemisection with a move toward the skin. The ankle should be held in maximum dorsiflexion to tension the AT while doing the hemisections. If the deformity is valgus, the cuts should be made lateral, medial, then lateral (distal to proximal), and if it is varus or neutral, the cuts should be made medial, lateral, and then medial. If the hemisections are complete and dorsiflexion tension is adequate, there will be a give and the dorsiflexion in the ankle will be restored. The posterior tibialis (PT) tendon is tight in varus and can be released through the TN approach. The peroneus brevis (PB) tendon is often tight in valgus and can be released or lengthened through the lateral incision.

23.6.2 Joint Exposure and Preparation

ST joint. For the double fusion, this joint can be exposed through a mini-approach that cuts down postoperative wound healing issue. The incision is made from the tip of the fibula and extends distal toward the fourth metatarsal base (**Fig. 23.3**). In most cases, the extensor digitorum brevis (EDB) muscle is present once through the fatty subcutaneous tissue (**Fig. 23.4**). Spend time saving the fascia on the EBD as it makes the closure more secure. If the muscle is large, it can split along the line of the skin incision and this exposes the sinus tarsi. If normal contours, the EDB can be elevated beginning on the plantar edge

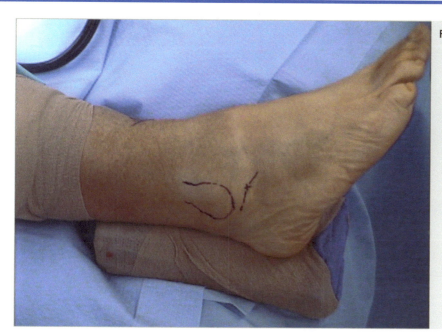

Fig. 23.3 Incision for the lateral incision.

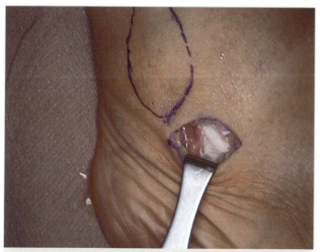

Fig. 23.4 The inferior edge of the extensor digitorum brevis muscle and the peroneal tendons are exposed.

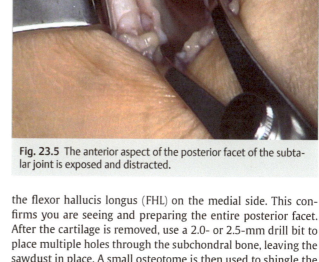

Fig. 23.5 The anterior aspect of the posterior facet of the subtalar joint is exposed and distracted.

just dorsal to the PB tendon. A corner of the muscle fascia can be created in the proximal portion of the incision to gain more exposure. The PB tendon can be released or lengthened from this exposure at any time if needed. The contents of the sinus tarsi can be removed sharply and with a rongeur. The anterior lateral edge of the posterior facet of the ST joint is accessible (**Fig. 23.5**). All of the periarticular osteophytes can be removed now. This allows distraction of the joint, first with an osteotome and when motion is gained by using a lamina spreader or a pin-based distractor. The cartilage is peeled off the bone (talus and calcaneus) with sharp osteotomes and curettes (**Fig. 23.6**). The goal is to maintain the joint contours to allow for easier reduction and deformity correction. In the ST joint, one must be careful to remove all of the cartilage, in particular on the far side (medial) talus as the joint curves away from the incision. You have not completed the joint preparation until you can see

the flexor hallucis longus (FHL) on the medial side. This confirms you are seeing and preparing the entire posterior facet. After the cartilage is removed, use a 2.0- or 2.5-mm drill bit to place multiple holes through the subchondral bone, leaving the sawdust in place. A small osteotome is then used to shingle the remaining subchondral bone to create a broad bleeding surface for the fusion (**Fig. 23.7**).

TN joint. For this joint, a second incision is made just medial to the distal anterior tibialis (AT) tendon, extending proximally from just distal to the anterior aspect of the medial malleolus and distally to the navicular cuneiform joint (**Fig. 23.8**). Once through the skin and subcuticular fat, the TN joint capsule is exposed. The capsule is split and the TN joint is exposed (**Fig. 23.9**). The joint is distracted with a pin-based distractor. The cartilage is removed in the identical way the ST joint was prepared (**Fig. 23.10**).

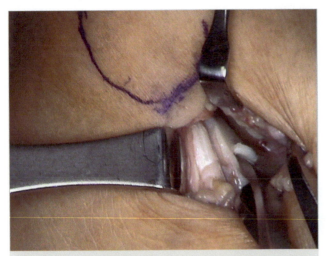

Fig. 23.6 The cartilage is removed with osteotomes and curettes while maintaining joint contours.

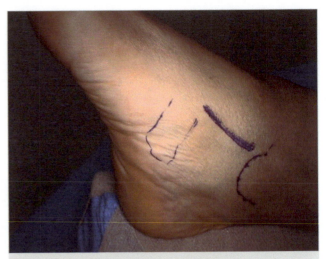

Fig. 23.8 Medial incision for talonavicular joint exposure.

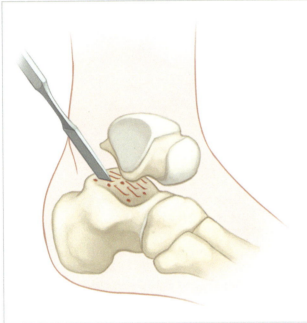

Fig. 23.7 Drawing showing preparation of the bone for fusion.

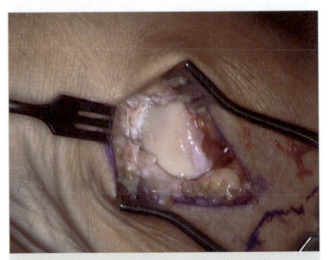

Fig. 23.9 Full thickness incision through the talonavicular capsule.

23.6.3 Graft the Fusion Sites

To maximize the chance of fusion, the joint surfaces should be augmented with some kind of grafting material. Choices for autograft are iliac crest and proximal tibia. If autograft cannot be used, there are a number of commercially available bone graft products that also have been shown to work to augment the fusion sites safely.

23.6.4 Correct the Deformities

The next step is to create a plantar grade foot by restoring more normal hindfoot architecture. If the joint surfaces were taken down in a manner that maintained the joint contours and the deforming soft-tissue barriers have been eliminated, the deformity can be corrected in a sequential manner. The first manipulation is to reduce the TN joint. In valgus, the talus is subluxed medial and the navicular is shifted laterally with the rest of the foot (**Fig. 23.11**). The navicular is easily rotated medial to cover the talar head. The ST joint will most often reduce out of valgus at the same time. The TN will also need to be rotated to bring the medial column down (to correct the forefoot varus). In valgus deformity, one will hold the TN reduction with temporary wire fixation and assess the calcaneus position. At this point, an on-table hindfoot alignment view helps confirm reduction and confirm the fibula is decompressed. In varus, the navicular will be swung laterally on the talar head. The ST joint reduction will also follow in most cases. If the heel does not swing into valgus, a lateral column shortening can be done through a CC joint fusion.

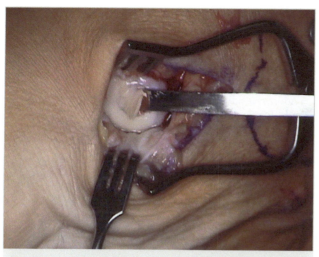

Fig. 23.10 Cartilage removal maintaining the joint contours.

23.6.5 Rigid Compressive Fixation with Radiographic Confirmation

Fusion of these joints requires more than one point of fixation, one to compress and the other to prevent rotation at the fusion site. The ST joint is secured first. The fixation of choice is one short threaded compression screw from the posterior heel into the anterior central talus. The second screw is fully threaded and is placed superior and posterior to the first into the center of the talar body (across the posterior facet of the ST joint). It is important to check a fluoroscopic lateral and axial of the foot and a mortise of the ankle to assure proper screw position. The TN joint can be fixed with a compression screw from the medial navicular into the talar neck and body. An attempt should be made to keep this screw in the plantar half of the talar head. Once the screw is in place, a compression plate with at least two screws on each side of the joint can be used. An anteroposterior (AP) and lateral X-ray of the foot can confirm the hardware placement (**Fig. 23.12a, b**).

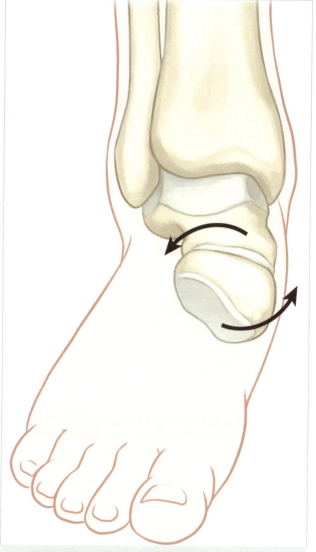

Fig. 23.11 Drawing showing the talonavicular and subtalar joints being reduced from valgus.

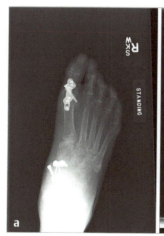
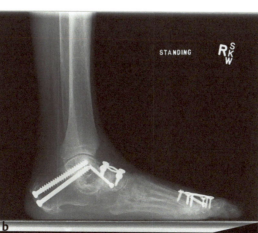

Fig. 23.12 (a) Anteroposterior view of the foot showing the fixation and the deformity reduction. (b) Lateral view of the foot showing the fixation and correction of the talonavicular collapse.

23.6.6 Layered Closure

The closure is simple and consistent. The lateral wound closure starts by repairing the EDB muscle to its bed. The edges can be tacked down with an absorbable interrupted stitch. The subcuticular layer is closed with the same absorbable stich and the skin with nylon suture. The TN incision is closed with only the subcuticular and the nylon. Rarely is the capsule able to be repaired. A soft sterile dressing with a rigid below-knee plaster splint is used as the initial postoperative dressing.

23.7 Tips and Pearls

- You must have full exposure of the joints in order to complete joint preparation.
- Preoperative planning is important to correct all pertinent deformities.
- Poor joint preparation bodes poorly for success.
- Leaving deformity undercorrected leads to worst function than preoperatively (must avoid fusion malunion).
- Careful full-thickness exposure can prevent wound complications.
- Grafting of the fusion sites can improve fusion rates.

23.8 Hazards and Pitfalls

- The CC joint should be evaluated preoperatively for arthritic changes; if present, this joint should be denuded and included in the fusion.
- The cuboid tends to drop plantarly in the severe flatfoot. This needs to be elevated dorsally in line with the calcaneus if this joint is included in the fusion.
- In severe chronic planovalgus deformities, correction can be difficult through the lateral incision. The PB (antagonist to the posterior tibial tendon [PTT] and major valgus deforming force) should be released through a longitudinal incision behind the fibular before approaching the ST joint to make the correction easier.
- The TN joint is the most common to develop a nonunion. Ensure adequate exposure of both the medial and the lateral aspects of the joint to ensure that any remaining cartilage is removed and bleeding bone exposed for the fusion.

23.9 Complications/Bailout/ Salvage

- Postoperative wound breakdown:
  - Early intervention with wound care and/or negative pressure wound management.
  - If deep infection can remove fixation and convert to small wire circular fixation for salvage.

- Nonunion:
  - The TN joint is most often involved.
  - Early CT scan can allow early intervention with earlier revision surgery, if needed, before collapse.
- Fusion malunion:
  - Difficult salvage.
  - Address residual deformities with osteotomies and revision fusion.

23.10 Postoperative Care

- Splint for 2 weeks.
- Cast non–weight-bearing for 4 weeks.
- Tall walker boot full–weight-bearing for 4 to 6 weeks.
- CT scan at 12 weeks to confirm fusion (**Fig. 23.13**).
- Therapy for gait training and edema control when confirmed fused.

23.11 Outcomes

The reason to resort to a fusion is for pain control and deformity correction. After the double fusion, the pain that arose from the hindfoot should be resolved. In addition, the deformity correction should be such that the foot should be plantar grade and aligned with the rest of the lower extremity. The fusion rate with this technique is near 90% and other complications (wound, infection, malunion) are rare. While the foot will be stiff, it is very stable.

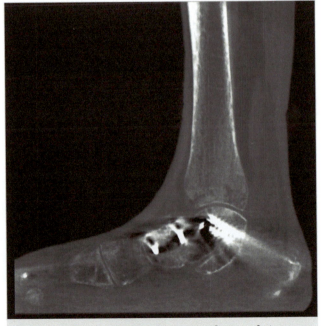

Fig. 23.13 CT scan at 12 weeks post-op confirming a fusion.

References

1. Anand P, Nunley JA, DeOrio JK. Single-incision medial approach for double arthrodesis of hindfoot in posterior tibialis tendon dysfunction. Foot Ankle Int 2013;34(3):338–344

2. Baumhauer JF, Pinzur MS, Daniels TR, et al. Survey on the need for bone graft in foot and ankle fusion surgery. Foot Ankle Int 2013;34(12):1629–1633

3. Brilhault J. Single medial approach to modified double arthrodesis in rigid flatfoot with lateral deficient skin. Foot Ankle Int 2009;30(1):21–26

4. Coughlin MJ, Grimes JS, Traughber PD, Jones CP. Comparison of radiographs and CT scans in the prospective evaluation of the fusion of hindfoot arthrodesis. Foot Ankle Int 2006;27(10):780–787

5. Moore BE, Wingert NC, Irgit KS, Gaffney CJ, Cush GJ. Single-incision lateral approach for triple arthrodesis. Foot Ankle Int 2014;35(9):896–902

6. Pell RF IV, Myerson MS, Schon LC. Clinical outcome after primary triple arthrodesis. J Bone Joint Surg Am 2000;82(1):47–57

7. Raikin SM. Failure of triple arthrodesis. Foot Ankle Clin 2002;7(1):121–133

8. Saltzman CL, Fehrle MJ, Cooper RR, Spencer EC, Ponseti IV. Triple arthrodesis: twenty-five and forty-four-year average follow-up of the same patients. J Bone Joint Surg Am 1999;81(10):1391–1402

9. Sammarco VJ, Magur EG, Sammarco GJ, Bagwe MR. Arthrodesis of the subtalar and talonavicular joints for correction of symptomatic hindfoot malalignment. Foot Ankle Int 2006;27(9):661–666

24 Flexor Digitorum Longus Transfer for Posterior Tibial Tendon Dysfunction

Martin J. O'Malley

Abstract

The flexor digitorum longus (FDL) transfer is an integral part of the adult flatfoot reconstruction for posterior tibial tendon dysfunction (PTTD). The posterior tibialis tendon (PTT) acts as an arch supporter main invertor for push off during gait. As the PTT fails due to tearing and degeneration, the foot falls into a more planovalgus configuration. It is crucial to reestablish the equilibrium of the foot to maintain proper force distribution. The FDL tendon is the most viable substitute for the torn PTT given it is isometric to the PTT. The operation for PTTD has evolved from a simple transfer of the FDL for the torn posterior tendon (which often failed because the flatfoot was not addressed) to one step of a major hindfoot procedure. The practice now is to reconstruct the arch with a series of osteotomies (medial slide calcaneal osteotomy, lateral column lengthening, and cotton osteotomy) in conjunction with an FDL transfer on the medial side for the torn tendon. The rationale for this approach is twofold. First, the FDL tendon is much weaker than the PTT (relative power is 1.8 for FDL and 6.4 for PTT), and as a stand-alone procedure it cannot support a valgus hindfoot. Second, the disease is often not limited to just the tendon, but falls on a spectrum of peritalar subluxation (spring ligament, PTT, and deltoid ligament) and correction of the hindfoot valgus and forefoot abduction is crucial for the tendon transfer to work. The only time a tendon transfer should be considered a stand-alone procedure is for an acute PTT laceration and in the rare case of a torn tendon in a cavus foot.

Keywords: *FDL transfer, posterior tibial tendon dysfunction, adult-acquired flatfoot*

24.1 Indications and Pathology

- Posterior tibial tendon dysfunction (PTTD) has been well documented as a distinct pathological entity. The tendon is particularly susceptible to attritional tears in the medial malleolar, because of attritional blood supply and with the watershed area being 2 to 3 cm proximal to the medial malleolus and is often the site of rupture (**Fig. 24.1**).
- As the disease progresses, the peritalar subluxation occurs with progressive deterioration of the medial hindfoot structures (spring ligament, deltoid) and the foot falls into abduction and hindfoot valgus.
- Four stages of PTTD have been described; most cases requiring a tendon transfer are stage 2 (**Table 24.1**).

24.1.1 Clinical Evaluation

- A standard exam of the foot and ankle is performed with the patient seated as well as standing. Palpation of the medial ankle will reveal tenderness and swelling along the course of the PTT (**Fig. 24.2**). The ankle and hindfoot should be put through a full range of motion to determine if there are any

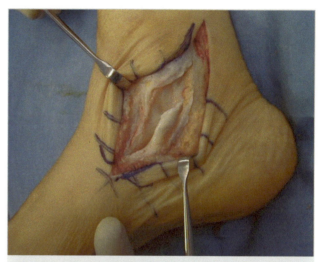

Fig. 24.1 Multiple longitudinal splits are seen in the inframalleolar region of this torn posterior tibial tendon.

Table 24.1 Stages of posterior tibial tendon dysfunction

Stage	Posterior tibial tendinopathy	Planovalgus foot description
1	Peritendinitis and/or degeneration	Minimal/No deformity
2	Tendon elongation	Minimal/No deformity
2b	Tendon elongation	Correctable deformity
3	Tendon elongation	Fixed planovalgus
4	Tendon elongation	Valgus tilt of talus within ankle with mortise with degenerative changes

fixed deformities. The patient is then examined as they stand. The amount of forefoot abduction and hindfoot valgus are determined and compared to the opposite side. The classic finding when viewing the heel from the rear is "too many toes sign" where you can see the fourth and fifth toes due to forefoot abduction (**Fig. 24.3**). The patient is asked to perform a single heel rise—inability to do so is pathognomonic for a ruptured PTT.

24.1.2 Radiographic Evaluation

- Preoperative magnetic resonance imaging (MRI) and standing X-rays of the foot and ankle are obtained for all patients undergoing flexor digitorum longus (FDL) transfer. A Saltzman rearfoot view is also obtained.
- X-rays are used to determine concomitant procedures, while the MRI is used to determine the status of the PTT and extent of the medial soft disease (spring ligament and deltoid).

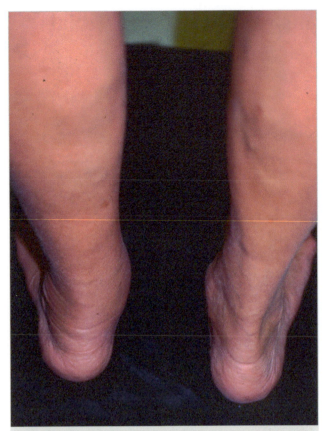

Fig. 24.2 Posterior view showing left medial ankle swelling due to posterior tibial tendon dysfunction.

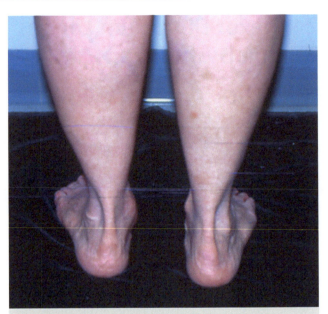

Fig. 24.3 Patient showing classic "too many toes sign" on left side due to posterior tibial tendon dysfunction.

- Weight-bearing cone computed tomography (CT) exams are becoming more commonly used to determine hindfoot position as well as lateral subluxation of the subtalar joint.

24.1.3 Nonoperative Options

- Rest, ice, and nonsteroidal anti-inflammatory medication are a first line.
- A cam walker boot is used for acute cases of tendinitis.
- An Arizona ankle–foot orthosis (AFO) or Richie brace is prescribed to control the hindfoot valgus.
- Steroid injections are almost never used given that they can cause rapid deterioration of the tendon. Platelet-rich plasma (PRP) injections will be used as an anti-inflammatory and possible regenerative therapy in conjunction with an Arizona type AFO for flexible cases early in the course of the disease.

24.1.4 Contraindications

- Stage 3 (fixed deformity) where the deformity is fixed and the foot requires a hindfoot arthrodesis or stage 4 as a stand-alone procedure.
- Relative conditions prohibiting the patient from undergoing FDL transfer are advanced age, obesity, and diabetes.
- Absolute contraindications prohibiting the patient from undergoing FDL transfer are Charcot's foot or vascular insufficiency.

24.2 Goals of Surgical Procedure

- Stable and pain-free plantigrade foot with inversion power. Additional goal are to produce a mobile (nonfused) hindfoot to lessen stress on the ankle.

24.3 Advantages of Surgical Procedure

- FDL is readily accessible in approaching the PTT as it lies directly behind the tendon in its own sheath.
- There is little function loss of toe flexion because of cross-connections between the FDL and flexor hallucis longus (FHL) in the midfoot.

24.3.1 Alternative Tendon Transfer Procedures

- FHL transfer: this tendon is much harder to harvest and results in weakness of the hallux and the tendon must be passed from posterior to anterior around the neurovascular bundle.
- Free tendon graft: allografts or autografts are not recommended because the disease is usually too extensive given the PTT with the segmental graft most likely will continue to degenerate.

24.4 Key Principles

- The FDL is fixed to the navicular through a drill hole from plantar to dorsal and fixed either by suturing back on itself or with interference screws or anchors, which should be available depending on surgeon's preference.

- Tension the FDL tendon in 15 degrees of plantar flexion and slight inversion but still able to get the ankle to neutral without the FDL transfer subluxing out of the posterior tibialis sheath.
- Medial calcaneal osteotomy, lateral column lengthening, or cotton osteotomies are performed prior to the tendon transfer.

24.5 Preoperative Planning and Patient Positioning

24.5.1 Anatomy

- The origin of the tibialis posterior is the lateral part of the posterior surface of the tibia, medial two-thirds of the fibula, interosseous membrane, intermuscular septa, and deep fascia.[1] The PTT runs in the deep posterior compartment, then crosses from lateral to medial beneath the tendon of the FDL and enters the foot immediately behind the medial malleolus.[2] It changes direction from vertical to horizontal posterior to the medial malleolus.[1] PTT splits before inserting on the navicular tuberosity. The anterior band inserts on the navicular, the medial band inserts on bones of the midfoot, and the posterior band inserts on calcaneus and cuboid.[3]
- The PTT is found just below the medial malleolus with the FDL tendon found behind the PTT and can easily be accessed through the PTT sheath (**Fig. 24.4**). Care must be taken to avoid the neurovascular bundle. The FDL is traced down past the master knot of Henry, where the FHL crosses, and is harvested deep in the midfoot to get enough length. The most difficult part of the harvest of the FDL is the vascular leash of vessels underneath the navicular, which must be cauterized to prevent excessive bleeding.

24.5.2 General

- Spinal or general anesthesia is used.
- A popliteal block will require heavy sedation because the popliteal block is not as effective along the medial ankle.

24.5.3 Positioning

- Patient is placed on a beanbag with the foot inverted for the lateral procedures (calcaneal osteotomy, lateral column) that are done first.
- The beanbag is deflated and removed (or hip rolled) to allow the foot to externally rotate to allow access to the medial foot.

24.6 Operative Technique

24.6.1 Surgical Approach

A medial incision extends along the course of the PTT. Depending on the degree of damage and amount of PTT that needs to be resected, the incision will begin either at the myotendinous junction 6 cm proximal to the medial malleolus or at the tip of the malleolus. The incision extends over the medial tubercle of the navicular and then curves plantarly and distally along the path of the FDL tendon toward the knot of Henry.

24.6.2 Surgical Procedure

The tendon sheath of the PTT is opened with iris scissors to inspect the tendon. Usually the tendon is too degenerated to

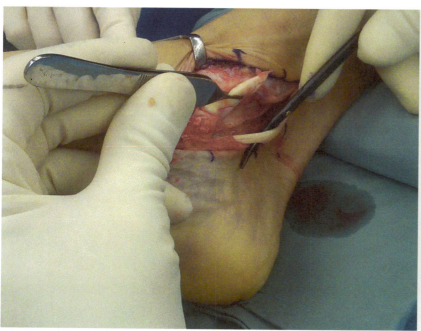

Fig. 24.4 Flexor digitorum longus tendon is harvested just behind the torn posterior tibial tendon.

incorporate into the repair, but some authors opt to include the PTT or muscle into the soft-tissue reconstruction. Options include repairing the PTT and supplementing with the FDL plantar to the PTT; weaving the FDL into the degenerated PTT; resecting and tenodesing the FDL to the PTT proximally at the myotendinous junction level; or resecting the PTT completely and transferring the FDL into navicular without any tenodesis. This decision is a combination of surgeon's preference and intraoperative and preoperative (MRI) appearance of the PTT. The tendon is the main pain generator medially, so the author tends to completely resect the torn PTT (take off the navicular and resect in the lower calf) tendon and rarely performs any of the tenodesing procedures, given the torn PTT can remain a pain generator (**Fig. 24.5**). We have found that tenodesis proximally to the PTT often results in retromalleolar pain and weaving distally often leaves a bulky, painful area just inferior to the navicular.

Once the PTT has been resected, the FDL is easily found in its sheath plantar and medial to the PTT posterior sheath, using iris scissors. The FDL tendon is allowed to fall into the PTT sheath, where it will remain for the reconstruction. The FDL is then traced down underneath the navicular into the midfoot. A major key in this dissection is hemostasis control directly under the navicular, given that there are many crossing veins that need to be tied off or cauterized during this approach.

Once the dissection gets past the navicular, the FHL is found and the two tendons cross each other at the knot of Henry, which is released and Penrose drains are placed around both tendons. The FHL is then pulled on to see how many toes flex (usually two, three, and sometimes four) to document cross-connections between the tendons to mitigate loss of the FDL. The FDL is then sharply cut just proximal to the soft-tissue connections of the FHL, and a whipstitch is placed in the end of the tendon for later passage (**Fig. 24.6**). Fluoroscopy is used to help direct a drill bit from dorsal to plantar and distal to proximal in the navicular, making sure there is an adequate bony bridge. Once this is confirmed, a 4.5-mm cannulated drill is drilled dorsal to plantar, over a guide wire through the navicular (**Fig. 24.6**). A suture passer is passed through the drill hole (alternatively a

standard metal suction tip can be used) and the whipstitch attached to the FDL is brought through the drill hole from plantar to dorsal (**Fig. 24.7a,b**). The foot is held in slight plantar flexion of 10 degrees and slight inversion of 15 degrees. The FDL is then sutured back onto itself or secured into the navicular bone tunnel with an absorbable interference screw (**Fig. 24.8a,b**). The previously opened posterior tendon sheath now is closed over the FDL tendon with a 2.0 Vicryl suture (**Fig. 24.9**).

24.7 Tips and Pearls

- Performing the lateral bony work first is the most efficient way to perform the reconstruction. Closing the lateral wounds first and then exposing the medial ankle also allows easy access for a gastrocnemius lengthening release if required.
- Using a cannulated 4.5-mm drill is easiest for the navicular tunnel. Use the guide wire and then check on fluoroscopy to make sure your bridge is adequate, then drill with the 4.5-mm drill. The FDL tendon will easily pass through this size tunnel and then you can suture back on itself or use an absorbable interference screw.
- Make sure you do not overtighten the FDL in the tunnel or the tendon will sublux from behind the medial malleolus or be a source of pain. The FDL should be fixed in slight inversion and plantar flexion but easily brought up to neutral without subluxing or undue pressure on the construct.
- In almost all cases, completely resect the posterior tibial tendon, because if left behind, it can remain a pain generator.

24.8 Hazards and Pitfalls

- Care must be taken when tightening the FDL transfer, as overtightening can lead to medial ankle pain and subluxation of the FDL behind the malleolus.
- The foot should be able to be brought to neutral dorsiflexion easily without the subluxation of the FDL out of the PTT grove.

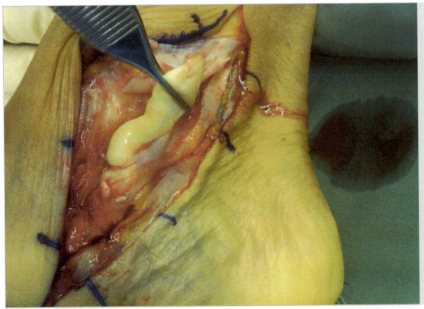

Fig. 24.5 The degenerated posterior tibial tendon is completely excised because it can remain a pain generator.

- There is risk for excessive bleeding postoperatively, if the vessels are not cauterized under the navicular during the dissection.
- Care must be taken during dissection of the two layers of the foot to avoid injuring the medial plantar nerve, which sits just below the knot of Henry.
- Use fluoroscopy to make the drill hole in the navicular so that it is not too medial.

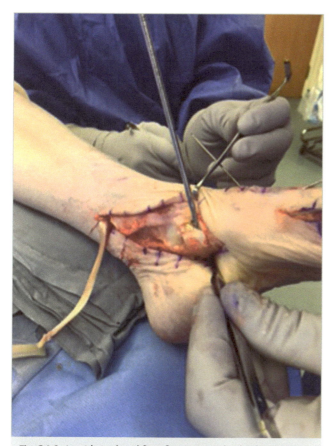

Fig. 24.6 A guide is placed first, fluoroscopy checks the position, and then a 4.5-mm cannulated drill is used to make the navicular tunnel.

24.9 Complications/Bailout/Salvage

- In the case that the FDL is not adequate as a segmental graft for the torn PTT, a free hamstring graft or the FHL tendon can be used. The hamstring autograft is the most accessible as a segmental graft. The peroneus brevis has also been reported as a transfer but would take the FHL over peroneals.
- All cases of failed FDL transfer plus hindfoot osteotomies are usually salvaged by a hindfoot arthrodesis.

24.9.1 Complications

- Most postoperative complaints postoperatively following a PTTD reconstruction involve the later bony procedures. There have been some cases of the navicular bridge through the FDL transfer passes fractures and the tendon graft fails.

24.10 Postoperative Care

- Patients are kept in a short leg, well-padded splint for 2 weeks and then at 2 weeks transferred to a non–weight-bearing CAM walker boot for an additional 6 weeks. Depending on the what other procedures are performed (and how the X-rays look), we then advance weight-bearing 25% per week with crutches until 10 weeks when the patient is allowed to bear full weigh in the boot.

24.11 Outcomes

- While full power is not restored to the PTT, most patients will be pain free medially and are able to go up on their toes for a double toe rise. We have found that patients who are operated on earlier in the stage of disease do better than patients with more severe deformities who require more extensive bony procedures.

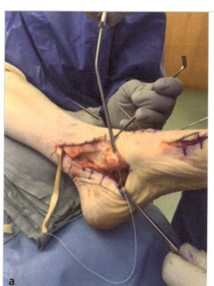
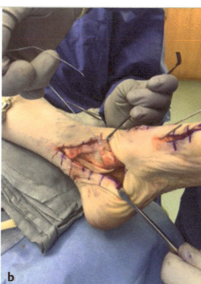

Fig. 24.7 (a) Standard metal suction tip used to pass the suture through the navicular drill hole. (b) The flexor digitorum longus tendon now passed from plantar to dorsal through navicular.

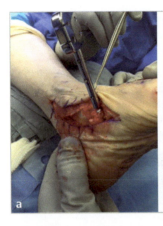
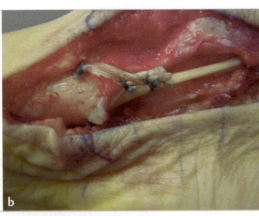

Fig. 24.8 **(a)** Fixation of flexor digitorum longus (FDL) with absorbable interference screw. **(b)** Fixation of FDL by suturing back onto itself after passing through navicular tunnel.

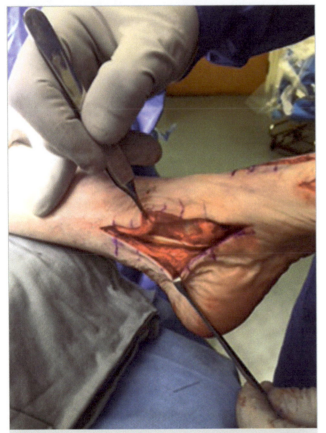

Fig. 24.9 The flexor digitorum longus (FDL) is fixed to the navicular in 10 to 15 degrees of plantarflexion and the sheath of the posterior tibial tendon now closed over the FDL transfer.

- Chadwick et al[3] reported an increase in mean American Orthopedic Foot and Ankle Society (AOFAS) score from 48.4 preoperatively to 90.3 at the final follow-up for 31 patients with stage 2 PTTD that underwent FDL transfer and medial displacement calcaneal osteotomy.[4]
- Niki et al[4] reported an increase in mean AOFAS score from 46.4 preoperatively to 89.5 1 year postoperatively for 38 patients (40 feet), with stage 2 PTTD, who underwent FDL transfer with medializing calcaneal osteotomy.

References

1. Plaass C, Fumy M, Claassen L, et al. Lecture Presented AO-FAS Summer Meeting 2014
2. Lapinksi B, Porcelli T. Adult acquired flatfoot: nonoperative treatment. In: Coetzee JC, Hurwitz SR, eds. Arthritis and Arthroplasty: The Foot and Ankle. Philadelphia, PA: Saunders Elsevier;2010:251–257
3. Chadwick C, Whitehouse SL, Saxby TS. Long-term follow-up of flexor digitorum longus transfer and calcaneal osteotomy for stage II posterior tibial tendon dysfunction. Bone Joint J 2015;97-B(3):346–352
4. Niki H, Hirano T, Okada H, Beppu M. Outcome of medial displacement calcaneal osteotomy for correction of adult-acquired flatfoot. Foot Ankle Int 2012;33(11):940–946

25 Medializing Calcaneal Osteotomy

Brian S. Winters and Joseph N. Daniel

Abstract

The medializing calcaneal osteotomy is a frequently performed procedure usually done in conjunction with a flexor tendon transfer as part of a flatfoot correction surgery. By sliding the posterior tuber of the calcaneus 1 cm medially, the mechanical axis of the limb is medialized, thereby decreasing the stress on the posterior tibial tendon's mechanics to invert the hindfoot. Additionally, the Achilles tendon insertion is medialized, converting the gastroc-soleus complex into a true plantar flexor and not a hindfoot evertor as occurs when the hindfoot is in valgus. This procedure has a high union rate and is technically reproducible.

Keywords: *calcaneal osteotomy, medializing, valgus*

25.1 Indications

- As part of flatfoot deformity correction:
  - Together with flexor digitorum longus (FDL) transfer for posterior tibial tendon reconstruction.
  - Stage 2A flatfoot.
- To medially shift mechanical axis of limb to unload lateral ankle joint.

25.1.1 Clinical Evaluation

- Standing patient viewed from behind: valgus hindfoot alignment > 5 degrees.
- Flexible hindfoot valgus: corrected with a reverse Coleman block test/passive hindfoot inversion of subtalar joint.

25.1.2 Radiographic Evaluation

- Weight-bearing anteroposterior and lateral radiographs of foot.
  - Flatfoot deformity with Meary's angle > 4 degrees but < 30 degrees.
  - Talonavicular (TN) uncoverage of 20 to 40%.
  - Absence of hindfoot (subtalar/TN) arthritis.
- Saltzman's alignment view demonstrating hindfoot valgus.

25.1.3 Nonoperative Options

- Medially posted orthotics.
- Ankle foot orthosis (Arizona brace).

25.1.4 Contraindications

- Hindfoot arthritis.
- Fixed flatfoot deformity.
- Severe flatfoot with Meary's angle >30 degrees/TN uncoverage >40%.

25.2 Goals of Surgical Procedure

- The goal of the procedure is to stably change the biomechanical axis of the hindfoot. By shifting the calcaneal tuber medially, the posterior leg of the tripod making up the foot is moved medially. This can change the weight-bearing axis of the lower extremity. By doing so, the forces placed across the subtalar joint and to a lesser degree the ankle joint can be changed. In addition, the line of pull of the Achilles tendon is medialized.

25.3 Advantages of Surgical Procedure

- Advantages of this procedure are that it is relatively easy to perform, has low morbidity, and has a high rate of success.

25.4 Key Principles

- Lateral incision over calcaneus inferior to the peroneal tendons.
- Oblique osteotomy of the posterior calcaneal tuberosity anterior to a line between the Achilles insertion and the plantar fascial insertion.
- Distraction of the osteotomy.
- Medial translation of the posterior calcaneal tuber 1 cm.
- Rigid fixation of the osteotomy with cannulated screw.

25.5 Preoperative Preparation and Patient Positioning

- Preoperative preparation should include the planning of the equipment to be used.
- A list of the equipment that may be required includes
  - Sagittal saw/micro-sagittal saw.
  - Self-retaining retractor.
  - Cannulated screws or a specially designed fixation plate.
  - Bone tamp.
  - Mallet.
  - Absorbable monofilament sutures.
  - Skin stapler.
- The patient is placed in a supine position on the operating table. A bump should be placed underneath the ipsilateral hip to facilitate internal rotation of the operative extremity. This type of positioning allows for the surgeon to work over both the lateral and the medial aspects of the foot. This is very useful when performing an acquired flatfoot deformity (AAFD) reconstruction involving both bony and soft-tissue work, such as tendon transfers.
- Alternatively, a lateral position can be used. This makes access to the medial aspect of the ipsilateral foot more difficult but in some cases, may be desirable if the medializing calcaneal osteotomy (MCO) is done without the need for additional procedures, and the amount of assistance available during the case is limited.

25.6 Operative Technique

- After the patient has been placed on the table, a bump is placed underneath the ipsilateral hip. This should allow easy access to the lateral heel. A stack of folded blankets for a commercially available foam ramp to the pool lower extremity above the nonoperative contralateral side can be helpful.

- The last step before prepping should be placement of a high thigh tourniquet on the ipsilateral lower extremity. Alternatively, a sterile tourniquet may be placed on the midportion of the leg if desired.

- The patient then undergoes a standard prep and drape of the lower extremity. The lateral hindfoot is then palpated in an effort to try and localize the superior and inferior orders of the calcaneal tuber. This is fairly easy on most patients but may be more difficult with in those with a high body mass index. Also, if possible, palpation of the sural nerve is performed. If the surgeon is able to identify the nerve, its path may be marked with a surgical marker. In the event that the sural nerve cannot be palpated, the line of the incision is made approximately midway between the tip of the fibula and the posterior border of the calcaneus. The incision should be aligned perpendicular to the long axis of the calcaneal tuber. The length of this incision does not need to be much longer than the superior/inferior thickness of the calcaneal tuber (**Fig. 25.1**).

- The skin is then incised. Care should be taken to identify the sural nerve in the subcutaneous tissues. Once this has been identified, the nerve is then retracted superiorly to give better access to the lateral wall of the calcaneus. Once the nerve has been protected and moved out of the way, dissection can be carried out straight to the lateral wall of the calcaneus.

- A small soft-tissue elevator can be used to create a 2-mm channel in the periosteum (**Fig. 25.1**). After this has been done, the sagittal saw is used to create the osteotomy. This should be perpendicular to the long axis of the calcaneal

tubercle. Care should be taken not to plunge through the medial cortex of the calcaneus. If possible, we choose to finish the osteotomy through the medial portion of the calcaneus using an osteotome.

- After completion of the osteotomy, the fragments need to be distracted to allow stretching of the soft tissues and compliance of the soft tissues. This greatly eases the translation of the posterior fragment. Osteotomes can be used to start this process (see below).

- A smooth laminar is inserted and the osteotomes are removed. Arms of the laminar spreader should be inserted deeply enough to allow the tip to slightly overhang the medial cortex of the osteotomy site. This allows for optimal cortical support of the arms of the laminar spreader during distraction of the osteotomy fragment and prevents compaction of the soft cancellous bone (**Fig. 25.2**). A second osteotome may also be placed within the osteotomy site. After both laminar spreaders have been inserted, they are expanded to allow distraction of the posterior calcaneal fragment from the main body of the calcaneus. Distraction should be at least 1-cm wide. This position is held for a few minutes to allow the soft tissues to gently stretch. This stretching will facilitate easy translation of the calcaneal fragment prior to fixation.

- After a few minutes of distraction, a guide pin may be inserted into the posterior calcaneal osteotomy fragment in preparation for provisional fixation of the osteotomy after translation has been obtained. If this is done, the pin is inserted

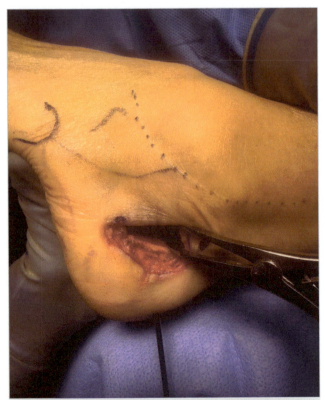

Fig. 25.2 Insertion of laminar spreader. The laminar spreader is inserted into the calcaneal osteotomy such that the arms are overhanging both the lateral and the medial cortices. This allows distraction and stretching of the surrounding soft tissues without compaction of the soft medullary cancellous bone of the calcaneal tuber.

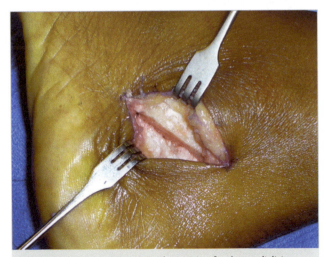

Fig. 25.1 Incision orientation. The incision for the medializing calcaneal osteotomy (MCO) is made approximately midway between the tip of the fibula and the posterior border of the calcaneus. The incision is aligned perpendicularly to the long axis of the calcaneal tuber. The periosteum has been advanced about 2 mm from the location of the osteotomy to avoid damage during the performance of the actual osteotomy.

approximately 5 to 7 mm medial to the lateral cortex of the posterior fragment and slightly inferior in the fragment as well (**Fig. 25.3**). This positioning allows for advancement of a lag screw beyond the osteotomy site and into the anterior process of the calcaneus without breaching the medial cortex and potentially harming the medial neurovascular structures. This screw position gives excellent purchase especially in patients who have a relatively short calcaneal tuber in which it may be difficult to fully advance all the threads of a partially threaded screw across the osteotomy site.

- Once the guide pin is advanced into the posterior fragment of the calcaneal tubercle, the laminar spreaders can be removed. The osteotomy is then translated approximately 1 cm medially from its native position (**Fig. 25.4**). Slightly less or more translation can be used depending on the amount of correction felt to be needed by the surgeon.

- After the osteotomy has been translated, the surgeon should ensure that the osteotomy surfaces lie flush to one another. At this point, the previously inserted guide wire is advanced across the osteotomy site into the main body of the calcaneus. Great care should be taken so as not to advance the guide pin across the posterior facet of the subtalar joint or the calcaneocuboid joint depending on what the orientation of the screw will be. Fluoroscopy should be used to confirm proper positioning of the guide wire. A lateral and axial view of the calcaneus should be obtained. At this point, a sterile ruler can be inserted at the osteotomy site to confirm that adequate translation of the osteotomy has been achieved. Once confirmation of proper positioning has been obtained, a second guide wire is placed across the osteotomy site to prevent rotation of the fragment during screw insertion.

- At this point, the surgeon measures the length of the guide wire for choosing the appropriate length of screw to be inserted. We have found that a transverse incision at the

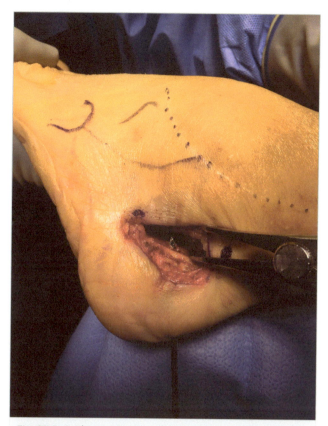

Fig. 25.3 Guidewire insertion. The cannulated screw guidewire is inserted approximately 5 to 7 mm medial to the lateral cortex of the posterior fragment and slightly inferior in the fragment as well. This positioning allows for advancement of a lag screw beyond the osteotomy site and into the anterior process of the calcaneus without breaching the medial cortex and potentially harming the medial neurovascular structures.

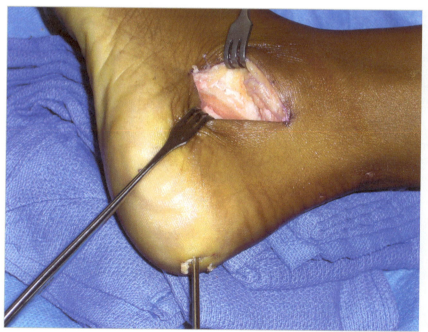

Fig. 25.4 Medial shift. A 1-cm medial shift of the calcaneal tuber is demonstrated. The translated osteotomy has been provisionally fixed with a guidewire for a cannulated screw. The bony overhang anterior to the osteotomy may be bluntly beveled using a bone tamp and mallet.

insertion point of the wire in the skin heals very well as the skin is compressed across this plane during weight-bearing. A depth gauge is then inserted over the wire to aid the surgeon in choosing the appropriate length for the lag screw. A cannulated drill is then advanced over the guide wire across the osteotomy site. Depending on the density of the calcaneal bone, the surgeon may want to drill the entire length of the guide wire or only a portion of it. In patients with low bone density, we choose to drill over the guidewire to, or just past, the osteotomy site, whereas in those with denser bone we will advance the drill almost the entire length of the guide wire. Discerning the depth of drilling can be aided with fluoroscopic imaging.

- A partially threaded 6.5- to 8.0-mm screw is then inserted either by hand or on power to achieve compression across the osteotomy site. The size of the screw is determined by the size of the patient. In patients with extremely soft bone, washers may be added over the screw if needed. We generally only insert one screw, but multiple screws can be used if needed.
- We prefer to place the screw in the inferior half of the calcaneal tuber and advance it in to the anterior process. This allows for a longer screw with greater thread length. This may need to be modified if a concomitant lateral column lengthening (LCL) through the anterior process is to be performed (**Fig. 25.5**).

25.7 Tips and Pearls

- Non-saw hand is placed medial to the heel while sawing to provide another tactile sensory input to prevent plunging of the blade and resultant possible damage of the neuromuscular bundle along the medal hindfoot.
- Straight osteotome wedging. Once the osteotomy has been completed, two straight osteotomes are inserted side by side in the calcaneal osteotomy. After this has been done, they are levered in opposite directions to allow separation of the osteotomy fragments and to start loosening of the soft tissues surrounding the calcaneus.
- In most cases, pure medial translation of the posterior fragment is all that is needed. In certain cases, translation in the superior or inferior plane may also be added by the surgeon to help in correcting high or low calcaneal pitch angles, respectively.
- Use fully threaded screws in a "lag-by-technique" mode if too little bone is present on the anterior portion of the calcaneus to allow full advancement of the threads of a partially threaded screw across the osteotomy site.

- To avoid the potential of soft-tissue irritation from the bony overhang produced by the displacement of the osteotomy a "crushplasty" can be performed. During performance of this step, it is recommended that the additional guidewire that was previously placed to prevent rotation of the bone placed across the osteotomy site be maintained to prevent loosening of the reduction and fixation. A bone tamp is then used to compact the overhanging bone anterior to the osteotomy. The surgeon needs to make sure that the superior and inferior portions have adequate beveling of the overhang before completion of the procedure (**Fig. 25.4**).
- If an LCL through the anterior process of the calcaneus is to be done in addition to the MCO, screw placement will need to be modified so as not to disrupt the LCL. To facilitate both procedures, the fixation screw can be angled more superiorly to lie along the longitudinal axis of the tuber (**Fig. 25.5**).

25.8 Hazards and Pitfalls

- The sural nerve lies directly in the region of the incision. The nerve needs to be protected to prevent painful neuroma formation or scar entrapment.
- The medial neurovascular bundle lies in close proximity to the medial cortex of the osteotomy. Great care is required when penetrating the medial border of the calcaneus and this should be done with an osteotome and not with the saw blade.
- Calcaneal bone compaction can occur when distracting with the laminar spreaders. This distraction should be done slowly and with care. The spreaders should be adjusted and placed deeply within the calcaneus to prevent this occurrence.
- Avoid varus tilting of the calcaneal tuber during the medial translation. This will limit contact area with resultant nonunion. This can also result in varus overcorrection of the osteotomy.

25.9 Complications/Bailout/Salvage

- The MCO is a very vascular osteotomy and as a result a low nonunion rate.
- Excess translation will limit bone contact area and can cause an unstable osteotomy or nonunion. Generally, no more than 1 cm of distraction is warranted. This needs to be assessed intraoperatively with an axial calcaneal view fluoroscopy and readjusted if needed.

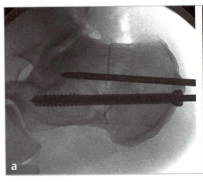 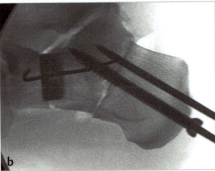

Fig. 25.5 Comparison of screw placement into anterior process of calcaneus and beneath posterior facet. Calcaneal osteotomies fixed with partially threaded screws placed into the **(a)** anterior process and **(b)** placed just inferior to the posterior facet of the calcaneus. In both cases, a second guidewire has been added to allow crushplasty to be performed without rotation through the plane of the osteotomy.

- Sural neuroma formation or scar entrapment may require surgical excision and burial of the nerve into muscle proximal to the ankle.
- Medial nerve injuries seem to be more likely if the osteotomy is made more anteriorly compared to those carried out posteriorly.
- Wound healing problems such as dehiscence and infection are uncommon and when occur can usually be successfully treated with local wound care and oral antibiotics
- Tibial nerve injury can be evaluated on electromyography (EMG) and may require surgical decompression and rarely nerve transection and burial or medical management of nerve pain.
- Occasionally the head of the fixation screw can cause pain with weight-bearing or shoe wear. Once the osteotomy has healed, the screw can be safely removed.

25.10 Postoperative Care

- This is determined by the requirement of the primary procedure associated with the MCO procedure.
- In most cases, this will require 6 weeks of non–weight-bearing in a cast or boot, followed by additional ambulation in a boot until bone consolidation occurs.

25.11 Outcomes

- The outcomes of this procedure are very reliable. The calcaneus osteotomy has a very high rate (>95%) of union.

- When done in conjunction with soft-tissue procedures, the calcaneal osteotomy contributes to a reliable correction of AAFD with increases in functional outcomes and improvement in radiographic parameters.

References

1. Bruce BG, Bariteau JT, Evangelista PE, Arcuri D, Sandusky M, DiGiovanni CW. The effect of medial and lateral calcaneal osteotomies on the tarsal tunnel. Foot Ankle Int 2014;35(4):383–388
2. Guyton GP, Jeng C, Krieger LE, Mann RA. Flexor digitorum longus transfer and medial displacement calcaneal osteotomy for posterior tibial tendon dysfunction: a middle-term clinical follow-up. Foot Ankle Int 2001;22(8):627–632
3. Niki H, Hirano T, Okada H, Beppu M. Outcome of medial displacement calcaneal osteotomy for correction of adult-acquired flatfoot. Foot Ankle Int 2012;33(11):940–946
4. Sammarco GJ, Hockenbury RT. Treatment of stage II posterior tibial tendon dysfunction with flexor hallucis longus transfer and medial displacement calcaneal osteotomy. Foot Ankle Int 2001;22(4):305–312
5. Wacker JT, Hennessy MS, Saxby TS. Calcaneal osteotomy and transfer of the tendon of flexor digitorum longus for stage-II dysfunction of tibialis posterior. Three- to five-year results. J Bone Joint Surg Br 2002;84(1):54–58

26 Evans Lateral Column Lengthening and Cotton Osteotomy

Jonathan Deland and Mackenzie Jones

Abstract

Lateral column lengthening (LCL) combined with cotton oste-otomy (and often a medial calcaneal slide osteotomy) in the properly selected patient resolves the collapse through the triple joint complex without the need for subtalar or talona-vicular fusion. The patient must not be so collapsed in the tri-ple joint complex that the foot cannot be tensioned by an LCL to accomplish good position of the talonavicular and subta-lar joints when the patient stands. Such a patient most often preoperatively does not have subfibular impingement but can certainly have subtalar impingement. Success with an LCL and cotton osteotomy is defined by achieving the right amount of correction with good alignment of the talonavicular and subta-lar joints, resolving subtalar impingement and abduction of the talonavicular joint yet avoiding an overly stiff adducted/lateral weight-bearing foot. The successful patient has near-normal eversion motion remaining in the hindfoot, and good alignment of the heel. If surgery has achieved these goals, the patient is likely to have a good functional outcome with minimal stiffness and minimal chance of recurrence of the collapsing foot.

Keywords: *lateral column lengthening, cotton osteotomy, best functional outcome, alignment*

26.1 Indications and Pathology

- Adolescent flexible flatfoot.
- Adult acquired flatfoot deformity 2B:
  - Posterior tibial tendon (PTT) dysfunction.

26.1.1 Clinical Evaluation

- Flatfoot deformity with medial arch collapse.
- Usually will have pain over the PTT.
- Too-many-toe sign when foot observed from behind in stand-ing position due to forefoot abduction.
- Hindfoot valgus.
- Inability to perform a single-leg heel raise (heel should invert).

26.1.2 Radiographic Evaluation

- Weight-bearing anteroposterior (AP), lateral and Saltzman's view radiographs are performed to assess degree of planoval-gus.
- Indication for this procedure is excessive eversion/abduction of the midfoot with collapse of the arch as evidenced by one of the following:
  - Forty percent or more talonavicular uncoverage on a standing AP X-ray of the foot.
  - Lateral incongruity of the talonavicular joint on a standing AP foot X-ray.
  - Borderline X-ray findings of one or two, but the patient has excessive pronation (eversion and abduction) seen clinically by a severe flatfoot with sag in the arch just distal to the ankle but not at the level of the tarsometatarsal or naviculocuneiform joints. Standing plain X-rays can underestimate deformity if patient is not allowing the arch to collapse, the patient is leaning back, or the X-ray is not properly centered over the talonavicular joint.
- If available, obtain a standing computed tomography (CT) scan in cases of severe deformity. This is helpful to assess possible lateral impingement at the subtalar joint and sub-fibular impingement. Also, on the coronal views of the CT scan, look for lateral subluxation of the subtalar joint, which probably indicates the need for a subtalar fusion.
- A magnetic resonance imaging (MRI) scan is not essential, but it can be helpful to assess the condition of the spring ligament in cases with severe deformity.

26.1.3 Nonoperative Options

- Boot or hinged ankle–foot orthosis (AFO) brace.
- Ritchie (ankle-level hinged brace with plantar orthotic com-ponent).
- Arizona brace.

Note: Any of these options may help symptoms and possibly slow down progression, but they do not halt progression. This should be explained to the patient.

26.1.4 Contraindications

- Unable to passively bring the talonavicular joint into an adducted or inverted position.
- Moderate to severe osteoporosis. In an osteoporotic patient with significantly weak bone, an Evans procedure is preferable to a step-cut osteotomy (see section "Lateral Column Length-ening Alternative Procedure: Step-cut Osteotomy") because of less chance of fracturing the bone with manipulation.
- Symptomatic arthritis of the subtalar, calcaneocuboid, or talonavicular joint.

26.2 Goals of Surgical Procedure

- Correct alignment so that each of the following is achieved:
  - No remaining subtalar or subfibular impingement.
  - Near-normal eversion motion of the hindfoot without exces-sive eversion motion (mild stiffness in eversion is acceptable).
  - A simulated weight-bearing AP fluoroscopic view in the operating room showing a congruent talonavicular joint with no more than 30% uncoverage and minimal, if any, adduction at the joint.
  - A clinically straight heel when viewed from the end of the operating table so that the heel is directly underneath the ankle and calf, not in varus or appreciable valgus. Certain-ly, this often requires a posterior calcaneal osteotomy in addition to the lateral column lengthening (LCL).

26.3 Advantages of Surgical Procedure

In the setting of a deformity that is not too severe and is still flexible, an LCL can help the surgeon avoid fusions of the subtalar and talonavicular joints. These joints are important for the patient being able to exercise on the foot and minimize the risk of ankle arthritis over time.

26.4 Key Principles of the Surgical Procedure

- Achieve the right amount of correction taking care not to overcorrect, which is the most common mistake.
- Perform compression fixation of the osteotomies, especially the LCL.
- Confirm that the heel alignment is good after temporary fixation of the LCL and the posterior calcaneal osteotomy. In cases with more than a little increased heel valgus, it is normally necessary to do a posterior calcaneal osteotomy as well as an LCL to obtain correct position of the heel.
- If the first metatarsal is elevated, it should be brought down to a good position in comparison to the second metatarsal head. Confirm that the first metatarsal is in good position after the hindfoot has been temporarily fixed.

26.5 Preoperative Preparation and Patient Positioning

- Use standing X-rays preoperatively, with the patient allowing the arch to collapse. Judge the abduction of the talonavicular joint on the AP foot X-ray and the plantar sag at the talonavicular joint on the lateral X-ray. Also, look for possible sags at naviculocuneiform and first tarsometatarsal joints on the standing lateral X-ray.
- Assess a standing AP view of the ankle to confirm no valgus of the talus in the ankle joint.
- Patient is positioned supine. A small bump can be placed under the ipsilateral hip to aid with the lateral column lengthening, although this may make the approach to the PTT more difficult during the tendon transfer procedure if the leg is rotated too internally. Best position is toes pointing to the ceiling with the foot at rest.
- A flexor digitorum longus tendon transfer is usually performed in combination with the osteotomies in adult acquired flatfoot deformity with associated PTT pathology.

26.6 Operative Technique

26.6.1 Lateral Column Lengthening: Evans Procedure

- Use a sinus tarsi incision extending from the tip of the fibula to the anterior process of the calcaneus (**Fig. 26.1**).
- Dissect at the midportion of the incision to find the floor of the sinus tarsi, taking care to avoid and stay above the peroneal tendons and sural nerve. Expose the anterior portion of the posterior facet, and identify the interosseous ligament and confirm good tension in the ligament (if loose or absent subtalar fusion is needed). Take care not to cut the ligament.
- Dissect laterally over the anterior calcaneus, from a point adjacent to the calcaneocuboid joint to the level of the posterior facet. Mobilize the peroneal tendons so that they can be retracted with a Bennett retractor to allow a saw cut into the lateral aspect of the anterior calcaneus.

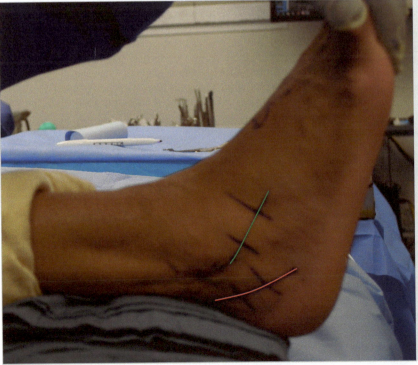

Fig. 26.1 Incisions for lateral column lengthening (LCL; green) and posterior calcaneal osteotomy (red).

- Place a K-wire 17 mm from the calcaneocuboid joint through the lateral cortex and into the medial cortex one-third the way down from the dorsal rim aiming in between the middle and posterior facets (**Fig. 26.2**). The interval between the facets can usually be identified bluntly with an elevator. Measure the depth of the K-wire when it has reached the medial cortex. This will give the surgeon a good idea of the depth for the saw blade cut. The depth of the saw cut can be marked on the saw with a marking pen.
- With the thin oscillating saw, make the osteotomy perpendicular to plantar aspect of the foot just distal to the K-wire into the medial cortex. Weaken the medial cortex so that the osteotomy can be hinged open with an osteotome (**Fig. 26.3**).
- Place a pin distractor with one pin right next to the calcaneocuboid joint and the other well posterior to the saw cut.
- Use an osteotome to hinge open the osteotomy. Use the pin distractor to hold open the osteotomy and try different amounts of lengthening to correct the deformity.
- Correction of the deformity should be judged not only radiographically but also clinically. Radiographically, the abduction should be corrected so that there is a normal amount of uncoverage of the talar head (30% or less), and no adduction of the talonavicular joint. Clinically, there should be near-normal eversion motion remaining, but mild stiffness is acceptable (**Fig. 26.4**).
- If, on a simulated AP weight-bearing view with the eversion stress, there is adduction at the talonavicular joint or there is almost no eversion in the hindfoot, the foot is overcorrected. Undercorrection is defined by excessive uncoverage with over 30% uncoverage of the talar head on the simulated weight-bearing view or by excessive eversion motion remaining in the hindfoot. Undercorrection can also be identified by everting the foot and seeing that there is

impingement or near impingement of the anterior aspect of the lateral talar process into the floor of the sinus tarsi. Too much correction can result in a good-looking X-ray and no impingement, but the hindfoot still too stiff. That situation will lead to an unsatisfied patient with lateral weight bearing. Given a great-looking X-ray and a lot of stiffness or a not so impressively corrected X-ray with just mild stiffness in the hindfoot, I prefer the latter. The most common amounts of LCL are in the range of 6 to 8 mm.
- Hold the osteotomy open to the desired amount of lengthening and fashion a tricortical allograft to fit that space. Another method (my preferred method) is to use trial wedges in 1-mm increments or some instrument with the desired amounts of lengthening to judge the foot.[1] Use the wedges or instrument inserted into the osteotomy to judge the correction. Fashion the graft according to the ideal amount of correction as shown by looking at the osteotomy held open to the desired amount. Take note of the shape of the opening, and replicate the shape. The wedge is usually trapezoidal in shape.
- Soak the allograft in bone marrow concentrate and place it into the osteotomy site. Make sure that the fit is good. If there is any space on either side between the graft and native bone, rotate or trim the graft slightly to achieve excellent apposition along the lateral and dorsal aspects of the osteotomy. When this is achieved, place a pin from the anterior calcaneus across the graft and into the posterior calcaneus.
- With the graft in place and pinned, confirm that the amount of correction is appropriate and that both clinical inspection and fluoroscopic views show good apposition of the graft to the native bone. Fix the osteotomy with two longitudinal 3.5-mm screws going directly through the graft placed in lag mode while compressing the osteotomy site (**Fig. 26.5**). Alternative fixation is with a lateral low-profile claw-type plate to provide compression.

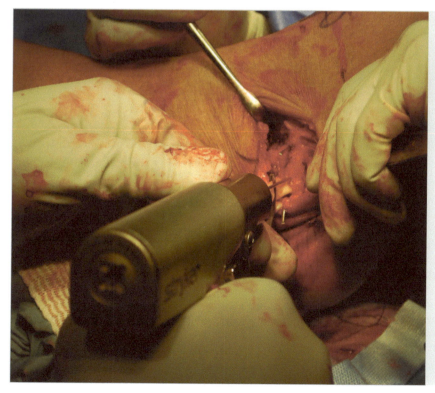

Fig. 26.2 Pin placement to guide cut for osteotomy. For Evans, it is 15 to 20 mm from the calcaneocuboid joint. For the step-cut, the distal horizontal arm starts 12 mm from the calcaneocuboid joint.

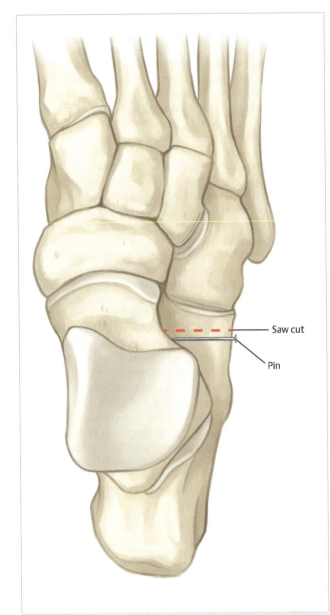

Saw cut

Pin

Fig. 26.3 First a pin is placed along the proposed osteotomy site. Second, a saw cut (red) is made perpendicular to the plantar aspect of the foot along the pin to, and partially through, the medial cortex.

- Check the alignment of the foot including heel valgus, correction of the midfoot, and elevation of the first ray (**Fig. 26.6**). In cases of significantly increased heel valgus, I make the posterior calcaneal osteotomy first, temporarily pinning it in just slightly less than the desired amount of correction, and then assess the amount of correction for the LCL. Remember the LCL will give just a small amount of correction to the hindfoot valgus. I do not fix the posterior calcaneal osteotomy with screws until after the LCL is judged. I like to judge the LCL, posterior calcaneal osteotomy, and cotton osteotomy or first tarsometatarsal fusion (if performed) all fixed with temporary fixation so that I know I have good position of the hindfoot and forefoot before proceeding with screw fixation of any of the sites. I look for good position of the hindfoot with a clinically straight

heel, near-normal eversion motion, and no elevation of the first metatarsal comparison to the second. If these are not present, the correction is adjusted accordingly.
- If there were severe elevation in the first ray or elevation with metatarsus primus varus, I would choose a first metatarsal–tarsal fusion having already temporarily fixed it with pins. Adjust it only if it is necessary once the hindfoot is temporarily fixed. Once all sites are temporarily fixed, the order of the final fixation is posterior calcaneal osteotomy, first tarsometatarsal fusion, and then the LCL. The exception to this order would occur when there is mild to moderate elevation of the first ray without metatarsus primus varus. For that situation, I would use a cotton osteotomy, preparing the osteotomy at the beginning of the case but fix it last with a 2.4-mm screw once the bone wedge has been placed.

26.6.2 Alternate Grafts and Fixation Techniques in Lateral Column Lengthening

- There are alternatives to allograft bone. Certainly one that I have used extensively is autograft bone, particularly in older adults. My experience is that donor site complications are rare and certainly nothing has been shown to heal better than autograft bone. However, allograft bone has not been shown to be statistically inferior when compared to autograft in terms of rate of union, and there are no donor site risks.[2,3] Fiber metal wedges instead of bone have been used. They are not my personal preference given they do not come in 1-mm increments for fine adjustment in the amount of lengthening, and adjusting the wedge at surgery or revision surgery could be problematic.
- For fixation, metal wedge plates or claw plates are an option. They should be low profile, and my personal preference is still screws because they can be placed so as not to abut on the peroneal tendons.

26.6.3 Lateral Column Lengthening Alternative Procedure: Step-Cut Osteotomy

Currently, I use the step-cut type of LCL[4] (**Fig. 26.7**). This is because it heals faster and, with its horizontal arm, is less likely to lose any correction in the unlikely event of difficulty healing the bone graft. This is admittedly a more difficult osteotomy to perform and takes some experience. Try it on a cadaver first, as plunging medially could cause nerve damage. Both osteotomies can achieve the same functional outcome as long as the proper amount of correction is achieved. With the step-cut osteotomy, it is particularly important to protect the peroneal tendons given they are at more risk for injury during the horizontal and posterior/inferior saw cuts. In bone that is osteoporotic, an Evans rather than a step-cut osteotomy is preferable because of less risk of fracturing the bone during manipulation. In severely osteoporotic bone, any osteotomy is problematic; a subtalar and/or talonavicular fusion is preferable.
- Do the exposure as it would be done for an Evans osteotomy, but expose the lateral calcaneus somewhat more posteriorly to allow for the inferior plantar cut (posterior to the peroneal tubercle and in line with the front edge of the posterior facet).

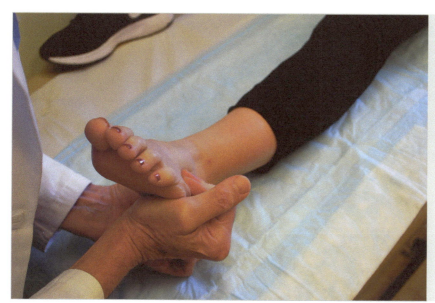

Fig. 26.4 Picture demonstrating intraoperative technique to confirm near-normal eversion in the hindfoot after trial of amount of lateral column lengthening.

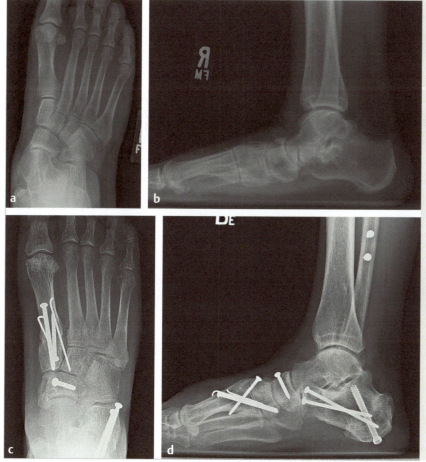

Fig. 26.5 Standing pre-op **(a)** anteroposterior (AP) and **(b)** lateral views. Standing post-op **(c)** AP and **(d)** lateral views. Screws in the navicular and fibula represent fixation of a spring ligament reconstruction with tendon graft. Note the two screws for the Evan osteotomy that are placed with lag technique.

- Dissect between the skin and peroneal tendons/sural nerve to a level below those structures so that a soft-tissue window can be created underneath peroneal tendons and sural nerve to access the lateral calcaneus in the region of the posterior vertical limb of the step-cut (**Fig. 26.8**).
- Retract the peroneal tendons and sural nerve posteriorly and inferiorly. Hold them maximally retracted with a pin just anterior to the retracted tendons. Keep them retracted with multiple pins and Bennett retractors while the horizontal and anterior vertical cuts are made.
- First, make the horizontal cut starting at a pin placed one-third the way down from the dorsal aspect of the lateral calcaneus 11 or 12 mm from the calcaneocuboid joint line (**Fig. 26.2**). Extend the cut to a pin that has been placed posteriorly so that the height of the posterior cut is just above the plantar third of the lateral calcaneus. The length of

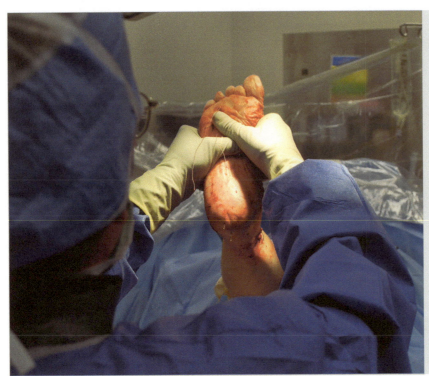

Fig. 26.6 Operative photograph showing optimal position of the heel, which is a straight heel directly underneath the calf without valgus or varus.

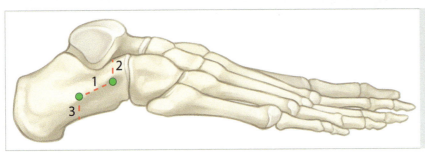

Fig. 26.7 Step-cut osteotomy: the "horizontal" line (1) is cut first in between two pins (green dots). The anterior vertical cut (2) is cut next, being careful not to extend the cut plantarly. After retracting the peroneal tendons dorsally and the skin plantarly with wide retractors, the posterior vertical cut (3) is done through the soft-tissue window, protecting the peroneal tendons and soft tissue with the large retractors (**Fig. 26.9**).

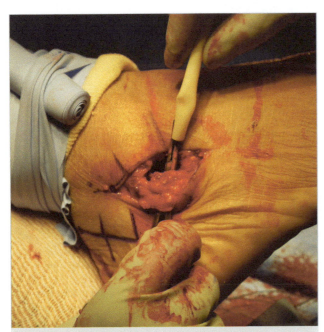

Fig. 26.8 Mobilization of the peroneal tendons and sural nerve as a unit in preparation for their dorsal retraction during the posterior vertical cut of the step-cut osteotomy.

the horizontal arm is 15 to 20 mm. Cut the lateral cortex of the horizontal arm first, then push the saw to the medial cortex and carefully perforate the medial cortex with the saw. Use two-hand control on the saw, so there is no plunging into the medial soft-tissue structures.

- Make the anterior/vertical cut by removing the distal pin and use it as the starting point and aim just anterior to the medial facet (identify the facet with a blunt elevator first).
- In some cases, it is possible to make the posterior vertical cut with the peroneal tendons already retracted posteriorly and inferiorly as described earlier. In many cases, this is not possible. If so, remove the pin and retract the peroneal tendons and sural nerve dorsally with a wide retractor underneath those structures and a Bennett retractor underneath the inferior cortex of the calcaneus (**Fig. 26.9**). Make the posterior vertical cut starting from the horizontal limb and exit plantarly, being careful to go through the medial cortex with two-hand control, and without plunging.
- Make sure the osteotomy is mobile once the cuts are made. If it is not, check the medial cortex with the saw blade not running. Usually, it is the corners that can be a problem with intact bone. Feel and cut those parts that are not cut.
- Using a pin distractor with the pins placed adjacent to the calcaneocuboid joint but below the horizontal limb and in the posterior fragment (**Fig. 26.10**) distract, being careful

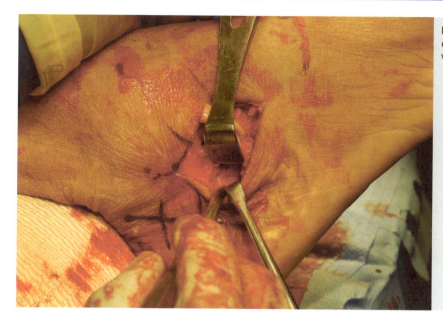

Fig. 26.9 Dorsal retraction of peroneal tendons and sural nerve to make the posterior vertical cut of the step-cut osteotomy.

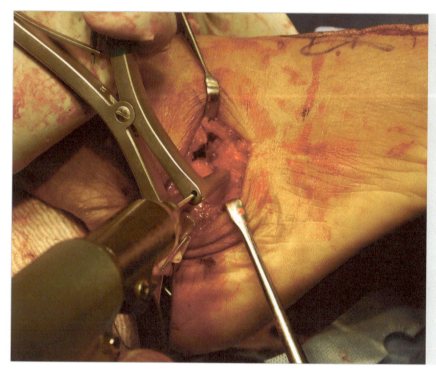

Fig. 26.10 Pin distractor used to distract the joint and allow insertion of wedge or object that holds the joint distracted. This allows for fluoroscopic assessment of correction and testing that eversion motion remains.

to keep the horizontal limb well opposed. Do not try to distract if the osteotomy does not move easily. Should the osteotomy not move easily, check for remaining bone to cut.

• Assess the amount of correction as in the case of an Evans osteotomy.
• Two cortical allografts are used, but only prepare the anterior one at this point according to the desired opening/lengthening of the osteotomy.
• Fit and temporarily fix the anterior allograft first. Confirm as described for the Evans osteotomy that the bone has an excellent fit against the native bone. Pin the osteotomy once good apposition is confirmed. Then place two screws as in the Evans osteotomy description. Originally, I had used one

dorsal-to-plantar screw at the lateral sinus tarsi (**Fig. 26.11**), but had discontinued that because of potential risk of peroneal tendon irritation. The two longitudinal screws will both need to start in the dorsal one-third of the calcaneus starting at the anterior process of the calcaneus. I usually overdrill the anterior process portion of the drill hole as in a lag screw technique and then compress the osteotomy as I put the first screw in.

• After both screws are in, fashion and place the posterior allograft in, making a snug fit (**Fig. 26.12**). It does not need to be super tight. Do not aggressively force the allograft in, given it could disrupt the fixation of the osteotomy and gap the important firm fit and compression at the anterior vertical limb. Trim the allograft as necessary for a not difficult insertion.

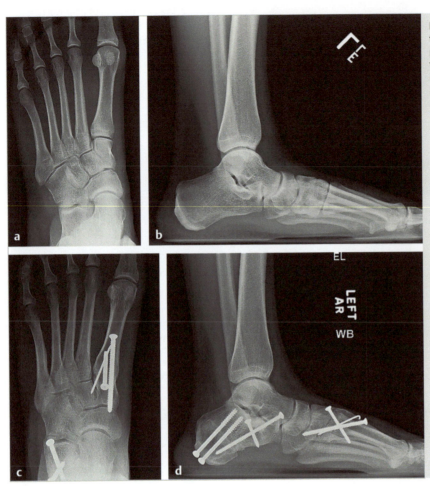

Fig. 26.11 Standing pre-op (a) anteroposterior (AP) and (b) lateral views. Standing post-op (c) AP and (d) lateral views. Note the two screw fixation of the step-cut. The more posterior of those screws can irritate the peroneal tendons. Therefore, a two-parallel screw technique similar to Evan's procedure is now used.

26.6.4 Osteotomy for Possible Remaining Subtalar Impingement

- If, after placing the graft, the anterior portion of the lateral process of the talus is at all close to the floor of the sinus tarsi with eversion stress, trim the talar process with an osteotome as shown in **Fig. 26.12**.

26.6.5 Cotton Osteotomy

- Incise over the lateral border of the medial cuneiform dorsally (**Fig. 26.13**). Take care not to injure the branch of the superficial peroneal nerve, which often can be seen medially or proximally once just the skin incision is made. Another nerve branch laterally is often present and should be protected.
- Expose the dorsal aspect of the medial cuneiform and retract the extensor hallucis longus (EHL) and nerve medially.
- Place one pin parallel to the first tarsometatarsal joint in the distal aspect of the medial cuneiform. Once good placement of this pin is confirmed by lateral fluoroscopy, place another pin parallel to the first pin in the proximal portion of the cuneiform. With retractors in place, cut the medial cuneiform from the dorsal cortex toward the plantar cortex parallel and in between the pins. Protect the EHL with a retractor during the saw cut. Do not incise the plantar cortex; go to 5 mm dorsal to the plantar cortex. This depth of cut can be

achieved by checking the length of the uncut pins adjusted down to the plantar cortex on the lateral view and appropriately marking the saw blade with a skin marker.
- Mobilize the osteotomy by placing an osteotome three quarters of the way down the osteotomy site. Gently hinge it open.
- A pin distractor can then be used over the pins to dorsally open the joint. Try different amounts of dorsal opening wedge to bring the first ray down. This can be done with the laminar spreader and/or trial wedges. A correction with a 5-, 6-, or 7-mm bone wedge is most often done.
- Fashion the allograft bone according to the shape of the opening wedge and desired amount of correction. Use the number of millimeters in the dorsal opening with the proper amount of correction as a guide.
- Soak the allograft bone in bone marrow concentrate. Once the graft is properly cut, place it in the osteotomy.
- Fix the osteotomy with a 2.4 screw placed from the proximal/dorsal to the plantar/distal aspect of the cuneiform.

26.7 Tips and Pearls

- Have a good method of trialing the amount of LCL. I use intraoperative wedges of different sizes so that the hindfoot and midfoot can be assessed for position, yet also have clinical confirmation in the OR (operating room) by everting the foot to confirm that adequate eversion hindfoot motion is remaining (**Fig. 26.14**). The method must allow testing

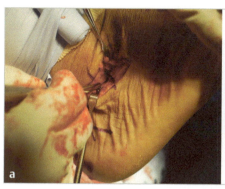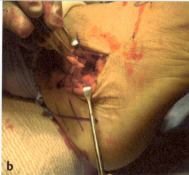

Fig. 26.12 **(a)** Exposure for osteotomy of anterior portion of the lateral talar process in cases of residual or near impingement once lengthening has been performed. **(b)** Size of bone removed.

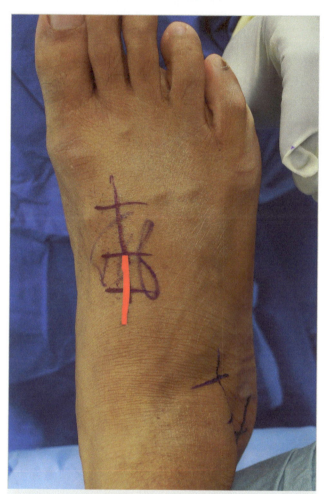

Fig. 26.13 Cotton osteotomy incision marked in red.

hindfoot eversion with manipulation. Confirmation can then be gained that there is no subtalar impingement by checking the sinus tarsi with full eversion. There should be no excessive stiffness in the hindfoot with minimal, if any, adduction of the midfoot (as measured by talonavicular joint with a simulated weight-bearing everted fluoroscopic AP of the foot).

- Although the size of the wedge varies according to laxity of the foot, most common size of LCL is 6 to 7 mm.
- For the cotton osteotomy, the most common sizes of the wedge to bring the first ray down into good position are 5 to 6 mm.

26.8 Hazards and Pitfalls

- Avoid over- and undercorrection. This can be done by carefully checking the intraoperative X-ray to be sure there is no adduction at the talonavicular joint with the osteotomy held open to the desired length. Make sure there is near-normal eversion motion remaining.
- Avoid delayed union or nonunion by checking that the bone graft has excellent apposition on the dorsal and lateral views and that the fixation is placed under compression.
- Make sure that, once in place, the grafts are not prominent dorsally into the sinus tarsi. If this is the case, carefully trim the graft dorsally with a saw once the osteotomy has been fixed.

26.9 Complications/Bailout/ Salvage

- If assessment in the operating room finds that there is over- or undercorrection, remove the temporary fixation, trim or take another graft and place the correctly sized graft. Do not leave the operating room with over- or undercorrection present.

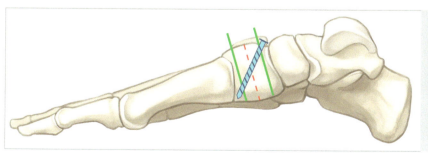

Fig. 26.14. Diagram for cotton procedure. First, pins (green) are placed perpendicular to the bone, ending at the plantar cortex. Second, saw cut (red) is made 5 mm from plantar cortex. Third, after opening the osteotomy, use pins with a pin distractor to distract and judge the wedge. Once wedge is in place, use screw (blue) in direction as shown.

- If apposition of the bone graft to the native bone is not good, trim the prominent portion of the graft or rotate it until there is excellent apposition. If necessary, use another graft.

26.10 Postoperative Care

The patient is toe-touch or non–weight-bearing for 6 weeks. At 2 or 4 weeks, depending on the condition of the wounds, a boot could be used so that the patient can remove it for range-of-motion exercises. The patient is instructed in ankle dorsiflexion/plantar flexion, inversion/eversion, and plantar flexion/dorsiflexion of the toes. At 6 weeks, X-rays or preferably a CT scan is taken. The CT scan allows the best assessment of bony healing. If good bony bridging is starting, then the patient progresses to partial weight-bearing first by standing during the first week and then 25, 50, 75, and finally 100% weight-bearing with walking by 10 to 11 weeks. Formal physical therapy is started between 6 and 8 weeks. At 10-11 weeks, using crutches for balance, the patient is instructed to walk barefoot (or with a sneaker) at home to encourage use of calf and foot muscles. After 12 weeks, the patient is gradually weaned out of the boot for walking outside of the house.

26.11 Outcomes

As patients can see and feel the better structure of their foot, they can be very satisfied patients. The exceptions are patients who are overcorrected or, less commonly, undercorrected. Gross overcorrection with visible lateral bearing, which does not improve over the 4 to 5 months from surgery, should be avoided given these patients may require additional surgery to decrease the amount of LCL and/or to slide the heel back if it is inverted. In the past 5 years, I have not had to perform such a surgery. Also, with the exception of one case with unusual flexibility, I have not had to go back to fuse a foot for undercorrection in 10 years. I attribute the avoidance of these problems to preserving, in the OR, near-normal hindfoot eversion motion (but not excessive eversion motion) and with simulated weight-bearing fluoroscopy avoiding adduction or abduction at the talonavicular joint (the articular surfaces should be lined up/congruent at the lateral aspect of the joint).

With the proper correction, it is highly likely that the patient will be able to get exercise on the foot. Running is clearly the biggest challenge in patients who have had an LCL. Running for exercise is not routinely achieved. The patients with the best chance of achieving running are the younger patients who have moderate deformity rather than severe failure of the spring ligament complex with a very pronated foot. What is told to the patient with severe deformity is that they will be able to get exercise by elliptical machine, biking, and moderate walking, but not necessarily hiking.

References

1. Ellis SJ, Williams BR, Garg R, Campbell G, Pavlov H, Deland JT. Incidence of plantar lateral foot pain before and after the use of trial metal wedges in lateral column lengthening. Foot Ankle Int 2011;32(7):665–673
2. Vosseller JT, Ellis SJ, O'Malley MJ, et al. Autograft and allograft unite similarly in lateral column lengthening for adult acquired flatfoot deformity. HSS J 2013;9(1):6–11
3. Dolan CM, Henning JA, Anderson JG, Bohay DR, Kornmesser MJ, Endres TJ. Randomized prospective study comparing tri-cortical iliac crest autograft to allograft in the lateral column lengthening component for operative correction of adult acquired flatfoot deformity. Foot Ankle Int 2007;28(1):8–12
4. Demetracopoulos CA, Nair P, Malzberg A, Deland JT. Outcomes of a stepcut lengthening calcaneal osteotomy for adult-acquired flatfoot deformity. Foot Ankle Int 2015;36(7):749–755

27 Spring Ligament

Johnny T.C. Lau, Rupesh Puna, and Joyce Fu

Abstract

The spring ligament complex is an important structure in the foot. In combination with the deltoid ligament, it provides major static stabilization of the medial longitudinal arch. The spring ligament is the primary restraint to talonavicular deformity, whereas the deltoid ligament provides the main restraint to valgus tilt and external rotation of the talus. There is a relative paucity of accepted methods of spring ligament reconstruction in current literature. This chapter will outline the evaluation of spring ligament pathology and detail our surgical reconstructive procedure of choice, which aims to simultaneously reconstruct both the spring ligament and deltoid given that both are often concurrently attenuated or pathologic, and we believe both should be addressed.

Keywords: *spring ligament, talocalcaneonavicular ligament, tibiospring ligament, medial longitudinal arch reconstruction, pes planus, planovalgus foot, posterior tibial tendon dysfunction*

27.1 Introduction

27.1.1 Pathology

- The spring ligament complex is an integral part of the foot.
- It provides static support to the medial longitudinal arch.
- Three bundles[1]:
  - Superomedial calcaneonavicular ligament.
  - Inferior calcaneonavicular ligament.
  - Third ligament.
- Pathology often noted in pes planus deformity.
- Commonly associated with posterior tibial tendon (PTT) dysfunction but can also be independent of PTT dysfunction in the context of pes planus deformity.[2,3]

27.2 Indications

- Failure of conservative treatment.
- More than 30 degrees of talonavicular (TN) uncoverage persisted on anteroposterior (AP) intraoperative fluoroscopic imaging.
- Ten degrees of plantar TN sag persisted on lateral intraoperative fluoroscopic imaging.[4]
- Repair may be performed if notable tear or laxity found in the ligament intraoperatively (usually performed in combination with flatfoot correction).

27.2.1 Nonoperative Options

- Orthotics:
  - Medial heel posting.
  - Medial arch support.

27.2.2 Clinical Evaluation of Pathology

- Inspection in stance:
  - Depression of medial longitudinal arch.
  - Valgus hindfoot alignment.
  - Pronation and abduction of the forefoot.
- Special examination maneuvers:
  - Single-leg heel rise:
    - ❖ Ability to perform with partial restoration of medial arch height indicates an intact PTT.
    - ❖ Inability to perform suggests PTT dysfunction.
    - ❖ Persistent forefoot abduction and valgus alignment of the hindfoot suggests spring ligament injury.[3]

27.2.3 Radiographic Evaluation

Weight-Bearing Radiographs of Bilateral Ankles and Feet

- Assessment of bony malalignment associated (i.e., pes planus deformity).
- Weight-bearing AP radiographs:
  - Talar-first metatarsal angle.
  - TN uncoverage.
  - Talocalcaneal angle.
  - Weight-bearing lateral radiographs.
  - Medial cuneiform height.
  - Meary's angle (lateral talar-first metatarsal angle).
  - Talocalcaneal angle.

Ultrasound

- Typical thickness of superomedial calcaneonavicular ligament is 4 mm (range 2.5–5.5 mm).
- Imaging of spring ligament insufficiency demonstrates
  - Increased thickness (>5.5 mm).
  - Loss of fibrillar echo pattern.
  - Increased vascularity.[3]
- This may represent chronic repetitive injury or a healing acute rupture.
- Dynamic ultrasound can also be used to evaluate PTT disorders.
- If PTT ruptured, suspect spring ligament attrition.[5]

Magnetic Resonance Imaging

- Moderately sensitive, highly specific.[6]
- Appropriate for patients with more ill-defined symptoms or suspected bone or joint pathology.[3]
  Injuries may appear widened on imaging, or can appear gapped from full-thickness rupture.[6]
- Evaluation of PTT should also be noted:
  - Degeneration at hypovascular portion of tendon, distal to medial malleolus.[7]

27.2.4 Contraindications to Operative Management

- Fixed deformity of TN joint.
- Residual TN subluxation > 50%.
- Degenerative TN joint.

27.3 Goal of Procedure

- Restoration of TN alignment.[8]
- To avoid hindfoot fusion.[4]
- Maintenance of transverse tarsal motion.
- Reduction in pain and improvement of function.

27.4 Advantages of the Procedure

- Direct repair of insufficient medial spring ligament supporting the TN joint.
- Addresses the medial and plantar band of the spring ligament.
- Augmented reconstruction prevents delayed stretching out and failure of the repair.

27.5 Key Principle to Surgical Procedure

- Tibiospring, or tibiocalcaneonavicular (TCN) ligament is one of the most consistently found components of the deltoid.[9]
- Superficial deltoid blends with dorsal aspect of superomedial spring ligament to provide medial tibiotalar and TN stability.
- It has the largest total attachment area and provides a significant portion of medial stability among other medial collateral and spring ligament complexes.[9]
- Our reconstructive procedure of choice aims to simultaneously reconstruct both the deltoid and spring ligaments.
- We believe both components must be addressed to sufficiently correct alignment.
- Bony realignment is imperative as an adjunct.

27.6 Preoperative Preparation and Patient Positioning

27.6.1 Preoperative Radiology

- Weight-bearing films of the foot and ankle obtained.
- Valgus stress films also completed to assess mortise and medial clear space (preoperative valgus tilt should be < 10 degrees).
- MRI (magnetic resonance imaging) is obtained to assess the PTT and spring ligament.

27.6.2 Reconstructive Graft Options

- Autograft (gracilis, semitendinosus, or peroneus longus[4,10]).
- Allograft (peroneus longus or semitendinosus).
- We prefer allograft to reduce donor site morbidity.

27.6.3 Positioning

- Patient positioned supine with the operative extremity resting in external rotation.
- Thigh tourniquet applied but not routinely inflated (senior surgeon's preference).
- Limb prepared with alcoholic chlorhexidine (70%/2%).
- Preoperative antibiotic prophylaxis administered.

27.7 Operative Technique

Our technique is essentially the same as that published by Grunfeld et al.[11] Our preference is to simultaneously reconstruct both the deltoid and spring ligament. Bony corrective procedures are initially performed (medial translational calcaneal osteotomy and/or first ray plantar flexion osteotomy and/or plantar flexion osteotomy of the first metatarsal).

27.7.1 Approach

- Universal medial longitudinal incision.
- PTT sheath is incised and the diseased portion of PTT is excised.
- Flexor digitorum longus (FDL) is harvested at master knot of Henry.
- One to five toes and ankle are maximally plantarflexed to maximize the length of FDL tendon harvested.
- FDL is tenodesed to flexor hallucis longus (FHL) prior to sectioning.
- Medial ligament complex is inspected and tears of native spring ligament are repaired and imbricated if possible.

27.7.2 Allograft Preparation

- Allograft peroneus longus is our preferred graft.
- Length of graft required is usually 25 cm (diameter ~ 6 mm).
- Allograft is folded in half to create two limbs (**Fig 27.1**).
- Folded portion of 2 cm is trimmed to allow easy passage through 7-mm sizer (**Fig 27.2**).
- No. 2 Ethibond is placed in folded portion, and also in distal 4 cm of each limb (**Fig 27.2**).

27.7.3 Tunnel Preparation

- Tunnels are drilled in navicular, medial malleolus, and sustentaculum tali (based on anatomic footprints of the tibionavicular, tibiospring, inferior calcaneonavicular, and tibiocalcaneal ligaments).

27.7.4 Tunnel Location (Fig. 27.3)

In brief, these locations are the following:
- Navicular tunnel at medial edge of navicular tuberosity in a dorsal to plantar direction.
- Medial malleolus tunnel made vertically at anterior portion of intercolliculus aimed toward medial side of distal tibia.

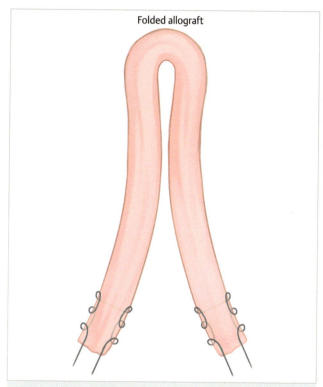

Fig 27.1 Allograft preparation: peroneus longus allograft is folded in half to create two limbs. No. 2 Ethibond locking Krakow suture placed in the distal 4 cm of each limb.

○ Sustentaculum tali tunnel centered 1 mm below sustentaculum tali directed 20 degrees plantarward away from subtalar joint.

27.7.5 Graft Passage and Tensioning

- All limbs are secured in their respective tunnels with an interference screw.
- Initially passed into the medial malleolar tunnel and secured.
- Two limbs are then passed into their respective calcaneal and navicular tunnels.
- Graft is passed from plantar to dorsal in the navicular (FDL also passed from plantar to dorsal in the navicular; **Fig 27.4**).
- Final tension is set in navicular midway between maximal and minimal tension to maintain excursion of transferred FDL.
- Calcaneal limb is secured in maximal tension.

27.8 Tips and Pearls

- Fix medial malleolar tunnel first, followed by navicular tunnel (preserve FDL excursion), and finally calcaneal tunnel.
- Do not overtighten or overconstrain.

27.9 Hazards and Pitfalls

- Be careful not to drill navicular tunnel too medial (avoid medial blowout).
- Take care when creating calcaneal tunnel to avoid calcaneal osteotomy site or fixation (so as not to compromise).

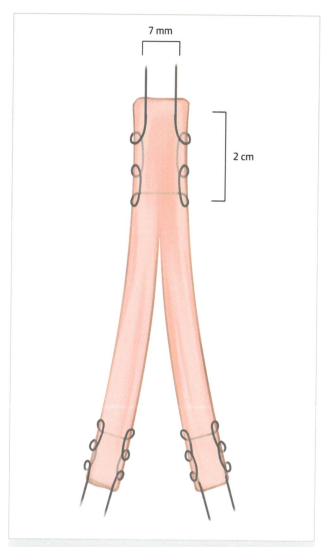

Fig 27.2 Allograft preparation: 2 cm of folded portion of allograft trimmed to allow easy passage through 7-mm sizer. No. 2 Ethibond locking Krakow suture also placed into folded portion.

27.10 Complications

- Infection (superficial or deep).
- Neurologic injury (tibial nerve during exposure of sustentaculum tali, sural nerve during calcaneal tunnel guidewire passage).
- Posterior tibial artery injury (during sustentaculum tali exposure).
- Peroneal tendon injury (passage of guidewire in calcaneal tunnel).
- Subtalar joint injury (during calcaneal tunnel preparation).
- Navicular tunnel blowout.
- Other general complications include deep vein thrombosis, stiffness, graft failure, and subsequent arthritis.

27.10.1 Salvage

- Where the navicular tunnel is too small for peroneus longus tendon, fixation is placed in the cuneiform.[4]
- Failure with ongoing symptoms and deformity may warrant arthrodesis.

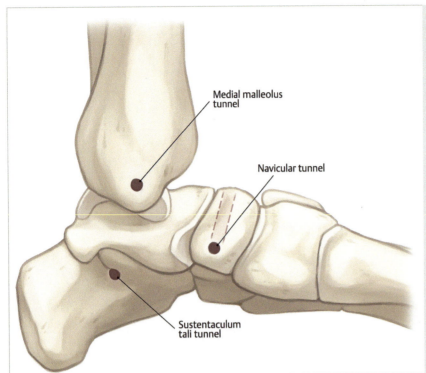

Fig 27.3 Tunnel placement: Medial malleolar tunnel vertical at anterior portion of inter-colliculus aimed toward medial side of tibia; navicular tunnel at medial edge of navicular tuberosity from dorsal to plantar (graft passed from plantar to dorsal); sustentaculum tali tunnel 1 mm below sustentaculum tali directed 20 degrees plantar so as to avoid subtalar joint.

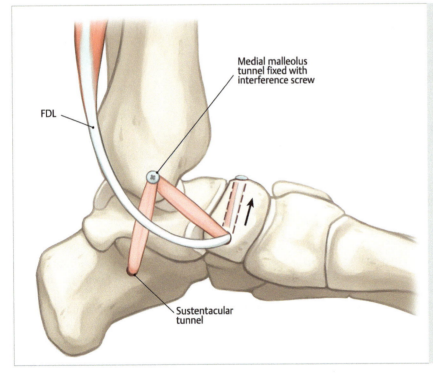

Fig 27.4 Graft passage and tensioning: Graft passed from plantar to dorsal in the navicular in a similar way in which flexor digitorum longus (FDL) is passed through the navicular tunnel. Ensure FDL is superficial to calcaneal limb of graft so excursion is not limited.

27.11 Postoperative Care

- Non–weight-bearing below knee splint for 2 weeks until sutures removed.
- Short leg fiberglass cast and non–weight-bearing for further 4 weeks.
- Gradual weight-bearing in aircast begun at 6 weeks with gentle range of motion.
- Therapy begun at 8 weeks focused on range of motion, strengthening, and proprioception.

Table 27.1 Summary of current literature reporting both radiographic results and patient-reported outcome measures of various spring ligament reconstruction techniques

Study	Number of patients	Concomitant bony or soft-tissue procedures	Radiographic parameters pre-op	Radiographic parameters post-op	Pre-op scores	Post-op scores
Johnson 2000[12]	16 patients	Yes	AP talo-first MT angle 24; TN coverage angle 34; Lat talo-first MT angle 18; Lat TC angle 55; MC to floor 12 mm	AP talo-first MT angle 18; TN coverage 17; Lat talo-first MT angle 8; Lat TC angle 34; MC to floor 18 mm		AOFAS hindfoot score 82; Maryland foot score 86
Williams et al 2010[4]	13 patients (14 feet)	Yes	AP first TMT angle 18.5; TN coverage angle 34.4; Lat calc pitch 3.9; Lat TN angle 12.0	AP first TMT angle 11.6; TN coverage angle 19.8; Lat calc pitch 8.7; Lat TN angle 0.30	AOFAS ankle hindfoot score	AOFAS ankle–hindfoot score 90; FAOS pain 83.7, symptoms 84.7, daily activities 91.8, sports activities 78.2, quality of life 75.9, stiffness 1.9, SF-36 77.3, VAS 2.1
Woo-Chun Lee 2014[13]	23 patients	No	AP talo-first MT angle 21.8; Lat talo-first MT angle 22.6; TN coverage angle 33.7	AP talo-first MT angle 13.3; Lat talo-first MT angle 9.0; TN coverage angle 20.8	AOFAS score 72.6	AOFAS score 86.4

Abbreviations: AOFAS, American Orthopaedic Foot and Ankle Society; AP, anteroposterior; calc, calcaneal; FAOS, Foot and Ankle Outcome Survey; Lat, lateral; MT, metat arsal; SF-36, 36-item short form health status survey; TC, talocalcaneal, TMT, tarsometatarsal; TN, talonavicular; VAS, visual analogue scale.

27.12 Outcomes

- There is limited literature (Johnson,[12] Williams,[4] Woo-Chun Lee,[13] Grunfeld et al[11]) detailing clinical and radiographic outcomes of various spring ligament reconstruction techniques.
- One limitation of these studies is that there is no one accepted reconstruction technique; in addition, all these studies except for one (Woo-Chun Lee[13]), report on spring ligament reconstruction as an adjunct to standard pes planus bony realignment surgery.
- To summarize the available literature, all of these series (Johnson,[12] Williams et al,[4] Williams,[14] Woo-Chun Lee,[13] Grunfeld et al[11]) have demonstrated an improvement in radiographic parameters, and those that have reported clinical outcomes (Woo Chun Lee,[13] Williams,[14] Williams et al[4]) have demonstrated improved patient reported outcome measures.
- Based on the available evidence, one must be cautious about drawing meaningful conclusions about the clinical benefit of spring ligament repair alone.

References

1. Taniguchi A, Tanaka Y, Takakura Y, Kadono K, Maeda M, Yamamoto H. Anatomy of the spring ligament. J Bone Joint Surg Am 2003;85-A(11):2174–2178

2. Orr JD, Nunley JA II. Isolated spring ligament failure as a cause of adult-acquired flatfoot deformity. Foot Ankle Int 2013;34(6):818–823

3. Tryfonidis M, Jackson W, Mansour R, et al. Acquired adult flat foot due to isolated plantar calcaneonavicular (spring) ligament insufficiency with a normal tibialis posterior tendon. Foot Ankle Surg 2008;14(2):89–95

4. Williams BR, Ellis SJ, Deyer TW, Pavlov H, Deland JT. Reconstruction of the spring ligament using a peroneus longus autograft tendon transfer. Foot Ankle Int 2010;31(7):567–577

5. Deland JT, de Asla RJ, Sung IH, Ernberg LA, Potter HG. Posterior tibial tendon insufficiency: which ligaments are involved? Foot Ankle Int 2005;26(6):427–435

6. Yao L, Gentili A, Cracchiolo A. MR imaging findings in spring ligament insufficiency. Skeletal Radiol 1999;28(5):245–250

7. Robinson SP, Hodgkins CW, Sculco P, et al. Spring ligament reconstruction for -posterior tibial tendon insufficiency: the Y-tendon reconstruction technique. Tech Foot & Ankle. 2006;5(3):198–203

8. Tan GJ, Kadakia AR, Ruberte Thiele RA, Hughes RE. Novel reconstruction of a static medial ligamentous complex in a flatfoot model. Foot Ankle Int 2010;31(8):695–700

9. Cromeens BP, Kirchhoff CA, Patterson RM, et al. An attachment-based description of the medial collateral and spring ligament complexes. Foot Ankle Int 2015;36(6):710–721

10. Choi K, Lee S, Otis JC, Deland JT. Anatomical reconstruction of the spring ligament using peroneus longus tendon graft. Foot Ankle Int 2003;24(5):430–436

11. Grunfeld R, Oh I, Flemister S, et al. Reconstruction of the deltoid-spring ligament: tibiocalcaneonavicular ligament complex. Tech Foot & Ankle. 2016;15:39–46

12. Johnson JE, Cohen BE, DiGiovanni BF, Lamdan R. Subtalar arthrodesis with flexor digitorum longus tendon transfer and spring ligament repair for treatment of posterior tibial tendon insufficiency. Foot Ankle Int 2000;21(9):722–729

13. Lee W, Young Y. Spring ligament reconstruction using the autogenous flexor hallucis longus tendon. Orthopaedics 2014;37(7):467–471

14. Williams BR, Ellis SJ, Deland JT. Spring ligament reconstruction in posterior tibial tendon insufficiency. Current Orthopaedic Practice 2010;21(3):268–272

28 Peroneal Tendon Repair

Christopher W. Reb and Gregory C. Berlet

Abstract

Peroneal tendon pathology is common. When this pathology includes a tear, nonsurgical treatment is unlikely to be successful. In the setting of surgical repair, peroneal tendon repair offers reliable pain relief and functional recovery. Careful patient evaluation is required to determine if the procedure should be performed alone or in combination with adjunct procedures to address underlying or related pathology. Often, multiple procedures can be achieved through a well-localized incision. Attention to detail during each step of the procedure key will help achieve the surgical goals while minimizing the risk to adjacent neurologic structures.

Keywords: *tendinosis, tendon tear, peroneal tendon, peroneus brevis, peroneus longus, reconstruction, surgical technique*

28.1 Indications and Pathology

- Acute peroneal tendon tear.
- Acute peroneal tendon rupture.
- Peroneal tenosynovitis.
- Peroneal tendinosis.
- Peroneal instability.

28.1.1 Clinical Evaluation

- History of pain and swelling along the course of the peroneal tendons.
- Ask about past trauma, including inversion ankle injuries.
- Mechanical symptoms may include snapping, subluxation, or dislocation around the fibula.
- Examine for hindfoot deformity that may only be present when weight-bearing.
- Evaluate all cavovarus feet for flexibility with weight-bearing and hindfoot correction with Coleman's block testing. Bear in mind that subtle cavovarus deformity may be contributing.
- Evaluate for ligamentous and functional ankle instability.
- Consider associated pathology such as posterior ankle impingement syndrome, anterolateral ankle impingement syndrome, ankle syndesmosis sprain, subtalar varus instability, talus osteochondral defect (OCD), fifth metatarsal base fracture, and symptomatic os peroneum.

28.1.2 Radiographic Evaluation

- Weight-bearing anteroposterior (AP), mortise, and lateral X-rays of the hindfoot to evaluate for deformity, ankle or hindfoot arthritis, and radiographic signs of past trauma, such as previous avulsion fractures.
- Magnetic resonance imaging (MRI) without contrast is indicated to confirm peroneal tendon rupture, to rule out alternative diagnoses, or when peroneal symptoms are refractory to an initial period of conservative treatment.
- Computed tomography (CT) with thin slice reconstruction may be used to confirm peroneal tendon rupture.

- Ultrasound is operator dependent, but can be used to confirm peroneal tendon rupture and is the best real-time modality for assessment of peroneal instability.

28.1.3 Nonoperative Options

- Protected mobilization, rest, ice, compression, elevation (PRICE).
- Oral or topical nonsteroidal anti-inflammatory drugs (NSAIDs).
- Local injection or short course of oral corticosteroids.
- Physical therapy focused on hip, knee, and ankle proprioceptive training and strengthening.
- Bracing.
- Activity avoidance, modification, or retraining.

28.1.4 Contraindications

- Active infection.
- Patient medically unfit for surgery.
- Patient noncompliance anticipated.
- Uncorrected hindfoot deformity.
- Complex regional pain syndrome.

28.2 Goals of Surgical Procedure

- Pain relief.
- Functional improvement.
- Preserve native tissues.

28.3 Advantages of Surgical Procedure

- Peroneal repair can be performed alone or in combination with other procedures.
- Single approach allows multiple procedures.

28.4 Key Principles

- Well-localized incision for adequate visualization.
- Meticulous anatomic dissection.
- Atraumatic soft-tissue handling.
- Address all pathology.
- Restore the superior peroneal retinaculum.

28.5 Preoperative Preparation and Patient Positioning

The patient is positioned laterally on a beanbag with nonsterile ipsilateral thigh tourniquet set to 250 or 300 mm Hg. The nonsurgical limb is outfitted with a pneumatic serial compressive device in a semiflexed position. All bony prominences are well padded.

The surgical limb is supported with a stack of blankets or foam platform. The limb is prepped and draped to above the knee.

28.6 Operative Technique

The limb is elevated, exsanguinated with an Esmarch bandage, and tourniquet is inflated. The lateral malleolus, lateral neck of the talus, and fifth metatarsal base are palpated. A curvilinear incision is drawn over the course of the peroneal tendons. If the surgical plan calls for ankle lateral ligament reconstruction, the incision can be modified by orienting it from the peroneal tendons proximal to the lateral malleolus, over the tip of the fibula toward the superior aspect of the anterior process of the calcaneus (**Fig. 28.1**).

After the skin is divided and hemostasis is achieved, branches of the sural nerve, particularly the dorsal lateral cutaneous nerve to the foot, should be sought and protected as best as possible.

The inferior peroneal retinaculum forms separate sheaths around the peroneus brevis and longus. The tendon sheaths can be longitudinally incised just distal to the tip of the fibula to create a window for evaluating the tendons. Thickened and inflamed tenosynovium is often present and must be excised for best visualization.

The peroneal brevis is often diseased or torn within the retrofibular groove of the fibula. Using this window, the brevis tendon can be distally retracted and inspected to confirm this pathology (**Fig. 28.2**). In the event that the tendon appears healthy, this maneuver allows the surgeon to avoid taking down the superior peroneal retinaculum.

When peroneal pathology is known or highly suspected in the retrofibular groove, or when peroneal instability is present and superior peroneal retinaculum reconstruction is indicated, it is important to divide the superior peroneal retinaculum, leaving a cuff of tissue on the fibula for later use when reconstructing it. A linear metallic instrument, such a freer elevator, can be used to localize the incision to divide the superior peroneal retinaculum and to protect the peroneal tendons below during this step.

At this point, the posterior leaf of the retinaculum often has tenosynovium adherent to its internal surface. The tenosynovium can be peeled off, revealing the glistening, striated undersurface of the retinaculum (**Fig. 28.3**). A stay suture is used to mark this posterior leaf for later retrieval.

If a low-lying peroneus brevis muscle belly or a peroneus quartus is present, acting as a space occupying lesion in the retrofibular space, the muscle belly can be dissected away prior to addressing the peroneal tendons.

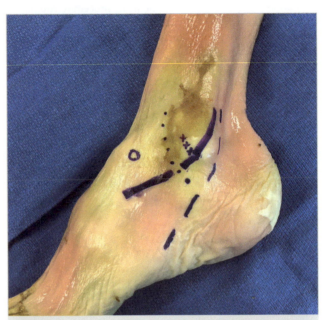

Fig. 28.1 The standard approach to the peroneals follows their course along the hindfoot (solid line). Alternatively, the incision can be modified by directing it distally over the superior aspect of the anterior process of the calcaneus to allow ankle joint and ligament procedures to be performed through the same incision (dashed line).

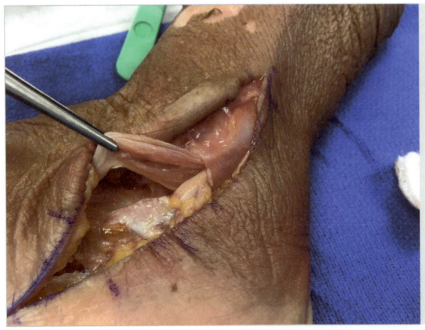

Fig. 28.2 Before committing to dividing the superior peroneal retinaculum, the peroneal sheath can be opened below the retinaculum and the tendon can be distally displaced to evaluate the appearance of the tendon lying in the retrofibular groove of the fibula.

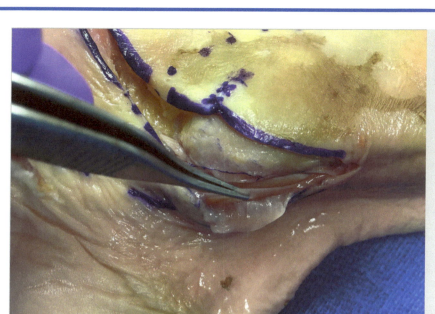

Fig. 28.3 Dissection of adherent tenosynovium from the internal surface of the superior peroneal retinaculum reveals the glistening, striated appearance of the retinaculum itself.

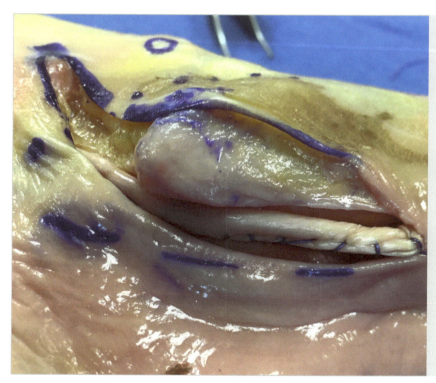

Fig. 28.4 After tendon debridement, tubularization can be achieved using an internally buried running stitch of absorbable suture.

Oftentimes, the tenosynovium can be excised as a single unit using the following sequence of dissection. First, the peroneal longus can be elevated out of the groove and the tenosynovial reflection is dissected away from the posterior margin of the tendon. Then, the peroneus brevis is elevated out of the groove and the tenosynovium is dissected away from its posterior margin. Finally, the tenosynovium is dissected from posterior to anterior off the retinaculum and finally the retrofibular groove.

At this point, the integrity of the calcaneofibular and posterior talofibular ligaments can be assessed with direct visualization.

Next, the peroneus brevis tendon can be debrided of tendinotic or torn tissue. It is generally recommended that if greater than 50% of the tendon remains after debridement, it may be preserved. Often the tendon is flattened and may be repaired by tubularization of the tendon.[1] To do this, a buried knot is tied at one end of the repair and a running stitch is used along the length of the repair and completed with another buried knot. Absorbable suture, such as 3–0 Monocryl or Vicryl, is preferred (**Fig. 28.4**).

In the setting of a split peroneal tendon tear, the location of the tear will guide the surgical strategy. A peripheral tear that occupies less than 30% of the tendon can either be repaired or excised. If excised, the residual tendon is repaired with Monocryl as a running suture. A central tear of the peroneal tendon needs to be repaired. The repair technique for a central tear is a running 2–0 Vicryl with buried knots followed by a Monocryl suture with buried knots on the periphery.

The peroneus longus is then evaluated, debrided, and repaired as needed using the same technique as above. At this point, adjunctive procedures may be completed such as calcaneofibular ligament repair, fibular groove deepening, anterolateral ankle arthrotomy, and lateral ankle ligament reconstruction.

Repair of the superior peroneal retinaculum is saved for the last step before skin closure. Generally, three horizontal mattress sutures based off the fibula are used to draw the posterior leaf of the retinaculum beneath the anterior leaf at the anterior margin of the fibula grove (**Fig. 28.5**). To achieve this, the horizontal mattress suture is passed posterior, first from the anterior leave, then the posterior leave, and then passed anteriorly through the posterior leave, and finally through the anterior leaf.

When the pathology is localized to the peroneal tubercle or cuboid groove, the lateral approach allows direct visualization of these structures. Following tendon debridement and repair, the inferior extensor retinaculum does not require repair.

Peroneal tubercle hypertrophy is common in the foot with a varus hindfoot. When present, the peroneal tubercle should be removed with an osteotome or ronguer, followed by a rasp to smooth the cut bone surface. Bone wax may be applied at the surgeon's discretion.

Skin closure is performed in a layered fashion with absorbable suture for the subcuticular layer and either nylon or Monocryl for the epidermis.

28.7 Tips and Pearls

When delivering the tendons out of the groove, a stack of towels under the medial forefoot relaxes tension so that the tendons can lay anteriorly without need for constant retraction.

When repairing the superior peroneal retinaculum, a freer elevator can be placed over top of the peroneal tendons both to serve a spacer so that the retinaculum is not overly constricting and to avoid inadvertent suture passage through one of the tendons.

Use of amniotic tissue derivatives in tendon repair is an area of interest in contemporary foot and ankle research. These products are marketed to regulate inflammation and decrease scarring. The tissue is applied as a wrap or in a particulate form. Given the added cost, the authors mainly utilize this technology when primarily repairing severely degenerative tendons and in revision cases.

28.8 Hazards and Pitfalls

The sural lateral cutaneous nerve has variable spatial anatomy at the level of the ankle. Great care must be taken when making the skin incision for the peroneal approach so as not to transect it.

It is important to tag the posterior leaf of the superior peroneal retinaculum so that it does not become retracted into the posterior ankle soft tissues, thus making it difficult to retrieve later. This could also lead to inadvertently utilizing subcuticular tissue or the pre-Achilles fat pad for the retinacular repair.

If ankle arthroscopy is performed before peroneal tendon dissection, minimizing diffusion of arthroscopy fluid into the anterolateral ankle soft tissues is important to minimize soft-tissue swelling. Strategies for this include making limited

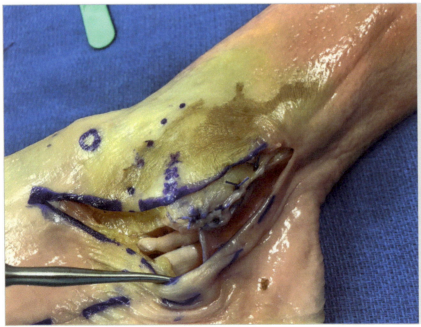

Fig. 28.5 The superior peroneal retinaculum can be reconstructed using a horizontal mattress suture that imbricates the posterior leaf below the anterior leaf.

capsular incisions and using minimum necessary pump pressure. If this occurs, the soft tissues can be desiccated using dry lap sponges and Esmarch compression after the peroneal incision has been made.

Failure to recognize and correct cavovarus deformity may be a cause for poor outcome. When cavovarus deformity does not correct with weight-bearing or with the use of a lateral hindfoot and forefoot posted orthotic with a first ray relief, correction should be planned.

28.9 Complications/Bailout/Salvage

Preoperative planning should include contingency strategies for when extensive tissue debridement is needed. These strategies include side-to-side tendon transfer, flexor hallucis longus transfer, and allograft reconstruction. For the latter, a staged procedure may be indicated by first implanting Hunter's rods and later performing the allograft reconstruction or tendon transfer.[2]

28.10 Postoperative Care

The wounds are dressed with nonadherent gauze, 4 × 4 gauze, an ABD (abdominal) pad, and sterile cast padding. Then, a well-padded short leg splint is fashioned with the foot held in neutral dorsiflexion and slight eversion. The stitches are removed at 2 weeks. The patient maintains non–weight-bearing for 4 to 6 weeks. Open chain active ankle range of motion is initiated at 4 weeks and ankle rehabilitation under the supervision of a physical therapist is initiated at 6 weeks.[3]

28.11 Outcomes

In general, pain relief, functional recovery, and patient satisfaction after peroneal tendon repair are expected in the long term.[4,5] Minor complications, such as wound infection or nerve injury, are infrequent, and major complications requiring reoperation are rare. Patients should be advised that return to unrestricted closed chain activities (e.g., elliptical training or biking) may be as long as 4 months and that open chain exercise (e.g., running and kicking) may take up to a year. Some degree of swelling may last for more than 1 year. Expectations should be tempered in higher demand patients or those whose pathology is more advanced at the time of presentation.

References

1. Krause JO, Brodsky JW. Peroneus brevis tendon tears: pathophysiology, surgical reconstruction, and clinical results. Foot Ankle Int 1998;19(5):271–279
2. Raikin SM, Schick FA, Karanjia HN. Use of a hunter rod for staged reconstruction of peroneal tendons. J Foot Ankle Surg 2016;55(1):198–200
3. van Dijk PA, Lubberts B, Verheul C, DiGiovanni CW, Kerkhoffs GM. Rehabilitation after surgical treatment of peroneal tendon tears and ruptures. Knee Surg Sports Traumatol Arthrosc 2016;24(4):1165–1174
4. Demetracopoulos CA, Vineyard JC, Kiesau CD, Nunley JA II. Long-term results of debridement and primary repair of peroneal tendon tears. Foot Ankle Int 2014;35(3):252–257
5. Steginsky B, Riley A, Lucas DE, Philbin TM, Berlet GC. Patient-reported outcomes and return to activity after peroneus brevis repair. Foot Ankle Int 2016;37(2):178–185

29 Peroneal Groove Deepening for Peroneal Subluxation

Gregory P. Guyton

Abstract

The peroneal tendons run within a concave groove in the retrofibular region as they cross behind the ankle, and are held in place by the superior peroneal retinaculum (SPR). Forceful firing of the peroneal tendons during an eversion injury can result in stretching, tearing, or avulsion of the SPR and dislocation or subluxation of the peroneal tendons out of the groove. This can be predisposed to by having a shallow or even convex retrofibular groove, but can occur even in patients with a relatively normal groove depth. There are two variations of peroneal subluxation, one where one or both of the tendons sublux or dislocate completely out of the groove and a variation where the peroneus longus and brevis sublux within the sheath—reversing their anatomic positions causing dysmotility and pain. This condition is addressed by a deepening procedure of the retrofibular peroneal groove as outlined in this chapter.

Keywords: retrofibular groove, groove deepening, fibular osteotomy, peroneal tendons, peroneal subluxation, peroneal dislocation

29.1 Indications

- The *primary* indication is subluxation or dislocation of the peroneal tendons associated with a convex groove on the posterior fibula.
- A *secondary* indication is the presence of any tear or pathology requiring reconstruction of the peroneal tendons passing through the retromalleolar space. Substantial pressure reduction on the peroneal tendons occurs with groove deepening even in the presence of normal fibular morphology; groove deepening has been advocated as a biomechanical adjunct to reconstructive procedures.[1]

29.1.1 Pathology

- The normal retromalleolar groove is concave. In the presence of a convex groove, subluxation of one or both tendons is more likely to occur around the posterolateral margin of the fibula.
- Subluxation may occur as a result of an acute injury or from chronic attrition of the insertion of the superior peroneal retinaculum (SPR) on the posterior margin of the distal fibula.
- Typically, the periosteum of the posterolateral fibula will also be elevated, resulting in a periosteal pouch in continuity with the peroneal sheath. Alternatively, a small avulsion of the fibular margin itself will be present and is seen as a "fleck sign" on plain radiographs.
- A longitudinal tear of one of the peroneal tendons may result in subluxation of only a portion of the tendon, creating an incarceration of the tear around the posterolateral fibula. The peroneus brevis is relatively flat as it passes through the retromalleolar space and is more commonly involved in this pattern.
- Subluxation may occur within the peroneal sheath (intrasheath subluxation) or the tendons may dislocate completely out from behind the fibular.

29.1.2 Clinical Evaluation

- Some acute peroneal subluxations are missed in the setting of ankle sprains. Complete irreducible dislocations may only be suspected based upon the presence of lateral fullness and peroneal weakness.
- Subacute or voluntary subluxation of the tendons may be elicited by having the patient forcibly evert the foot against resistance while simultaneously moving from a plantarflexed to a dorsiflexed ankle position. Marked lateral prominence will result.
- Voluntarily induced snapping of the tendons at or above the retromalleolar space may indicate intrasheath subluxation of the peroneal tendons. The tendons dynamically cross over each other within the sheath without passing around the posterolateral corner of the fibula. Most patients can reproduce the snapping with forcible circumduction of the hindfoot.

29.1.3 Radiographic Evaluation

- Internally rotated (mortise) views of the ankle may demonstrate a "fleck sign" indicating avulsion of the insertion of the SPR.
- Magnetic resonance imaging (MRI) of the ankle may be very useful in evaluation of peroneal pathology because it allows evaluation of the morphology of the groove (**Fig. 29.1**) and detection of tears or an accessory peroneus quartus. The false-negative rate, however, is high, and a high index of suspicion must be maintained for subtle longitudinal peroneal tears in patients with associated ankle instability even in the presence of a negative study.[2]
- Dynamic evidence of peroneal subluxation can be documented through ultrasound or dynamic computed tomography (CT). In practice, MRI is typically preferred as a readily interpretable modality, and these are necessary only when the combination of MRI and clinical examination is equivocal.

29.1.4 Nonoperative Options

- True dislocation of the peroneals is best considered a surgical problem.
- Historical precedent exists for cast immobilization of relocatable peroneal tendons following an acute trauma. The success rate is less than 50% and the required immobilization will delay rehabilitation of other associated injuries (typically an anterior talofibular ligament [ATFL] tear).[3] Cast treatment is recommended only for patients that are poor surgical candidates.
- Chronic dynamic posterolateral subluxation of the peroneal tendons eventually leads to further peroneal degeneration as the tendon forcibly passes around the posterior margin of the fibula. Surgical intervention is recommended.
- Intrasheath subluxation alone has not been demonstrated to lead to chronic degeneration. The problem may be made more symptomatic by the presence of inflamed tenosynovium. Immobilization, physical therapy, or modalities may be safely attempted as alternative to surgical intervention.

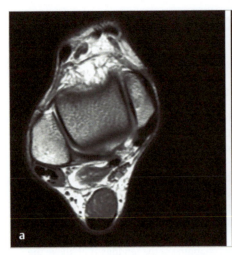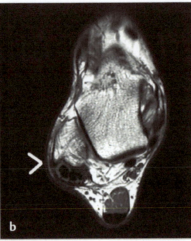

Fig. 29.1 Convex peroneal groove **(a)** before and **(b)** after (*arrow*) groove deepening.

29.1.5 Contraindications

- Groove deepening is relatively benign and contraindications are minimal.
- Care must be exercised if the patient has had a prior tenodesis procedure for augmented lateral ankle ligament reconstruction because the prior bone tunnels may be too extensive to allow a standard trapdoor deepening procedure.

29.2 Goals of Surgical Procedure

- The primary goal of the procedure is to eliminate subluxation of the peroneal tendons around the posterolateral corner of the fibula.
- The secondary goal of the procedure is to create a more capacious retromalleolar space, reduce the pressure on the tendons themselves, and eliminate any extraneous sources of impingement that may contribute to pain or intrasheath subluxation.[1,4]

29.3 Advantages of Surgical Procedure

- A groove deepening procedure utilizing a cortical trapdoor allows for extensive deepening of the retromalleolar groove if necessary. If properly performed, the result is minimal exposure of the tendon to a raw bony surface.
- The most common alternative to the trapdoor procedure is the indirect method in which a drill from the distal tip of the fibula is used to remove the cancellous bone underneath the posterior cortex. A tamp is used to forcibly impact the posterior bone.[5] The overall degree of dissection is similar to the traditional technique, but any redundancy of the SPR is not as readily addressed.
- Simple retinacular repair without groove deepening has also been advocated. Although equivalent results have been reported in small retrospective selected series,[6] no randomized controlled prospective trial has compared the two techniques. The secondary benefits of creating space for and reducing pressure on the tendons remain attractive.

- Tendoscopic groove deepening with creation of a raw bony surface has been reported,[7] but does not allow access to associated peroneal pathology and has significant potential for postoperative adhesion.
- Posterior sliding bone block techniques are effective at eliminating subluxation, but have considerable potential for adhesion and do not provide decompression of the tendon in the retromalleolar space.[8] They remain a viable option for rare cases with severely dysplastic fibulae.

29.4 Key Principles

- Adequate decompression of the sheath is mandatory.
- Redundancy in the SPR must be eliminated along with any periosteal elevation.
- Early motion is always indicated for any peroneal reconstruction.

29.5 Preoperative Preparation and Patient Positioning

- A bolster is used under the ipsilateral buttock to internally rotate the operative leg.
- Thigh tourniquet control is used.

29.6 Operative Technique

- An extensile incision along the peroneal sheath is mandatory because peroneal tears may be encountered extending distally or proximally. MRI alone is not adequate to exclude this possibility.
- Chronic ankle instability often coexists with peroneal pathology, and ligament reconstruction may be required. Both sites may be readily addressed with an extensile incision placed over the midline of the fibula.
- The critical portion of the SPR is usually visible as a condensation of fibers attaching to the posterior margin of the fibula and beginning at the distal tip (**Fig. 29.2**). The first 1.5 cm of the sheath is the most mechanically important portion. Open the peroneal sheath below this level with a gentle spreading technique.

- The SPR is now divided *directly off its posterior attachment to the fibula* (**Fig. 29.2** inset). If a periosteal pouch and/or an avulsed bony fragment is present, manipulate the tendons back into position and divide the SPR at the site that would be expected to attach to the posterior margin of the bone.
- The peroneal tendons are now separately inspected. **Table 29.1** provides an algorithm for addressing peroneal pathology in the retromalleolar region.
- Excess tenosynovium and peroneus brevis muscle belly extending into the retromalleolar space is excised. If a peroneus quartus is present, it will have a small muscle belly in the sheath and a separate tendon blending into the calcaneal periosteum (**Fig. 29.3**). It is nonfunctional and should be excised.
- The peroneals are now dislocated anteriorly.
- A microsagittal saw is used to create a posterior to anterior cut just behind the posterolateral margin of the distal fibula. The cut must extend approximately 5 mm around the tip of the fibula and proximally for 2.5 cm (**Fig. 29.4**).
- Transverse counter cuts are made at the proximal and distal ends of the trapdoor cut (**Fig. 29.5**).

- An 8-mm Hoke osteotome is used to gently crack open the posterior cortex of the fibula, hinging on the uncut medial margin (**Fig. 29.6**).
- A rongeur or burr is used to remove cancellous bone from the posterior fibula as necessary to deepen the groove (**Fig. 29.6** inset).
- A bone tamp is used to reposition the trapdoor into place (**Fig. 29.7**). Deepening of at least 4 to 6 mm is typically expected. No fixation is needed; impaction and pressure from the relocated peroneal tendons will be adequate.
- Two 0.062 K-wire holes are drilled from the lateral cortex into the groove just posterior to the now-impacted trapdoor of cortical bone. A 2–0 Ethibond suture is used in mattress fashion to advance the previously divided SPR into the groove (**Fig. 29.8** and inset). This maneuver covers the raw bone of the overhanging lip of posterolateral fibula and eliminates any redundancy in the SPR itself.
- Free gliding of both tendons is confirmed. The remaining proximal portion of the SPR is repaired with 2–0 Vicryl suture.

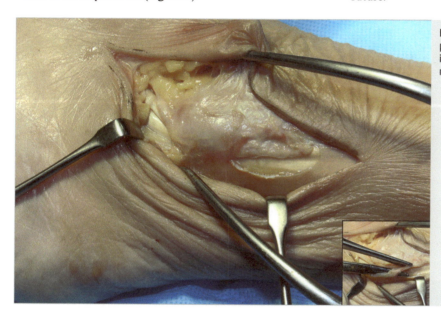

Fig. 29.2 The critical portion of the superior peroneal retinaculum (SPR). Inset: the SPR is now divided directly off its posterior attachment to the fibula.

Table 29.1 Strategies for addressing retromalleolar peroneal pathology based on extent of tear

Extent of tear		
Less than 25%	**25–50%**	**Over 50%**
Debridement and tubularization 6–0 Prolene suture in a running baseball stitch pattern is minimally reactive and has adequate strength to invert the tendon margins on themselves	*Repair* For simple longitudinal split tears *Debridement and tubularization* For extensive fibrillation	*Semitendinosus allograft reconstruction* For the brevis or brevis and peroneal tendon tears only Proximal to the SPR running to the fifth metatarsal base *FDL transfer* For patients with inadequate proximal muscle Restores balance of the foot but less effective strength *Proximal tenodesis* Alternative for peroneus longus-only tears or less active patients

Abbreviations: FDL, flexor digitorum longus; SPR, superior peroneal retinaculum.

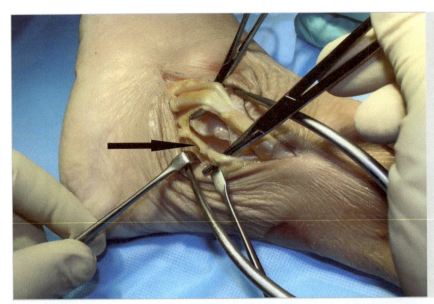

Fig. 29.3 A peroneus quartus (arrow) may be encountered and should be excised.

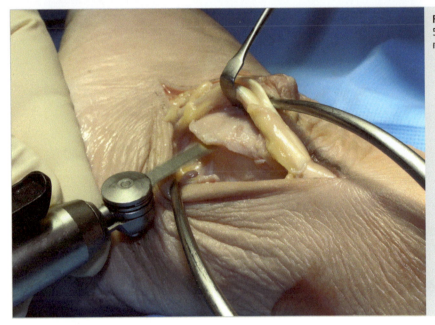

Fig. 29.4 The cut must extend approximately 5 mm around the tip of the fibula and proximally for 2.5 cm.

29.7 Tips and Pearls

- Combining peroneal groove deepening with a Broström procedure is straightforward. If an augmented lateral ankle ligament reconstruction is considered necessary because of recurrence or tissue insufficiency, tenodesis bone tunnels may present a challenge. Consider augmentation using a nonabsorbable suture brace.
- Allograft reconstruction of the peroneal tendons is a viable option for high-grade pathology of the tendons even if a groove deepening is necessary. No undue scar formation appears to occur.
- Early motion is mandatory for all peroneal tendon reconstructions, and groove deepening is no exception. Supervised motion in physical therapy is recommended within the first 10 days.

- SPR reconstruction is critical, but reconstruction of the inferior peroneal retinaculum is not. At this level around the peroneal tubercle, both tendons enter separate restrictive sheaths. Have a low threshold to take down and open both sheaths as well as remove the septum between them to decompress, expose, and mobilize the tendons if necessary.
- A prominent peroneal tubercle on the calcaneus may be a separate nidus of peroneal pathology. If present, it can be readily debulked with a rongeur. Careful preoperative examination will assist in determining whether this area is also symptomatic.
- The peroneus quartus is often mistaken for a torn peroneus brevis on MRI. Do not mistake the extratendinous slip of the peroneus quartus for a split tear of the peroneus brevis. The peroneus quartus must be excised from a symptomatic retromalleolar space.

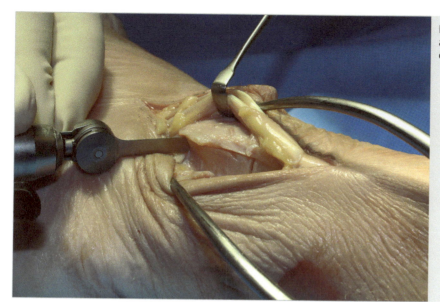

Fig. 29.5 Transverse counter cuts are made at the proximal and distal ends of the trap-door cut.

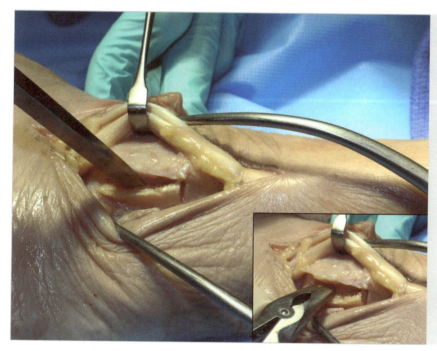

Fig. 29.6 An 8-mm Hoke osteotome is used to gently crack open the posterior cortex of the fibula, hinging on the uncut medial margin. Inset: a rongeur or burr is used to remove cancellous bone from the posterior fibula as necessary to deepen the groove.

29.8 Hazards and Pitfalls

- *Avoid nonextensile incisions.* This point especially holds true for peroneal pathology. In particular, the archaic "J" incision for the Broström procedure is difficult to extend.
- *Avoid attempting peroneal reconstruction, lateral ankle ligament reconstruction, and calcaneal osteotomy through one long incision.* The rate of sural nerve dysfunction is remarkably high. A lateralizing calcaneal osteotomy should be accomplished through a minimal incision technique or short (3- to 4-cm) parallel incision, leaving the sural nerve undisturbed. A 4-cm skin bridge is adequate if the calcaneal incision is limited.
- *Do not divide the SPR over the middle of the sheath.* Adequate advancement of the SPR under the posterolateral lip of bone may be possible only if it is taken *directly off the posterior margin of the fibula*.

- *Ensure free gliding of the peroneal tendons at the end of the case.*

29.9 Complications/Bailout/Salvage

- An irreparable peroneal tendon is the most commonly encountered problem. In the presence of suspected high-grade pathology, allograft may prove to be a more straightforward salvage procedure than tendon transfer or repair.
- Fragmentation of the posterior cortex may occur. In a worst-case scenario, the posterior cortex can be discarded and aggressive early motion performed. Although the tendon will be gliding against a denuded cancellous surface, historical precedent exists for this approach.

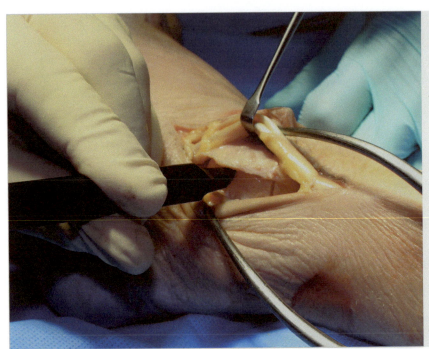

Fig. 29.7 A bone tamp is used to position the trapdoor into place.

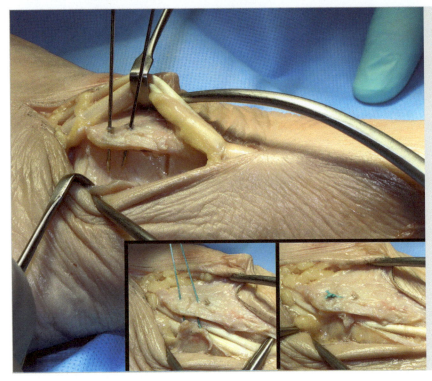

Fig. 29.8 Two 0.062 K-wire holes are drilled from the lateral cortex into the groove just posterior to the now-impacted trapdoor of cortical bone. Insets: a 2–0 Ethibond suture is used in mattress fashion to advance the previously divided superior peroneal retinaculum (SPR) into the groove.

Fracture of the distal fibula is a rare complication. Screw fixation should be available if necessary.

29.10 Postoperative Care

- Peroneal reconstructions should be moved as early as the wound allows.
- Avoid active eversion past 5 degrees for the first 3 weeks, but encourage passive motion and active inversion.
- Weight-bearing in a boot is allowed at 3 weeks, with weaning to a functional ankle brace at 6 weeks.

- Sports activities may be resumed once peroneal tendon strength returns. This may vary between 3 to 6 months depending on the activity.

29.11 Outcomes

- The advantages of groove deepening over simple retinacular repair are difficult to demonstrate because of the relative rarity of the condition.[8]
- A recent systematic review of extant level IV studies[9] provides moderate support for the addition of groove

deepening based on rates of return to sport, but level I evidence is lacking. Reported pooled study outcomes include a rate of return to sport following groove deepening of 91 to 100% and time to return to sport of 4.6 ± 2.6 months with overall incidence of re-dislocation of the peroneal tendons following the procedure of 1.5%.[9]

References

1. Title CI, Jung H-G, Parks BG, Schon LC. The peroneal groove deepening procedure: a biomechanical study of pressure reduction. Foot Ankle Int 2005;26(6):442–448

2. O'Neill PJ, Van Aman SE, Guyton GP. Is MRI adequate to detect lesions in patients with ankle instability? Clin Orthop Relat Res 2010;468(4):1115–1119

3. Escalas F, Figueras JM, Merino JA. Dislocation of the peroneal tendons. Long-term results of surgical treatment. J Bone Joint Surg Am 1980;62(3):451–453

4. Raikin SM, Elias I, Nazarian LN. Intrasheath subluxation of the peroneal tendons. J Bone Joint Surg Am 2008;90(5):992–999

5. Ogawa BK, Thordarson DB, Zalavras C. Peroneal tendon subluxation repair with an indirect fibular groove deepening technique. Foot Ankle Int 2007;28(11):1194–1197

6. Cho J, Kim JY, Song DG, Lee WC. Comparison of outcome after retinaculum repair with and without fibular groove deepening for recurrent dislocation of the peroneal tendons. Foot Ankle Int 2014;35(7):683–689

7. Vega J, Batista JP, Golanó P, Dalmau A, Viladot R. Tendoscopic groove deepening for chronic subluxation of the peroneal tendons. Foot Ankle Int 2013;34(6):832–840

8. Ferran NA, Oliva F, Maffulli N. Recurrent subluxation of the peroneal tendons. Sports Med 2006;36(10):839–846

9. van Dijk PA, Gianakos AL, Kerkhoffs GM, Kennedy JG. Return to sports and clinical outcomes in patients treated for peroneal tendon dislocation: a systematic review. Knee Surg Sports Traumatol Arthrosc 2016;24(4):1155–1164

30 Cavovarus Reconstruction

Chuanshun Wang and Selene G. Parekh

Abstract

The deformity of cavovarus foot is typically a result of muscular imbalance with an underlying neurologic disorder. The most common cause of symptomatic cavovarus deformity is hereditary motor sensory neuropathies including Charcot–Marie–Tooth disease. Other causes include trauma, tumor, stroke, poliomyelitis, and idiopathic problems. Classical pathologic changes such as forefoot pronation, high arch, hindfoot varus, and Achilles contracture may lead to abnormal load distribution resulting in ankle instability, peroneal tendonitis, lateral column overload or stress fracture, and finally degenerative arthritis. Surgical treatment is indicated in symptomatic and/or progressive cavovarus deformity. Many procedures are available for foot and ankle surgeons to employ in the surgical correction of the equinovarus foot. In this chapter, we will discuss the tricks of the trade of cavovarus deformity correction.

Keywords: *cavovarus deformity, surgery, Charcot–Marie–Tooth disease, calcaneal osteotomy, first metatarsal osteotomy, tendon transfer, Achilles lengthening, arthrodesis*

30.1 Indications and Pathology

- Cavovarus deformity occurs as a result of muscle imbalance around the foot and ankle. As it is the most discussed, the Charcot–Marie–Tooth (CMT) disease is a good example for understanding the pathology of cavovarus deformity.
- The tibialis anterior and peroneus brevis muscles are usually affected first, which is followed by dysfunction of the intrinsic muscles. Their muscular antagonists, the peroneus longus and tibialis posterior muscles, are relatively stronger, leading to plantar flexion of the first ray and medialization of the navicular, which results in pronation and adduction of forefoot.
- As the deformity progresses, forefoot-driven hindfoot varus may develop. The deformity of cavovarus foot is often flexible in the early phase, which may gradually become rigid over time. Peroneal tendonitis and lateral instability can be present due to overloading.
- Contracture of plantar fascia and Achilles tendon is often found.
- A great toe cock-up deformity can develop with compensation of the relatively normal extensor hallucis longus (EHL) to dorsiflex the ankle.
- With the intrinsic muscles weakened, the stronger pull of the extrinsic extensor digitorum longus (EDL) and flexor digitorum longus (FDL) tendons can lead to claw toe formation. Painful arthritic change can be presented in late stage cases.

30.1.1 Clinical Evaluation

- The patient should be examined standing and walking with bare feet.
- The peek-a-boo sign (**Fig. 30.1**), a common finding, is present when the examiner can see the medial aspect of the heel when viewed from the front.

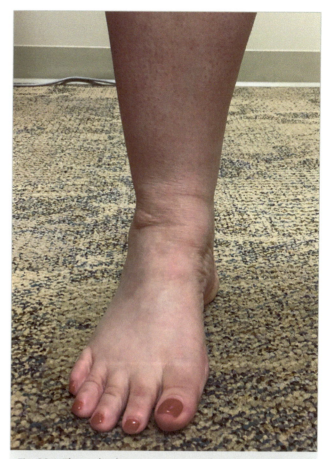

Fig. 30.1 The peek-a-boo sign, a common finding, is present when the examiner can see the medial aspect of the heel from the front.

- Forefoot pronation along with adduction, cock-up great toe, clawed lesser toes, elevated longitudinal arch, hindfoot varus, and calf atrophy can be seen.
- Foot drop and balance problems can be observed during walking as the anterior tibial muscle continues to weaken.
- With the patient seated, range of motion and tenderness are accessed for the ankle, hindfoot, midfoot, and forefoot to evaluate for possible arthritis and rigid deformities.
- It is essential to perform a complete neurologic examination to evaluate muscle strength and sensory deficits, and to differentiate an upper motor neuron versus a lower motor neuron–based pathology.

Coleman Block Test

- The Coleman block test can be used to evaluate whether the hindfoot deformity is flexible or fixed.
- If the heel reduces into valgus by weight bearing on a block supporting only the lateral column of the foot (**Fig. 30.2**), the cavovarus deformity is defined as forefoot driven or flexible and can be corrected by addressing the forefoot deformity alone.

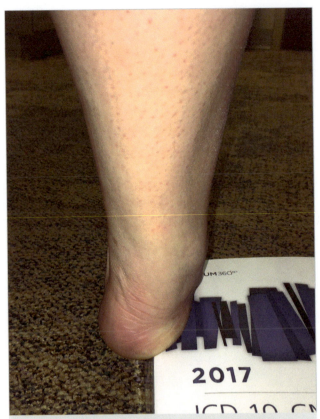

Fig. 30.2 Coleman block test showed fixed hindfoot varus.

• If not, then the deformity is rigid and a bony correction of the hindfoot varus may be necessary.

Silfverskiöld's Test

• If ankle equinus is observed only with extension of the knee, a gastrocnemius contracture is diagnosed, and it should be treated by a gastrocnemius recession.
• If contracture is found throughout the complete range of motion of the knee, then a formal Achilles tendon lengthening is indicated.

30.1.2 Radiographic Evaluation

• Weight-bearing anteroposterior (AP) and lateral X-rays are necessary cavovarus deformity evaluation.
• An increased calcaneal pitch, Meary's angel, and Hibbs' angles can be found on the lateral view. A posterior fibula and a flat-topped talus may also be found.
• A Saltzman view is essential to evaluate the degree of hindfoot varus and the angle of the subtalar joint.
• The talar tilt can be assessed on the AP view.
• Computed tomography and magnetic resonance imaging (MRI) can be helpful to find joint degenerative changes and possible tarsal coalitions.

30.1.3 Nonoperative Options

• Laterally posted custom orthotic inserts, with posting extended out to the midfoot.
• Accommodative shoe wear.
• Custom ankle foot orthosis (Arizona brace, Richie brace, and molded ankle–foot orthosis [MAFO] brace).
• Physical therapy.

30.1.4 Contraindications

• The contraindications include severe cardiovascular diseases, poor vascularization of the lower extremity, heavy smokers, local infection, and noncompliant patients.
• For children younger than 8 years, arthrodesis should be avoided because it may result in growth arrest of more than 25% compared to the contralateral foot.

30.2 Goals of Surgical Procedure

Soft-tissue balancing procedures are often effective for mild to moderate cases with flexible deformity. Combining bony correction procedures may help with those having rigid deformities. Joint sparing correction is always the first choice until arthritic changes develop, which indicates necessary arthrodesis. The goal of surgical correction is to reconstruct a plantigrade foot without pain.

30.3 Advantages of Surgical Procedure

• Recreating balance between muscular agonist/antagonist groups.
• Realignment of the bony structures of the foot through osteotomies.

30.4 Key Principles

• Joint preservation through tendon transfers and osteotomies to try to avoid arthrodesis procedures whenever possible.
• Rebalance the muscle groups of the foot.
• Recreate a balanced bony tripod of the foot to create a plantargrade foot for ambulation.

30.5 Operative Technique

30.5.1 Surgical Procedure: Plantar Fascia Release

The contracted plantar fascia plays an important role in keeping the high arch and the hindfoot varus; hence, plantar fascia release is usually indicated for cavovarus deformity reconstruction. The plantar fascia should be released completely from the origin on the calcaneus. This procedure allows further forefoot cavus correction and lowering the longitudinal arch.

Preoperative Preparation

The patient is placed in the supine position with the lower limb externally rotated for better visualization of the foot. A thigh-level tourniquet is applied.

Operative Technique

Either an oblique incision or a longitudinal one may work to expose the insertion of the plantar fascia as well as the fascia of the abductor hallucis. A transection is then performed at the origin of the plantar fascia, taking care to protect the neurovascular bundle. In addition, the fascia of the abductor hallucis muscle is released (**Fig 30.3**).

Tips and Pearls

Tensioning the windlass mechanism with dorsiflexion of the metatarsal phalangeal joints may facilitate the release of the plantar fascia. With some cases of severe cavus deformity, releasing the fascia of the abductor hallucis may be necessary.

Hazards and Pitfalls

The surgeon must be cautious to protect the lateral plantar nerve that passes through the medial side of the heel.

30.5.2 Surgical Technique: Achilles Tendon Lengthening

Achilles contracture can often be found in cavovarus feet. Lengthening the Achilles may help reduce the stress of the forefoot and improve gait pattern by regaining normal dorsiflexion of the ankle. The modified Strayer procedure is performed for Achilles contracture with a positive Silfverskiöld's test (gastrocnemius contracture only). Otherwise, the Hoke procedure is utilized.

Preoperative Preparation

The patient is placed in the supine position with the lower limb externally rotated. A bump under the contralateral hip can help visualize the posteromedial part of the leg. A thigh-level tourniquet is applied.

Operative Technique

The Modified Strayer Procedure

Flex the knee with the hip flexed and externally rotated. A longitudinal 3-cm posteromedial incision is made over the junction of the gastrocnemius–soleus complex, either posteromedially or directly posterior. After incising the fascia in line with the skin incision, the gastrocnemius tendon can be identified. The fascia is identified. This is carefully incised transversely, taking care to avoid injury to the sural nerve. The foot is then maximally dorsiflexed elongating the gastrocnemius.

Using a speculum, either vaginal or nasal, or malleable retractors can be helpful for visualization in a modified Strayer procedure.

The Hoke Procedure

This is a three-step hemicut within the distal Achilles tendon. An assistant holds the elevated limb while dorsiflexing the ankle. The first incision is placed about 2 cm proximal to the insertion into the heel. A no. 15 or 11 blade is used to pierce through the skin at the middle of the width of the tendon. The blade

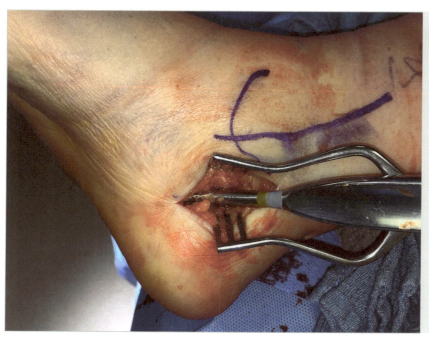

Fig. 30.3 Plantar fascia release: a joker elevator is used to protect the neurovascular bundle.

is inserted parallel with the tendon fibers. Once through, the scalpel is turned 90 degrees medially and the medial half of the tendon fibers are severed. The next incision is made about 3 cm proximal to the first. The tendon is again stabbed centrally; this time the lateral half of the tendon is severed. A third and the final incision is placed another 3 cm proximal to the second stab with the medial half of the tendon being transected. Dorsiflex the ankle joint with the knee extended and Achilles lengthening of up to 1.5 cm can be achieved.

A Z-lengthening may be necessary for severe Achilles contracture.

30.5.3 Surgical Technique: First Metatarsal Osteotomy

A first ray plantar flexion deformity can result from the overpull of the peroneus longus muscle against the weak anterior tibialis muscle. This is termed forefoot-driven cavovarus and needs to be corrected through a dorsiflexing (dorsal closing wedge) osteotomy of the first ray to lower the longitudinal arch. The effect is to neutralize Meary's angle on the lateral foot X-ray.

Preoperative Preparation

The patient is placed in a supine position. An Esmarch or thigh-level tourniquet is applied. Review the radiographs to plan the location of the dorsiflexion osteotomy.

Operative Technique

A dorsal longitudinal incision is made to visualize the proximal first metatarsal and the tarsometatarsal joint. The proximal cut is usually 1 to 1.5 cm distal from the tarsometatarsal joint and should be perpendicular to the long axis through the talus and the navicular. The distal cut is made perpendicular to the axis of the first metatarsal (**Fig. 30.4**). The plantar cortex is left intact and greensticked to close the osteotomy after the wedge

of bone has been removed. Care should be taken not to over-shorten or overdorsiflex the first ray for it may cause transfer metatarsalgia. Fixation should be stable for bone healing utilizing either a screw, staple, or plate.

An osteotomy of the second and third rays may be necessary for severe forefoot cavus deformity. A midfoot osteotomy should be considered when the apex of the high arch is at the level of the midfoot. This will usually require a fusion at the level of the midfoot wedge resection.

30.5.4 Surgical Technique: Calcaneal Osteotomy

In the hindfoot-driven varus deformity (rigid deformity), a valgus creating calcaneal osteotomy is needed. This can be a powerful technique to correct the hindfoot varus into normal valgus alignment.

Preoperative Preparation

The patient is placed in a lateral or supine position with a bump under the ipsilateral hip for adequate visualization of the lateral aspect of the calcaneus. An Esmarch or thigh-level tourniquet is applied.

Operative Technique

Dwyer Osteotomy

An oblique incision is made from about 2 cm posterior to the tip of lateral malleoli, parallel with the peroneals, toward the plantar aspect of the calcaneocuboid joint, perpendicular to the axis of the calcaneus. Deep dissection is performed posterior to the peroneal tendon sheath. Place a Hohlman retractor on the dorsal and plantar aspects of the calcaneus and strip back the periosteum to expose the area of bone to be resected. The first transverse cut is placed about 2 cm posterior to the posterior

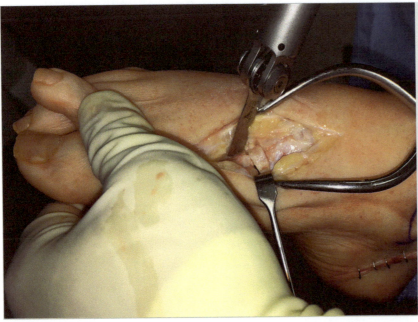

Fig. 30.4 First metatarsal osteotomy: a dorsal wedge is removed.

facet of subtalar joint in line with the skin incision. The more posterior second cut is made to remove a bone wedge usually 5 to 7 mm wide. K-wires can be inserted and checked under fluoroscopy to ensure that the osteotomy is appropriately positioned. Once again the deep medial cortex should be left intact and greensticked to create a stable hinge. After resecting the wedge, close the osteotomy and make sure the correction is adequate before fixation. One or two 6.5- or 7.0-mm screws are used to fix the osteotomy.

Lateral Sliding Osteotomy

The same exposure is utilized as for the Dwyer osteotomy. Here the single osteotomy cut is about 2 cm posterior to the posterior facet of subtalar joint and parallel to the skin incision. The medial cortex penetration should be posterior to the sustentaculum tali in order to protect the neurovascular bundle. Mobilize the calcaneal tuberosity and slide it laterally. The distance of translation is determined by the degree of varus deformity, which is usually 1 to 1.5 cm. This may be limited by prominence of the lateral bone under the skin laterally. One to two 6.5- or 7.0-mm screws are used to fix the osteotomy. Trim the lateral aspect of the calcaneus before irrigation and wound closure.

In many cases, a combination of a Dwyer closing wedge and a lateral sliding osteotomy can be performed to optimize correction.

Malerba's Z Osteotomy

The approach to the lateral calcaneal wall is as described earlier. The anterior vertical cut is 1 to 2 cm posterior and parallel to the calcaneocuboid joint, while the posterior vertical cut is 1 to 2 cm anterior to the Achilles insertion. A horizontal cut is made in the middle of the calcaneus and in line with the plantar fascia. A second horizontal cut is made obliquely to meet the medial

extent of the first horizontal cut. The lateral wedge of bone can be removed from the horizontal osteotomy and the osteotomy reduced (**Fig 30.5**). In addition, if further correction is needed, the calcaneal tuberosity can be translated laterally to correct the hindfoot varus. The Malerba Z osteotomy can provide multiplanar correction, which is ideal for severe deformities.

For any of the calcaneal osteotomies, an AP, lateral, and calcaneal axial views of the ankle should be taken intraoperatively. The surgeon must attempt to line up the calcaneus with the long axis of the leg when trying to decide if a sufficient degree of correction has been achieved. Trim the lateral aspect of the calcaneus before irrigation and wound closure.

Hazards and Pitfalls

Care should be taken to protect the sural nerve, which passes through the lateral aspect of the heel (**Fig. 30.6**). Sometimes the Dwyer osteotomy may not be able to achieve a full correction. It should be reserved for mild hindfoot varus deformities. Care should be taken to protect the medial neurovascular bundle.

30.5.5 Surgical Technique: Tendon Transfers

A tendon transfer is indicated for a dynamic cavovarus deformity and is often useful with the combination of bony procedures to maintain the correction. It is an effective way to regain a balanced foot and is especially successful for young patients.

There are several general principles for tendon transfers that must be considered:
- The tendon to be transferred should have enough strength (4+ better) given there will be a loss of 1 degree of strength after transfer.

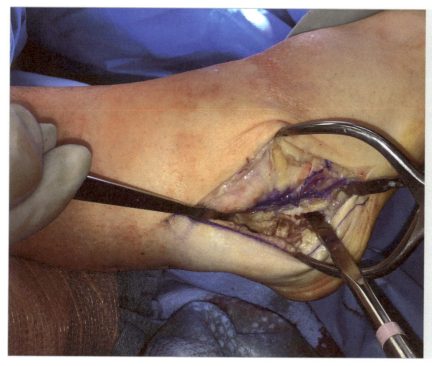

Fig. 30.5 Malerba's Z-shaped calcaneal osteotomy.

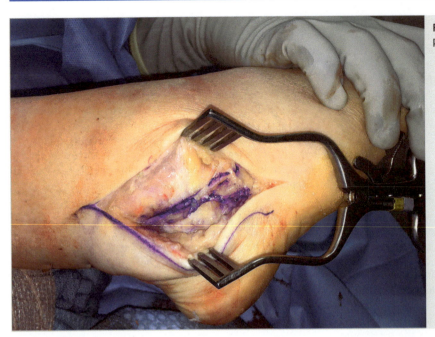

Fig. 30.6 The sural nerve is marked and protected.

- The transferred tendon should be inserted close to the tendon function to be replaced and routed without angulation.
- There should be flexibility of the joints involved with the tendon transfer.
- Fixation of the tendon should be to the bone directly or indirectly to another tendon.
- Agonists are preferable to antagonists.
- Tension should be performed at half of the tendon excursion.

Preoperative Preparation

The patient is placed in a lateral or supine position. A bump under the ipsilateral hip can be used for adequate visualization of the lateral aspect of the foot with the peroneal tendon transfer. A thigh-level tourniquet is applied.

Operative Technique

Peroneus Longus to Peroneus Brevis Transfer

Transferring the peroneus longus to brevis may correct the hyper-plantarflexion of the first ray and strengthen the function of the weakened peroneus brevis.

An incision is made from the tip of the fibula to the base of the fifth metatarsal. Carefully open the tendon sheath of both tendons. Cut the peroneus longus as distal as possible and weave it to the peroneus brevis with the Pulvertaft technique or in a side-to-side fashion with the foot held in an everted position (**Fig. 30.7**).

Posterior Tibialis Transfer

The posterior tibialis tendon (PTT) transfer may provide the strength for dorsiflexion of the ankle instead of the failed anterior tibialis while removing the deforming force caused by the unopposed pull of the PTT against the weak peroneus brevis muscle.

The first incision is made at the medial side of the navicular tuberosity where the posterior tibial tendon is released from its insertion. The tendon is brought out through a second incision, which is made at the level of the junction between the middle and distal third of the leg. The third incision is made above the level of the syndesmosis, in the interosseous membrane. A large enough window is made in the membrane to avoid impingement of the tendon. Through the second incision, a Cobb elevator is then used to elevate all of the soft tissues from the posterior aspect of the tibia. The tendon is then gently inserted into this portal and directed anteriorly through the interosseous membrane. The last dorsal incision is made over the lateral cuneiform. A hole is made central in the cuneiform. The tendon is bought through a subcutaneous tunnel, superficial to the extensor retinaculum. A tenodesis is made through the bone tunnel in the lateral cuneiform with an interference screw.

If combined with other procedure, the final tensioning and suture of the tendon should be done after bony corrections. Tenodesis of the posterior tibial tendon can also be made either medially or laterally to balance the foot with inversion and eversion depending on the nature of the deformity.

30.5.6 Surgical Technique: Triple Arthrodesis

Triple arthrodesis indicated for severe rigid cavovarus deformity or the presence of arthritis within the hindfoot joints. The goal is to restore a stable plantargrade foot by fusing the subtalar joint, talonavicular joint, and calcaneocuboid joints in an anatomic valgus alignment.

While arthrodesis should ideally be avoided, in severe cases with a fixed deformity, the results of a well-done arthrodesis are superior to those of a joint-sparing surgery that preserves a limited amount of motion but fails to gain complete correction.[1]

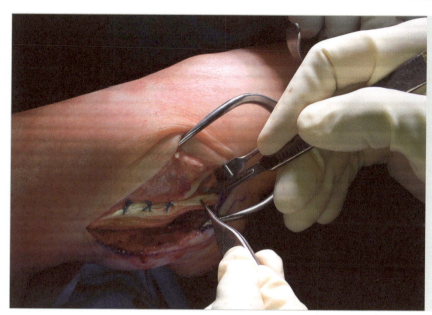

Fig. 30.7 Peroneus longus to peroneus brevis transfer.

Preoperative Preparation

The patient is placed in the supine position with the lower limb externally rotated for better visualization of the foot. A bump under the ipsilateral hip may help for adequate visualization of the lateral aspect of the foot. A thigh-level tourniquet is applied.

Operative Technique

A lateral incision is made from the tip of the fibula to the base of the fourth metatarsal. Retract the peroneal tendons along with the sural nerve plantarward and the extensor digitorum brevis dorsally to visualize the sinus tarsi, subtalar joint, and the calcaneocuboid joint. After stripping the soft tissue in the sinus tarsi, the interosseous ligament is cut by the scalpel to allow access to the posterior and middle facets of the subtalar joint. The cartilage in both joints is removed by a curette. Micro-fracture of the subchondral bone is done with a 2-mm drill bit and 0.25-inch osteotome.

The medial incision is made from the tip of the medial malleolus to the tubercle of the talus, which is about above the posterior tibial tendon. With the talonavicular capsule opened, the cartilage is removed by a curette and followed by micro-fracture of the subchondral bone.

Adequate correction is confirmed under fluoroscopy and provisional pins are used to hold the joints in position. One or two 6.5- or 7.0-mm screws are used for subtalar joint from the calcaneus to the talus. Either screws or staples can be used for fixation of talonavicular joint or calcaneocuboid joint. Locking plates may provide more stability with osteoporotic bones. Anteroposterior and lateral view images are taken before irrigation and wound closure.

Tips and Pearls

Since the medial column is often short in cavovarus foot, the bony structure should be preserved as much as possible at the talonavicular joint. A Hintermann distractor can be very helpful to visualize the joints need to be fused.

Hazards and Pitfalls

The entry of the subtalar screws should be away from the weight-bearing zone of the calcaneus or postoperative pain may develop. Care should be taken to protect the sural nerve when making the lateral incision. A single medial incision may hardly expose the subtalar joint in cavovarus deformity, so bilateral incisions are recommended. Recurrence of deformity may happen with triple arthrodesis alone, so it should be combined with soft-tissue balancing procedures.

30.5.7 Surgical Technique: Jones' Procedure

An overpowered peroneus longus with the contracted plantar fascia and the excessive compensating EHL for the weak anterior tibialis are the causes for a cock-up deformity of the great toe, or a claw hallux. The Jones procedure transfers the EHL to first metatarsal neck, so as to elevate the first ray, and fused the hallux interphalangeal joint fusion to prevent or correct flexion contracture. Alternatively, the flexor hallucis longus (FHL) tendon can be transferred to the base of the proximal phalanx while maintaining flexibility of the first interphalangeal joint.

Preoperative Preparation

The patient is placed in the supine position. A thigh-level tourniquet is applied.

Operative Technique

Jones' Procedure

A dorsal transverse incision is made over the first interphalangeal joint. Release the EHL tendon from its attachment and the collateral ligaments of the first interphalangeal joint to visualize the articular surface. Two flat surfaces are then created by saw cut. A 4.0- or 5.5-mm cancellous lag screw is used to fix the arthrodesis with mild plantar flexion on sagittal plane and neutral on axial plane. The screw is placed in a retrograde fashion from the tip of the distal phalanx into the base of the proximal phalanx. Alternatively, two staples can be placed across the joint.

The second incision is made longitudinally over the dorsal aspect of the distal first metatarsal. A transverse drill hole is made in the distal part of the first metatarsal neck. The EHL tendon is passed through the bone tunnel. Then the tendon is sutured to itself with tension while holding the ankle in dorsiflexion.

Flexor Hallucis Longus Transfer

A plantar incision is made under the great toe. The FHL is identified and released from its insertion. If contractured, the plantar plate of the interphalangeal joint is released. A second incision is made over the dorsal proximal phalanx of the great toe. The EHL tendon is retracted and a drill hole is made in a plantar to dorsal direction at the base of the proximal phalanx. With the toe held 20 degrees of plantar flexion, the FHL is transferred through the proximal phalanx and tenodesed to the EHL. Auxiliary pining of the interphalangeal joint for 4 weeks may help maintain the rotational stability. The more distal the EHL tendon is transferred, the more dorsiflexion strength can be gained.

30.5.8 Surgical Technique: Claw Toe Correction

With the intrinsics weakened, the unopposed EDL hyperextends the unstable lesser toes at the metatarsophalangeal level while the FDL and brevis flex the phalanges.[2] The Girdlestone–Taylor procedure is indicated when the claw toe deformities are flexible. The additional DuVries arthroplasty may help with fixed claw toes.

Preoperative Preparation

The patient is placed in the supine position. A thigh-level tourniquet is applied.

Operative Technique

Girdlestone–Taylor Procedure/Flexor Digitorum Longus Transfer

A transverse incision is made in the flexor crease on the plantar aspect of the proximal phalanx to expose the FDL tendon, which can be identified by its midline raphe. A curved mosquito hemostat is inserted between the tendon and the proximal phalanx to keep the tendon under tension. A percutaneous transverse incision is made at the level of the distal interphalangeal joint to release the FDL tendon from its insertion. The tendon is brought through the proximal incision and split along the raphe to create two tails as proximally as possible. Then a longitudinal incision is made on the dorsal aspect of the proximal

phalanx. A mosquito hemostat is passed subperiosteally along the extensor hood to the plantar incision. The tendon should be passed just along the extensor hood to avoid compromising the neurovascular bundle. Both the tails of the tendon are brought dorsally along the medial and lateral side of the extensor hood. The tendon is sutured to the EDL with mild tension by holding the toe in 20 degrees of plantar flexion at the metatarsophalangeal joint.

DuVries' Arthroplasty

A longitudinal or transverse elliptical incision is made over the proximal interphalangeal joint and the extensor tendons, and the dorsal capsule and the collateral ligaments are excised. The plantar aspect of the capsule is also released. The condyles of the proximal phalanx are resected perpendicular to the long axis of the phalanx. The proximal base of the middle phalanx can be excised if interphalangeal joint fusion is expected. The toe is pinned by a 1.5-mm Kirschner wire through the interphalangeal joints and sometimes it may be necessary to pin through the metatarsophalangeal joint to maintain the proper alignment.

The DuVries arthroplasty is recommended to be used in combination with the Girdlestone–Taylor procedure to gain satisfactory correction. Metatarsophalangeal capsule release or metatarsal shortening osteotomy may help when the metatarsophalangeal joint is still hyperdorsiflexed after claw toe correction.

30.6 Complications/Bailout/Salvage

In general, tendon transfers result in a decrease in their overall strength. Occasionally, the sural nerve becomes entrapped in scar tissue or disrupted, which can create a problem for the patient. Transient and irreversible tibial nerve palsy after lateralizing calcaneal osteotomies has also been described.[3] Delayed union or nonunion can happen with the bony procedures.

The most common complication is the recurrence of the cavovarus deformity, which may necessitate revision surgery.

30.7 Postoperative Care

The patient is placed into a short-leg compression dressing along with plaster splints. A popliteal block can be useful in controlling postoperative pain. The sutures are removed 14 days after surgery, and a CAM boot is applied. Partial weight-bearing is permitted in the boot 4 weeks after surgery. At 8 to 10 weeks postoperatively, walking with daily shoes can be started if radiographic bony union is confirmed.

30.8 Outcomes

A wide variety of procedures for the treatment of cavovarus foot deformities have been described, but no single combination of the procedures has gained wide acceptance.[4] Few studies have been published for outcome assessment. Foot pressure distribution is improved after plantar fascia release combined with first metatarsal osteotomy by dynamic pedobarographic study.[5] Both radiographic and clinical improvements are achieved by Dwyer osteotomy of the calcaneus for cavovarus deformity with different causes.[6] Short- to mid-term results with 90% satisfactory rate for 52 feet treated by first ray dorsiflexion osteotomy combined with tendon transfers were reported by Leeuwesteijn et al.[7] Ward et al reported long-term results that first metatarsal osteotomy combined with soft-tissue rebalancing procedures had better outcomes than those with triple arthrodesis.[8] Favorable results were reported by Maskill et al with different combination of procedures including lateral displacement calcaneus osteotomy, peroneus longus to brevis transfer, dorsiflexion first metatarsal osteotomy, and Achilles tendon lengthening.[9] Posterior tibial tendon transfer was proved to be effective at correcting the foot drop component of cavovarus foot deformity by three-dimensional gait analysis.[10]

References

1. Zide JR, Myerson MS. Arthrodesis for the cavus foot: when, where, and how? Foot Ankle Clin 2013;18(4):755–767
2. Aminian A, Sangeorzan BJ. The anatomy of cavus foot deformity. Foot Ankle Clin 2008;13(2):191–198, v
3. Krause FG, Pohl MJ, Penner MJ, Younger AS. Tibial nerve palsy associated with lateralizing calcaneal osteotomy: case reviews and technical tip. Foot Ankle Int 2009;30(3):258–261
4. VanderHave KL, Hensinger RN, King BW. Flexible cavovarus foot in children and adolescents. Foot Ankle Clin 2013;18(4):715–726
5. Kwon YU, Kim HW, Hwang JH, Park H, Park HW, Park KB. Changes in dynamic pedobarography after extensive plantarmedial release for paralytic pes cavovarus. Yonsei Med J 2014;55(3):766–772
6. Barg A, Hörterer H, Jacxsens M, Wiewiorski M, Paul J, Valderrabano V. Dwyer osteotomy: lateral sliding osteotomy of calcaneus. Oper Orthop Traumatol 2015;27(4):283–297
7. Leeuwesteijn AE, de Visser E, Louwerens JW. Flexible cavovarus feet in Charcot-Marie-Tooth disease treated with first ray proximal dorsiflexion osteotomy combined with soft tissue surgery: a short-term to mid-term outcome study. Foot Ankle Surg 2010;16(3):142–147
8. Ward CM, Dolan LA, Bennett DL, Morcuende JA, Cooper RR. Long-term results of reconstruction for treatment of a flexible cavovarus foot in Charcot-Marie-Tooth disease. J Bone Joint Surg Am 2008;90(12):2631–2642
9. Maskill MP, Maskill JD, Pomeroy GC. Surgical management and treatment algorithm for the subtle cavovarus foot. Foot Ankle Int 2010;31(12):1057–1063
10. Dreher T, Wolf SI, Heitzmann D, Fremd C, Klotz MC, Wenz W. Tibialis posterior tendon transfer corrects the foot drop component of cavovarus foot deformity in Charcot-Marie-Tooth disease. J Bone Joint Surg Am 2014;96(6):456–462

31 Local Bone Graft

David N. Garras

Abstract

The use of bone graft in foot and ankle surgery is critical to the success of many of our everyday procedures. With the rising number of readily available allografts and biological augments, autograft use has decreased. However, autograft bone remains the gold standard in many fusions and nonunion repairs. In this chapter, we demonstrate technique for local autograft from the calcaneus, distal tibia, and proximal tibia.

Keywords: *bone graft calcaneus, distal tibia, proximal tibia, nonunion, malunion*

31.1 Indications

• Bone grafting is the general technique of placing new bone into spaces around a broken bone or an area where a bone defect is present. It is often used to fuse joints and fill gaps that have sustained bone tissue loss, or to repair other areas of the bone that have failed to heal properly.

• When bone graft is necessary, it can be either an autograft or an allograft. Autograft is bone taken from the patient's healthy bone, while an allograft is donated bone that has been processed and frozen, typically from a cadaver. The autograft bone is the preferred option because there is less of a chance of cellular rejection, a greater number of viable cells, and a greater chance for proper adhesion (hatch). Autograft is osteogenic, osteoinductive, and osteoconductive.

• The surgeon has options in terms of where the autograft is harvested locally. Typically, cancellous bone harvest is taken from the proximal tibia, distal tibia, or the calcaneus. Alternative site—such as the iliac crest, femoral canal, distal femur—may be beneficial for large volumes or cortical bone grafts but are not considered local autograft. Local autografts provide usable osteoblasts, bone morphogenic proteins, and a scaffold to aid in a fusion, a malunion, or a nonunion of a fracture. In this chapter, we will cover the proximal tibia, distal tibia, and calcaneus cancellous autograft procedures.

31.2 Goals of Surgical Procedure

The goals of an autograft procedure are to safely harvest viable bone from the patient in order to use in an operation aimed to repair a bony defect, aid in an arthrodesis, or a nonunion. This is done with the aim of improving the patient's quality of life and the rate of a successful procedure. Local bone harvesting procedures are simple, generally safe, and fairly well tolerated.

31.3 Advantages of Surgical Procedure

Autograft remains the gold standard for the treatment of nonunions and malunions, as well as to aid in arthrodeses. Autograft is preferred over allograft because of the lower rate of infection, lower revision rates, and a faster time to healing.[1] Proximal tibial autograft provides a higher number of viable cells and the largest amount of bone. However, it is typically associated with some postoperative pain. Distal tibial autograft may be used in hindfoot procedures where the calcaneus is involved and when proximal to the autograph is not an option such as with revision total knee arthroplasties. Calcaneal autograft is a readily available source of bone graft that can be used in a variety of midfoot and forefoot fusions or nonunion repairs and is very well tolerated.

31.4 Key Principles

• The three key principles of harvesting autograft bone are as follows:
  ○ Choosing the appropriate location for harvesting the autograft.
  ○ Meticulous dissection and soft-tissue protection to avoid any neurovascular or soft-tissue compromise.
  ○ Care not to weaken or fracture the harvest site.

• When deciding on the appropriate site to harvest the autograft, the surgeon must consider the volume of bone needed and possible future surgical procedures associated with the current procedure. For example, when performing a triple arthrodesis, it would be advisable to obtain bone graft from the proximal tibia because this gives you more graft for all three joints. This also avoids any defects within the distal tibia, given the need for ankle fusion or replacement in the future may be necessary.

31.5 Preoperative Preparation and Patient Positioning

31.5.1 Proximal Tibia

The patient is positioned supine. Anesthesia may be with a femoral and sciatic nerve block, a spinal, or general anesthetic. The leg is prepped and draped to above the knee.

31.5.2 Distal Tibia

The patient is positioned supine. Anesthesia may be with a popliteal and saphenous nerve block or a general anesthetic. The leg is prepped to the musculotendinous junction of the gastrocnemius muscle.

31.5.3 Calcaneus

The patient is positioned supine with a small bump under the ipsilateral hip. Anesthesia may be with a regional nerve block, an ankle block, or a general anesthetic. The leg is prepped to the musculotendinous junction of the gastrocnemius muscle.

31.6 Operative Technique

Local bone graft can be obtained by either creating a small cortical window using an osteotome or small saw in the metaphyseal bone and using a curette or gauge to obtain the graft or by using readily available bone harvesting equipment. When using an osteotome or saw created cortical window, care should be taken to avoid creating a stress riser in the bone where a fracture could potentially occur. The author's personal preference is using a cylindrical trephine harvester, which avoids the risk of fracture propagation. Different diameter trephines are available for bone harvesting procedures.[2]

31.6.1 Proximal Tibia

Approximately 1 cm distal and 1 cm lateral to the insertion of the patellar tendon on the tibia, a 2-cm incision is made in the skin (**Fig. 31.1**). Blunt dissection is carried down to the anterior compartment fascia. The fascia is opened and an elevator is used to elevate the anterior compartment musculature off the lateral surface of the tibia. The trephine is then inserted directly on the bone. The position of the trephine should be checked flu-

oroscopically to ensure that the anterior and posterior cortices are not accidentally reamed. The trephine is then drilled into the proximal tibia in a radial clockwise direction. Multiple passes may be performed using the same entry hole by directing the trephine in different directions to obtain a larger quantity of graft. The trephine is then detached from the power equipment and a plunger is used to obtain the graft. Gelfoam is used to decrease bleeding from the cortical defect. The fascia is closed with interrupted Vicryl suture and the skin is closed in standard layered fashion.

31.6.2 Distal Tibia

An incision is made over the medial aspect of the distal tibia 2 cm above the ankle joint (**Fig. 31.2**). Care should be taken to avoid the saphenous nerve and vein. Blunt dissection is carried down to the bone. The periosteum is elevated off the medial tibia. The trephine is then inserted directly on the bone. The position of the trephine should be checked fluoroscopically to ensure that it is well above the ankle joint. The trephine is then drilled into the distal tibia in a radial clockwise direction. Multiple passes may be performed using the same entry hole by

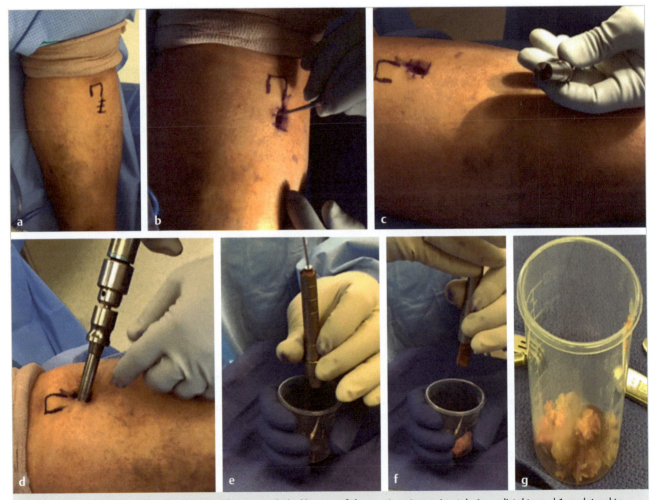

Fig. 31.1 Proximal tibia. (**a**) The incision used for proximal tibial bone graft harvesting. Approximately 1 cm distal to and 1 cm lateral to the tibial tuberosity. (**b**) After the fascia is opened, an elevator is used to elevate the anterior compartment musculature off the lateral tibia. (**c**) The graft harvesting trephine. (**d**) Reaming of the lateral tibial surface with the trephine. (**e**) The plunger used to obtain the graft. (**f**) The graft being delivered out of the trephine. (**g**) The graft obtained through this technique.

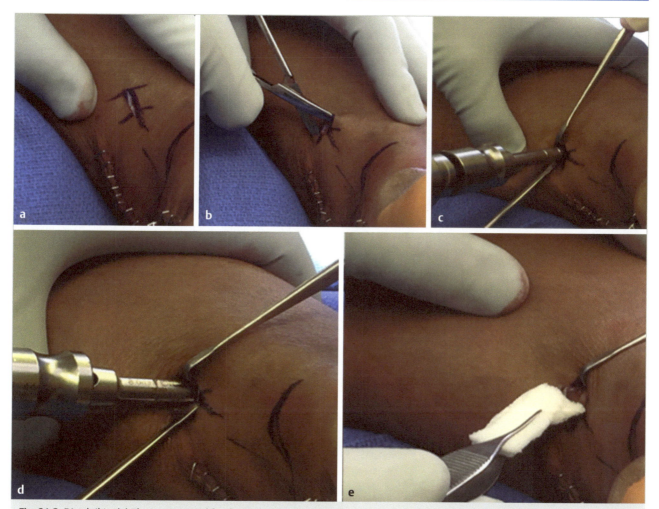

Fig. 31.2 Distal tibia. **(a)** The incision used for distal tibial bone graft is about 2 cm proximal to the joint line. **(b)** Blunt dissection to avoid injury to the saphenous nerve and greater saphenous vein. **(c)** Reaming with the trephine to obtain the bone graft. **(d)** Changing directions with the trephine for a second pass to obtain more graft. **(e)** Gelfoam being inserted to control postoperative bleeding.

directing the trephine in different directions to obtain a larger quantity of graft. The trephine is then detached from the power equipment and a plunger is used to obtain the graft. Gelfoam is used to decrease bleeding from the cortical defect. The skin is closed in standard layered fashion.

31.6.3 Calcaneus

An incision is made over the lateral calcaneus between the superior aspect of the calcaneal tuberosity and the inferior lateral calcaneal process. Blunt dissection should be carefully performed down to the periosteum to avoid injury to the sural nerve and its many branches (**Fig. 31.3**). The periosteum is elevated off the lateral calcaneus. The trephine is then inserted directly on the bone. The position of the trephine should be checked fluoroscopically to ensure that it is in the middle of the tuberosity and not near the superior or inferior edges of the bone. The trephine is then drilled into the calcaneus in a radial clockwise direction. Multiple passes may be performed using the same entry hole by directing the trephine in different directions to obtain a larger quantity of graft. The trephine is then detached from the power equipment and a plunger is used to

obtain the graft. Gelfoam is used to decrease bleeding from the cortical defect. The skin is closed in standard layered fashion with care not to encircle any branches of the sural nerve.

31.7 Tips and Pearls

If using an osteotome to create a cortical window for your harvest, ensure that your osteotomes are thin, small, and very sharp. Fracture propagation usually occurs if the bone is entered bluntly. A small sagittal saw may also be used, but be conscious of the side cutting of the sagittal motion of the saw so that a stress riser does not occur at the corners of the window. A trick that the author has often used when he had to use these techniques is to use a rongeur on the corners of the window to make the corners more rounded. Finally, when obtaining the graft, avoid levering on the cortex with your curette or gauge to avoid an accidental fracture.

If using a bone harvesting trephine, the cortical window is typically created by the trephine. However, the trephines tend to slip off the bone easily, so be careful and support the trephine by placing your other hand on the patient's leg for support. In dense bone, it may be beneficial to make a pilot hole with a 3.5-mm

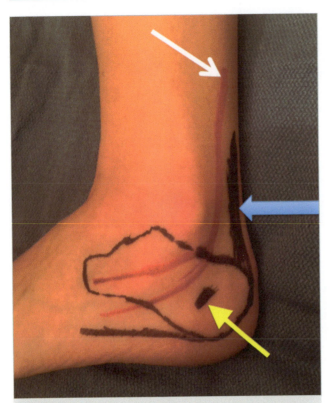

Fig. 31.3 A lateral photograph of a patient's ankle showing the typical trajectory of the sural nerve (red line with white arrow). The incision is in the middle of the tuberosity (yellow arrow). Blue arrow indicates the Achilles tendon.

drill bit first and then use the trephine to enter the bone to avoid accidental slipping off the bone. Once the window is created, avoid going through the opposite side of the bone because you may inadvertently injure the neurovascular structures on the opposite side and unnecessarily weaken the bone. Finally, cancellous bone graft sites tend to bleed and bruise profusely. Using a small piece of Gelfoam in the bone helps decrease this dramatically.

31.8 Hazards and Pitfalls

During proximal tibial bone graft harvesting, the anterior recurrent tibial artery and motor branches to the tibialis anterior from the deep peroneal nerve lie deep within the anterior compartment and may be at risk. Once the fascia is entered, care should be taken to remain very superficial within the compartment. Blunt finger dissection should be performed between the tibialis anterior and the fascia until the lateral tibia is reached. The genicular artery and nerves are above the tibial tuberosity and should not be encountered using this technique.

The saphenous nerve, which travels with the greater saphenous vein at the medial ankle, may be injured during distal tibial graft harvesting procedures. Careful dissection and retraction should be sufficient to avoid this complication. The same is true of the calcaneal bone harvesting procedure and the sural and the lateral dorsal cutaneous nerves. Accidental reaming or piercing of the medial cortex of the calcaneus with the trephine or a curette could lead to a plantar nerve or posterior tibial artery injury within the tarsal tunnel.

31.9 Complications/Bailout/Salvage

Fractures during bone graft harvesting procedures are extremely rare. However, a treatment plan should be prepared in case of fracture. Avoiding a fracture is much easier to accomplish that treatment of said fractures. Most fractures caused by a bone harvesting procedure can be treated nonoperatively with limited weight-bearing and immobilization. Calcium phosphate cement or polymethyl methacrylate may be used to fill the defect of the harvest site or support a small fracture.

31.10 Postoperative Care

Postoperatively, the patient should have no additional restrictions as a result of the bone graft procedure. When using the trephines, the circular window created allows for no weight-bearing restrictions postoperatively. The restricted weight-bearing is typically due to the concomitant procedures that required the graft.

31.11 Outcomes

The use of local autograft in foot and ankle surgery is a vital part of our treatment of the various pathologies that we encounter regularly. Autograft has been shown to have very low risk of rejection, reduced time to union, and less revision rates than allograft.[1] Patients should still be advised that there is a possibility of nonunion even with the use of autograft. Generally, most local bone graft procedures are very well tolerated with minimal postoperative pain or dysfunction.

References

1. Flierl MA, Smith WR, Mauffrey C, et al. Outcomes and complication rates of different bone grafting modalities in long bone fracture nonunions: a retrospective cohort study in 182 patients. J Orthop Surg 2013;8:33
2. Acumed. Acumed Bone Graft Harvesting System Surgical Technique www.acumed.net. Published 2015. Accessed November 23, 2016

32 Open Achilles Rupture Repair

Steven M. Raikin

Abstract

The overall incidence of acute Achilles tendon rupture has been steadily rising with the Achilles being the third most commonly injured tendon in the body. These occur most commonly in male recreational "weekend warrior" athletes in their fourth decade, with injury occurring during sports participation. The Achilles tendon experiences the highest tensile loads of any tendon in the body, often up to 10 times the body weight during athletic activity. Rupture can lead to significant functional morbidity if not adequately treated. Optimal treatment of acute Achilles tendon ruptures remains controversial between formal open repair, limited more percutaneous surgical repair, and nonoperative treatment. While the details of this debate are beyond the realms of this chapter, the major concern with open repair remains the risk of wound healing complications, which range from 3% for deep infections to more than 10% for overall complications. This chapter aims to present surgical tips and pearls to limit the risk of wound complications while optimizing strength of the tendon repair and allowing for an early and aggressive rehabilitation process.

Keywords: *Achilles tendon, Achilles rupture, open Achilles repair, Achilles rupture rehabilitation*

32.1 Indications

- Acute rupture of the Achilles tendon:
  - Less than 4 weeks from the injury.
  - Less than 3-cm retraction gap.

32.1.1 Pathology

- Patients may have symptoms of Achilles tendonitis prior to the acute rupture, with degenerative changes see in micro-pathological evaluation of the ruptured tendon ends in the majority of cases.[1]
- Sports participation is involved in about 70% of injuries:
  - Basketball is the most commonly causative sport in the United States.
  - Soccer is the most common causative sport in Europe.
- Injury most commonly occurs in the watershed hypovascular zone of the tendon, approximately 5 to 7 cm from the calcaneal insertion.
- Ruptures usually occur during eccentric contracture of the tendon during forceful ankle dorsiflexion.

32.1.2 Clinical Evaluation

- Patients often give a history of hearing a pop at the time of the injury.
- The feeling is described as being kicked, hit with a bat, or being shot in the back of the ankle.
- A high degree of suspicion is required so as not to miss an Achilles tendon rupture, which is reported to occur in 10 to 20% of times in the emergency room, particularly in older patients (> 55 years old), obese and diabetics patients, and those not participating is sports at the time of the rupture.
- Patient should be evaluated prone with both legs exposed, and with their knees bent at 90 degrees and both limbs examined.
- There are three cardinal findings of an acute Achilles tendon rupture. When all three are present, the diagnosis is present in 100% of cases.[2] These are as follows:
  - Diminished resting tension of the ankle compared to the unaffected side (which usually rests at 20 degrees of equinus with the knee flexed).
  - Gentle palpation along the tendon will usually detect a defect within the tendon—most commonly 5 to 7 cm from the calcaneal insertion.
  - Thompson's test (gentle squeezing of the gastrocnemius-soleus calf muscle) will result in plantar flexion of the ankle with an intact tendon. In a case where the tendon is ruptured, a small "flicker" of plantar flexion motion may occur due to intact deep compartment flexors, but will be less than/asymmetric to the uninvolved normal limb.
  - The ability of the patient to actively plantarflex the ankle does not exclude an acute Achilles rupture.

32.1.3 Radiographic Evaluation

- In most cases, no radiographic studies are required.
- Plane radiographs are only indicated if an insertional rupture (evaluate for a Haglund process and insertional spurs), or calcaneal avulsion fracture is suspected.
  - Subtle signs on plane radiographs include the following:
    - Loss of sharp contour of Kager's fat pad.
    - Anterior translation of the Achilles tendon shadow (no longer parallel to the skin): Arner's sign.
- Tertiary studies such as MRI or ultrasound are usually unnecessary when the clinical evaluation is consistent with an acute rupture.
  - These studies are costly and may delay time to treatment.
  - Indications for magnetic resonance imaging (MRI)/ultrasound:
    - Inconsistent clinical examination.
    - Prior rupture or Achilles surgery.
    - Chronic rupture more than 4 weeks old or to quantify suspected gap greater than 3 cm.
    - Known chronic Achilles tendinosis.

32.1.4 Nonoperative Options

- Many different nonoperative treatments have been described. These include the following:
  - Cast treatment with the ankle in plantar flexion.

○ Boot immobilization.
○ Functional bracing with early weight-bearing:
   ❖ This has been shown to have the best outcomes of non-operative treatment.
   ❖ Requires close vigilance and monitoring.
• Nonoperative treatment has been shown to have a significantly higher rerupture rate.[3,4]

32.1.5 Contraindications

• Medical comorbidities (high anesthesia risk).
• Infection at/near surgical site.
• High risk of incision-related complications:
  ○ Uncontrolled diabetes.
  ○ Steroid use.
  ○ Poor circulation.
• Inability to comply with postoperative instructions.
• Low functional demand.

32.2 Goals of Surgical Procedure

• To provide a contiguous Achilles tendon with adequately strong repair to allow rapid rehabilitation and long-term return to prerupture functional levels of activity.

32.3 Advantages of Surgical Procedure

• Ability to debride tendinotic edges of rupture.
• End-to-end anastomosis of Achilles tendon.
• Allows multiple locking suture loops at each end of the ruptured tendon.
• Full visualization of tendon.
• Allows early weight-bearing and rehabilitation.
• Lower rerupture rates than nonoperative treatment.
• Stronger muscle function.
• Low incidence of sural nerve injury.

32.4 Key Principles

• Limit wound complications by performing full-thickness incision, deep compartment fasciotomy, limited retraction, and adequate wound closure.
• Stable fixation with locking Krackow's stitches on each end of tendon.
• Rigid repair at the rupture site with multiple knot repair.
• Ensuring strong enough repair to allow early rehabilitation.

32.5 Preoperative Preparation and Patient Positioning

• Supine with a large hip bump under the contralateral hip (Author's preference; **Fig. 32.1**).
• Can be positioned prone on chest rolls:

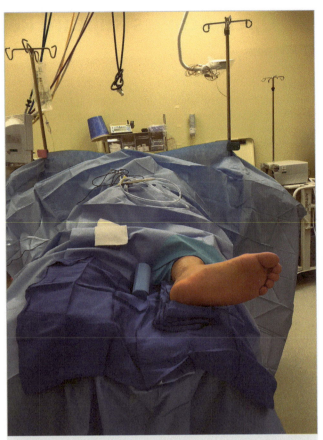

Fig. 32.1 Supine positioning with hip bump under contralateral hip and surgical leg internally rotated.

  ○ This requires patient to be intubated, and has a longer setup time.
• Thigh tourniquet (calf tourniquet will squeeze the gastrocnemius-soleus calf muscle making assessment of Achilles length at repair difficult).
• Leg should be elevated for exsanguination:
  ○ Preferable not to use Esmarch, which may lead to DVT (deep vein thrombosis)/PE (pulmonary embolism).

32.6 Operative Technique

32.6.1 Surgical Approach

• Full thickness 6- to 8-cm longitude incision over the medial border of the Achilles tendon (**Fig. 32.2**):
  ○ Through skin subcutaneous tissue down to and through the paratenon.
• Incision centered over the region of the Achilles tendon rupture.
• Digitally mobilize both ends of the tendon (especially proximally) to free any adhesions or contractures that may have occurred since the rupture (**Fig. 32.3**).
• Tendon ends are then debrided by sharp dissection resecting nonviable and tendinotic tissue usually found at the rupture ends (**Fig. 32.4**). Minimize the amount of tendon being resected.

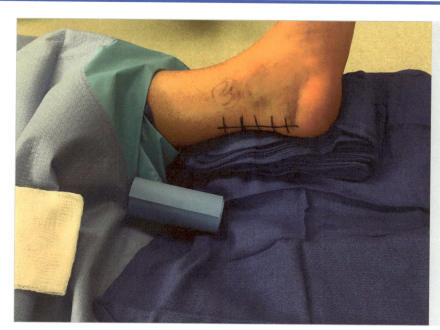

Fig. 32.2 Medial para-Achilles incision, Esmarch's bandage not used.

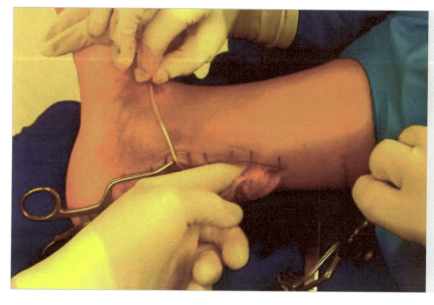

Fig. 32.3 Digitally freeing up proximal ruptured stump of Achilles tendon.

- A deep posterior compartment fasciotomy is performed over the flexor hallucis longus muscle belly anterior to the Achilles tendon (**Fig. 32.5**). This will free up the paratenon, making closure easier at the end of the procedure.
- Skin retraction should be limited as much as possible, and self-retaining retractors should only be used at one end of the incision at a time, limiting skin traction.

32.6.2 Achilles Tendon Repair

- A 1- to 3-cm gap is usually present due to tendon retraction, which can easily be mobilized to obtain end-to-end repair.
- A no. 2 nonabsorbable braided suture is used for the repair. We recommend using FiberWire suture (Arthrex, Naples, FL), which has more than double the load to failure (Newtons [N]) and stiffness (N/mm) than Ethibond suture (Ethicon, Bridgewater, NJ).

- A multilooped Krakow locking suture technique is performed on each end of the ruptured tendon.
- Four to five locking loops are ideally performed on each end of the tendon medially and laterally.
- The ends of the suture should enter and exit within the ruptured end of the tendon.
- If there is a gap between the ruptured ends, traction is applied to the proximal stump mobilizing the muscle and allowing end-to-end approximation of the ruptured tendon ends.
- The ankle should be placed in a neutral resting position (20–30 degrees of plantar flexion) during the repair.
- The knot is the weakest point of the repair. We use 10 locking surgical knots in each matching pair of the suture for repair.
- Knots are placed intratendinous—that is, within the ends of the ruptured tendon.

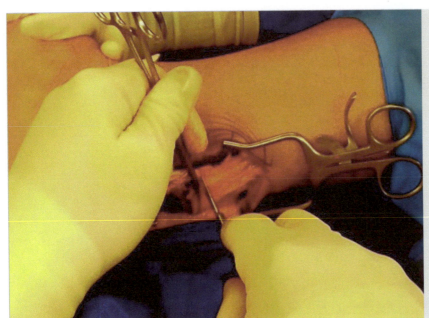

Fig. 32.4 Trimming tendinosis ruptured ends of Achilles.

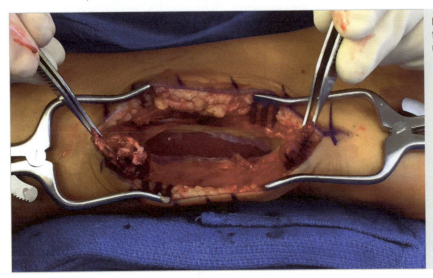

Fig. 32.5 Deep posterior compartment fasciotomy over flexor hallucis longus (FHL) muscle to mobilize paratenon.

- To prevent knot irritation, the ends of the suture are then passed under the tendon to the opposite side, thereby burying the knots deep (anterior) to the tendon (**Fig. 32.6**).
- An absorbable braided no. 0 suture is then used to perform an epitendinous type running suture circumferentially around the repair site (**Fig. 32.7**):
  - This will help bury the suture knots within the substance of the repaired Achilles tendon.
  - This will additionally limit the bulkiness at the repair end of the tendon (tubularize the tendon).
  - Based on the literature, this adds strength to the repair, but this has not been proved in the ruptured (as opposed to the lacerated) tendon.
- Resting tension of the repair is assessed with the knee bent to 90 degrees, and compared to the nonruptured side.
- Before closure, the ankle should be dorsiflexed to 5 to 10 degrees to ensure that the tendon repair remains intact without diastasis between the tendon ends.

32.6.3 Closure

- This is a very important part of the procedure.
- The paratenon needs to be closed as a separate layer over the Achilles tendon:
  - This will limit tendon-to-skin adhesions and improve tendon gliding.
  - Improves the vascularity to the Achilles tendon.
  - Adds an extra layer of tissue over the tendon in the event of skin breakdown.
- As a result of the performed deep compartment fasciotomy, the paratenon can be easily mobilized to cover the Achilles tendon repair.
- We use a running continuous suture of no. 0 braided absorbable suture for this layer of closure.
  - The repair is initially performed loosely preventing cutout of the suture in this thin tissue layer (**Fig. 32.8**).
  - Ensure that none of the sutures are locked.

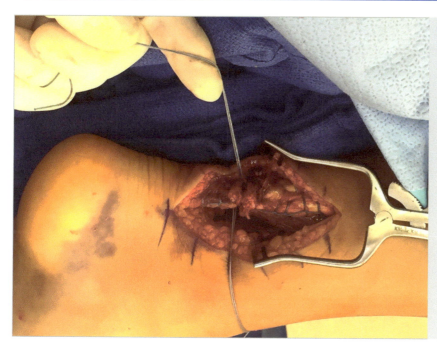

Fig. 32.6 Burying suture knots anterior to the tendon.

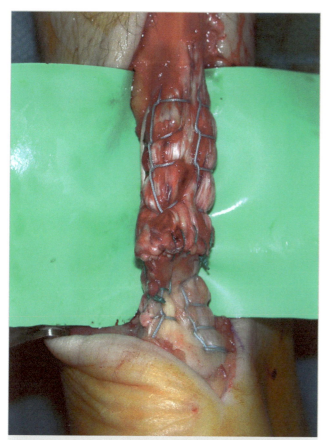

Fig. 32.7 The repaired Achilles tendon with multiple locked Krakow sutures. The circumferential epitendinous suture is shown rounding off the rupture level.

○ Once the length of the repair has been completed, the end of the suture is pulled longitudinally allowing the paratenon to close like a zipper, evenly distributing the tension throughout the length of the repair and preventing cutting out of the suture (**Fig. 32.9**).

• The subcutaneous layer is then closed over the paratenon with absorbable interrupted suture.
• Skin closure can be performed with 2–0 nylon sutures or skin staples:
  ○ We have had no problems using skin staples.
• A well-padded posterior and U splint is then applied.
  ○ This is applied with the ankle in 20 degrees of equinus to optimize skin end vascularity.
• Tourniquet use has not been shown to cause any problems, but the tourniquet time should be kept to a minimum.

32.7 Tips and Pearls

• Surgery should be performed within 2 weeks of rupture.
• Avoiding wound complications improves outcome.
• Do not overlengthen tendon at repair.
  ○ A little too tight is better (more rehabilitationable) than too loose a repair.
• Ensure adequate strength of the repair to allow early weight-bearing and rehabilitation:
  ○ If not happy with strength of repair, weight-bearing/rehabilitation should be delayed.

32.8 Hazards and Pitfalls

• Tight skin closure and inadequate postoperative elevation results in higher wound complications.

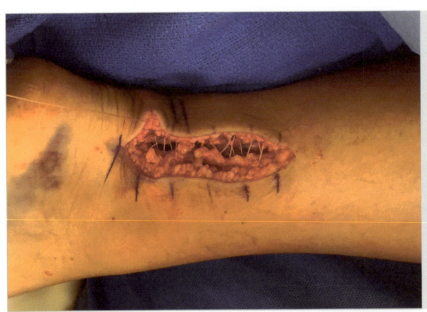

Fig. 32.8 Loose reapproximation of paratenon layer.

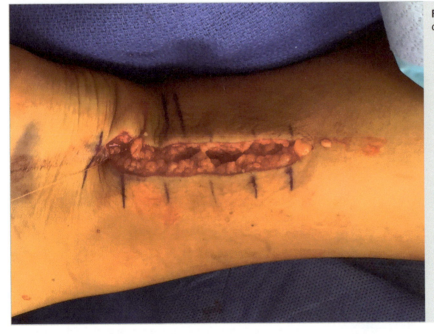

Fig. 32.9 Paratenon repair after "zipper" closure.

- If a larger gap (usually > 3 cm) is present that cannot be approximated, a lengthening procedure should be added to bridge the gap.
- If severe tendinosis is present, an FHL tendon transfer can be utilized through the same incision to augment the repair.

32.9 Complications/Bailout/ Salvage

- Skin wound complications:
  - About 10 to 15% of cases will have some wound healing problem.
  - Most are minor and do not require additional treatment or require local care.
    - Can be avoided or limited with careful surgical technique.
- Deep infection:
  - Occurs in 0.5 to 5% of cases.
  - Requires open surgical debridement and antibiotic treatment.
  - Do not ignore a deep infection.
- Nerve injury:
  - Rare when using medial para-Achilles approach.
  - Sural nerve more commonly injured with percutaneous techniques.
- Overlengthened tendon:
  - Very difficult to treat.
  - Results in weakness of the tendon, which does not improve with therapy:
    - Difficulty on inclines/stairs (particularly downward).

❖ Weakness in push-off phase of gait.
○ Usually requires revision shortening surgery.
• Rerupture:
  ○ 1.5% with open repair.
  ○ Much higher with nonsurgical treatment.
• DVT/PE:
  ○ Negatively affects outcome when this occurs.
  ○ Higher risk with chronic rupture (> 4 weeks) treatment.[5]
  ○ Higher risk with high BMI (body mass index).
  ○ Higher risk age greater than 40 years.[6]
  ○ High index suspicion required.

32.10 Postoperative Care

• Procedure is usually performed on an outpatient basis:
  ○ Strict elevation is crucial (above heart level) for the first 2 weeks following surgery:
    ❖ This significantly diminishes wound complications.
  ○ Non-weight-bearing for the first 2 weeks.
• At 2-week postoperative visit, sutures are removed if adequate wound healing is present:
  ○ Patients are placed in a three-wedge plantarflexed walking boot (30 degrees).
  ○ Patients can be weight-bearing as tolerated, with crutch support for the next 2 weeks.
• At 4 weeks (no visit required), one wedge is removed from the boot (ankle now at 20 degrees equinus) and patients are encouraged to ambulate without external support.
  ○ Patients are instructed on home eccentric strengthening of the tendon without dorsiflexion beyond 0 degrees.
• At 6 weeks, the second wedge is removed and ambulation in boot continued.
  ○ Physical therapy is formally started—this is done out of the boot and includes Achilles eccentric strengthening, Alfredson's step protocol, stretching, and progressive treadmill ambulation out of the boot.
• At 8 weeks, the final wedge is removed:
  ○ Under the guidance of the therapist, the boot is weaned between 8 and 12 weeks.
• Between 12 weeks and 6 months, progressive strengthening and activity are allowed.
  ○ Continued physical therapy (formal or on own).
  ○ Limited jumping, cutting, or aggressive acceleration activities.
• At 6 months, patients are allowed activity as tolerated.
• Often it takes 12 months to resume full preinjury activity level.

32.11 Outcomes

• Sixty-five percent of professional athletes (football, basketball, soccer) return to professional sports:[7–10]
  ○ Decreased performance and longevity of career.[7–10]
• Wound complications rate of 2.5% requiring additional care:[11]
  ○ Wound complications of 0.5% require additional surgery.
• Never regains 100% strength of contralateral uninjured leg:
  ○ Usually 70 to 90%.[12–14]

References

1. Cetti R, Junge J, Vyberg M. Spontaneous rupture of the Achilles tendon is preceded by widespread and bilateral tendon damage and ipsilateral inflammation: a clinical and histopathologic study of 60 patients. Acta Orthop Scand 2003;74(1):78–84
2. Garras DN, Raikin SM, Bhat SB, Taweel N, Karanjia H. MRI is unnecessary for diagnosing acute Achilles tendon ruptures: clinical diagnostic criteria. Clin Orthop Relat Res 2012;470(8):2268–2273
3. Möller M, Movin T, Granhed H, Lind K, Faxén E, Karlsson J. Acute rupture of tendon Achilles. A prospective randomised study of comparison between surgical and non-surgical treatment. J Bone Joint Surg Br 2001;83(6):843–848
4. Erickson BJ, Mascarenhas R, Saltzman BM, et al. Is Operative treatment of Achilles tendon ruptures superior to nonoperative treatment?: a systematic review of overlapping meta-analyses. Orthop J Sports Med 2015;3(4):2325967115579188
5. Bullock MJ, DeCarbo WT, Hofbauer MH, Thun JD. Repair of chronic Achilles ruptures has a high incidence of venous thromboembolism. Foot Ankle Spec 2016:1938640016679706
6. Arverud ED, Anundsson P, Hardell E, et al. Ageing, deep vein thrombosis and male gender predict poor outcome after acute Achilles tendon rupture. Bone Joint J 2016;98-B(12):1635–1641
7. Amin NH, Old AB, Tabb LP, Garg R, Toossi N, Cerynik DL. Performance outcomes after repair of complete Achilles tendon ruptures in national basketball association players. Am J Sports Med 2013;41(8):1864–1868
8. Minhas SV, Kester BS, Larkin KE, Hsu WK. The effect of an orthopaedic surgical procedure in the National Basketball Association. Am J Sports Med 2016;44(4):1056–1061
9. Mai HT, Alvarez AP, Freshman RD, et al. The NFL Orthopaedic Surgery Outcomes Database (NO-SOD): the effect of common orthopaedic procedures on football careers. Am J Sports Med 2016;44(9):2255–2262
10. Parekh SG, Wray WH III, Brimmo O, Sennett BJ, Wapner KL. Epidemiology and outcomes of Achilles tendon ruptures in the National Football League. Foot Ankle Spec 2009;2(6):283–286
11. Marican MM, Fook-Chong SM, Rikhraj IS. Incidence of postoperative wound infections after open tendo Achilles repairs. Singapore Med J 2015;56(10):549–554
12. Arslan A, Çepni SK, Sahinkaya T, May C, Mutlu H, Parmaksızoğlu AS. Functional outcomes of repair of Achilles tendon using a biological open surgical method. Acta Orthop Traumatol Turc 2014;48(5):563–569
13. Kadakia AR, Dekker RG II, Ho BS. Acute Achilles tendon ruptures: an update on treatment. J Am Acad Orthop Surg 2017;25(1):23–31
14. Rosenzweig S, Azar FM. Open repair of acute Achilles tendon ruptures. Foot Ankle Clin 2009;14(4):699–709

33 Direct Posterior Midline Approach for Treatment of Insertional Achilles Tendonitis

Taggart T. Gauvain and William C. McGarvey

Abstract

Posterior midline approach for the treatment of insertional Achilles tendonitis is a highly reproducible surgical procedure that has good results with long-term follow-up. Patient satisfaction has reached 96% in some studies and most patients report that they would recommend the procedure to family and/or undergo it again if needed. Few complications occur with respect to the soft tissues due to the position of the incision in between two separate angiosomes. Excellent visualization and access is provided for the Achilles tendon debridement. Up to 70% of the tendon insertion can be safely elevated without increased risk of delayed rupture. This provides for adequate debridement and re-establishment of native resting tone following repair. This approach provides direct access for flexor hallucis longus tendon transfer if indicated. Haglund's deformity can be adequately resected to decompress the posterior heel with this approach. Double row suture bridge repair provides large surface area of tendon–bone interface allowing for rapid healing and early mobilization in most cases.

Keywords: *insertional Achilles tendonitis, Haglund's deformity, Fowler–Philip angle, Pavlov's parallel pitch lines, intratendinous spur, nonoperative treatment, surgical approach*

33.1 Indications and Pathology

- Degenerative process at the insertion of the Achilles tendon onto the posterior calcaneus.
- Painful condition commonly seen as a chronic overuse issue. It is also seen in sedentary patients as a degenerative process.
- Painful inflammation and degeneration occurs both at the tendon insertion and within the local substance of the Achilles tendon.
- Patients present with heel pain that is exacerbated by mechanical irritation from closed shoe wear, presence of bony impingement, and local bursitis causing inflammation.
- This condition represents 10 to 20% of all Achilles pathology.
- Ten percent of patients are recalcitrant to nonsurgical intervention.[1]
- The posterior midline approach for debridement and repair of the insertion of the Achilles tendon is a successful and reproducible means to treat this condition.

33.1.1 Anatomy

- The Achilles tendon (confluence of the gastrocnemius and soleus tendons) is the largest tendon in the body. It connects the triceps surae (two heads of the gastrocnemius and the soleus muscle) to the calcaneus bone in the foot.
- Its primary function is to plantarflex the foot.
- The tendon bears up to 10 times the body weight during single leg stance while running.
- It inserts broadly on the posterior calcaneus covering the entirety of the distal tuberosity and extends to the medial and lateral plantar borders of the bone.

- Anterior to the tendon lies the retrocalcaneal bursa. This bursa can become a source of inflammation and pain especially when a large Haglund's deformity is present (superolateral calcaneal prominence).
- Deep to the retrocalcaneal bursa lies the deep posterior compartment of the leg encased in its fascial layer. Structures within the deep posterior compartment include flexor hallucis longus (FHL), the posterior tibial artery and vein, the tibial nerve, and flexor digitorum longus. These structures lie in this order from lateral to medial starting at the medial border of the distal tibia within the deep posterior compartment.

33.1.2 Clinical Evaluation

- Palpation of the tendon insertion often elicits pain, most commonly over the superolateral corner of the calcaneus where a visible prominence may be present.
- Patients often have a contracture of the Achilles tendon and have limited dorsiflexion.
- The intratendinous spur is often painful and palpable on physical exam.
- Thickening and nodularity of the tendon is common.
- Occasionally there will be crepitus or even an actual squeak with motion.
- Shoe wear is mostly limited to backless or soft-heeled types.

33.1.3 Radiographic Evaluation

- Lateral radiographs will often show a large Haglund's deformity (superolateral calcaneal prominence), ossific changes within the distal portion of the tendon, and traction spur formation at the insertion of the Achilles tendon (**Figs. 33.1**).
- The Haglund deformity can be diagnosed using radiographic parameters including Fowler–Philip angle, Pavlov's parallel pitch lines, and calcaneal pitch angle.
  - A Fowler–Philip angle greater than 75 degrees (normal is 44–69 degrees).[2]
  - Posterior bone prominence above the superior parallel pitch line.[3]
  - Combined pitch angle and Fowler–Philip angle greater than 90 degrees.
- Magnetic resonance imaging (MRI) is indicated preoperatively in select cases (**Fig. 33.2**).
  - Prior Achilles surgery.
  - Suspicion of infection.
  - Atypical pain and presentation.
  - Defining the extent of degenerative tendon in noncalcification tendinopathy.

33.1.4 Nonoperative Options[1,4-6]

- Icing regimens.
- Activity modification.

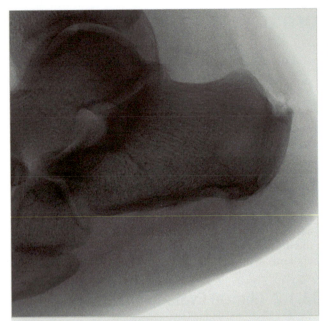

Fig. 33.1 Lateral radiograph demonstrating large posterior calcaneal spur, tuberosity deformity, and Haglund's deformity.

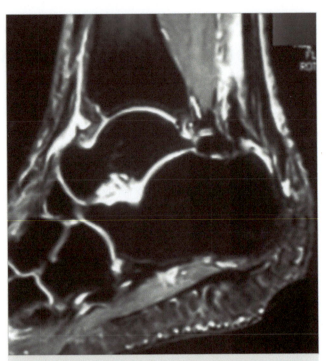

Fig. 33.2 Sagittal magnetic resonance imaging (MRI) of the heel. Note increased uptake surrounding the distal insertion of the Achilles and the deterioration at the bone-tendon interface. This is a severe case of this disorder.

- Boot immobilization.
- Oral anti-inflammatory medication.
- Physical therapy including eccentric strengthening, iontophoresis, and aggressive Achilles tendon stretching exercises.
- Extracorporeal shock wave therapy.
- Nitroglycerine patches.
- Platelet-rich plasma (PRP) injections.
- Almost 90% of patients will respond well to nonoperative intervention.

33.1.5 Contraindications

- Presence of adjacent scars/incisions that may be utilized to approach the Achilles tendon.
- Posterior skin ulceration or wound.
- Dysvascular extremity.
- Active infection.
- Large, thick callosities.

33.2 Goals of Surgical Procedure

- Goals of the surgery are to remove damaged and diseased tendon tissue, inflamed bursal tissue, bone prominences causing impingement, and painful osteophytes as well as calcified areas in and around the insertion of the Achilles tendon.
- By removing the degenerative and inflamed tissue, the patient may find great relief of pain and the ability to resume desired activities and normal shoe wear.

33.3 Advantages of Surgical Procedure

- The direct posterior midline approach provides direct access to the Achilles tendon and calcaneus. Ninety-five percent of patients have central tendon disease that needs to be removed. Exposure of this area is generous and uncomplicated with good technique.
- The midline incision gives you healthy tissue flaps by not requiring division or disruption of the blood supply to the skin. The incision is in between angiosomes of the posterior leg with the medial flap supplied by the calcaneal branches of the posterior tibial artery and the lateral flap supplied by the calcaneal branches of the peroneal artery.
- The incision also keeps the sural nerve and vein safely in the tissues lateral to the surgical wound. There is almost no loss of sensation following this incision because it is placed at the border of the medial saphenous nerve dermatome and the lateral sural nerve dermatome.
- This approach is indicated for insertional Achilles tendonitis, Achilles tendinosis, posterior compartment access, tibiotalar joint fusion, subtalar joint fusion, and tibiotalocalcaneal fusion.

33.4 Key Principles

- Prone positioning.
- Direct midline approach over the distal Achilles tendon.
- Split the Achilles insertion and remove all tendonotic portions of the tendon.
- Resect the Haglund's deformity.
- Reattach the Achilles back to the tuberosity with suture anchors.
- FHL tendon transfer augmentation is performed if greater than 50% of the Achilles tendon is debrided.

33.5 Preoperative Preparation and Patient Positioning

- Operative limb is appropriately shaved with an electric clipper in the pre-op holding area.
- General endotracheal anesthesia should be applied with the patient still on the hospital gurney.
- Tourniquet should be placed high on the thigh of the operative limb prior to turning prone.
- The patient is turned prone on the OR (operating room) table with gel rolls supporting the chest and padding for all bony prominences. The arms should be in the "superman" position with the shoulders abducted less than 90 degrees.
- The feet should be hanging just off the edge of the bed with a pillow under the anterior ankles.
- A bump can be placed under the nonoperative side hip to adjust rotation of the operative limb to have the posterior midline ankle facing directly to the ceiling.

33.6 Operative Technique

- A 6-cm incision is made directly in the posterior midline of the heel. Incision starts 2 to 3 cm above the insertion of the Achilles tendon on the calcaneus and ends just distal to the glabrous–nonglabrous skin junction (**Fig. 33.3**).

- Full-thickness dissection down to the level of the paratenon, which is then incised vertically along the tendon midline.
- Tendon and its insertion are split in the midline with the scalpel the length of the skin incision.
- The tendon insertion is reflected with subperiosteal dissection off the calcaneus medially and laterally, but be sure to leave some far medial and far lateral tendon insertion intact to maintain natural resting tone and tension for the repair later.
- Small Weitlaner self-retainer is then placed within the split portion of the tendon proximally. Be careful not to place any excessive retraction directly on the skin flaps (**Fig. 33.4**).
- Sharply excise degenerative and calcific portions within the tendon and along the insertion with the scalpel. You can feel these portions of the tendon as lumps and grainy areas along the tendon.
- Deep to the tendon layer is the tissue of the retrocalcaneal bursa. There is fatty tissue and small veins present in this area. This tissue should be removed with the assistance of electrocautery given it is a fairly vascular tissue. You are safe in the midline and superficial to the deep posterior compartment fascial layer (**Fig. 33.4**).
- Any posterior spur on the calcaneus can be removed with osteotome or oscillating saw.
- The Haglund's deformity can now be removed using osteotome or oscillating saw. Be sure to angle your cut so that you do not violate the posterior facet of the calcaneus. The goal is to remove the triangular bony prominence and leave a flat surface behind (**Fig. 33.5**).

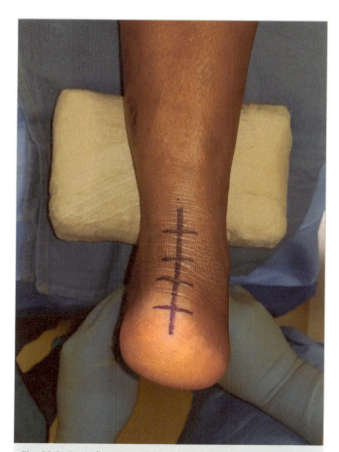

Fig. 33.3 Central position of the incision marked on the heel. 6-cm incision starting 2 cm above the insertion of the Achilles on the calcaneus and ending just distal to the glabrous-nonglabrous skin junction.

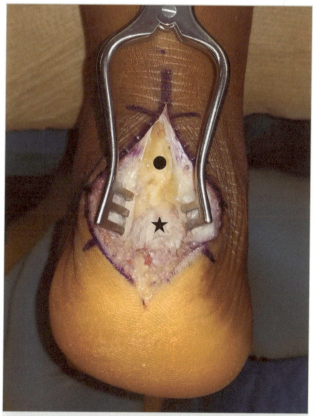

Fig. 33.4 Careful placement of retractor within the tendon split. Retrocalcaneal bursa and fatty tissue noted deeper in the wound (*black circle*). Haglund's deformity can now be visualized as well (*black star*).

- The calcaneus can then be shaped with a power rasp to round and smooth the medial and lateral edges as well as the convexity of the posterior calcaneus (**Fig. 33.6**).
- Palpate the heel through the incision and the skin for any prominent bony areas that should be addressed. Fluoroscopy can be used to ensure adequate resection (**Fig. 33.7**).
- Irrigate area and suction all debris from the operative field.

- Inspect the remaining Achilles tendons. Transfer of the FHL should be considered if 50% or more of the native tendon has been debrided during the procedure.[7]
- Suture anchor fixation with a double row is used to reattach the tendon to the calcaneus.
- Predrill and tap two anchor holes on the superior calcaneus surface at the proximal insertion point of the tendon onto the bone (**Fig. 33.8**). Predrill and tap two additional anchor

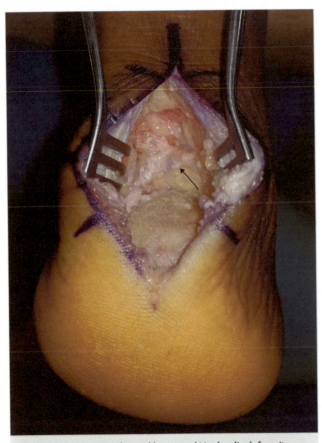

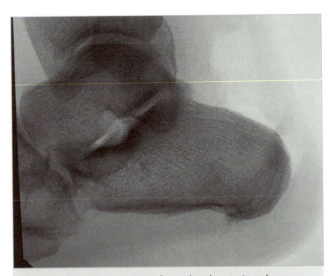

Fig. 33.7 Fluoroscopic image of completed posterior calcaneus bony resection.

Fig. 33.5 Note retrocalcaneal bursa and Haglund's deformity are now resected. Deeper fascial layer seen now is the fascia of the deep compartment (*black arrow*).

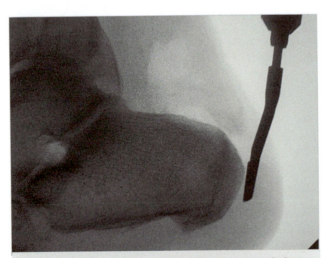

Fig. 33.6 Aggressive resection of posterior calcaneus including, but not limited to spur and Haglund's deformity. Up to 1 cm of bone is sometimes removed to decompress the heel.

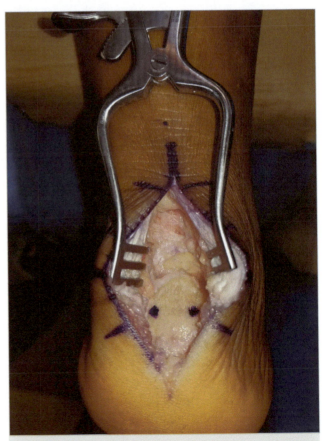

Fig. 33.8 Planned insertion sites for the superior anchor row. All pilot holes are drilled and tapped.

holes just distal to the apex of the convexity of the posterior calcaneus.

- Two double loaded suture anchors should be placed in the superior calcaneus anchor pilot holes, one medial and one lateral. Bring the suture through the medial and lateral tendon portions at the area that corresponds to the proximal insertion contact point when the tendon is pulled back down on to the calcaneus.
- Take one suture from each side and secure into the two posterior anchor spots creating the double row and bringing the Achilles tendon securely into contact with the calcaneus (**Figs. 33.9–33.11**).
- Vancomycin powder can be placed into the space deep to the tendon if desired.
- The tendon should be closed side to side with a dissolvable suture in interrupted or running fashion. Knots should be buried within the tendon (**Fig. 33.12**).
- Resting tension can be assessed by comparing to the contralateral side and is critical at this point to avoid overlengthening.
- Close the paratenon layer using a running monofilament suture. Do not neglect this step given the Achilles tendon can scar the skin layer, causing skin issues if the paratenon is not properly repaired (**Fig. 33.13**).
- Close the subcutaneous tissue and skin with interrupted sutures.
- Place a well-padded posterior splint with the foot in resting equinus.

33.7 Tips and Pearls

- Ensure all tendenotic portions of the tendon are removed.
- Inadequate resection of the Haglund's deformity can cause recurrence of insertional tendonitis.
- Ensure good tendon to bone contact when reattaching the tendon down to the calcaneal bone to ensure appropriate ingrowth.
- Do not repair/reattach the Achilles in a lengthened position— match to the opposite side.
- An FHL transfer can be performed through the same midline posterior incision to augment the Achilles without adding to the morbidity of the procedure.

33.8 Hazards and Pitfalls

- An overlengthened tendon is harder to rehabilitate than an overtight tendon.
- In severe cases, most of the distal tendon—often up to 2 cm—may need to be resected. This can be accommodated for by adding a Strayer gastrocnemius recession to mobilize the myotendinous region and deliver the distal tendon down to the calcaneus for reinsertion.
- The posterior heel (area of the incision) should be protected from pressure postoperatively to avoid wound complications.

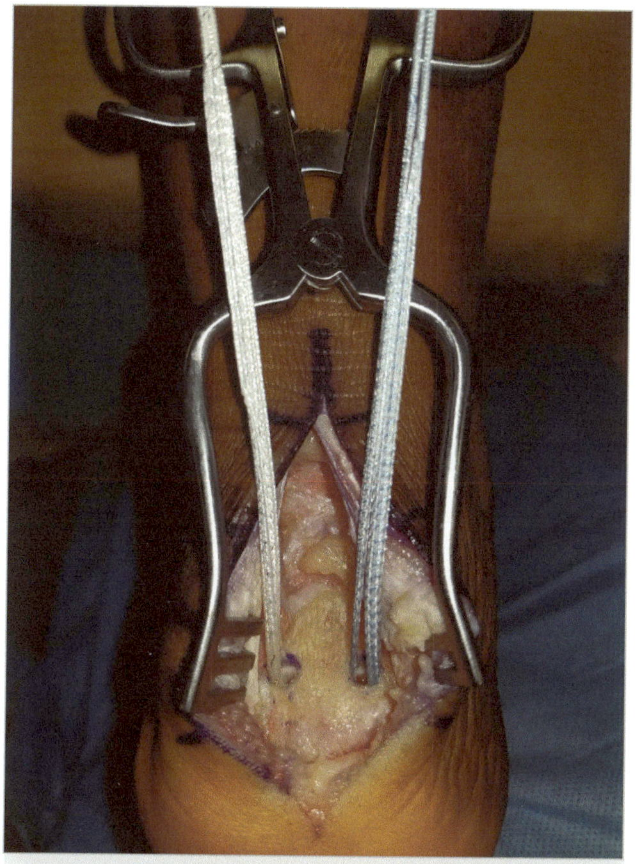

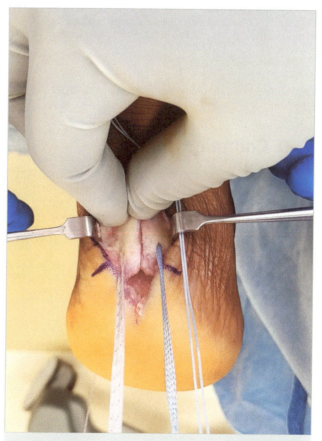

Fig. 33.9 Insertion of first row of planned double row of suture anchors. If tendon transfer is performed, that should be done first and the anchors placed beside or more posterior on the tuberosity (closer to the surgeon) to the tenodesis screw.

Fig. 33.10 Sutures are brought through the limbs of the tendon at the appropriate level to bring the tendon down into contact with the calcaneus at the appropriate tension.

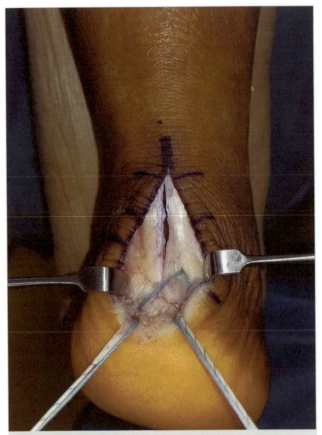

Fig. 33.11 One limb of each suture is crossed over and then fixed into the distal anchor row with the remaining limb on the opposite side.

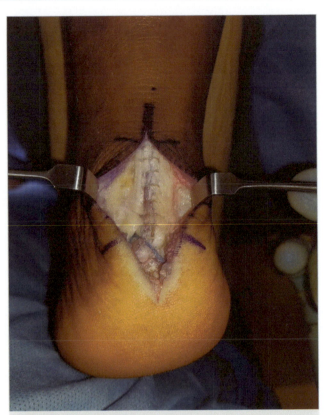

Fig. 33.12 Midline Achilles split is repaired side to side with a running suture.

Elevating pillows should be positioned under the calf and not the heel.

33.9 Complications

- Wound complications are the most common problem following this procedure. This is at greatest risk in obese patients, those with diabetes, suboptimal circulation, and if pressure is applied directly over the heel area during recovery.
- Failure of the tendon to obtain adequate ingrowth into the calcaneal bone.
- Recurrent tendinosis of the insertion.
- Achilles insertional rupture. This is rare and usually associated with a traumatic event (fall) during the perioperative period.

33.10 Postoperative Care

- Patient should be seen at 2 weeks post-op for suture removal and transition to either a cast or tall boot with a 2-inch heel lift.

- If patient is placed into a boot, allow TDWB (touchdown weight-bearing) for the following 2 weeks.
- At 4 weeks post-op, full weight-bearing is allowed in a tall boot with a 2-inch lift. Lift is removed layer by layer until foot is returned to neutral in the boot by 6 weeks post-op.
- Begin formal physical therapy at 6 weeks post-op with non-impact strengthening exercise as tolerated. Begin transition to normal shoe wear by week 8 to 10 post-op.
- At 3 months post-op, full-impact activity is allowed and patient is given full clearance for sports activity.

33.11 Outcomes

- Overall patient satisfaction for surgical intervention is 82% at 33 months.[1]
  - Ninety percent in patients under 50 and 75% in patients older than 55 years.[1]
  - Four- and 7-year follow-up data have shown 96% overall satisfaction rates.[8]
- Ninety percent younger than 50 years return to work/activity by 3 months.[1]
- Fifty percent older than 55 years return to work/activity by 3 months.[1]

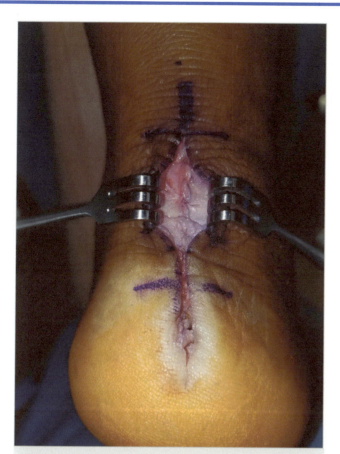

Fig. 33.13 Paratenon layer is closed with a running monofilament. Care is taken to reapproximate this very important layer to avoid wound complications of the skin scarring directly to the Achilles tendon.

- Average time to maximum symptomatic improvement is approximately 10 months.[1]
  - Pain resolution occurs on average at approximately 5 to 6 months.[8]
- Average Visual Analog Scale pain scores improved 7.2 points, from 7.5 to 0.3.[9]
- Average American Orthopaedic Foot and Ankle Society (AOFAS) Ankle Hindfoot scores improved 39.9 points, from 56.3 to 96 .2.[9]

- Patients who have undergone debridement of the Achilles tendon using these methods are likely to recommend the procedure to family and/or undergo the procedure again if needed.[10]

References

1. McGarvey WC, Palumbo RC, Baxter DE, Leibman BD. Insertional Achilles tendinosis: surgical treatment through a central tendon splitting approach. Foot Ankle Int 2002;23(1):19–25
2. Fowler A, Philip JF. Abnormality of the calcaneus as a cause of painful heel. Br J Surg 1954;32:494–500
3. Pavlov H, Heneghan MA, Hersh A, Goldman AB, Vigorita V. The Haglund syndrome: initial and differential diagnosis. Radiology 1982;144(1):83–88
4. DeOrio MJ, Easley ME. Surgical strategies: insertional Achilles tendinopathy. Foot Ankle Int 2008;29(5):542–550
5. Hunte G, Lloyd-Smith R. Topical glyceryl trinitrate for chronic Achilles tendinopathy. Clin J Sport Med 2005;15(2):116–117
6. Rompe JD, Furia J, Maffulli N. Eccentric loading compared with shock wave treatment for chronic insertional Achilles tendinopathy. A randomized, controlled trial. J Bone Joint Surg Am 2008;90(1):52–61
7. Hunt KJ, Cohen BE, Davis WH, Anderson RB, Jones CP. Surgical treatment of insertional Achilles tendinopathy with or without flexor hallucis longus tendon transfer: a prospective, randomized study. Foot Ankle Int 2015;36(9): 998–1005
8. Nunley JA, Ruskin G, Horst F. Long-term clinical outcomes following the central incision technique for insertional Achilles tendinopathy. Foot Ankle Int 2011;32(9):850–855
9. Elias I, Raikin SM, Besser MP, Nazarian LN. Outcomes of chronic insertional Achilles tendinosis using FHL autograft through single incision. Foot Ankle Int 2009;30(3): 197–204
10. Watson AD, Anderson RB, Davis WH. Comparison of results of retrocalcaneal decompression for retrocalcaneal bursitis and insertional Achilles tendinosis with calcific spur. Foot Ankle Int 2000;21(8):638–642

34 Midsubstance Achilles Tendinosis

Christopher Diefenbach, Christopher Kreulen, and Eric Giza

Abstract

Midsubstance Achilles tendonosis is a painful chronic condition that has many associated factors. This chapter details a concise and thorough review of the pathology, appropriate workup and conservative management, operative technique including pertinent tips/tricks/bailouts, postoperative rehabilitation, and outcomes of midsubstance Achilles tendonosis treatment. Operative repair is indicated after thorough evaluation and work-up, and the patient has failed conservative management, which occurs in approximately 24 to 45% of cases. The goals of open excision and repair of midsubstance Achilles tendinopathy are to excise fibrotic adhesions, remove degenerated nodules, identify and resect intratendinous lesions, and restore vascularity to remaining healthy tendinous tissue to help stimulate a healing response. The ultimate goal is to restore function and strength of the Achilles tendon. The operative technique described within this chapter reflects the most current knowledge of the disease process and optimal technique for complete resolution of symptomatology, restoration of function, and timely rehabilitation. Excellent patient outcomes and satisfaction can be obtained, and hinge on the extent of disease as well as meticulous surgical technique followed by thorough rehabilitation.

Keywords: midsubstance Achilles tendinosis, Achilles tendon, tendinosis, tendinopathy, operative repair, open repair, surgical technique, Achilles rehabilitation, Achilles repair

34.1 Indication and Pathology

- Tendinopathy of the midsubstance of the Achilles tendon.
- Associated factors (not necessarily causative).
- Intrinsic: overuse vascularity, gastrocnemius–soleus dysfunction, age, gender, BMI (body mass index), metabolic factors, foot malalignment, ankle instability.
- Extrinsic: quinolone antibiotics, training pattern changes, poor technique, footwear, environmental training factors (hard, slippery, slanted surface).[1]

34.1.1 Clinical Evaluation

- Pain localized 2 to 6 cm proximal to the calcaneal insertion, particularly with exercise (**Fig. 34.1**).
- Pain increased at the beginning and end of exercise sessions, with intermediate period of minimized discomfort.
- Hindfoot inspected for malalignment, deformity, tendon asymmetry, thickening, Haglund's deformity, previous scarring.
- Palpable tenderness, heat, thickening, nodularity, crepitus.
- "Painful range of motion" characterized by movement of the nodule within paratenon during plantar/dorsiflexion.[2-7]

34.1.2 Radiographic Evaluation

- Plain film lateral radiograph is useful because it may show an associated bony abnormality or intrasubstance calcification (**Fig. 34.2**).

- Magnetic resonance imaging (MRI)/ultrasound provides information on the internal tendon morphology and is useful for preoperative planning, extent of degeneration, peritendinitis versus tendinosis.
- Sagittal and axial MRI images are helpful to determine the percentage of tendon involvement as augmentation may be necessary if greater than 50% of the tendon is removed (**Fig. 34.3**).
- Disorganized tissue appears as intrasubstance intermediate signal intensity.

34.1.3 Nonoperative Options

- A trial of conservative treatment is typically recommended prior to indicating a patient for surgical intervention.

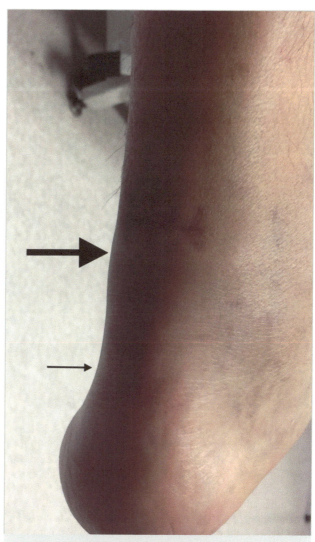

Fig. 34.1 Clinical photograph demonstrating a fusiform swelling of an Achilles tendon 4 cm proximal to the calcaneus (*large arrow*) contrasted with the normal width of the Achilles tendon (*small arrow*).

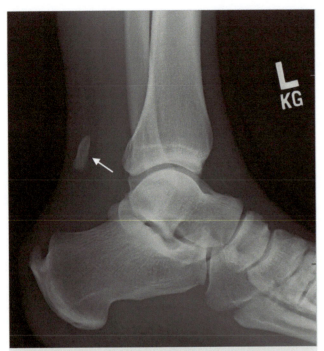

Fig. 34.2 Lateral radiograph of the ankle demonstrating an intrasubstance calcification in the center of an area of midsubstance tendinopathy (*arrow*).

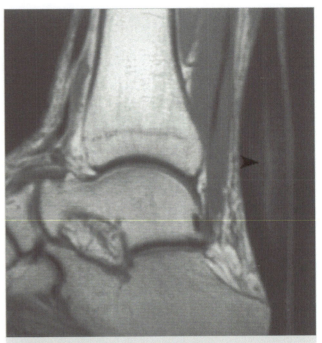

Fig. 34.3 Sagittal T1-weighted MRI (magnetic resonance imaging) demonstrating a thickened Achilles tendon with altered signal intensity within the central tendon.

- Boot immobilization.
- Nonsteroidal anti-inflammatory drugs can help alleviate acute symptoms.
- Eccentric loading and low-energy shockwave therapy show comparatively beneficial results.[8,9]
- Other controversial options: gastrocnemius–soleus recession, peritendinous aprotinin, or topical glyceryl trinitrate.[10-12]
- Platelet-rich plasma injection can provide pain relief and decreased tendon circumference for many patients, and remains an option prior to surgical intervention. The injection is best performed under ultrasound guidance to provide direct visualization of the diseased fibers.[13]

34.1.4 Contraindications

- Elderly or sedentary patients.
- Significant medical comorbidities including diabetic neuropathy and severe vascular disease.

34.2 Goals of Surgical Procedure

Operative repair is indicated after the patient has failed 6 months of conservative management, which occurs in approximately 24 to 45% of cases.[10] The goals of open excision and repair of midsubstance Achilles tendinopathy are to excise fibrotic adhesions, remove degenerated nodules, identify and resect intratendinous lesions, and restore vascularity to remaining healthy tendinous tissue to help stimulate a healing response. The ultimate goal is to restore function and strength of the Achilles tendon.[9]

34.3 Advantages of Surgical Procedure

The advantages of an open midsubstance Achilles tendinopathy repair can be attributed to the resultant healing response to the operative procedure in general, as well as the specific technique. Operative repair has been shown to yield successful results in patients who have otherwise failed conservative management. Complete debridement of tendinopathic tissue allows for viable tendon healing and restoration of function and strength. This meticulous technique maintains the soft-tissue envelope as much as possible. This confers less scar and adhesion formation and significantly decreased incidence of wound complications. Less peritendinous disruption may enhance speed of healing and quality of tissue through preserved circulation. Ensuring that the procedure is performed inside the paratenon also reduces the chance of sural nerve injury. This method offers the benefit of operative intervention while minimizing the associated risks, and thus maximizing patient benefit and satisfaction.[14]

34.4 Key Principles

- Meticulous skin and soft-tissue handling.
- Preservation of the paratenon.
- Excision of all diseased tissue.
- Construct stability via durable suture fixation.
- Postoperative protocol that allows for healing and revascularization of viable tendon.

34.5 Preoperative Preparation and Patient Positioning

- Following diagnosis and appropriate workup, the preoperative preparation is crucial for optimal patient outcomes. A compressive elastic or cohesive tape wrap can be placed for significant swelling. Allow ambulation in a CAM walker boot to promote circulation and prevent venous thrombosis. Preoperative imaging will guide incision placement. Ensure resolution of any existing wounds near this area.
- Once in the operating room, proper patient positioning is important. The patient is positioned prone with an Achilles bump or over the edge of the table, allowing for plantar flexion and dorsiflexion of the ankle during the procedure.
- Pillows are not recommended given they can soften during the procedure and make exposure difficult.
- The operation is performed under anesthesia with use of a thigh tourniquet.
- The resting tension of the uninjured side should be noted in case a segment of tendon requires resection.
- Intravenous antibiotics and regional anesthesia is administered.
- Place well-padded thigh tourniquet prior to prone positioning.
- Proper positioning on the operating table in a prone position with all bony prominences padded.
- Position legs with Achilles bump or over the edge of the table, resting position (**Fig. 34.4**).
- The operative extremity is prepped and draped in standard sterile fashion.
- The area of diseased tissue is palpated and correlated to preoperative imaging for site and length of incision.

34.6 Operative Technique

- Posterior incision slightly medial to the midline is utilized to minimize risk of injury to sural nerve, saphenous vein, and discomfort from external pressure.
- Full-thickness flaps are developed to expose and preserve the paratenon.
- The use of excessive or constant retraction with rakes or self-retainers is avoided to prevent tension on the skin, which could lead to wound complications.
- The paratenon is then incised and an attempt is made to dissect the paratenon as a separate layer for closure at the completion of the procedure (**Fig. 34.5**).
- Coexisting paratendinopathy or scarring will require excision of the scarred and thickened tissue.
- Any adhesions are then released from the paratenon using a small Cobb elevator or freer for blunt dissection. Dissection on the ventral surface is performed only when there is severe scar of the tendon to the paratenon. If the tendon still glides, the ventral paratenon can be preserved to aid in blood flow to the tendon (**Fig. 34.6**).
- The tendon is then incised longitudinally in line with its fibers directly overlying the diseased segment (**Fig. 34.7**).
  - The longitudinal tenotomy should follow the 90-degree rotation of tendon fibers as they course distally.
- Tendinopathic tissue is identified by disorganized fiber bundles, "crab meat appearance" (**Fig. 34.8**).
- Thorough intraoperative tendon evaluation is essential for complete disease elimination. Visualization of the axial MRI during the procedure can help find the diseased tendon given the pathologic fibers are not always apparent on initial visual inspection.

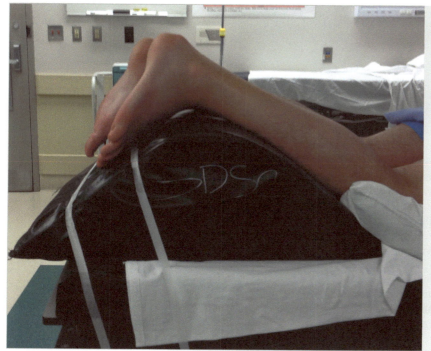

Fig. 34.4 Prone positioning with a firm Achilles bump.

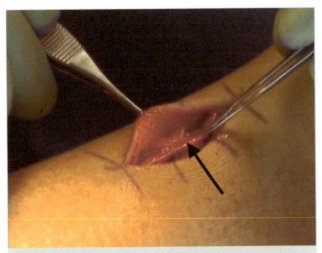

Fig. 34.5 Posterior and slightly medial incision demonstrating the paratenon dissected as a separate layer (*arrow*).

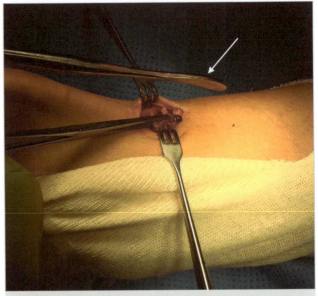

Fig. 34.6 Adhesions can be released from the paratenon using a small Cobb elevator for blunt dissection (*arrow*).

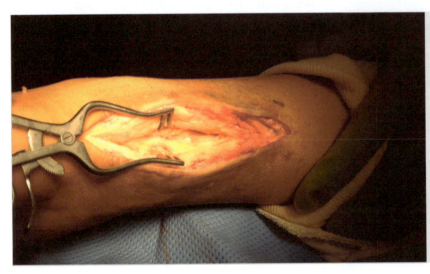

Fig. 34.7 The tendon is then incised longitudinally in line with its fibers directly overlying the diseased segment.

- The tendinopathic tissue is then excised in its entirety (**Fig. 34.9**).
  - Significant tendon loss (> 50%) following debridement may necessitate tendon augmentation or transfer.
    - Gastrocnemius turndown, plantaris weave, and flexor hallucis longus (FHL) transfer are options for this purpose.
    - Wrapping of the defect with dermal allograft that is sutured to the proximal and distal healthy tendon can be done to strengthen the repair and provide the potential of collagen ingrowth.[15]
- Depending on the preference of the surgeon, the tendon can be augmented with biologics prior to closure. Platelet-rich plasma or bone marrow aspirate concentrate mixed with thrombin can be placed in the tendon. Alternatively, live or cryopreserved allograft amniotic tissue can be placed longitudinally into the defect.
- The remaining gap is then repaired using a buried side-to-side, nonabsorbable suturing technique.
- Paratenon is then closed with absorbable suture.

- Skin and subcutaneous tissues are reapproximated in layers.
- A well-padded posterior and U splint is applied with the ankle in 20-degree equinus.

34.7 Tips and Pearls

- A surgical technician with knowledge or experience in this procedure is invaluable.
- Meticulous soft-tissue handling is critical to prevent complications of wound healing.
- Proper mobilization of the tendon with a Cobb elevator increases the technical ease of the procedure and optimizes outcomes by helping eliminate adhesions and promote tendon excursion.
- Thorough intraoperative evaluation and excision of tendinopathic tissue in its entirety decreases risk of continued symptoms.
- If there is a large amount of pathologic tissue evident on the MRI (> 30–40%), then it is necessary to properly counsel the

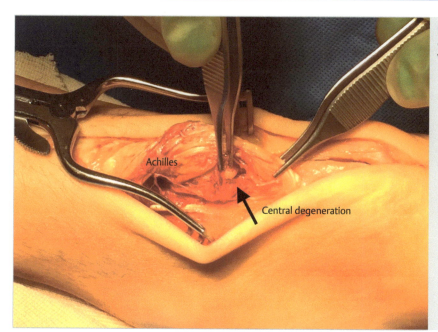

Fig. 34.8 Tendinopathic tissue: centralized degeneration with disorganized fiber bundles with a "crab meat appearance."

Achilles

Central degeneration

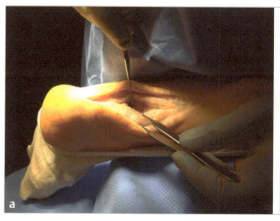
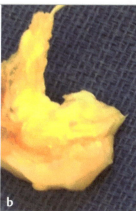

Fig. 34.9 Longitudinal incision in a midsubstance tendinosis **(a)** after removal of an intrasubstance calcification **(b)**.

patient on the need for augmentation procedures such as tendon transfer. The surgeon should ensure that the possible procedures on the surgical consent form and the proper equipment are present in the surgical suite.

34.8 Hazards and Pitfalls

- Sural nerve injury: minimized by posteromedial incision and knowledge of approximate nerve location at the lateral Achilles tendon border 9.8 cm proximal to the calcaneal attachment.[16]
- Residual tendinopathic tissue: minimized by thorough intraoperative evaluation.
- Wound dehiscence: prevented by meticulous soft-tissue management.

34.9 Complications/Bailout/Salvage

- Inadequate healthy tendon length for apposition or inability to reapproximate tendon edges after tendinopathic tissue resection.

  - Minimized or preoperatively planned for with proper preoperative workup (i.e., MRI if concern).
  - Consider Strayer gastrocnemius recession, V-Y lengthening, turndown flap, or FHL transfer.
  - A chevron excision of segments 2 to 3 cm can be performed and a biologic augmentation can be added (**Fig. 34.10**).
- Wound complications: skin necrosis, wound dehiscence, infection.
  - Depending on the size of the skin defect: local wound care, myocutaneous flap, or free flap.
  - Leaving sutures in place until wound is fully healed.
  - Initiation of oral broad-spectrum antibiotics for signs of cellulitis/infection.[17]

34.10 Postoperative Care

The postoperative protocol is tailored to the extent of tendon debridement, particularly if tendon augmentation or transfer is required. The following protocol reflects postoperative care of patients requiring less than 50% tendon debridement, therefore not including augmentation or transfer. The operative extremity is immobilized non-weight-bearing in a plantarflexed

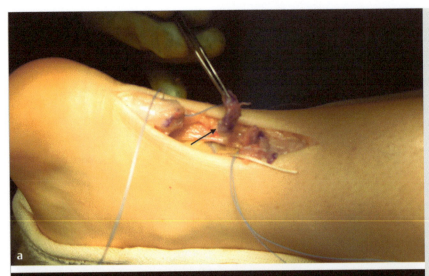

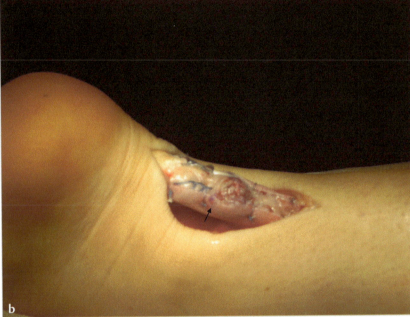

Fig. 34.10 Intraoperative photos of a patient with chronic tendinopathy requiring a 1.5-cm excision of the tendon (**a**, *arrow*). Final approximation of the tendon with an allograft augmentation (*arrow*) of the direct tendon repair (**b**).

position for 2 weeks before the first postoperative visit. This provides optimal conditions for wound healing and to allow postoperative pain and swelling to subside. At 2 weeks, the immobilization is removed, the wound is assessed, and sutures are removed. Weight-bearing as tolerated in a CAM walking boot with one to two plantar flexion wedges is then initiated. The patient is instructed to perform daily active and passive motion exercises in accordance with physical therapy instruction. After 6 to 8 weeks, the initial tendon healing is complete and more intensive strengthening can be performed. The patient is permitted to remove the boot for weight-bearing physical therapy at this point. A regular shoe is then worn. A follow-up appointment 3 months postoperatively will allow clinical re-evaluation of the patient's progress and typically will allow the patient to return to full activity. Sport-specific physical therapy, eccentric strengthening, and progressive physical therapy are initiated. Final follow-up is at 6 months to ensure the patient has returned to the desired level of activity.[9,18,19]

34.11 Outcomes

This repair technique allows for early mobilization and weight-bearing. Observations of improved patient experience due to comfort and function have been described. Patients have the potential for early return to sport, and low rates of wound complication, nerve injury, or postoperative rupture. Patient expectations should be managed appropriately for potential failure of the procedure, risk of wound complications, and the length of recovery (6–12 months).[6] Appropriate rehabilitation is critical and should be focused on early motion and limited strengthening until after the initial healing phase of the tendon. Finally, ensuring that patients receive the appropriate and timely physical therapy will help with improved outcomes and satisfied patients.

References

1. Maffulli N, Longo UG. Open management of Achilles tendinopathy. In Operative Techniques in Orthopedic Surgery. Philadelphia, PA: Lippincott Williams & Wilkins;2011:4443–4446/bok

2. Maffulli N. Re: Etiologic factors associated with symptomatic Achilles tendinopathy. Foot Ankle Int 2007;28(5):660–661, author reply 660–661

3. Maffulli N, Kader D. Tendinopathy of tendo Achilles. J Bone Joint Surg Br 2002;84(1):1–8

4. Maffulli N, Kenward MG, Testa V, Capasso G, Regine R, King JB. Clinical diagnosis of Achilles tendinopathy with tendinosis. Clin J Sport Med 2003;13(1):11–15

5. Maffulli N, Khan KM, Puddu G. Overuse tendon conditions: time to change a confusing terminology. Arthroscopy 1998;14(8):840–843

6. Maffulli N, Sharma P, Luscombe KL. Achilles tendinopathy: aetiology and management. J R Soc Med 2004;97(10):472–476

7. Maffulli N, Testa V, Capasso G, Bifulco G, Binfield PM. Results of percutaneous longitudinal tenotomy for Achilles tendinopathy in middle- and long-distance runners. Am J Sports Med 1997;25(6):835–840

8. Rompe JD, Nafe B, Furia JP, Maffulli N. Eccentric loading, shock-wave treatment, or a wait-and-see policy for tendinopathy of the main body of tendo Achillis: a randomized controlled trial. Am J Sports Med 2007;35(3):374–383

9. Sayana MK, Maffulli N. Eccentric calf muscle training in non-athletic patients with Achilles tendinopathy. J Sci Med Sport 2007;10(1):52–58

10. Maffulli N, Testa V, Capasso G, et al. Surgery for chronic Achilles tendinopathy yields worse results in nonathletic patients. Clin J Sport Med 2006;16(2):123–128

11. Molund M, Lapinskas SR, Nilsen FA, Hvaal KH. Clinical and functional outcomes of gastrocnemius recession for chronic Achilles tendinopathy. Foot Ankle Int 2016;37(10):1091–1097

12. Owens RF Jr, Ginnetti J, Conti SF, Latona C. Clinical and magnetic resonance imaging outcomes following platelet rich plasma injection for chronic midsubstance Achilles tendinopathy. Foot Ankle Int 2011;32(11):1032–1039

13. Monto RR. Platelet rich plasma treatment for chronic Achilles tendinosis. Foot Ankle Int 2012;33(5):379–385

14. Lim J, Dalal R, Waseem M. Percutaneous vs. open repair of the ruptured Achilles tendon—a prospective randomized controlled study. Foot Ankle Int 2001;22(7):559–568

15. Giza E, Frizzell L, Farac R, Williams J, Kim S. Augmented tendon Achilles repair using a tissue reinforcement scaffold: a biomechanical study. Foot Ankle Int 2011;32(5):S545–S549

16. Webb J, Moorjani N, Radford M. Anatomy of the sural nerve and its relation to the Achilles tendon. Foot Ankle Int 2000;21(6):475–477

17. Bluman EM, Chiodo C, Calhoun J. Acute repair of the Achilles tendon rupture: open and limited open. Foot Ankle Int 2013:713–726

18. Maffulli N, Tallon C, Wong J, Lim KP, Bleakney R. Early weightbearing and ankle mobilization after open repair of acute midsubstance tears of the Achilles tendon. Am J Sports Med 2003;31(5):692–700

19. Chiodo CP, Glazebrook M, Bluman EM, et al; American Academy of Orthopaedic Surgeons. Diagnosis and treatment of acute Achilles tendon rupture. J Am Acad Orthop Surg 2010;18(8):503–510

35 Flexor Hallucis Longus Tendon Transfer for Achilles Reconstruction

Milap S. Patel, Mauricio P. Barbosa, and Anish R. Kadakia

Abstract

The use of tendon transfer to treat deficiency of a pathologic motor unit is a fundamental skill for the practicing orthopaedic surgeon. New concepts with regard to autograft/allograft reconstruction have been noted; however, the ability of a traditional tendon transfer to restore function is proven and effective. For reconstruction of the Achilles tendon, whether for chronic tendinosis or rupture, the transfer of the flexor hallucis longus to the calcaneus is a proven, effective, and reliable method to restore a patient's ability to ambulate without significant difficulty or pain. Modern fixation techniques allow for a single posterior incision approach with decreased morbidity to the midfoot, with minimal functional loss of hallux plantar flexion strength for an overwhelming majority of patients. The use of the flexor hallucis longus is an excellent option for Achilles reconstruction, with good functional outcomes noted after 1 year. In the high-level athlete, however, consideration for graft reconstruction or use of the peroneal tendons may be considered to avoid the morbidity of the loss of hallux strength.

Keywords: *flexor hallucis longus, Achilles tendinosis, Achilles reconstruction, tendon transfer*

35.1 Indications and Pathology

- Flexor hallucis longus (FHL) transfer is indicated to reconstruct the Achilles tendon in its entirety, or augment an insufficient Achilles tendon.
- On rare occasions, FHL transfer can be utilized in the setting of an acute Achilles tendon rupture where primary repair is not possible. This is most common in the setting of an insertional rupture given that most noninsertional ruptures are amenable to nonoperative or operative repair.
- Chronic Achilles tendon ruptures are associated with contracture of the triceps surae with difficulty to obtain a direct repair in most settings. FHL tendon transfer is utilized to augment a reconstruction (V-Y, turndown, allograft) that both improves power and provides a new vascular bed.
- If reconstruction is not possible in chronic Achilles tendon rupture, then an FHL transfer in isolation can be performed with the understanding that a 20 to 30% functional loss of power will occur.[1]
- Advanced insertional and noninsertional Achilles tendinosis that requires operative debridement of greater than 50% of the viable tendon may benefit from FHL augmentation.

35.1.1 Clinical Evaluation

- Clinical evaluation of Achilles pathology has been previously described in detail in chapters 32 to 34.
- Chronic Achilles tendon rupture results in insufficient plantar flexion power that significantly affects the ability to navigate inclines and stairs in addition to athletic activity. The greatest difficulty in activities of daily living may occur with descending stairs giving the inability of the Achilles to generate sufficient power to control the descent.
- Plantar flexion is present, but weak due to compensatory involvement from posterior tibial tendon (PTT), FHL, flexor digitorum longus (FDL), peroneus longus, and peroneus brevis (PB).
- Clinical evaluation for an intact and adequately strong FHL tendon is essential before choosing this tendon for a transfer. This is performed by evaluating interphalangeal flexion strength of the hallux with the ankle in flexion and extension. Palpation behind the ankle for tenderness is important to exclude an FHL tear or entrapment within the fibro-osseous tunnel.

35.1.2 Radiographic Evaluation

- A lateral weight-bearing radiograph of the ankle is important when evaluating Achilles tendon pathology.
  - Radiographs of the ankle may demonstrate avulsion of the Achilles tendon insertion.
  - Significant calcific tendinosis of the midsubstance or insertion of the tendon should alert the surgeon to the possible need for an FHL transfer.
  - In most cases, the radiograph will be nondiagnostic given the soft-tissue nature of Achilles tendon disorders.
- Magnetic resonance imaging (MRI) or ultrasound can provide added diagnostic value and localize level of the tear in the acute setting; however, this is not routinely required.
  - This can be used if there is concern about FHL tendon pathology or integrity.
  - In chronic/neglected Achilles rupture, MRI will provide further information regarding degree of gastrocnemius and soleus muscle fatty infiltration.
  - If a significant, greater than 50%, fatty infiltration is noted, isolated reconstruction of the Achilles without augmentation will be unlikely to achieve a satisfactory clinical outcome without an additional tendon transfer.
- In the setting of tendinosis, MRI is useful in analyzing the quality of the tendon. An FHL tendon transfer is beneficial where more than 50% of the Achilles is abnormal, given that this is predictive of the amount of tendon resection that will be required.

35.1.3 Nonoperative Options

- Nonoperative treatment options regarding the various Achilles pathology are explained in detail in Chapters 32 to 34.

35.1.4 Contraindications

- Athletic patients who rely on unaffected hallux motion such as ballerinas, soccer, or volleyball players may benefit from peroneal tendon augmentation instead of FHL transfer.[2]

• Four percent of patients will complain of constant balance loss and this should be discussed prior to surgery.[3]

35.2 Goals of Surgical Procedure

• Restore plantar flexion power to the affected lower extremity to enable functional ambulation.
• Improve plantar flexion power in the setting of a reconstruction of the Achilles tendon (V-Y, turndown, allograft) to enable high-impact activity.

35.3 Advantages of Surgical Procedure

• Strength.
  ○ The FHL is twice as strong as the FDL and is a stronger plantar flexor than the PB.
  ○ FHL is active during the same phase as triceps surae, which is helpful in maintaining normal ankle biomechanics.
• Anatomic location:
  ○ Proximity to the Achilles tendon making it convenient for harvesting and may be performed through a single incision.
• Vascular:
  ○ The large muscle belly may improve the overall environment for healing of the reconstructed Achilles tendon (V-Y, turndown, allograft).
• Viability:
  ○ FHL has a very low rate of intrinsic disease, making this a very reliable choice and resilient tendon transfer.
• Hypertrophy:
  ○ Clear data have demonstrated hypertrophy of the FHL muscle following tendon transfer, improving the overall function over time.[4]

35.4 Key Principles

• Prone position facilitates the harvest and transfer of the FHL; however, a supine approach with external rotation of the affected limb may also be performed if desired.
• Thorough understanding of the proximity of the tibial nerve immediately medial to the FHL is required to avoid iatrogenic injury.

35.5 Preoperative Planning and Patient Positioning

• Preoperative imaging to determine the relative amount of tendinosis or fatty atrophy (chronic rupture) should be performed to determine the likely need for an FHL transfer.
• Equipment:
  ○ Interference screw fixation is preferred for the single incision technique:
    ❖ Appropriate reamers and interference screws should be available. A 6.5- to 7.25-mm screw is commonly utilized.
  ○ Fluoroscopy:
    ❖ Use of a large C-arm facilitates placement of the calcaneal bone tunnel and facilitates removal of any calcaneal spurs.

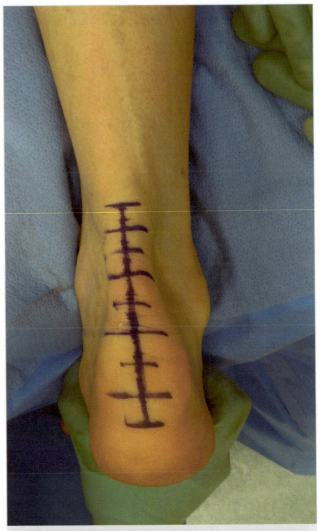

Fig. 35.1 Patient is positioned prone with a centrally placed incision. In cases of insertional disease, the incision must be carried distally in order to ensure removal of the insertional calcific spur.

• Positioning:
  ○ Patient lying prone with both feet just off the end of the surgical table facilitates the harvest and placement of the transfer.
    ❖ If the patient cannot be placed prone, then the surgery can be performed supine with a beanbag or large bump used to externally rotate the affected leg. Placement of multiple blankets underneath the affected leg places the foot in a "figure 4" position, which improves the externally rotated position of the foot.
• This position may be preferred if a long harvest from the midfoot is chosen. However, given the modern fixation methods available, a long harvest is not required for most cases.
  ○ Regional anesthesia is preferred if possible.
  ○ Our preference is not to utilize a tourniquet in nearly all surgical cases. If a tourniquet is preferred, make sure to place a thigh tourniquet and have the tubing face posteriorly if placed while the patient is supine in order to prevent pressure-related skin problems. A calf tourniquet will limit full muscle mobilization and excursion and is therefore not advised.
  ○ Lower extremity is prepped and draped up to the knee.

35.6 Operative Technique

35.6.1 Surgical Approach

- Prone position:
  - A direct midline approach is made between the posterior tibial and peroneal artery angiosomes (**Fig. 35.1**).
- Supine:
  - A medially based incision is made 1 cm anterior to the posterior border of the Achilles tendon, with the dissection directed laterally.

35.6.2 Surgical Procedure: Posterior Ankle FHL Harvest

- Care should be taken to avoid creating large subcutaneous planes superficial to the crural fascia to minimize unnecessary soft-tissue trauma. The fascia is then incised allowing visualization of the Achilles tendon:

- In the setting of tendinosis, adhesions may be present, obliterating the normal plane between the fascia and the Achilles tendon.
  - All nonviable tissue is excised prior to accessing the FHL (**Fig. 35.2**).
- Deep posterior compartment fascia is incised to gain access to FHL anterior to the Achilles tendon.

Flexor Hallucis Longus Harvest

- Correct identification of the FHL is critical as the posterior neurovascular structures run immediately medial to the FHL. Therefore, dissection and exposure is performed centrally with attention directed to identification of the lateral aspect of the FHL tendon.
- FHL sheath is incised and dissection is performed along the lateral edge down to posterior aspect of the medial malleolus into its fibro-osseous tunnel. FHL muscle extends distally to tibiotalar joint before transitioning into tendon and is another visual clue to avoiding iatrogenic injury to the tibial nerve.

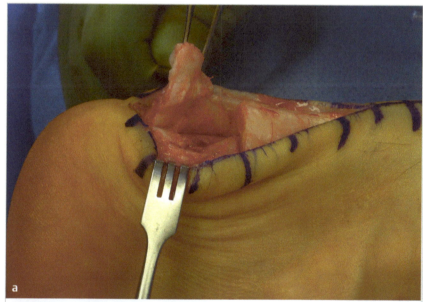

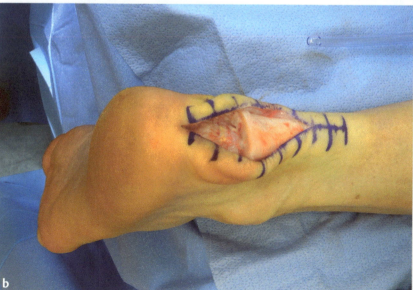

Fig. 35.2 All nonviable tissue (**a**) is excised to ensure maximal pain relief. Following aggressive excision (**b**), a large defect may be present, which required FHL (flexor hallucis longus) augmentation.

- Once the FHL is identified, a digit or right angle retractor is hooked deep to muscle belly and retracted. A secondary confirmation can be visualized by hallux flexion when traction is placed on the FHL tendon (**Fig. 35.3**).
- Once distal aspect of tendon is exposed, ankle and hallux are maximally plantarflexed while placing traction on FHL proximally in order to obtain maximum amount of tendon for transfer.
- The tendon is transected as distal as possible in order to ensure adequate length is obtained.
- A knife is taken from medial to lateral to avoid injury the neurovascular structures.
- Diameter of the tendon stump is measured for accurate tunnel size.
  - The tendon stump is secured with a locking whipstitch with no. 0 suture in order to facilitate tendon passage through the bone tunnel.

Calcaneal Bone Tunnel

- Bone preparation.
  - The posterior aspect of the calcaneus is prepared by excising any Haglund's deformity or insertional calcific

tendinosis. In the setting of noninsertional disease or acute rupture, this is typically not required.
- A Beath pin is taken from the posterior aspect of the calcaneus, immediately anterior to the insertion of the native Achilles tendon. The tunnel should be placed centrally to avoid inadvertent inversion or eversion pull. Distally, the pin should exit proximal to the tuberosity to avoid damage to the lateral plantar nerve (**Fig. 35.4**).
  - A bone tunnel is created using a cannulated size-specific reamer (**Fig. 35.5**).

Proximal Tenodesis

- The FHL can be weaved through the proximal aspect of the remaining Achilles tendon. In cases of a residual gap that remains after tendon debridement, this is preferred to maximize the plantar flexion power for the patient.

Tendon Transfer to Calcaneus

- The tendon is passed through the tunnel by placing the whipstitch sutures through the Beath pin eyelet and pulling the pin out from plantar aspect of the foot (**Fig. 35.6**).
- Traction is applied to the suture to shuttle tendon into the bone tunnel.
  - In some cases, excess tendon length may be present and distal translation of the tendon may be arrested by the soft tissue.
    - ❖ If this is encountered, a small incision should be made on the plantar aspect of the heel with blunt dissection

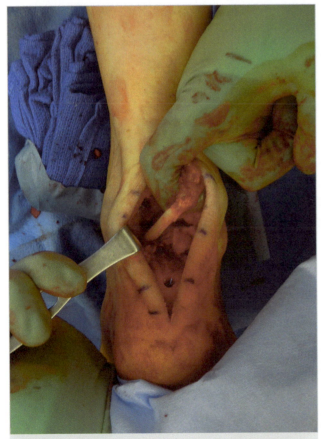

Fig. 35.3 The FHL (flexor hallucis longus) is identified lateral to the tibial nerve and is grasped with a finger with to place tension on the tendon prior to distal transection. Note the low level of the muscle belly, clearly differentiating this tendon from the tibial nerve.

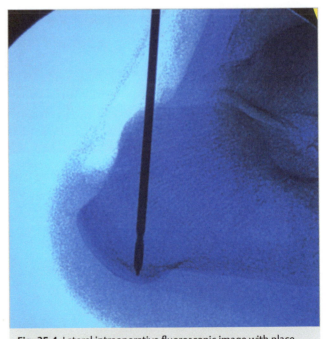

Fig. 35.4 Lateral intraoperative fluoroscopic image with placement of the calcaneal bone tunnel in the setting of an overly aggressive resection of the superior calcaneal tuberosity. In this case, the tunnel was placed anteriorly in order to achieve fixation. Note that inferiorly the Beath pin exits within the center of the tuberosity to avoid damage to the lateral plantar nerve.

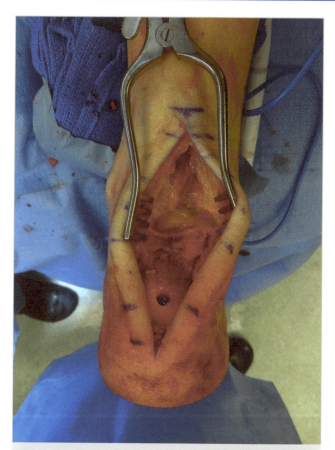

Fig. 35.5 Following resection of the prominent superior calcaneal tuberosity, a smooth dorsal calcaneus should be achieved. The tunnel for the FHL (flexor hallucis longus) should begin immediately anterior to the posterior calcaneal cortex to maximize the strength of fixation.

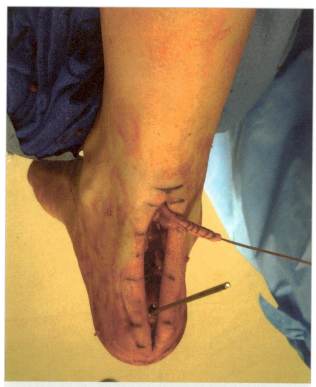

Fig. 35.6 The whipstitch suture for the FHL (flexor hallucis longus) is placed through the eyelet of the Beath pin to facilitate transfer into the bone tunnel.

taken to the tuberosity. The tendon is then pulled through the plantar skin incision in order to obtain appropriate tension.

Tensioning

- The suture that exits the plantar aspect of the heel is secured with a needle driver at the desired level of tension. The needle driver can be rotated after securing the driver to the suture to increase the tension on the tendon.
  - The senior author's experience is that the tendon should be secured with the foot in 5 degrees of plantar flexion with maximum tension on the tendon. Once secure, the foot is reliably able to dorsiflex to neutral with excellent tension on the FHL (**Fig. 35.7**).
    - ❖ The tendon is secured with an interference screw, avoiding metallic screws to decrease the risk of iatrogenic transection of the tendon (**Fig. 35.8**).
    - ❖ Screw size is dependent on the tendon diameter; however, in most cases, a 6.5- to 7.25-mm screw is required. Given the cancellous nature of the calcaneus, the screw size should be slightly larger than the drill hole as opposed to choosing a small screw when performing tendon transfers in hard cortical bone.

35.6.3 Surgical Procedure: Long FHL Harvest

- FHL tendon can also be harvested from the midfoot if additional length of tendon is required.
  - Given the reproducible nature of the single incision technique combined with the strength of fixation, this is not routinely required.
    - ❖ However, if interference screw fixation is not available, or the surgeon preference is to loop the tendon back to the native Achilles, a long harvest is required.
- A separate incision is made on the plantar medial aspect of the midfoot from talonavicular joint extended toward the first tarsometatarsal joint distally.
- The abductor hallucis is taken inferiorly exposing the FDL in the proximal aspect of the incision. The dissection is taken distally, with care taken to identify the knot of Henry. Multiple venous vasculatures must be identified and cauterized to avoid postoperative bleeding and hematoma formation. The tissue constituting the knot of Henry is incised, which exposes the FHL as it crosses over and medial to the FDL to insert on the distal phalanx.
- Multiple cross-tendinous connections exist between the FHL and FDL and must be transected to allow a complete release of the FHL. The distal stump of the FHL and FDL may be sutured together to minimize the effect of the loss of the FHL to the distal phalanx. This is not required with a single incision technique given that the tendon is taken proximal to the cross-connections and the FDL is still able to exert force to the distal phalanx.

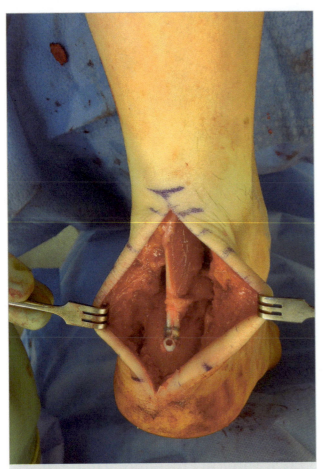

Fig. 35.7 Final intraoperative appearance of the FHL (flexor hallucis longus) tendon transfer following fixation with an interference screw. Note the level of the muscle belly at or near the calcaneal tuberosity. If significant tendon is visible, the tendon may not be sufficiently tensioned.

- The medial plantar nerve is at risk during this exposure and is best avoided by transecting the FHL distally and releasing all the cross-connections to the FDL prior to pulling the tendon proximally.
- The FHL is now retracted proximally from the posterior incision.
  - Fixation can be obtained by creating a transverse drill hole within the calcaneal tuberosity and securing the tendon to itself or the remaining Achilles tendon with no. 0 suture.

35.7 Tips and Pearls

- Proximal release of FHL fascia is required to transfer the tendon into superficial compartment from the deep compartment.
- Tension: The author's preference is to place maximum tension with 5 degrees of plantar flexion—one should be able to dorsiflex the ankle to neutral intraoperatively following fixation.
- Beath pin should not exit distal to the calcaneal tuberosity to avoid damage to lateral plantar nerve.

35.8 Hazards and Pitfalls

- Tibial nerve injury.
  - This can be avoided by performing the deep dissection centrally and identifying the FHL muscle belly and tendon prior to attempting harvest.
  - The FHL tendon should be pulled at the posterior incision while observing for hallux interphalangeal flexion to ensure that one has the tendon and not the adjacent tibial nerve.
- Insufficient length: To avoid this complication with a single incision harvest, the tendon should be transected as distally as possible within the fibro-osseous tunnel. Alternatively, overly aggressive resection of the posterior calcaneus functionally requires more length of the tendon to engage bone and should be avoided if possible. If this cannot be avoided, then a long harvest should be considered.
  - Fixation can be obtained and compensated for the insufficient length by placing the tendon more anteriorly. Although this may achieve bony fixation, some mechanical advantage is lost because the tendon is now placed closer to the center of rotation.
  - Suture anchors can also be used to supplement or replace interference screw fixation if required.
    - ❖ Two 3.5-mm anchors should be used to achieve sufficient strength of fixation as compared to an interference screw.
- Failure to tension properly: This can be from a graft that is too long as the graft bottoms out on the inferior calcaneus or the plantar soft tissue.
  - To avoid this, we recommend drilling bicortically and making a small counter incision to properly tension the graft as required.

35.9 Postoperative Care

- Immediately postoperatively, the leg is immobilized in a splint placed in 20 degrees of plantar flexion to maximize perfusion to the posterior skin. The patient is kept non-weight-bearing.
- Two weeks:
  - Surgical incisions are evaluated in office and sutures are removed. Lower extremity is placed in a Controlled Ankle Motion (CAM) boot with two 1-inch heel wedges and kept non-weight-bearing; however, active range of motion is allowed. Boot is to remain on during sleep.
- Four weeks:
  - Weight-bearing in the boot with two 1-inch heel wedges is initiated.
- Six weeks:
  - Office evaluation is performed to ensure integrity of the Achilles tendon and a formal physical therapy program is prescribed. Weight-bearing is allowed with only one heel lift. Boot is not required during sleep.
- Eight weeks:
  - Transition to weight-bearing in the boot without any heel wedges.
- Nine weeks:
  - Ambulation in an athletic shoe with a 1-inch heel wedge in each shoe to decrease stress on the transfer.

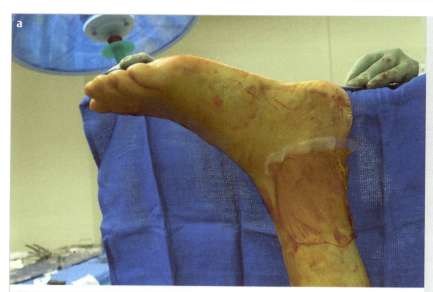

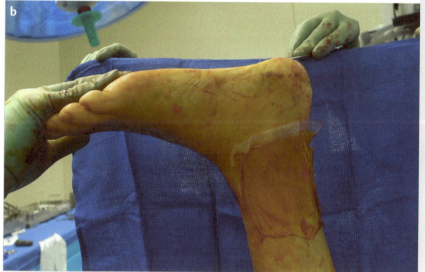

Fig. 35.8 Intraoperative tensioning of the tendon transfer should create approximately 5 to 10 degrees of resting plantar flexion. (a) With dorsally directed tension upon the forefoot, the foot should not go past neutral (b).

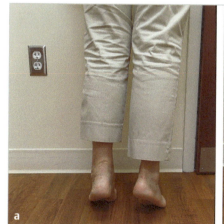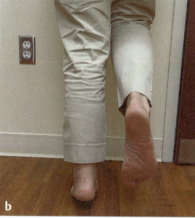

Fig. 35.9 One year following isolated FHL (flexor hallucis longus) transfer for a chronic insertional Achilles rupture. The patient is able to perform a double limb heel rise (a), in addition to a single limb heel rise (b). Although the patient may be able to perform a single limb heel rise, the patient may not be able to perform aggressive athletic activities.

- Eleven weeks: The heel wedge is removed from both shoes.
- Twelve weeks: Office evaluation is performed to ensure integrity of the repair.
  - Physical therapy is continued as needed for the patient with the understanding that a single limb heel rise may not

be achievable in some patients. Despite this fact, patients will typically achieve an excellent functional outcome for nonimpact activities, but they may always be limited with regard to running and jumping (**Fig. 35.9**).

35.10 Outcomes

- Multiple small clinical retrospective studies have demonstrated satisfactory outcomes following FHL tendon transfer.
  - Will and Galey reviewed 19 patients with Achilles tendinopathy treated with a single-incision FHL transfer.[5]
    - They noted improvement in the VAS (visual analog scale) score from 7.5 to 0.6 at final postoperative exam with a mean AOFAS (American Orthopaedic Foot and Ankle Society) score of 96.4.
  - Martin et al demonstrated an 86% satisfaction and 95.5% rate of minimal to no pain in 56 patients treated with an FHL transfer for insertional Achilles tendinosis with complete excision of the distal Achilles stump.[1]
    - However, a 28.6% strength deficit at 30 degrees/s and a 22.8% deficit at 60 degrees/s were noted.
  - Elias et al performed a V-Y lengthening with associated FHL transfer in 15 patients for chronic Achilles tendon ruptures.[6]
    - Despite the combined reconstruction, a persistent deficit of 22.3% was noted at 60 degrees and a 13.5% deficit at 120 degrees.
  - Richardson et al evaluated the morbidity on hallux plantar flexion following a single-incision technique in 22 patients.[7]
    - Despite a significant pedographic decrease in pressure beneath the distal phalanx, patient function as measured by the SF-36 (36-Item Short Form Survey) score and AOFAS hallux score was high. The authors concluded that the functional loss demonstrated in the lab was not clinically relevant.

References

1. Martin RL, Manning CM, Carcia CR, Conti SF. An outcome study of chronic Achilles tendinosis after excision of the Achilles tendon and flexor hallucis longus tendon transfer. Foot Ankle Int 2005;26(9):691–697
2. Maffulli N, Spiezia F, Longo UG, Denaro V. Less-invasive reconstruction of chronic Achilles tendon ruptures using a peroneus brevis tendon transfer. Am J Sports Med 2010;38(11):2304–2312
3. Schon LC, Shores JL, Faro FD, Vora AM, Camire LM, Guyton GP. Flexor hallucis longus tendon transfer in treatment of Achilles tendinosis. J Bone Joint Surg Am 2013;95(1):54–60
4. Oksanen MM, Haapasalo HH, Elo PP, Laine HJ. Hypertrophy of the flexor hallucis longus muscle after tendon transfer in patients with chronic Achilles tendon rupture. Foot Ankle Surg 2014;20(4):253–257
5. Will RE, Galey SM. Outcome of single incision flexor hallucis longus transfer for chronic Achilles tendinopathy. Foot Ankle Int 2009;30(4):315–317
6. Elias I, Besser M, Nazarian LN, Raikin SM. Reconstruction for missed or neglected Achilles tendon rupture with V-Y lengthening and flexor hallucis longus tendon transfer through one incision. Foot Ankle Int 2007;28(12):1238–1248
7. Richardson DR, Willers J, Cohen BE, Davis WH, Jones CP, Anderson RB. Evaluation of the hallux morbidity of single-incision flexor hallucis longus tendon transfer. Foot Ankle Int 2009;30(7):627–630

36 Arthroscopic Microfracture and Drilling for Osteochondral Lesions of the Talus

Eric I. Ferkel and Richard D. Ferkel

36.1 Introduction

- Osteochondral lesions of the talus (OLTs) are a somewhat uncommon injury to the ankle but can often be associated with other pathologies such as ankle sprains, chronic instability, and ankle fractures.[1,2]
- Majority of OLTs are traumatic in nature.
- The medial side of the talus is most commonly involved.
- Most OLTs are within the equatorial zone of the talus.

36.2 Indications

- Most success in patients with lesions <107.4 mm² in area and/or 10.2 mm in diameter[3-6].

36.2.1 Clinical Evaluation

- Frequently has a history of a twisting/spraining injury to the ankle.
- Complaint of activity-related pain, catching and giving way of the ankle.
- Nonspecific clinical examination:
  ○ Tenderness at joint line.
  ○ Location of tenderness may not correspond to that of lesion.

36.2.2 Radiographic Evaluation

- Plain radiographs may show a fracture, loose body, or cavity in the area of OLT.
- Utilize X-ray, magnetic resonance imaging, and computed tomographic scans to best understand the osteochondral lesion prior to surgery. Each modality can offer insight into the staging of the lesion and knowledge of the cartilage, subchondral and bony anatomy, location, and pathology.

36.2.3 Nonoperative Options

- Brace immobilization.
- Activity modification.

36.2.4 Alternate Procedures

- Nonoperative management with biologic adjuncts, pharmacotherapy, and immobilization with constant range of motion exercises.
- Lavage and debridement with or without drilling and microfracture.
- Open ankle arthrotomy with or without osteotomy.
- Repair of an acute defect.
- Osteochondral autograft.
- Osteochondral allograft.
- Matrix-induced autologous chondrocyte implantation (MACI).
- Juvenile cartilage allograft.
- Allograft cartilage extracellular matrix.
- Metal resurfacing implant.

36.2.5 Contraindications

- >107.4 mm² in area and/or 10.2 mm in diameter.
- Large cysts under the osteochondral lesion.
- Degenerative joint disease.
- Failed previous microfracture.

36.3 Goals of Surgical Procedure

- Restore the cartilaginous anatomy of the surface of the talus.

36.4 Advantages of Surgical Procedure

- Arthroscopic-only treatment.
- Higher rate of success with the correct indications.
- No bridges burned to do other procedures in the future.

36.5 Key Principles

- Stimulate the bone marrow and remove any loose or unstable bone or cartilage.
- Allow for mesenchymal stem cells to create a clot at the lesion to assist in the formation of fibrocartilage (type I) and small amounts of type II cartilage for the noncystic and smaller lesion of the talus.

36.6 Preoperative Preparation and Patient Positioning (Fig. 36.1)

- Remove pad from the end of operative table for better access to posterior portals.
- Nonoperative leg on well-padded area, stabilized with a strap, and heel should be at table's edge.
- Supine with the thigh secured in a well-padded nonsterile thigh holder.
- Knee flexed at 65 degrees with popliteal fossa free and patella and ankle facing ceiling.
- Nonsterile tourniquet placed on proximal thigh.
- Thigh post at greater trochanter.
- Water should be gravity on the same side as the operative ankle.
- Mark out the superficial peroneal nerve before prepping and draping the patient.

243

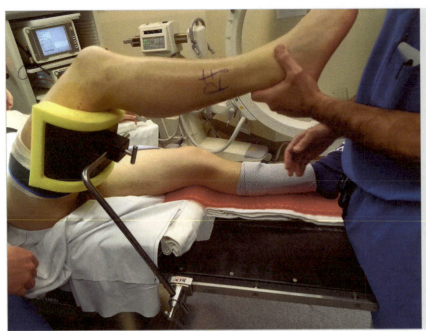

Fig. 36.1 The thigh is supported by a well-padded holder attached via a clamp to the rail of the table. The tourniquet is placed around the proximal thigh and the thigh support itself is placed proximal to the popliteal fossa to avoid injury to the neurovascular structures.

- After distraction, the anterior tibialis, fibula, and tibia/medial malleolus should be marked out.
- Tourniquet inflation per surgeon's preference.
- Distract the joint with noninvasive strap.

36.7 Operation Technique

36.7.1 Equipment

- Small joint arthroscopes.
- 1.9-mm 30-degree arthroscope.
- 2.7-mm 30-degree and 70-degree arthroscopes.
- 2.9-mm associated cannulas.
- 2.0-, 2.9-, and 3.5-mm shavers and burrs.
- 3.5- and 4.5-mm ring and cup curettes.
- 1.5-mm probes.
- 2.9- and 3.5-mm graspers and baskets.
- 2.9-mm osteotomes.
- Pituitary rongeurs.
- Microfracture picks.
- Nanofracture picks.
- K-wires (Kirschner wires; 0.045 and 0.062 inches)—smooth with trochar tips.
- Noninvasive ankle distractor, thigh holder, adjustable IV pole for gravity fluid management.
- 22-gauge 1.5-inch needle, 18-gauge spinal needle.
- 10-mL syringe with extension IV tubing.
- 2- to 50-mL syringes.

36.7.2 Anesthesia

- General plus a popliteal block with a saphenous block placed locally by the surgeon at the conclusion of the case with 10 mL of 0.5% bupivacaine without epinephrine.
- Patient should be completely "paralyzed" if possible for best distraction.

36.7.3 Incisions/Preferred Portals

- Always use the "nick-and-spread" technique to avoid neurovascular injury.
- Anteromedial portal—medial to the tibialis anterior with saphenous vein and nerve, anterior tibialis tendon, and extensor hallucis longus at risk (**Fig. 36.2**).
- Anterolateral portal—lateral to the peroneus tertius with the superficial peroneal nerve branch, extensor digitorum communis, and peroneus tertius at risk (**Fig. 36.2**).
- Posterolateral—at the soft spot lateral to the Achilles tendon, 1.2 cm above the tip of the fibula with the sural nerve and small saphenous vein at risk (**Fig. 36.3**).
- Transmalleolar for K-wire microfracture drilling through the fibula or tibial for entrance into the talar defect.
- Establish the anteromedial portal first by inserting a 22-gauge needle just medial to the anterior tibialis tendon, which is palpated with the outside hand. Once the proper trajectory is noted with the needle aiming just superiorly over the dome, inject 10 mL of sterile saline into the joint evaluating the backflow and joint distention laterally.
- Then use an 11-blade scalpel to make a vertical incision with the anterior tibial tendon palpated with the outside hand.
- Dissect bluntly with the mosquito, then insert the blunt trochar with the arthroscopic cannula attached.
- Once the scope is in the joint, initially use the side port of the cannula to inject fluid using the 50-mL syringes and extension tubing.
- Use a 22-gauge needle to locate the anterolateral portal and with the nick-and-spread technique enter the joint and insert the inflow cannula.
- Begin the initial joint assessment, then create the posterolateral portal by using a 18-gauge spinal needle at the soft spot, as described earlier, while viewing through the notch of Harty. Aim the needle 45 degrees toward the medial malleolus and just under the transverse tibiofibular ligament until there is backflow.

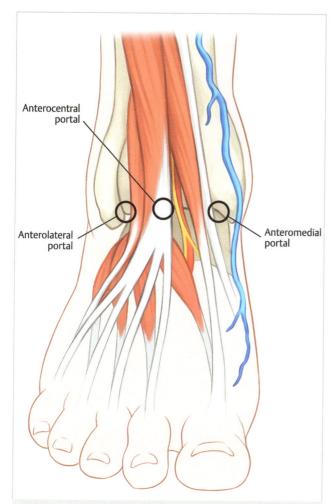

Fig. 36.2 The anteromedial and anterolateral portals are most commonly used for ankle arthroscopy. The anterocentral portal is rarely used.

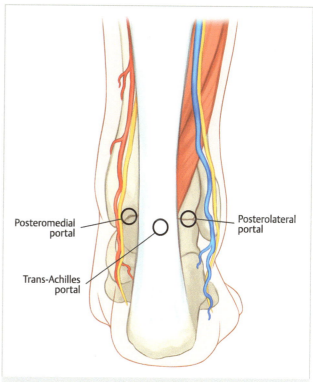

Fig. 36.3 The primary portal for ankle arthroscopy posteriorly is the posterolateral portal. The trans-Achilles or posteromedial portals are rarely utilized.

- The goal is to place the cannula just medial to the PITFL and inferior to the transverse tibiofibular ligament.
- At this point, switch the inflow to the posterolateral portal and finish the 21-point examination as described below.

36.7.4 21-Point Exam[7]

- The 21-point exam for a diagnostic ankle arthroscopy, as described by Richard Ferkel,[7] requires the surgeon to stop at each point of the exam to study the patient's anatomy.
- The order in which one evaluates each area is not as important as it is because the surgeon thoroughly evaluates each structure in an efficient manner.
- The structures visualized include the following:
  With the scope in the anteromedial portal (**Fig. 36.4**):
  1. Deltoid ligament.
  2. Medial gutter.
  3. Medial talus.
  4. Central talus and central overhang.
  5. Lateral talus.
  6. Trifurcation with the talus, tibia, and fibula, including anterior inferior tibiofibular ligament.
  7. Lateral gutter, including anterior talofibular ligament.

8. Anterior gutter.
   The central and posterior structures of the ankle are visualized from the anteromedial or anterolateral portal.
9. Medial tibia/talus.
10. Central tibia/talus.
11. Lateral tibia/talofibular articulation.
    The arthroscope is then maneuvered more posteriorly from either of the anterior portals to visualize the posterior structures. These include:
12. Posterior inferior tibiofibular ligament.
13. Transverse tibiofibular ligament.
14. Reflection of the flexor hallucis longus.
    The arthroscope is then changed to the posterolateral portal to complete the exam, visualizing the following (**Fig. 36.5**):
15. Posteromedial gutter.
16. Posteromedial talus.
17. Posterocentral talus.
18. Posterolateral talus.
19. Posterior talofibular articulation.
20. Posterolateral gutter, including the posterior talofibular ligament.
21. Posterior gutter.

36.7.5 Debridement

- Debride loose cartilage and bone and make firm and sharp cartilage walls to prepare the site with curettes and shavers. The calcified cartilage layer must be removed to allow for the clot to adhere well, thus improving the chance of repair.

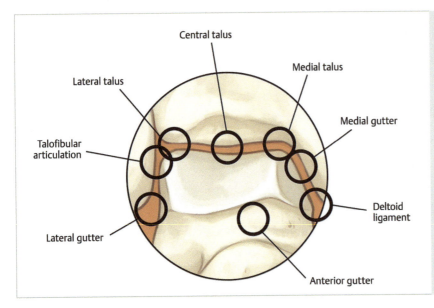

Fig. 36.4 Anterior ankle 8-point examination through the arthroscope.

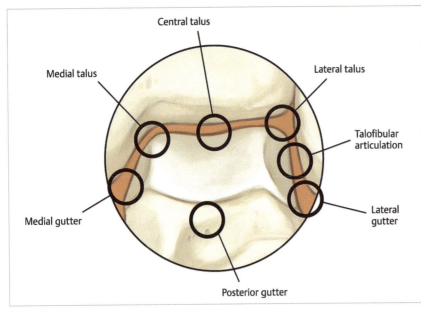

Fig. 36.5 Posterior ankle 7-point examination through the arthroscope.

36.7.6 Microfracture/Drilling

- Place the microfracture openings approximately 5 mm apart from each other and at a 2- to 6-mm depth with either a pick or thin K-wire (1.6 mm).
- This can be done through a portal, transmalleolar or transtalar (**Fig. 36.6**).

36.7.7 Biologic Adjuncts (Unproven Efficacy)

- Platelet-rich plasma—leukocyte poor.
- Bone marrow aspirate concentrate.

36.7.8 Closure and Splinting

- 4-0 Nylon in vertical mattress fashion.
- Short leg well-padded splint or cast of choice in neutral dorsiflexion.

36.8 Tips and Pearls

- Keep anteromedial portal close to the anterior tibial tendon.
- Move anterolateral portal more centrally.
- Take the pad out from the bed so that you have good separation of the ankle from the table.
- Angle the posterolateral portal toward the posteromedial osteochondral lesion and under the transverse tibiofibular ligament.
- Correct equipment availability: 30- and 70-degree scopes, curettes, and hoe (**Fig. 36.7**).

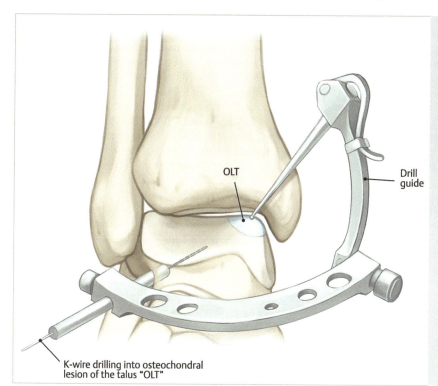

Fig. 36.6 Transtalar drilling of an osteochondral lesion of the medial talar dome. Illustration demonstrates the K-wire being inserted through the sinus tarsi using the MicroVector guide to drill up into the osteochondral lesion of the medial talar dome.

OLT

Drill guide

K-wire drilling into osteochondral lesion of the talus "OLT"

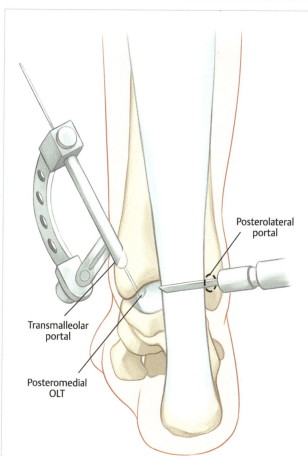

Posterolateral portal

Transmalleolar portal

Posteromedial OLT

Fig. 36.7 Treatment of posteromedial osteochondral lesion of the talus in a right ankle. The arthroscope visualizes the osteochondral lesion of the talus from the posterolateral portal, while the drill guide is brought in through the anteromedial portal.

36.9 Hazards and Pitfalls

• Neurovascular injury.
• Infection.
• Iatrogenic cartilage injury.
• Arthrofibrosis.

36.10 Complications/Bailout/Salvages

• Cartilage transplant surgery (autograft or allograft).

36.11 Postoperative Care

• Portal sutures can be removed at 7 days and covered with Steri-Strips and converted to a removable fiberglass splint or CAM boot to begin ROM exercises.
• Patient should remain non–weight bearing for approximately the first 4 weeks (depending on the size and location of the OLT) and advance to full weight bearing as tolerated in the boot and off crutches by week 5 and out of the boot at week 6.

36.12 Outcomes

• Clanton et al looked at patients with an average 70 mm lesions that were Outerbridge grades 3 and 4 and treated with microfracture. They found that, an average of 26 months' follow-up mean patient satisfaction was 8/10 with patients reporting considerably lower satisfaction if they had previously had ankle surgery.[8]
• van Bergen et al evaluated patients treated with microfracture at 12-year follow-up and showed good and excellent

Ogilvie-Harris scores in 78% of the patients, with 94% of patients returning to work and 88% resuming sports activities.[9]

- Ferkel et al evaluated their OLT patients at an average follow-up of 71 months and found 72% had excellent to good results. They looked at a smaller subgroup of 17 patients and evaluated them using the same measures 5 years earlier and found 35% had their results decreased one grade, suggesting that the results of microfracture for an osteochondral lesion may deteriorate with long-term follow-up in some cases.[10]
- Long-term results of return to sports after arthroscopic debridement and bone marrow stimulation found that 76% of patients continued to participate in sports at a mean follow-up of 118 months (range, 46–271). However, the median Ankle Arthritis Score before surgery of 8 significantly decreased to 4 at final follow-up.[11]

References

1. Saxena A, Eakin C. Articular talar injuries in athletes: results of microfracture and autogenous bone graft. Am J Sports Med 2007;35(10):1680–1687
2. Hintermann B, Regazzoni P, Lampert C, Stutz G, Gächter A. Arthroscopic findings in acute fractures of the ankle. J Bone Joint Surg Br 2000;82(3):345–351
3. Ramponi L, Yasui Y, Murawski CD, et al. Lesion size is a predictor of clinical outcomes after bone marrow stimulation for osteochondral lesions of the talus: a systematic review. Am J Sports Med 2017;45(7):1698–1705
4. Choi WJ, Choi GW, Kim JS, Lee JW. Prognostic significance of the containment and location of osteochondral lesions of the talus: independent adverse outcomes associated with uncontained lesions of the talar shoulder. Am J Sports Med 2013;41(1):126–133
5. Choi WJ, Park KK, Kim BS, Lee JW. Osteochondral lesion of the talus: is there a critical defect size for poor outcome? Am J Sports Med 2009;37(10):1974–1980
6. Chuckpaiwong B, Berkson EM, Theodore GH. Microfracture for osteochondral lesions of the ankle: outcome analysis and outcome predictors of 105 cases. Arthroscopy 2008;24(1):106–112
7. Ferkel RD. Foot and Ankle Arthroscopy. 2nd ed. Philadelphia, PA: Wolters Kluwer;2017
8. Clanton TO, Johnson NS, Matheny LM. Outcomes following microfracture in grade 3 and 4 articular cartilage lesions of the ankle. Foot Ankle Int 2014;35(8):764–770
9. van Bergen CJ, Kox LS, Maas M, Sierevelt IN, Kerkhoffs GM, van Dijk CN. Arthroscopic treatment of osteochondral defects of the talus: outcomes at eight to twenty years of follow-up. J Bone Joint Surg Am 2013;95(6):519–525
10. Ferkel RD, Zanotti RM, Komenda GA, et al. Arthroscopic treatment of chronic osteochondral lesions of the talus: long-term results. Am J Sports Med 2008;36(9):1750–1762
11. van Eekeren IC, van Bergen CJ, Sierevelt IN, Reilingh ML, van Dijk CN. Return to sports after arthroscopic debridement and bone marrow stimulation of osteochondral talar defects: a 5- to 24-year follow-up study. Knee Surg Sports Traumatol Arthrosc 2016;24(4):1311–1315

37 Arthroscopic Microfractures for Osteochondral Lesions of the Talus

Rocco Papalia, Guglielmo Torre, Vincenzo Denaro, and Nicola Maffulli

Abstract

Arthroscopic microfracture is a routine and safe procedure for managing osteochondral lesions of the talus. No special expertise is required to perform this technique and results are satisfactory when good preoperative planning is carried out. The main focus must be put on the size and location of the lesion, with appropriate assessment of imaging features, activity level, and age of the patient. Great attention must also be paid to postoperative rehabilitation, to ensure full healing of the microfracture site, before allowing the patient to load the ankle.

Keywords: osteochondral, talus, microfracture, marrow stimulation

37.1 Introduction

Osteochondral defects are common in sports medicine practice, involving major joints such as knee, elbow, hip, and ankle. The lesion consists of a full-thickness defect of the cartilage, also with the involvement of the subchondral bone. Osteochondral lesions of the talus (OLTs) are relatively uncommon in the general population, but increasingly common in athletes.[1] OLTs are mainly caused by trauma, but can also be subsequent to ischemia, abnormal ossification, genetic predisposition, and severe osteoarthritis.[2,3] These lesions cause pain with athletic activities, and also make walking and weight bearing difficult. A number of OLTs are asymptomatic and are revealed by imaging studies carried out for different complaints.[4] Therefore, the mere presence of a lesion at imaging can be a chance finding, and does not mandate surgical treatment.

37.2 Indications

- Primary indication for microfractures is a small, largely frayed, noncystic lesion.
- However, in all the cases in which advanced cartilage softening, fraying of the cartilage, and instability of the osteochondral fragment are present, microfractures are recommended.
- OLTs < 150 mm^2 in surface area.
- Unstable OLTs recalcitrant to nonoperative modalities.

37.2.1 Pathology

- During sport activities, inversion of the foot, forced dorsiflexion, plantar flexion, and external tibial rotation are the most common injuries causing these lesions.[5] About 50% of ankle sprains and about 70% of fractures are associated with osteochondral defects.[6] Trabecular bone fractures affect vascularization of the area and, as a consequence, subchondral bone is affected, developing OLT.[7]

37.2.2 Clinical Evaluation

- When isolated OLT occurs, common symptoms include pain, catching, and stiffness of the joint, with effusion and swelling of the ankle. As these symptoms are nonspecific and are commonly reported in ankle trauma and sprain, OLTs are often not diagnosed, and hence not treated.
- In general, patients mainly report pain on weight bearing and walking, and the ankle is painless at rest. This is caused by the increase in fluid pressure when the joint is loaded on weight bearing.[5] Moreover, ankle sprain pain resolves spontaneously in 4 to 6 weeks, while persisting pain is more commonly associated with osteochondral defects.
- Clinical presentation is often nonspecific, with complaints of vague activity-related ankle pain and swelling. Patients may complain of a feeling of instability of the ankle. The location of the patients' subjective pain often does not correlate with the location of the OLT.
- On clinical evaluation, patients will usually have joint-line ankle tenderness, particularly at the location of the lesion. Given most lesions are at the equatorial region of the talus, and not anteriorly, plantarflexion of the ankle during palpation may help deliver the lesion into the clinical field and increase the accuracy of palpation locating the lesion. In most cases, the ankle joint is stable without clinical evidence of ligamentous dysfunction, despite the common symptom of subjective ankle instability. There is, however, a subset of patients with combined ankle instability and an OLT. These patients will have both clinical laxity of their lateral ligaments on anterior drawer testing and pain in the ankle joint—and are best correlated with magnetic resolution imaging (MRI) examination.

37.2.3 Radiographic Evaluation

- Standard three-view weight-bearing radiographs of the ankle are initially performed. The OLT may not be seen in all cases, but may be visualized as a lytic shadowing or as a loose fragment over the affected area of the talar dome.
- In most cases, additional studies are required to evaluate the bioactivity and anatomic configuration of the lesion. MRI is the best initial study to confirm the diagnosis in unclear cases of OLTs, or to confirm that a lesion seen on plain radiographs is in fact the cause of the patient's symptoms. This is demonstrated by the presence of bone marrow edema at the site of the OLT on MRI. An MRI is additionally useful to exclude other commonly associated pathologies such as tears of the lateral ankle ligaments, and peroneal or posterior tibial tendon pathology.
- MRI, however, is inaccurate at determining the exact size of the lesion because of the presence of bone marrow edema. When the size of the lesion may influence treatment choice, a fine-cut computed tomographic (CT) scan should be added to confirm that anatomy, size, location, and the presence of microcysts adjacent to the OLT.

37.2.4 Nonoperative Options

- Conservative management includes immobilization, antalgic therapy with nonsteroidal anti-inflammatory drugs, oral supplementation of cartilage components (chondroitin and glucosamine), intra-articular injections of hyaluronic acid or platelet-rich plasma, physical therapy, and strengthening of the calf muscles.
- However, these treatments do not address the structural lesion, and, when pain persists or intra-articular loose bodies are detected, arthroscopic surgery is indicated.

37.2.5 Classification of OLTs

Ferkel et al[8] proposed a CT-scan–based classification of the lesions (**Fig. 37.1**), composed of four grades of lesion severity (**Table 37.1**).

Each of the different grades has a different prognosis and treatment. For grade 1 lesions, conservative treatment may reduce symptoms and restore function, although the defect is not filled. Grade 2 to 4 lesions are usually treated by surgery. The Bristol classification is comparable with Ferkel's classification, although bone cysts are considered as a grade 5. At MRI,[9] there is a greater frequency of medial lesions (62%), compared with lateral lesions (34%). The center of the talus was also frequently involved (80%), while involvement of the anterior and posterior edges was less common (6 and 14%, respectively). Concerning location, there is a statistically significant association of medial lesion with poorer prognosis.[10] Moreover, lesions greater than 150 mm² have been associated with poorer prognosis.[11] In addition, the prognosis is also influenced by the age of development of the OLT. Lesions developed during childhood and adolescence have a significantly better prognosis when compared to those occurring during adulthood or in the elderly.[12]

37.2.6 Contraindications

- Diffuse ankle arthritis.
- Large cystic type 5 OLTs.
- Surface area >150 mm² (relative contraindication).
- Septic arthritis/infection of the ankle.
- Recurrent OLTs/failed previous microfracture surgery.

37.3 Goals of Surgical Procedure

Microfracture is a bone marrow stimulation technique, performed to induce bleeding of the subchondral bone and promote fibrocartilage formation. As the cartilage is avascular, spontaneous regeneration cannot be expected. The stimulation of the osteochondral bone to release growth factors contained in the marrow and marrow blood promotes cartilage repair through the formation of an initial cloth, which organizes into fibrocartilage. This is also achieved by migration of bone marrow mesenchymal stem cells, which are mainly responsible for tissue growth at the site of lesion. The average time for fibrocartilage to mature is about 6 weeks, although complete maturation occurs in 12 to 24 weeks. Two major phases can be distinguished, with an initial inflammatory phase (weeks 1–2) with fibrin cloth formation and growth factors release, and a subsequent remodeling phase (weeks 3–12) with proliferation of mesenchymal stem cells and tissue architecture organization.[13] However, fibrocartilage does not have the physical, biochemical, and biomechanical properties of native articular cartilage, because of its lower content in collagen type II, and higher content in collagen type I. Therefore, the site of lesion will remain a *locus minoris resistentiae* of the joint. To improve tissue regeneration, some authors advocate the use of intraoperative platelet-rich plasma or fibrin glue for further delivery of growth factor concentrates at the microfracture site.[5] Given the cartilage environment is detrimental to the outcome of the surgery, in cases of chondromalacia, stability of the osteochondral fragment, minimal fraying of the surrounding cartilage, and microfractures should be avoided, and simple debridement or radiofrequency ablation is recommended.[7] In addition,

Grade	CT scan findings
1	Cystic lesion with intact walls
2a	Cystic lesion in communication with talar dome
2b	Full-thickness lesion with overlaying fragment
3	Undisplaced lesion with lucency
4	Free loose fragment

Table 37.1 Ferkel's classification of OLT

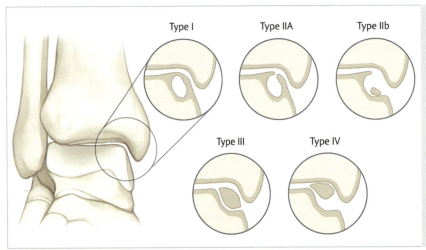

Fig. 37.1 Ferkel's classification of OLT. The five stages are visualized on CT scan of the ankle. (Adapted from Ferkel et al.[8])

microfractures are preferred to other marrow stimulation techniques with radiofrequencies or drilling, to avoid thermal necrosis of the surrounding tissues.

37.4 Advantages of Surgical Procedure

Among surgical techniques used for osteochondral lesions, the most common are microfractures, which are part of the bone marrow stimulation techniques family; autologous chondrocytes implantation, with and without matrix (ACI/MACI); and osteochondral transplantation. Regenerative medicine specialists are developing hydrogels to deliver stem cells or autologous blood elements for cartilage regeneration in osteochondral defects. However, microfracture remains the most effective, safe, and simple technique for osteochondral defect treatment. In this chapter, an overview on microfracture techniques is presented, and surgical technique is proposed, with a discussion of the results available in the literature.

37.5 Key Principles

- Full diagnostic arthroscopy of the ankle joint.
- Adequate visualization of the OLT.
- Debridement of the OLT to a stable cartilaginous rim.
- Debridement of the entire surface area of the base of the OLT of loose bone and cartilage.
- Microfracture of the OLT perpendicular to the base of the lesion.
- Microfracture holes need to be through the subchondral bone 2 to 4 mm deep (**Fig. 37.2**).
- Microfracture holes need to be at least 3 mm apart (**Fig. 37.2**).
- Ensure adequate egress of marrow after completing the microfracture.

37.6 Preoperative Preparation and Patient Positioning

The procedure is performed with the patient supine, after appropriate anesthesia has been induced. Some authors advocate the use of a leg holder at thigh, to fully relax calf muscles.[4] Temporary extraskeletal distraction is applied during arthroscopy. An arthroscopic fluid pump is useful to keep the joint distracted and to maintain an optimal fluid pressure during arthroscopy to maximize visualization. Two standard arthroscopic anteromedial and anterolateral portals are produced using the nick-and-spread technique. The anteromedial portal is produced about 1 cm distal to the joint line, and just medial to the tibialis anterior tendon. The anterolateral portal is produced at the same level, lateral to the common extensor tendon. If the location of the lesion requires access posteriorly, a posterolateral portal is produced, between the Achilles's tendon and peroneal tendons, slightly below the joint line. Arthroscopic exploration of the joint is carried out, through a 2.5- or 2.7-mm arthroscope with a 30-degree angle lens. In some cases, a 70-degree angle lens may be useful.[4] The entire joint should be evaluated with a diagnostic arthroscopy before addressing the lesion to avoid missing additional intra-articular pathology not seen on preoperative evaluation studies.

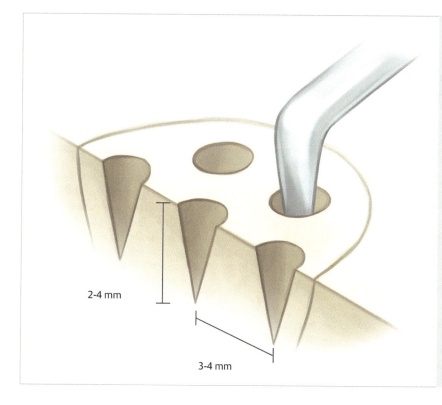

2-4 mm

3-4 mm

Fig. 37.2 Microfractures are traditionally made to a depth of 2 to 4 mm at a distance of 3 to 4 mm from each other. The awl tip must be placed perpendicular to bone surface before perforation.

37.7 Operative Technique

Bony and cartilage debridement is performed using a shaver and, if needed, a radiofrequency probe, along with partial synovectomy, and the osteochondral defects are identified. If loose bodies are present, they are removed arthroscopically. The cartilage surrounding the lesion is prepared with well-defined sharp margins of healthy tissue. This can be done using a 5–0 small arthroscopic curette to ensure a sharp border at the rim of the OLT. The edges should be probed to ensure healthy cartilage that will not delaminate postoperatively. Subsequently, the bony bed is completely cleaned from residual fragments of cartilage. The lesion is then measured using a probe. To carry out microfractures, an awl is introduced into the joint, and the tip is placed exactly perpendicular to the subchondral bone surface. Different angle awls or pick tips are available to assist in obtaining this perpendicular positioning prior to microfracture. Additionally, to achieve an exactly perpendicular position, a superomedial portal may also be made, 1 cm above the joint line and medially to the tibialis anterior.[4] The holes are traditionally made to a depth of 2 to 4 mm at a distance of 3 to 4 mm from each other. To avoid early bleeding of the holes, small increase in irrigation pressure can be made. In this way, a clear and blood-free arthroscopic view can be achieved. After completion of the microfracturing, decreasing the irrigation pressure allows the marrow to bleed, and small fat droplets are visible. No drainage is placed, and the portals are closed in the standard fashion. A light compression bandage is applied.

37.8 Tips and Pearls

- Before making an incision, the ankle joint can be injected with 20 to 30 mL of Ringer's lactate to distend the joint. This will help protect the cartilage during initial joint penetration with the arthroscope.
- When making the skin incision, do not penetrate into the ankle capsule. This will allow the injected fluid to drain out, decompressing the joint, prior to insertion of the arthroscope.
- Initially, the arthroscope should be inserted into the portal opposite to the site of the OLT. This will allow optimal visualization, and the working portal will allow direct access to the lesion.
- Availability of small joint arthroscopic equipment is essential in these cases. Standard knee-sized instruments will create unnecessary iatrogenic damage to the ankle joint cartilage and excessive microfracture of the lesion.
- Slowly reducing the arthroscopic pump pressure, while allowing drainage from the joint with an 18-gauge needle, will allow controlled decrease in joint pressure and visualization of bleeding from the microfracture holes.

37.9 Hazards and Pitfalls

- There are branches of the superficial peroneal nerve, saphenous nerve, and sural nerve immediately over the regions of the anterolateral, anteromedial, and posterolateral portals,

respectively. Injury to these must be avoided by making the skin incision very superficial utilizing a no. 11 scalpel blade, and then spreading the skin with a hemostat down to the ankle capsule, pushing the nerve branches out of the surgical field.
- Microfracture holes should be adequately spread apart (3–4 mm) to prevent coalescence of adjacent pick holes into one large cavity. If this occurs, curette out the loose bone fragments and reperform the microfracture procedure with a stable OLT base.
- If no bleeding/marrow is seen egressing from the awl/pick holes, repeat the process to a depth of 4 to 6 mm to ensure penetration through the subchondral bone. Failure of marrow cells to fill the base of the lesion will prevent the formation of fibrocartilage, and will produce failure of the procedure.

37.10 Complications/Bailout/Salvage

- Complications of the procedure are the same of standard arthroscopy of the ankle and include peroneal nerve palsy, superficial or deep infections, and thrombosis.

37.11 Postoperative Care

After surgery, an ankle brace or a walking boot could be used for immobilization of the ankle. Although traditionally an initial period of non–weight bearing of at least 6 weeks was advocated, no consensus has been reached concerning exact duration of non–weight-bearing period. A recent trial compared postrehabilitation outcomes of patients who had undergone microfractures for small defects. A 6-week non-bearing group was compared with a 2-week non-bearing group, with tolerance weight bearing after 2 weeks. Comparable outcomes were found at last follow-up, in terms of AOFAS score.[6] During the period of non-weight bearing, strengthening exercises for leg muscles must always be performed, to avoid atrophy, which is associated with longer recovery time. Therefore, strengthening and stretching exercise must be started the day after the surgery. After a period of non–weight bearing or partial weight bearing, gradual exercises for load transfer on the operated ankle should be carried out. Furthermore, rehabilitation to normal gait and recover of passive and active ROM of the ankle is fundamental for return to activities. After 4 to 6 months from surgery, patients should return gradually to normal activities. For full return to contact sports, further maturation of the tissue should be achieved. Therefore, return to full sports activities can be accorded in 8 to 10 months. A retrospective investigation by Ventura et al[14] reported outcomes of patients affected by OLTs of a mean size of 1 cm². At an average follow-up of 4 years, the study reported excellent improvement of AOFAS score, Tegner activity level evaluation, Karlsson–Peterson score, and Sefton scale. Furthermore, MRI assessment at 18 months from surgery revealed 27 completely healed lesions, 9 light bone edema, and only 2 non-healed lesions.

37.12 Outcomes

Of 44 athletes treated by microfractures for 46 OLTs, all, but two, returned to preinjury sport level in a mean time of 15.1 weeks, with a mean AOFAS score increasing from 54.6 to 94.4 at last follow-up.[15] These patients were compared with patients with grade 5 lesions (Hepple's classification) who were treated by autologous bone grafting, without any statistical difference in terms of AOFAS score. However, in the second group, the mean time to return to sport activities was 19.6 weeks.

The outcome of small lesions (<15 mm^2) was presented by Chuckpaiwong et al,[16] showing no failure. In the same study, patients with lesion greater than 15 mm^2 did not show successful outcomes, and were reoperated with the same unsuccessful results (AOFAS improved by mean of 17.2 points). A recent comparison study[17] showed no difference in clinical results in patients treated by microfractures or subchondral drilling. The mean preoperative AOFAS score was 66.5 and 66.0, respectively, improving to 90.1 and 89.0, respectively. Postoperative VAS and AAS scores did not differ significantly, and radiographic and MRI assessment showed improvement of the lesion.

Osti et al[18] presented the results of ankle arthroscopy and microfractures in 15 former professional soccer players, with a mean improvement in AOFAS score from 48 to 86 points. Furthermore, Kaikkonen's score improved similarly, from 43 to 85 points, as did VAS for pain. Of the 15 patients, 8 returned to recreational contact sport, 6 returned to light noncontact activities, and 1 did not return to activities.

References

1. Vannini F, Costa GG, Caravelli S, Pagliazzi G, Mosca M. Treatment of osteochondral lesions of the talus in athletes: what is the evidence? Joints 2016;4(2):111–120
2. van Dijk CN, Reilingh ML, Zengerink M, van Bergen CJ. Osteochondral defects in the ankle: why painful? Knee Surg Sports Traumatol Arthrosc 2010;18(5):570–580
3. van Dijk CN, Reilingh ML, Zengerink M, van Bergen CJ. The natural history of osteochondral lesions in the ankle. Instr Course Lect 2010;59:375–386
4. Thermann H, Becher C. Microfractures for osteochondral lesions of the talus, In: Wiesel SW, ed. Operative Techniques in Orthopaedic Surgery. Philadelphia, PA: Lippincott Williams & Wilkins;2011:4222–4228
5. Mei-Dan O, Carmont MR, Laver L, Mann G, Maffulli N, Nyska M. Platelet-rich plasma or hyaluronate in the management of osteochondral lesions of the talus. Am J Sports Med 2012;40(3):534–541
6. Grambart ST. Arthroscopic management of osteochondral lesions of the talus. Clin Podiatr Med Surg 2016;33(4):521–530
7. Choi WJ, Jo J, Lee JW. Osteochondral lesion of the talus: prognostic factors affecting the clinical outcome after arthroscopic marrow stimulation technique. Foot Ankle Clin 2013;18(1):67–78
8. Ferkel RD, Zanotti RM, Komenda GA, et al. Arthroscopic treatment of chronic osteochondral lesions of the talus: long-term results. Am J Sports Med 2008;36(9):1750–1762
9. Elias I, Zoga AC, Morrison WB, Besser MP, Schweitzer ME, Raikin SM. Osteochondral lesions of the talus: localization and morphologic data from 424 patients using a novel anatomical grid scheme. Foot Ankle Int 2007;28(2):154–161
10. Yoshimura I, Kanazawa K, Takeyama A, et al. Arthroscopic bone marrow stimulation techniques for osteochondral lesions of the talus: prognostic factors for small lesions. Am J Sports Med 2013;41(3):528–534
11. Choi WJ, Park KK, Kim BS, Lee JW. Osteochondral lesion of the talus: is there a critical defect size for poor outcome? Am J Sports Med 2009;37(10):1974–1980
12. Schenck RC Jr, Goodnight JM. Osteochondritis dissecans. J Bone Joint Surg Am 1996;78(3):439–456
13. van Eekeren IC, Reilingh ML, van Dijk CN. Rehabilitation and return-to-sports activity after debridement and bone marrow stimulation of osteochondral talar defects. Sports Med 2012;42(10):857–870
14. Ventura A, Terzaghi C, Legnani C, Borgo E. Treatment of post-traumatic osteochondral lesions of the talus: a four-step approach. Knee Surg Sports Traumatol Arthrosc 2013;21(6):1245–1250
15. Saxena A, Eakin C. Articular talar injuries in athletes: results of microfracture and autogenous bone graft. Am J Sports Med 2007;35(10):1680–1687
16. Chuckpaiwong B, Berkson EM, Theodore GH. Microfracture for osteochondral lesions of the ankle: outcome analysis and outcome predictors of 105 cases. Arthroscopy 2008;24(1):106–112
17. Choi JI, Lee KB. Comparison of clinical outcomes between arthroscopic subchondral drilling and microfracture for osteochondral lesions of the talus. Knee Surg Sports Traumatol Arthrosc 2016;24(7):2140–2147
18. Osti L, Del Buono A, Maffulli N. Arthroscopic debridement of the ankle for mild to moderate osteoarthritis: a midterm follow-up study in former professional soccer players. J Orthop Surg 2016;11:37

38 Posterior Ankle Arthroscopy

James D.F. Calder

Abstract
Posterior ankle arthroscopy was first published by van Dijk in 2000[1] who described using a two-portal endoscopic approach, making it possible to appropriately visualize the posterior ankle structures and safely manage these. Since then, the spectrum of different pathologies involving the posterior ankle that can be addressed arthroscopically has grown significantly. This chapter outlines these pathologies and describes how they can be addressed arthroscopically through minimal incisions, with limited soft-tissue disruption, allowing faster return to activities and athletic function.

Keywords: *posterior ankle, arthroscopy, impingement*

38.1 Indications and Pathology

- Posterior ankle impingement (PAI)—soft tissue or bone (os trigonum, avulsed bone fragments, and loose bodies).
- Release of flexor hallucis longus (FHL) tendon.
- Soft-tissue release for restricted ankle dorsiflexion (DF).
- Treatment of ankle osteochondral lesion (OCL).
- Achilles tendon (AT) pathology—noninsertional Achilles tendinopathy (NIAT) with release of plantaris tendon and insertional AT symptoms with Haglund's deformity and retrocalcaneal bursitis.
- Hindfoot arthritis—subtalar joint (STJ) fusion and also posterior ankle joint fusion when there is concern regarding anterior soft-tissue envelope (e.g., following trauma).

38.1.1 Clinical Evaluation of Pathology

- PAI—posterior ankle pain on forced plantar flexion of the ankle with or without restricted plantarflexion.
- FHL pathology—posteromedial (P/M) ankle pain with or without crepitus or "ratcheting" of the FHL tendon during FHL movement.
- Restricted ankle DF—usually several months following severe ankle trauma such as ankle dislocation. No obvious tightness of Achilles/gastrocnemius but a block coming up into DF frequently associated with anterior ankle pain but without obvious bone impingement anteriorly on imaging.
- OCL ankle—deep ankle pain during activities.
- Insertional AT pathology—swelling and tenderness medial and lateral to AT sometimes with "ballotable" bursa palpable.
- Hindfoot arthritis—generalized swelling and stiffness around hindfoot. Important to assess quality of soft tissues and scarring in relation to AT for planning of incisions for fixation.

38.1.2 Radiographic Evaluation

- Weight-bearing X-rays (anteroposterior [AP]/lateral). Os trigona are more easily demonstrated on lateral views with 20-degree internal rotation. AP ankle in 30 degrees may demonstrate OCL posterior talus. Lateral view of calcaneus will demonstrate bone spur within the AT and this may not

be amenable to endoscopic excision but may suggest open surgery if indicated.
- Magnetic resonance imaging (MRI). Useful for assessment of OCL and presence of active pathology in subchondral bone rather than just an incidental finding. Soft-tissue PAI is demonstrated well as is pathology surrounding the FHL. Bone marrow edema in the synchondrosis of the os trigonum and posterior talus demonstrates whether there is active bone pathology contributing to PAI symptoms (**Fig. 38.1**), and pathology such as ganglion cyst may be identified (**Fig. 38.2**). Assessment of AT pathology is important—if there is significant degenerative change with multiple partial tears, fissures, or incomplete avulsions from the tendon insertion, then endoscopic treatment of the Haglund or retrocalcaneal bursitis alone may be unsuccessful and a formal open procedure should be considered.
- Computed tomography (CT). Very useful to confirm the presence of fragmentation of an os trigonum and avulsed fragments or loose bodies. Small fragments from avulsion of the posterior inferior tibiofibular ligament (PITFL) may be more easily demonstrated on CT (**Fig. 38.3**).
- Ultrasound (US). Accurate assessment of presence and degree of tendinosis of AT.

38.1.3 Nonoperative Options

- PAI—strapping to prevent excessive plantarflexion and proprioceptive training and strengthening to reduce lateral ankle ligament instability which may exacerbate PAI symptoms. US-guided injections of corticosteroid and local anesthetic may reduce PAI—more effective and even curative in soft-tissue PAI but frequently only temporary benefit in bone PAI (os trigonum), and reports suggest longer recovery and less successful outcome following multiple injections for bone PAI.[2]

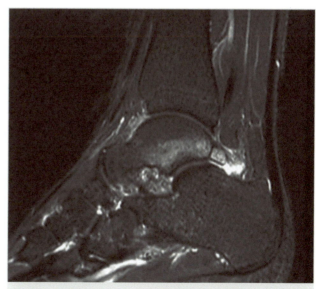

Fig 38.1 MRI scan demonstrating bone marrow edema in the os trigonum, the synchondrosis and the adjacent talus.

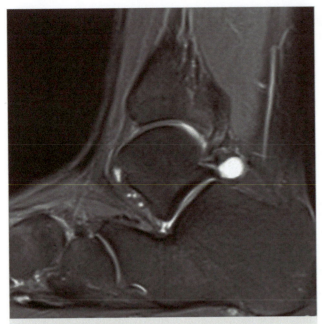

Fig 38.2 MRI demonstrating ganglion cyst in patient with posterior ankle impingement.

- OCL ankle and hindfoot arthritis—modification of activities and use of oral analgesics. Hyaluronic acid injections.[3,4]
- AT pathology—eccentric stretching and strengthening exercises, heel raise, oral analgesics. Avoid deep DF eccentric exercises in insertional AT pathology given this may exacerbate irritation of bursitis. Extracorporeal shockwave therapy. US-guided paratenon stripping injections (high-volume injection of local anesthetic without corticosteroid) may help with paratendinitis and NIAT. US-guided corticosteroid injection into a retrocalcaneal bursitis is controversial because of the risk of AT rupture but may be considered in the absence of significant AT tendinosis, and consider temporary protection in a boot for 2 weeks.[5]
- FHL pathology—US-guided injection of corticosteroid and local anesthetic.
- Soft-tissue contractures—physiotherapy stretching and night splints. US-guided injections tend to be unhelpful.

38.1.4 Relevant Contraindications

- Usual medical and vascular assessment.
- Local scar tissue from previous trauma and surgery (particularly important around the AT where there is a poor blood supply to local soft tissues).
- Smoking and diabetes are significant risk factors for soft-tissue complications following surgery related to the AT; however, endoscopic/posterior ankle arthroscopy has the advantage of less soft-tissue dissection compared to open procedures.

38.2 Goals of Surgical Procedure

- Reduce symptoms of pain or stiffness.
- Enable predictable and earlier return to activities than seen with open procedures.
- Reduce risk of complications seen with open procedures.

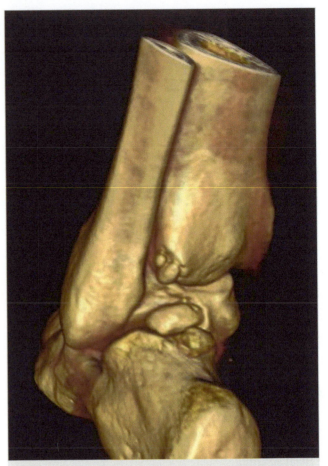

Fig 38.3 CT scan demonstrating avulsed fragments from avulsion of PITFL resulting in posterior ankle impingement.

38.3 Advantages of Surgical Procedure

- Clear views of pathology—it is easier to visualize the posterior ankle with an arthroscope than through a small incision.
- Minimal soft-tissue dissection and less scarring—improves wound healing and enables rehabilitation to commence earlier with improved speed of recovery.

38.4 Key Principles

- A standard 4-mm 30-degree knee arthroscope is routinely used. The cannula is 6 mm, which allows for good fluid flow and excellent vision. The small joint (2.7 mm × 67 mm) 30-degree arthroscope may be used, but with the 2.9-mm cannula, the fluid flow is more restricted and thus less optimal views are obtained. The author prefers the longer small joint 30-degree arthroscope (2.7 mm × 120 mm) using the 4.6-mm cannula given that this gives the best fluid flow and good views (Smith & Nephew, Boston, MA).
- A fluid management system is not a perquisite but is preferred by the author, ensuring pressure is kept to 35 mm Hg.

38.5 Operative Technique

38.5.1 Preoperative Preparation and Patient Positioning

- Fully informed consent and appropriate marking of the leg (the author insists on an "X" on the heel to avoid any confusion of site of surgery when the patient is turned).
- Thigh tourniquet is applied prior to turning the patient—it is more difficult to apply after turning.
- Spinal or general anesthesia.
- Patient is turned semi-prone into the "recovery position" with the operated leg lowermost.[6] This reduces the need for intubation and paralysis during general anesthetic, and a laryngeal mask may be used. A bolster is placed to support the chest in three-fourths turned position but the pelvis should be flat on the table so that the foot points vertically down. The foot should be supported with a gel pad under the ankle to raise it from the table and the foot placed over the end of the bed. It is important to ensure that the ankle may be fully dorsiflexed during the procedure and it is not restricted by the end of the table.

38.5.2 Surgical Procedure

Universal Technique for Posterior Ankle Arthroscopy

- Identify sites for posterior portals—medial and lateral to AT (**Fig. 38.4**).
- Standard positioning of the portals as described by van Dijk et al.[1]
- Use a hemostat through the posterolateral (P/L) portal to dissect toward the posterior talar process using "push and spread" technique. It is important to aim for the first web space as deviation may injure neurovascular structures medially or peroneal tendons laterally (**Fig. 38.5**).
- Introduce the arthroscope and then use a hemostat through the P/M portal perpendicular to the arthroscope. Once it reaches the arthroscope, follow along to the end of the arthroscope, and under direct vision, spread the hemostat to create a working space in the hindfoot into which a 4.5 or 5.5-mm shaver may be introduced (e.g., Incisor or Bone Cutter blades, Dyonics, Boston, MA).
- Ensure that the blade is pointing directly toward the camera and use suction to bring tissue into the blade in oscillating mode with a sweeping action proximally and distally to clear tissue from the posterior ankle/STJ. Normally, the STJ is first to be seen. Clear tissue from the superior surface of the posterior talar process until the FHL comes into view, always keeping the blade toward the camera.
- Therefore, the arthroscope is kept "extra-articular" as only rarely does it need to be placed "inside" the ankle.

FHL Release and Excision of Os Trigonum

- Once the FHL is observed, ensure that dissection is not made medial to this, as this may compromise the neurovascular bundle.

- The FHL tendon sheath may be released with the shaver or sharp cutting instruments.
- Occasionally, loose bodies become trapped in the FHL sheath causing irritation of the FHL and pseudolocking of the ankle. The may be "milked" digitally from the distal sheath (around the inferior sustentaculum tali) and then removed arthroscopically (**Fig. 38.6**).
- The os trigonum can be shaved away. The synchondrosis may be identified with a small osteotome or periosteal elevator loosening the os trigonum enabling it to be removed whole.

Treatment of Ankle OCL

- Gaining access to the ankle joint for treatment of an OCL or fusion of the ankle requires excision of the posterior intermalleolar ligament.[7] The 30-degree angle of the arthroscope may then be used to gain excellent vision of the posterior talar and tibial surfaces by rotating the camera.
- Standard techniques of debridement and microfracture are used.

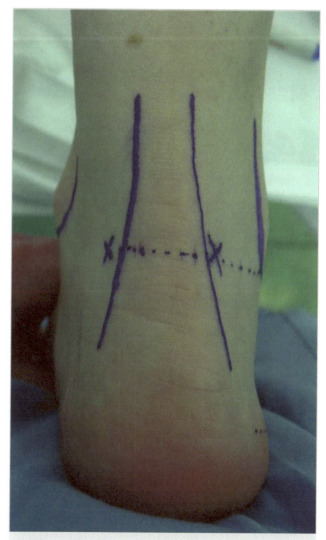

Fig 38.4 Marking incision for arthroscopy portals.

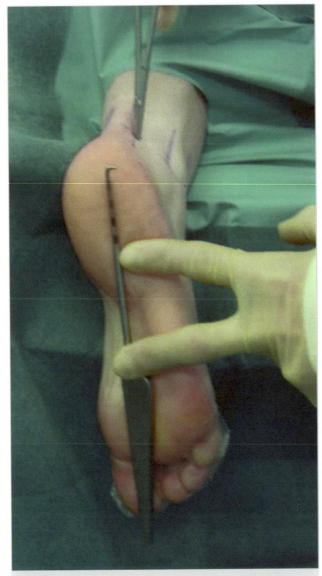

Fig 38.5 Demonstrating direction of the hemostat and subsequently the arthroscope toward the first web space.

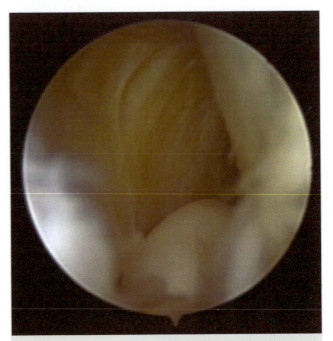

Fig 38.6 Loose body within the flexor hallucis longus tendon sheath.

cross-screws from medial and lateral tibia or two screws from the medial tibia.

Achilles Tendon Pathology

- Endoscopic excision of Haglund requires soft-tissue dissection across to the retrocalcaneal bursa and the removal of the posterosuperior bony prominence of the calcaneus and the bursa. A 4-mm Acromioniser (Dyonics, Boston, MA) may be used rather than the Bone Cutter shaver. Swopping portals is necessary to ensure that the medial and lateral edges of the calcaneus are removed, and using intraoperative image intensifier may help to assess that adequate bone has been resected. Poor results are associated with insufficient resection of bone.[9]
- In endoscopic treatment of NIAT, the distal-lateral portal placement is the same as for hindfoot arthroscopy as described earlier but the hemostat is used to penetrate the paratenon medially and then used in a sweeping action within the paratenon to release the AT. The second portal is then more easily placed over the medial edge of the AT 6 cm proximal (**Fig. 38.7**). Adhesions between the paratenon and the AT may be resected endoscopically and the ventral aspect of the AT debrided of scar tissue and neovascularization. The plantaris tendon may be identified and sectioned if this is thought to be have a frictional or compressive effect on the AT (**Fig. 38.8**).

Release of Constrictive Posterior Soft Tissues for Posttraumatic Restriction of Ankle DF

- The soft-tissue dissection described earlier is performed but it is more extensive. The entire posterior FHL sheath needs to be resected along with the intermalleolar ligament and

Arthroscopic Hindfoot Fusion

- During an arthroscopic STJ fusion, making the portals 1 cm more proximal than described earlier can help with placement of the shaver and the instruments along the posterior facet joint surface, which is sloped downward from posterior to anterior. two parallel screws are placed across the fusion under X-ray control.
- The posterior 60% of the talar articular surface may be removed using the posterior arthroscopic approach but the most anterior articular surface and anterior tibial osteophytes that may prevent adequate ankle DF and appropriate alignment for fusion may mean that additional portals are paced along the anterior ankle joint to enable debridement.[8] Although many screw configurations are described, the posterior approach is excellent for placing a "home-run" screw from the P/L tibia into the neck of the talus, ensuring the talus is pulled back against the posterior rim of the tibia. This is then supplemented either by two

the posterior tibial slip, all of which may contribute to ankle stiffenss.[7] The excision needs to be extensive to release the posterior structures adequately—this tissue is normally markedly thickened and hard once mature.

38.6 Tips and Pearls/Expert Suggestions

- Distraction of the ankle joint may be needed to aid visualization of an OCL. The easiest way is to use a commercial ankle strap with in-line traction using a crepe bandage around the surgeon's waist.
- The advantage of using the 2.7 mm × 120 mm arthroscope with the 4.6-mm diameter cannula is that fluid flow is maintained and also if traction needs to be applied for a tight ankle during treatment of an OCL and a true "intra-articular" arthroscopy is required, then the cannula may be changed to 2.9 mm, enabling easier access into the ankle joint itself.
- OCLs of the P/L talus may be difficult to approach and swapping the arthroscope to the P/M portal may provide better access.
- During an arthroscopic STJ fusion, a Steinmann pin may be introduced into the sinus tarsi and then used to lever open the joint, allowing easier preparation of the joint surfaces.
- During Haglund's resection, the distal posterior bone prominence just proximal to the AT insertion can be difficult. Plantar flexion of the ankle takes tension off the AT and provides more space for the shaver to resect this bone.
- During endoscopic treatment of NIAT, the ankle may be flexed up and down to bring the pathology into the shaver and enable adequate visualization of the tendon.

38.7 Hazards and Pitfalls

- Injury to the tibial neurovascular structures (ensure foot is vertically placed over the end of the operating table, the direction of portals is accurate, and careful initial dissection is performed to identify the FHL).
- An accessory FHL tendon, usually posterior to the main tendon, and a flexor digitorum accessorius longus have also been described, both of which may lead to confusion in local anatomy during dissection.[10]

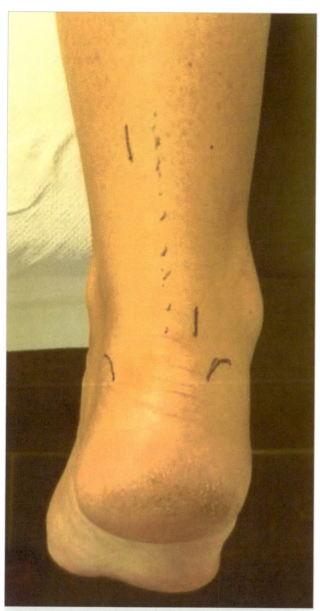

Fig 38.7 Incision sites for the Achilles tendoscopy portals.

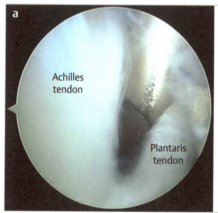
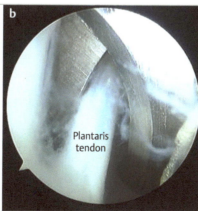

Fig 38.8 Identifying plane between the Achilles (a) and plantaris tendon with division of the plantaris under direct vision (b).

- Injury to the FHL due to incorrect orientation of the shaver.
- Injury to the sural nerve if P/L portal is placed too far laterally. There is a branch of the sural nerve which may be injured during portal placement, and patients should be warned that a small patch of numbness may be noticed over the P/L heel.

38.8 Complications/Bailout/Salvage

- Stiffness of the STJ during fusion despite using leverage of a Steinmann pin may make debridement of the joint surface difficult, and conversion to an open procedure may be required.
- If there is significant subfibular impingement from a "lateral wall blowout" following calcaneal fracture, an open STJ fusion may be preferred because clearing the lateral space may be difficult.
- In severe NIAT, developing a plane between the paratenon and AT may be difficult due to adhesions, and conversion to an open procedure extending the medial incision required.

38.9 Postoperative Care

- Arthroscopy portals should always be closed with sutures—the effect of gravity means that articular fluid will collect under the portals and risks sinus formation if not closed formally.
- Firm crepe bandage is left in place for 72 hours and the leg elevated. An elastic stocking is used to reduce swelling for 3 weeks.
- Except for hindfoot fusion, mobilize non-weight-bearing for 1 week, 50% weight-bearing for 1 week, and then weight-bear as able. Encourage FHL movements immediately postoperatively and ankle range of movements under physiotherapy supervision from 1 week. I routinely prescribe 1 month of nonsteroidal anti-inflammatory drugs (NSAIDs) with proton-pump inhibitor to reduce the inflammatory response and scar tissue/bone formation that can result in postoperative stiffness following hindfoot procedures.
- Following hindfoot fusion, NSAIDs are avoided and patients mobilized in a boot weight-bearing as able following 2 weeks non-weight-bearing and 4 weeks 50% weight-bearing.

38.10 Outcomes

- Arthroscopic treatment of PAI and FHL release—95% return to professional sport at a mean of 41 days.[2] Quicker return to ballet is achieved with arthroscopic than for open excision of os trigonum (9.8 vs. 14.9 weeks, $p = 0.001$).[11]
- NIAT—significant improvement in AOS and SF-36 scores have been reported following Achilles tendoscopy and endoscopic release and division of the plantaris tendon.[12]
- Insertional Achilles problems—Jerosch reported excellent or good results following endoscopic calcaneoplasty in 155/164 patients and a systematic review reported better results with endoscopic than open treatment.[9,13]

- Hindfoot fusion—excellent clinical results reported in 40 patients undergoing posterior arthroscopic ankle fusion with union within 3 months in all patients.[8] Arthroscopic STJ fusion has a low reported incidence of complications and fusion in 91 to 100% individuals.[14]

References

1. van Dijk CN, Scholten PE, Krips R. A 2-portal endoscopic approach for diagnosis and treatment of posterior ankle pathology. Arthroscopy 2000;16(8):871–876
2. Calder JD, Sexton SA, Pearce CJ. Return to training and playing after posterior ankle arthroscopy for posterior impingement in elite professional soccer. Am J Sports Med 2010;38(1):120–124
3. Witteveen AG, Hofstad CJ, Kerkhoffs GM. Hyaluronic acid and other conservative treatment options for osteoarthritis of the ankle. Cochrane Database Syst Rev 2015(10):CD010643
4. Henrotin Y, Raman R, Richette P, et al. Consensus statement on viscosupplementation with hyaluronic acid for the management of osteoarthritis. Semin Arthritis Rheum 2015;45(2):140–149
5. Wijesekera NT, Chew NS, Lee JC, Mitchell AW, Calder JD, Healy JC. Ultrasound-guided treatments for chronic Achilles tendinopathy: an update and current status. Skeletal Radiol 2010;39(5):425–434
6. Odutola A, Clarke A, Harries W, Robinson S, Hepple S, Soar J. Clinical tip: semi-prone position for Achilles tendon surgery. Foot Ankle Int 2007;28(10):1104–1105
7. Golanó P, Vega J, de Leeuw PAJ, et al. Anatomy of the ankle ligaments: a pictorial essay. Knee Surg Sports Traumatol Arthrosc 2010;18(5):557–569
8. de Leeuw PA, Hendrickx RP, van Dijk CN, Stufkens SS, Kerkhoffs GM. Midterm results of posterior arthroscopic ankle fusion. Knee Surg Sports Traumatol Arthrosc 2016;24(4):1326–1331
9. Wiegerinck JI, Kok AC, van Dijk CN. Surgical treatment of chronic retrocalcaneal bursitis. Arthroscopy 2012;28(2):283–293
10. Batista JP, Del Vecchio JJ, Golanó P, Vega J. Flexor digitorum accessorius longus: importance of posterior ankle endoscopy. Case Rep Orthop 2015;2015:823107
11. Ballal MS, Roche A, Brodrick A, Williams RL, Calder JD. Posterior endoscopic excision of os trigonum in professional national ballet dancers. J Foot Ankle Surg 2016;55(5):927–930
12. Pearce CJ, Carmichael J, Calder JD. Achilles tendinoscopy and plantaris tendon release and division in the treatment of non-insertional Achilles tendinopathy. Foot Ankle Surg 2012;18(2):124–127
13. Jerosch J. Endoscopic calcaneoplasty. Foot Ankle Clin 2015;20(1):149–165
14. Tuijthof GJ, Beimers L, Kerkhoffs GM, Dankelman J, Dijk CN. Overview of subtalar arthrodesis techniques: options, pitfalls and solutions. Foot Ankle Surg 2010;16(3):107–116

39 Autologous Osteochondral Transplantation

Yoshiharu Shimozono, Youichi Yasui, Andrew W. Ross, and John G. Kennedy

Abstract

Autologous osteochondral transplantation (AOT) is an osteo-chondral replacement technique to restore the biologic and anatomic function of the articular cartilage and subchondral bone. This procedure is typically indicated for large (>100–150 mm²) or cystic lesions. The surgical approach is determined by the location of the lesions, and adequate exposure of the lesions is essential for optimal results. Both medial and lateral tibial osteotomies have been utilized to obtain exposure of the lesions for perpendicular insertion of grafts. The osteochondral graft is typically harvested from the non-weight-bearing portion of the ipsilateral femoral condyle. Graft implantation should be flush with the adjacent native cartilage surface. Concentrated bone marrow aspirate may be utilized to promote bone healing and integration between the graft and host tissue cartilage. The clinical outcomes after AOT are promising in the short to medium term. In the athletic population, 90% of professional athletes returned to preinjury sports activity. Donor-site morbidity and postoperative cyst formation have been reported in several studies. However, donor-site knee pain does not appear to be a significant issue and its incidence is reported to be less than 5%, and most cysts are asymptomatic and resolve over time.

Keywords: *osteochondral lesion, ankle, talus, autograft, malleolar osteotomy*

39.1 Indications

- Osteochondral lesions of the talus (OLTs) with persistent ankle pain following 3 months of conservative treatment.
- Operative techniques can be broadly divided into two procedures: reparative, including bone marrow stimulation (BMS), and replacement procedures, including autologous osteochondral transplantation (AOT).
- The clinical criteria to decide which operative technique should be indicated are the following:
  - Lesion size:
    Large OLTs, traditionally characterized as lesions greater than 150 mm² in area or 15 mm in diameter, are candidates for AOT.[1,2] However, a recent systematic review study demonstrated that lesions greater than 107.4 mm² in area and/or 10.2 mm in diameter are the optimal for AOT.[3]
  - Previously failed BMS.[4,5]
  - Cystic lesions:
    OLTs with large cystic subchondral defects may be optimal candidates for AOT, although there are no clearly established criteria regarding cyst depth or size.[6]

39.1.1 Pathology

- Damage to the cartilage and underlying bone in the talar dome.

- Most commonly traumatic in nature.
- Most commonly seen in younger adult athletes.

39.1.2 Clinical Evaluation

- Patient usually complains of pain on weight-bearing on the ankle:
  - Usually pain-free when not weight-bearing.
- May have symptoms of ankle instability with clinically stable ligamentous complex.
- Tenderness at the ankle joint line:
  - Tenderness and location of reported pain does not always correspond with location of the lesion.

39.1.3 Radiographic Evaluation

- Weight-bearing anteroposterior, lateral, and mortise views of the ankle:
  - A shadowing or defect may be seen in the bone in the region of the lesion.
  - Loose body or fragment may be seen within or separate from the lesion base.
- Magnetic resonance imaging (MRI):
  - Useful in screening for OLTs.
  - Presence of associate bone marrow edema confirms bioactivity of the lesion.
  - Not reliable for determining the true size or anatomic configuration of the lesion.
- CT scan (fine cut)—with axial, coronal, and sagittal cuts:
  - Best study to determine the size and configuration of the bony lesion.
  - Accurate in determining presence of cysts and microcysts adjacent to the OLT.

39.1.4 Contraindications

- Rheumatoid disease.
- Posttraumatic ankle osteoarthritis with grade II or greater lesions.
- Uncorrected ankle malalignment.
- Moderate to severe medical comorbidities (e.g., diabetes, autoimmune disease, active infection).

39.2 Goals of Surgical Procedure

The goal of AOT is to restore the biologic and anatomic function of talar articular cartilage and subchondral bone. To achieve this, AOT includes replacement of the damaged cartilage and subchondral bone with one or more autologous grafts that have similar mechanical, structural, and biochemical properties of native hyaline articular cartilage.

39.3 Advantages of Surgical Procedure

The advantage of AOT is that this technique can replace the lesions with viable hyaline cartilage and subchondral bone without the need for two-staged procedure. Intraoperative damage of subchondral bone during BMS procedure is of growing concern. The role of the local subchondral environment has been shown to be integral to cartilage repair, and failed functional outcomes following BMS may be due to impairment of subchondral bone. Unlike BMS, AOT replaces local subchondral bone and may result in the restoration of the native biological environment leading to better functional outcomes.

AOT has several potential disadvantages, including donor-site morbidity, the possible need for an osteotomy while accessing the talar dome, differences of cartilage biology between the host and graft tissues, and poor potential for integration at the cartilage interface.

39.4 Key Principles

AOT involves cylindrical osteochondral grafts harvested from a donor site, typically a non-weight-bearing portion of the ipsilateral knee. These are transplanted into a recipient site at the location of the cartilage defect on the talus. The procedure is typically carried out in the following steps:

1. Tibial osteotomy.
2. Preparation of the recipient site for the insertion of the osteochondral graft.
3. Harvesting of osteochondral graft from ipsilateral lateral femoral condyle.
4. Insertion of osteochondral graft into the created recipient site of the talus.
5. Fixation of tibial osteotomy fragment.

39.5 Preoperative Preparation and Patient Positioning

Numerous commercial instruments are available for AOT of the talus. While several instruments are available, the authors utilize the Osteochondral Autograft Transplant System (OATS; Arthrex, Naples, FL). The utilized core sizes are 6, 8, and 10 mm.

A recipient sizer, recipient harvester, donor harvester, and tamp are basic instruments for AOT. Standard surgical instruments for the tibial osteotomy and exposure of the ankle joint are also required. Kirschner wires (K-wires), cannulated drill set and screws (3.5/4.0 mm), and fluoroscopy are used for fixation of the osteotomy site. Titanium screws are optimal for fixation of the osteotomy to allow for potential postoperative MRI evaluation with minimal metallic interference.

Under general or spinal anesthesia, the patient is placed in the supine position. The authors prefer to use a thigh tourniquet.

39.6 Operative Technique

39.6.1 Tibial Osteotomy

It is imperative to create a direct path for perpendicular insertion of the osteochondral graft in order to construct a congruent articular surface. The acceptable range between graft surface and native articular surface is only 1.0 mm sunken to 0.4 mm proud.[7]

Due to the majority of medial OLTs being located in the central or posterior position in talus, a medial malleolar chevron osteotomy is often required to provide adequate exposure. First, a longitudinal skin incision is made over the medial malleolus. The posterior tibial tendon is then retracted with extra care taken to avoid iatrogenic neurovascular damage. The medial corner of the anterior aspect of tibia is exposed in order to establish the anatomical landmark for the osteotomy line. Caution is taken to minimize periosteum stripping of the medial malleolus. A provisional K-wire is then inserted under fluoroscopy to determine a precise osteotomy line (**Fig. 39.1**). After the decision of the osteotomy line is complete, two parallel fixation holes in the medial malleolus are predrilled for later anatomic fixation with 4.0-mm titanium screws. A medial malleolar chevron osteotomy is then performed using an oscillating saw. A chevron-type osteotomy is preferred in order to provide appropriate anatomic alignment, stability after fixation, and a large surface area for greater healing and visualization. At the level of the subchondral bone, the saw is stopped and the osteotomy is completed with an osteotome. The osteomized medial malleolus is reflected in the plantar direction on the deltoid ligament hinge to allow exposure of the medial aspect of the talar dome. The authors employ a retractor to maintain visualization (**Fig. 39.2**).

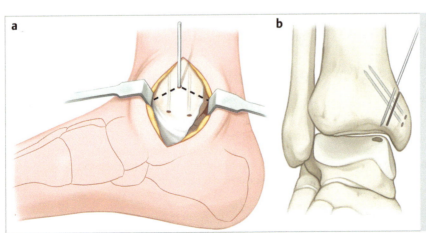

Fig. 39.1 (a) A provisional K-wire is drilled to visualize the osteotomy site fluoroscopically. (b) The remainder of osteotomy is completed with an osteotome.

Lateral OLTs are often located in the anterior aspect of the talar dome, which allows for anterolateral access with ankle plantarflexion and avoids the need for an osteotomy. In cases of central or posterior lesions, a tibial or fibular osteotomy can be required. Centerolateral and posterolateral lesions can be accessed with an anterolateral tibial trapezoid osteotomy (**Fig. 39.3**). This osteotomy is superior to a fibular osteotomy due to the avoidance of the need to reconstruct the lateral ligament complex following fibular osteotomy. Similar to the medial chevron osteotomy previously described, the site of proposed osteotomy should be predrilled for 4-mm titanium screw fixation (**Fig. 39.3**). In cases requiring a fibular osteotomy, anterior talofibular ligament or/and calcaneofibular ligament release should be performed.

39.6.2 Preparation of the Recipient Site for the Insertion of the Osteochondral Graft

Damaged unstable articular cartilage over the talus is first debrided using a curette and a rongeur until a stable and viable cartilage rim surrounding the lesions is exposed. The lesion size, subsequent graft size, and number of required grafts are determined and the appropriate-sized recipient trephine is placed in the talar defect. To reconstruct a smooth articular surface, it is crucial to maintain the recipient harvested trephine perpendicular to the lesion. If necessary, eversion or inversion may improve access. If the lesion requires two grafts,

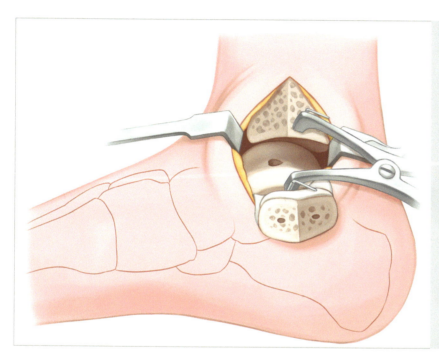

Fig. 39.2 A retractor is used to allow exposure of the medial aspect of the talar dome.

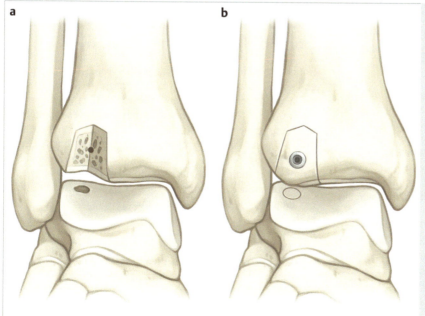

a   b

Fig. 39.3 (a) An anterolateral tibial trapezoidal osteotomy. (b) Final fixation of the osteotomy following the osteochondral graft implantation.

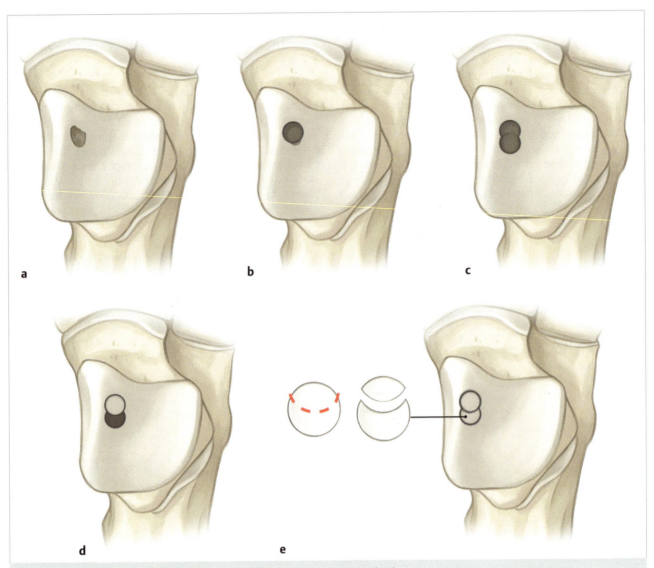

Fig. 39.4 (a–e) Figure-eight "nested" technique. Two plugs are contoured to each other.

a figure-eight "nested" technique in which two plugs are contoured to each other should be utilized (**Fig. 39.4**). This technique minimizes the empty space that would be filled with fibrocartilage.[8]

After removal of the lesion, the base of the recipient site should be deepened by an additional 2 mm using an acorn-shaped drill tip achieving a total created hole depth of 12 mm. This can additionally be done utilizing the appropriate-sized "recipient" harvesting trephine from the OATS system. Care should be taken to maintain a perpendicular alignment while the trephine is malleted into the lesion to the chosen depth. The trephine is then spun 90 degrees clockwise and counterclockwise to free the plug, which is then removed. Additionally, the recipient site should be observed carefully to ensure that any cystic lesions have been removed. Then, a 0.045-inch diameter K-wire is used to create multiple small holes in the wall of the recipient site. This may potentially improve the graft and native host tissue integration by providing neovascular channels. The acorn drill tip creates a bullet shape to the base of the talar hole. This will provide additional graft stability and maintains graft surface congruity throughout the maturation process (**Fig. 39.5**).[9]

39.6.3 Harvesting Osteochondral Graft from Ipsilateral Femoral Condyle

Donor osteochondral graft plug(s) are harvested from the ipsilateral knee. The authors prefer the non-weight-bearing portion of the lateral femoral condyle above the level of the sulcus terminalis (**Fig. 39.6**). The lateral femoral condyle provides topographic variations, which closely match the talar dome. A mini-open arthrotomy with a lateral parapatellar approach is performed to access the lateral femoral condyle. The "donor" trephine should be 1 mm larger than the recipient trephine because this allows for both interference and press fit. This is harvested using the same technique as the trephine bone removal from the recipient site in the talus, but using the "donor" trephine. After osteochondral graft harvest, the cancellous bone at the distal end of the graft is measured and trimmed to form "bullet-shape" to match the depth of the recipient site using a rongeur (**Fig. 39.6**). The authors then prefer to soak the graft in concentrated bone marrow aspirate (CBMA) in order to potentially improve integration between the osteochondral graft and narrative articular cartilage.

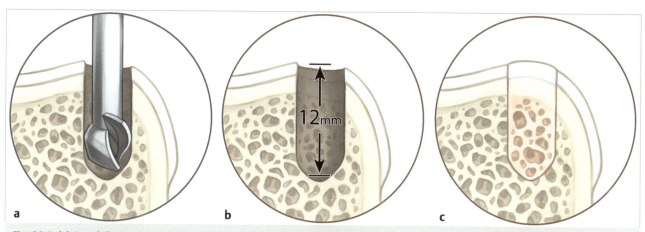

Fig. 39.5 (a) Overdrill is performed with an acorn-shaped drill tip. (b) The created recipient site is 2 mm longer than the harvested graft. (c) This technique may prevent incongruence of the graft surface throughout the incorporation process.

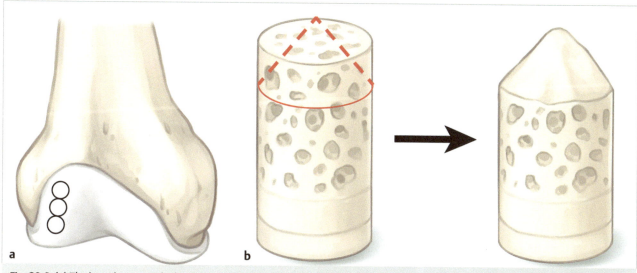

Fig. 39.6 (a) The lateral non-weight-bearing aspect of the femoral condyle. (b) The graft is trimmed in a "bullet" fashion using a rongeur.

The donor site can be backfilled with a synthetic bone plug or allograft. This procedure may allow for bone and fibrocartilage infill at the donor site and potentially prevent hemarthrosis by reducing excessive bleeding, which minimizes postoperative scar formation. The authors previously used the OBI TruFit plug (Smith & Nephew, Andover, MA)[10] but currently use allograft because OBI TruFit plug was removed from market in the United States.

39.6.4 Insertion of Osteochondral Graft into the Recipient Site

The osteochondral graft plug is transferred to the created recipient site. Prior to the graft placement, the authors inject CBMA into the recipient site. The graft is handled with a mosquito snap and the highest point of the graft is marked, as well as the highest point of the surrounding talar cartilage. The osteochondral graft is then implanted in the recipient site so that both marks are in alignment (**Fig. 39.7**). When the graft is in acceptable alignment, the graft is tapped into a final position with a tamp. If the graft is sunken, a K-wire can be inserted in the graft and use as a joy stick to elevate. The final graft position should be as flush as possible with surrounding articular surface.

39.6.5 Fixation of Malleolar Osteotomy

The osteotomized medial malleolus is anatomically reduced to the original position. Once the anatomical reduction is achieved, two partially threaded cancellous screws are inserted using two predrilled holes. A third transverse screw with a washer should be used to obtain rigid fixation and prevent possible proximal migration of the malleolus (**Fig. 39.8**).

39.7 Tips and Pearls

- Adequate exposure of OLTs through an osteotomy is essential for operative success. Perpendicular access to OLTs should be achieved. Therefore, in cases of medial lesions, the osteotomy should be adequate enough to access the most lateral margin of the OLTs.

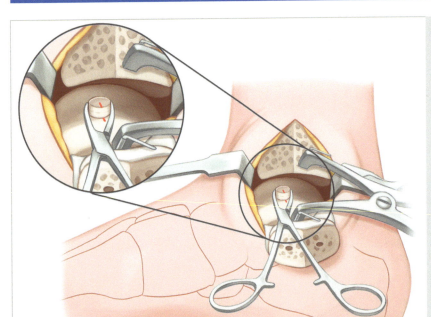

Fig. 39.7 A mosquito snap is utilized to rotate the graft gently until marks are in line.

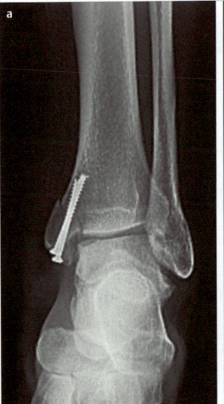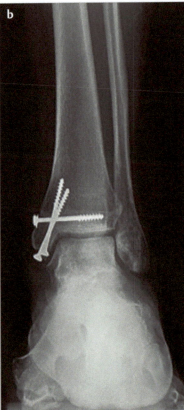

a

b

Fig. 39.8 **(a)** The medial malleolar fixated with two screws is shifted postoperatively. **(b)** Adding a third transverse screw prevents this potential. (Reproduced with permission from Kennedy and Murawski.[8])

- The graft site can be prepared using an acorn-shaped drill and the end of the graft can be fitted into "bullet-shape" using a rongeur to maintain graft congruency.
- The placement of the graft should be flush to the surrounding native cartilage surface for optimal results. For this, the highest point of the graft is aligned with the highest point of the surrounding talar cartilage.

- CBMA is utilized to promote the bone healing and the integration between the graft and host tissue cartilage.
- The chevron medial malleolar osteotomy is fixated with three titanium screws including one transverse screw to prevent the potential shifting during fixation.

39.8 Hazards and Pitfalls

- During malleolar osteotomy, the oscillating saw is stopped at the level of the subchondral bone and the final cut should be completed using a sharp osteotome rather than a saw. This avoids violation of the articular surface and protects the posterior tibial tendon.
- Care should be taken when the lateral patella retinaculum is repaired following graft harvesting. Too tight of a repair results in patella maltracking and may cause postoperative knee pain.
- The osteochondral autograph should neither be left proud of, nor countersunk below the level of the talar cartilage. Due to the thicker cartilage found in the lateral femoral condyle as compared to that of the talus, radiographic evaluation can be misleading as to the alignment of the articular cartilage. The tidemark seen on radiographs is usually lower than that of the talar dome; however, this is not due to cartilaginous level mismatch.

39.9 Complications/Bailout/Salvage

Knee pain after AOT is a concerning complication, but the rates of donor-site morbidity vary between authors. The most recent studies report less than 5% incidence with good functional outcomes.[10] Donor-site knee pain does not appear to be a cause for long-term concern. Cyst formation following AOT has been reported as high as in 75% of patients, but the clinical influence of cyst formation around the grafts was not found to be clinically significant in short-term to medium-term follow-up.[11]

Other minor complications include malunion and nonunion at the osteotomy site and soft-tissue impingement around the ankle joint. A chevron-type osteotomy can reduce the potential risk of malunion and nonunion given this provides better stability and healing potential compared to a straight-cut osteotomy.[8]

Range-of-motion (ROM) exercises are important to prevent soft-tissue impingement and should be started at 2 weeks postoperation. If it occurs, physical therapy including deep-tissue massage and extracorporeal shock-wave therapy are useful.

39.10 Postoperative Care

The ankle is immobilized in a well-padded splint with a non-weight-bearing status. At 2 weeks postop, the splint is replaced with a CAM walker boot and continued non-weight-bearing. At this point, the patient should start ROM exercises of the ankle. Ankle motion promotes cartilage metabolism and reduces soft-tissue edema and scar formation. At 4 weeks following surgery, weight-bearing is increased by 10% per day. Full weight-bearing is achieved approximately 6 weeks after surgery. If there are signs of healing of osteotomy site, physical therapy is started at this point. Sports-specific physical therapies are considered at 10 weeks. Normal daily activity can be resumed at 8 to 10 weeks. It usually takes 5 to 6 months to return to high-demand sports activity.

39.11 Outcomes

Approximately 85% of patients have successful clinical outcomes in short- and midterm periods.[6,8] A case series of 85 patients who underwent AOT found improved Foot and Ankle Outcome Score from 50 to 81 at a mean 47-month follow-up. This outcome was mirrored morphologically with a mean postoperative magnetic resonance observation of cartilage repair tissue (MOCART) score of 86 at a mean 25-month follow-up.[12] In the athletic population, a recent case series reported that American Orthopaedic Foot and Ankle Society scores were improved to 89.4 at a final follow-up of 24 months and 90% of professional athletes had returned to preinjury sports activity.[13] T2 MRI-mapping post-op demonstrates restoration of the radius of curvature of the talar dome with color stratification matching the native hyaline cartilage.[12]

References

1. Chuckpaiwong B, Berkson EM, Theodore GH. Microfracture for osteochondral lesions of the ankle: outcome analysis and outcome predictors of 105 cases. Arthroscopy 2008;24(1):106–112
2. Choi WJ, Park KK, Kim BS, Lee JW. Osteochondral lesion of the talus: is there a critical defect size for poor outcome? Am J Sports Med 2009;37(10):1974–1980
3. Ramponi L, Yasui Y, Murawski CD, et al. Lesion Size Is a Predictor of Clinical Outcomes After Bone Marrow Stimulation for Osteochondral Lesions of the Talus: A Systematic Review. Am J Sports Med 2017;45(7):1698–1705
4. Yoon HS, Park YJ, Lee M, Choi WJ, Lee JW. Osteochondral autologous transplantation is superior to repeat arthroscopy for the treatment of osteochondral lesions of the talus after failed primary arthroscopic treatment. Am J Sports Med 2014;42(8):1896–1903
5. Ross AW, Murawski CD, Fraser EJ, et al. Autologous Osteochondral Transplantation for Osteochondral Lesions of the Talus: Does Previous Bone Marrow Stimulation Negatively Affect Clinical Outcome? Arthroscopy 2016;32(7):1377–1383
6. Scranton PE Jr, Frey CC, Feder KS. Outcome of osteochondral autograft transplantation for type-V cystic osteochondral lesions of the talus. J Bone Joint Surg Br 2006;88(5):614–619
7. Fansa AM, Murawski CD, Imhauser CW, Nguyen JT, Kennedy JG. Autologous osteochondral transplantation of the talus partially restores contact mechanics of the ankle joint. Am J Sports Med 2011;39(11):2457–2465
8. Kennedy JG, Murawski CD. The Treatment of osteochondral lesions of the talus with autologous osteochondral transplantation and bone marrow aspirate concentrate: surgical technique. Cartilage 2011;2(4):327–336
9. Kock NB, Van Susante JL, Buma P, Van Kampen A, Verdonschot N. Press-fit stability of an osteochondral autograft: Influence of different plug length and perfect depth alignment. Acta Orthop 2006;77(3):422–428

10. Fraser EJ, Savage-Elliott I, Yasui Y, et al. Clinical and MRI donor site outcomes following autologous osteochondral transplantation for talar osteochondral lesions. Foot Ankle Int 2016;37(9):968–976

11. Savage-Elliott I, Smyth NA, Deyer TW, et al. Magnetic resonance imaging evidence of postoperative cyst formation does not appear to affect clinical outcomes after autologous osteochondral transplantation of the talus. Arthroscopy 2016;32(9):1846–1854

12. Flynn S, Ross KA, Hannon CP, et al. Autologous osteochondral transplantation for osteochondral lesions of the talus. Foot Ankle Int 2016;37(4):363–372

13. Fraser EJ, Harris MC, Prado MP, Kennedy JG. Autologous osteochondral transplantation for osteochondral lesions of the talus in an athletic population. Knee Surg Sports Traumatol Arthrosc 2016;24(4):1272–1279

40 Allograft Management Osteochondral Lesion of the Talus (OLT): Juvenile Cartilage

Samuel B. Adams

Abstract

Particulated juvenile cartilage allograft transplantation (PJ-CAT) is a technique of transplantation of multiple fresh juvenile cartilage allograft tissue pieces (1 mm^3 cubes), containing live chondrocyte cells within their native extracellular matrix, with fibrin adhesive securing the tissue pieces to the base of the osteochondral lesion of the talus (OLT). PJCAT is viable treatment option for OLTs that have failed prior operative management or primary OLTs that are likely to be unresponsive to marrow stimulation techniques. Reports of early follow-up demonstrate patient improvement. Basic science evidence demonstrates that this technique can restore hyaline cartilage. PJCAT delivery can be performed through all-open, arthroscopically assisted open, and all-arthroscopic techniques. The current evidence, indications, and surgical technique for the use of particulated juvenile cartilage allograft transplantation in the management of osteochondral lesions of the talus will be discussed in this chapter.

Keywords: *juvenile cartilage, transplantation, osteochondral lesion, talus, allograft*

40.1 Indications and Pathology

- Primary osteochondral lesion of the talus (OLT)[1] that is larger than 15 mm in one dimension[2] or surface area larger than 107 mm[2,3]
- Previously failed a marrow stimulation technique with continued symptoms.
- Currently, there is no evidence to exclude shoulder and cystic lesions. However, it is difficult to restore the native shoulder anatomy with this technique.

40.1.1 Clinical Evaluation

- Anterior ankle pain and joint line tenderness.
  - Plantarflex the ankle to expose the OLT during deep palpation.
  - Usually, but not always, located over the region of the OLT.
- May present with symptoms of ankle instability, but with a clinically stable ankle.

40.1.2 Radiographic Evaluation

- Weight-bearing anteroposterior (AP), lateral, and mortise views of the ankle:
  - A shadowing or defect may be seen in the talar dome in the region of the lesion.
  - Bone fragments may be seen within the base or separate from the OLT, especially in acute osteochondral fractures.
- Magnetic resonance imaging (MRI):
  - Useful in screening for OLTs.
  - Presence of associate bone marrow edema confirms bioactivity of the lesion.
  - Not reliable for determining the true size or anatomic configuration of the lesion.
- Computed tomography (CT) scan (fine cut)—with axial, coronal, and sagittal cuts:
  - Best study to determine the size and configuration of the osseous aspect of the lesion.
  - Accurate in determining presence of cysts and microcysts adjacent to the OLT.

40.1.3 Nonoperative Options

- Activity modification.
- Unloading bracing.

40.1.4 Contraindications

- Active ankle joint infection.
- Large deep cystic lesions without a stable bony base.
- Immunocompromised host:
  - Immune-deficient disease.
  - Medications cause immune compromise.

40.2 Goals of Surgical Procedure

- The goal of the procedure is to restore hyaline cartilage (cells plus extracellular matrix) to the OLT. Other methods used to deliver intact hyaline cartilage to an OLT are limited to osteochondral autograft transfer (OAT) and allograft transplantation, yet neither of these options provides juvenile cartilage.
- Basic science data support the use of juvenile cartilage. Adkisson et al[1] compared the chondrogenic activity of human juvenile and adult chondrocytes.
  - Chondrocytes from juvenile (<10 years) donors showed significantly greater extracellular matrix synthesis (sulfated glycosaminoglycan [S-GAG]) than chondrocytes from mature donors.
  - Moreover, the rate of S-GAG synthesis was greater than 100-fold for the juvenile chondrocytes. The authors also demonstrated 100- and 700-fold decreased amounts of mRNA (messenger ribonucleic acid) for type and type IX collagen, respectively, in mature chondrocytes compared to the juvenile chondrocytes. They speculate that the decreased gene expression directly affects the ability of adult chondrocytes to form neocartilage in vivo.
  - Likewise, they demonstrated a significantly increased growth rate for juvenile chondrocytes and that this cell population did not illicit an immunogenic reaction when transplanted into a xenogeneic goat model, indicating immunoprivilege for juvenile chondrocytes.

40.3 Advantages of Surgical Procedure

- The surgical procedure is less technically demanding than other cartilage replacement procedure because of the following:
  - Particulated juvenile cartilage allograft transplantation (PJCAT) does not need graft press-fitting/contouring (as needed for osteochondral autograft or allograft transplantation).
  - It does not require perpendicular access to the base of the OLT. Therefore, it does not require an osteotomy (as often needed for OAT or allograft transplantation) and can be performed arthroscopically or through a minimally invasive anterior ankle arthrotomy.
  - It is a single-stage procedure unlike autologous chondrocyte implantation (ACI).
  - There is no donor site morbidity unlike OAT.
  - The graft is readily available; therefore, there is no donor wait time as is the case for allograft transplantation.
  - There is minimal theoretical and no clinically documented chance for immunological reaction (cartilage is considered immune privileged) or disease transmission.

40.4 Key Principles

- Debride the OLT until a stable cartilaginous rim and stable bony base are obtained.
- Penetrate the subchondral plate, but ensure a dry bed before graft insertion.
- Fill at least 50% of the base of the lesion with allograft.
- Apply prethawed fibrin glue to seal the allograft squares into the OLT.
- Before the fibrin glue fully sets, contour the surface to match that of the talar dome articular cartilage.

40.5 Preoperative Preparation and Patient Positioning

- Determination of the appropriate amount of graft to be preordered is necessary. Per the manufacturer, one pack of DeNovo NT Natural Tissue graft (Zimmer Biomet, Inc., Warsaw, IN) is recommended to treat each 2.5 cm^2 of lesion surface area, with a recommended fill ratio of at least 50% of the lesion size (e.g., each pack contains enough graft to solidly fill 1.25 cm^2 of surface area). In practice, the author attempts to nearly completely fill the lesion's surface area to the depth of the surrounding healthy cartilage. Prior to the start of the procedure, inspect the packaging for expiration date.
- It is imperative that the patient understands the source of the transplanted tissue and is amenable to the transplantation. Currently, the only graft material available for this procedure is DeNovo NT Natural Tissue graft. The cartilage pieces of this product are obtained, in compliance with Good Tissue Practice, from donors ranging in age from newborn to 13 years; however, it is typically obtained from neomorts under the age of 2 years.[2] No stillborn or fetal tissue is used. Standard disease screening is performed on each lot (one lot of tissue comes from a single donor).

- Regardless of open or arthroscopic technique (see below), position the patient supine with an ipsilateral proximal thigh bump so that the toes point to the ceiling.
- Place an ipsilateral thigh tourniquet.

40.6 Operative Technique

- PJCAT can be performed via arthroscopic or open techniques. The open technique is typically an anterior medial or lateral arthrotomy. Rarely is an osteotomy needed because perpendicular access to the OLT is not needed. An open technique should be performed until the surgeon is experienced with the technique. Both techniques will be described.

40.6.1 Open Technique

- Even with an open technique, the author recommends a diagnostic arthroscopy to confirm the lesion location and size and to identify and treat any concomitant pathology.
- Use either an anteromedial arthrotomy (medial lesions) or an anterolateral arthrotomy (lateral lesions) based on the lesion location.
  - Anteromedial arthrotomy:
    - Make a longitudinal incision over the ankle joint and just medial to the tibialis anterior tendon. Incise the extensor retinaculum in line with the incision.
    - Retract the tibialis anterior tendon laterally and incise the joint capsule in line with the skin incision.
    - Place a deep retractor, typically a Gelpi retractor is best suited.
    - Plantarflex the ankle to identify the lesion.
  - Anterolateral arthrotomy:
    - Make a longitudinal incision just lateral to the peroneus tertius tendon and medial to the anterior border of the fibula.
    - Carefully identify and protect any branches of the superficial peroneal nerve.
    - Incise the extensor retinaculum, retract the peroneus tertius medially, and incise the ankle joint capsule longitudinally.
- Regardless of the approach, place a deep retractor inside the joint capsule. Typically, a Gelpi retractor works best. Plantarflex the ankle and determine the extent to which the lesion can be visualized.
- Perpendicular access is not needed, but access to the posterior portion of the OLT is needed for debridement. If additional access to the posterior OLT is needed, perform a plafondplasty.
  - Plafondplasty:
    - Use a curved 0.25-inch osteotome to remove the superior and medial or lateral aspect of the anterior tibial plafond. Place a Joker or Freer retractor into the joint space to protect against further damage to the talar cartilage. Careful attention should be paid not to remove more than 1 cm of the nonarticular tibia in any dimension.
    - Smaller plafondplasties are generally not repaired. If the plafondplasty approaches 1 cm in any dimension or loss of structural integrity is a concern, use a small fragmentary screw for fixation.

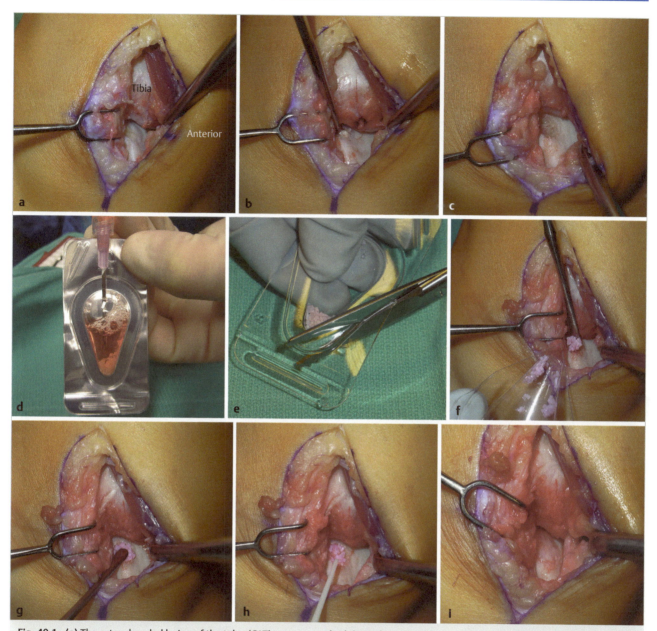

Fig. 40.1 **(a)** The osteochondral lesion of the talus (OLT) was approached through an anterolateral arthrotomy. **(b)** Debride the OLT using a scalpel, beaver blade, and curette. **(c)** The author prefers to violate the subchondral plate. **(d)** Place the juvenile cartilage packet vertically so all of the pieces fall to the bottom. Then inset a 16- to 21-gauge, 1.5-inch needle connected to a 10-mL syringe through the plastic and aspirate the media. **(e)** Cut the plastic package to a point to serve as a delivery vehicle. **(f)** Carefully take the plastic package with the pieces to the arthrotomy site and use a Freer elevator to deliver the pieces to the base of the OLT. **(g)** Use a Freer elevator to distribute and mold the pieces throughout the base of the OLT. **(h)** Apply fibrin glue over the juvenile cartilage pieces. **(i)** Allow the fibrin glue to set for about 5 minutes prior to joint manipulation or closure.

- Additional joint visualization can be obtained with a Hintermann pin type distractor in the tibia and talar neck.
- Identify (**Fig. 40.1a**) and debride the lesion to circumferential stable margins with a no. 15 blade, beaver blade, and small curette (**Fig. 40.1b**).
- If possible, leave a cartilage wall on the medial or lateral shoulder to contain the juvenile cartilage pieces.
- Prepare the base of the lesion. The author prefers to violate the subchondral plate. This may occur when using the curette to remove the cartilage (**Fig. 40.1c**). If the subchondral plate has not yet been violated, then use microfracture awls or a 0.045-inch K-wire with cold water irrigation.

Graft Preparation and Delivery

- The juvenile cartilage pieces are packaged with a proprietary chondrocyte survival media. This must be removed to properly handle the pieces. Take the packet and place it vertically with the pointed end faced up. The pieces will fall to the bottom. From the top, insert a 16- to 21-gauge, 1.5-inch needle connected to a 10-mL syringe through the plastic and aspirate the media. The cartilage pieces will not fit through the needle (**Fig. 40.1d**).
- Now, completely remove the foil cover and carefully use a sponge to remove any remaining media without losing any

pieces. Bend the foil in half lengthwise and narrow one end to a point with scissors. This creates a trough-shaped delivery device for the cartilage pieces. Alternatively, carefully cut the end of the plastic package to a point to act as a delivery vehicle (**Fig. 40.1e**).

- Carefully take the packet of juvenile cartilage pieces to the arthrotomy site. Use a Freer elevator to push the pieces into the base of the OLT until it is completely covered (**Fig. 40.1f, g**).
- Apply a small amount of fibrin glue to cover the cartilage pieces (**Fig. 40.1h**).
- Apply additional cartilage pieces and fibrin glue, in layered fashion until the depth of the lesion is completely filled.
- Before the fibrin glue completely sets, use a Freer elevator to contour the surface of the lesion.
- Also before the fibrin glue completely sets, remove any retractors and dorsiflex the ankle and apply axial compression to use the contour of the tibial plafond to mold the cartilage pieces. Hold in this position for 5 minutes (**Fig. 40.1i**).
- With the ankle held in dorsiflexion by an assistant, close the capsule, retinaculum, and skin in layered fashion and apply a splint.

40.6.2 Arthroscopic Technique

- The operative leg is placed in a leg holder to keep the hip and knee flexed. Use noninvasive distraction around the foot to allow working room for graft application.
- Perform routine arthroscopy through standard anteromedial and anterolateral portals.
- Take extra time to carefully debride the synovium and capsule around the working portal to prevent obstruction of the camera and graft delivery instruments.
- Carefully define the OLT and use various standard and ring curettes to debride the cartilage to stable margins (**Fig. 40.2a, b**). As with the open technique, leave a vertical cartilage wall on the medial or lateral shoulder to contain the juvenile cartilage pieces.
- Temporarily shut off the inflow. This allows the surgeon to assess for soft-tissue invagination at the working portal site that might interfere with graft insertion. Inflow is restored for further soft-tissue debridement.
- Prepare the graft as described earlier.

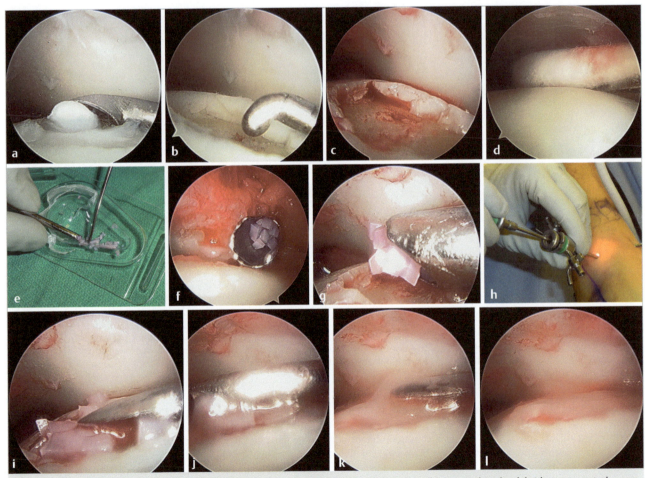

Fig. 40.2 (a) Identify and debride the osteochondral lesion of the talus (OLT) with curettes. (b) Ensure that the debridement created stable margins. (c) A dry arthroscopy is performed to deliver the juvenile cartilage pieces. (d) A cotton-tipped applicator can be used cautiously to perform additional fluid evacuation. (e) Insert one-third to half of the pieces into a 2.7-mm cannula in retrograde fashion. (f) Make sure the pieces are recessed so that they do not get caught on the capsule and synovium during delivery. Insert the cannula with the bevel faced up. (g) Rotate the bevel faced down when over the lesion. (h) Slowly insert the trocar into the cannula to deliver the pieces. (i) Use a Freer elevator to distribute and contour the juvenile cartilage pieces. (j) Apply fibrin glue. (k) Use a Freer elevator to contour the fibrin glue while it is setting. (l) The final construct should match the contour of the surrounding cartilage surface.

- It is imperative to have a dry environment for graft delivery (**Fig. 40.2c**). Shut off the inflow and evacuate the joint of fluid with the use of a small suction catheter and the arthroscopic shaver.
- Dry the base of the lesion with an epinephrine-soaked Weck-Cel sponge or cotton-tipped applicator to achieve hemostasis, followed by a dry cotton-tipped applicator to soak up the excess fluid (**Fig. 40.2d**).

Arthroscopic Graft Insertion

- Insert one-half to one-third of the graft material in a retrograde fashion into the tip of a 2.7-mm arthroscopic cannula using a Freer elevator and recess it with the trocar so that the pieces do not get caught on the synovium when going through the portal (**Fig. 40.2e, f**).
- Insert the loaded cannula, initially bevel up (**Fig. 40.2f**), then rotate so that the bevel is facing down when it is over the lesion (**Fig. 40.2g**). Use the trocar to push the pieces into the lesion (**Fig. 40.2h**).
- Remove the cannula and insert a freer or probe to distribute the graft uniformly throughout the base of the lesion (**Fig. 40.2i**).
- Insert the fibrin glue tip through the arthroscopic portal and apply a small amount of fibrin. Occasionally, the tip provided with the fibrin glue is too short and flimsy to get through the arthroscopic portal. Therefore, a needle can be used instead (**Fig. 40.2j**).
- Repeat in layered fashion until the lesion is completely filled.
- Use a Freer elevator to contour the cartilage pieces while the fibrin glue is setting (**Fig. 40.2k, l**).
- Remove the distractor and dorsiflex the ankle. Hold in this position while the fibrin glue is setting. The arthroscopic portals can be closed and a splint placed while in this position.

40.7 Tips and Pearls

- Make sure to thaw the fibrin glue at the start of the procedure. Rapid thawing of the fibrin glue in a hot water bath immediately before it is needed results in unfavorable handling characteristics.
- If the base of the OLT requires bone grafting, the bone from the plafondplasty can be used. Alternatively, trephine obtained bone from the calcaneus, tibia, or iliac crest can be used.
- Regardless of open or arthroscopic technique, do not deliver all of the pieces at once. If the delivery mechanism (foil trough or trocar) is accidentally dropped, all of the pieces will not have been lost.
- It is important to have extra fibrin delivery tips available because they can become clogged in between applications of fibrin glue to the defect.
- For arthroscopic delivery, bleeding can cause a problem for visualization and graft adherence to the base of the lesion. Therefore, the author does not recommend extensive synovial debridement or additional procedures that could cause excessive bleeding during the dry portion of cartilage allograft delivery.

- When evacuating the joint for arthroscopic delivery, suction can pull additional blood into the joint. Therefore, place a 16-gauge needle through the posterior lateral portal to suck air into the joint and not additional blood.

40.8 Hazards and Pitfalls

- Careful dissection and arthroscopic skills are needed to not create nerve damage or additional cartilage damage.
- The author recommends performing the procedure via an open approach for the first time using the PJCAT technique. One can practice the debridement with the scope equipment and then perform an extended portal arthrotomy to deliver the juvenile cartilage.

40.9 Complications/Bailout/Salvage

- Preoperative OLT sizing and ordering the correct number of juvenile cartilage packets (one vs. two) can be difficult. The product is very expensive and in the vast majority of cases, the author has only used one packet. The technique of PJCAT is relatively new and there are no data to determine which variable is more important: depth of fill or completely covering the base. In a scenario where there are not enough juvenile cartilage pieces to achieve both depth and complete coverage, the author recommends complete coverage over depth of fill. In theory, this will better seal off the subchondral bone at the base of the lesion.
- Care must be taken to not "lose" the majority of the cartilage pieces in the posterior recess of the ankle joint. Unfortunately, there is no bailout for this. Should this happen in an arthroscopic approach, one should convert to an open arthrotomy and apply a distraction device to see if the cartilage pieces can be retrieved. If not, the joint should be thoroughly irrigated. The author recommends microfracture to the base of the lesion. A postoperative discussion with the patient is necessary and an additional PJCAT procedure can be planned if warranted.

40.10 Postoperative Care

- There is no consensus on postoperative rehabilitation.
- The authors' postoperative rehabilitation protocol is as follows:
  ○ Postoperative non-weight-bearing splint for 2 weeks.
  ○ Controlled ankle motion (CAM) boot with progressive weight-bearing over the next 6 weeks. Weight-bearing allows for compression and contouring of the graft in this highly constrained joint. The patient may perform gentle active ankle motion. The author does not like full range of motion to be performed in anterior or posterior lesions so that they are not uncovered from underneath the tibial plafond.
  ○ At 2 months, the patient may start physical therapy.
  ○ The postoperative rehabilitation protocol is also dependent on associated procedures such as lateral ligament repair.

40.11 Outcomes

- There are limited data on the use of PJCAT for OLTs.
- Coetzee et al[3] presented a retrospective case series of 23 patients (24 ankles) treated with PJCAT at a mean follow-up of 16.2 months.
  - The mean lesion surface size was 125 mm^2 (range: 50–300 mm^2) with a mean depth of 7 mm (range: 3–20 mm). All lesions had at least one dimension ≥10 mm.
  - The lesions were accessed via an open approach in 12 cases, an arthroscopic approach in 3 cases, and through an extended portal open approach in 9 cases. Bone grafting was performed on lesions deeper than 5 mm.
  - Postoperative outcome scores were similar to published reports on patients who were treated with bone marrow stimulation, ACI, and matrix-induced autologous chondrocyte implantation.

References

1. Adkisson HD IV, Martin JA, Amendola RL, et al. The potential of human allogeneic juvenile chondrocytes for restoration of articular cartilage. Am J Sports Med 2010;38(7):1324–1333

2. Adams SB, Yao J, Schon LC. Particulated juvenile articular cartilage allograft transplantation for osteochondral lesions of the talus. Tech Foot Ankle Surg 2011;10(2):92–98

3. Coetzee JC, Giza E, Schon LC, et al. Treatment of osteochondral lesions of the talus with particulated juvenile cartilage. Foot Ankle Int 2013;34(9):1205–1211

41 Fresh Allograft for Osteochondral Lesions of the Talus (OLT)

Mary Kate Thayer and Michael Brage

Abstract

Osteochondral lesions of the talus (OLT) are defects of the cartilage and subchondral bone often as a result of prior trauma. When painful, these can cause significant disability to the patient and considerably affect the patient's quality of life. Here we discuss the use of fresh allograft to treat OLTs. This can be a powerful option to improve pain and maintain function of the ankle when used in the appropriate patient population.

Keywords: *osteochondral lesion, talus, fresh allograft*

41.1 Indications

- Indications for surgery.
- Large osteochondral lesions of the talus (OLTs) with surface area >107 mm^2 or any diameter >15 mm.
- Deep OLTs with large cystic components.
- Failed previous arthroscopic microfracture of OLT.
- Failed previous autograft or allograft treatment for OLTs (osteochondral autologous transplantation surgery [OATS] or juvenile cartilage).
- Lesion size too large for management with autograft harvest from patient's knee.
- Patient with a large OLT with severe knee arthritis or knee arthroplasty.
- Patients unwilling to accept donor site morbidity associated with autograft.

41.1.1 Pathology

- OLTs are lesions of the articular cartilage and underlying subchondral bone that can be described based on location and size, whether they are stable or unstable, and whether they are displaced or nondisplaced.[1,2]
- They are found often after even minor trauma, occurring most frequently in patients previously sustaining ankle sprains.[3]
- The exact pathogenesis and cause of OLT is not quite understood to date, but acute trauma, repetitive microtrauma, systemic host factors, vascular abnormalities resulting in avascular necrosis, anatomic variation or malalignment, and congenital abnormalities are thought to play a role.[1-3]

41.1.2 Clinical Evaluation

- Inspection: look for signs of acute injury such as swelling or ecchymosis.
- Palpation: evaluate for areas of focal tenderness.
- Ligamentous exam: anterior drawer, inversion, and eversion stress test.
- Hindfoot alignment exam with the patient standing and supine.
- Evaluation for equinus contracture.

- Evaluation for instability, malalignment, and contracture is especially critical, given that these should be corrected before or during allografting to prevent abnormal loading of the graft.

41.1.3 Radiographic Evaluation

- Radiographs in every patient—anteroposterior (AP), lateral, and mortise views with a radiographic marker to assist in future planning for graft size (**Fig. 41.1**).
- Advanced imaging in select patients provides further detail for preoperative planning.
  ○ Computed tomography (CT) scan provides bony detail.
  ○ Magnetic resonance imaging (MRI) provides information about the cartilage and soft tissues (**Fig. 41.1**).

These should be used with caution, however, as the OLT tends to appear less significant on CT and more exaggerated on MRI than it will appear in the operating room.

41.1.4 Nonoperative Options

- Asymptomatic lesions should be treated nonoperatively with serial radiographs.
- Symptomatic, acute, and nondisplaced lesions should have a trial of nonoperative treatment with non–weight-bearing in a cast or boot.
- Pediatric OLTs should be treated nonoperatively prior to surgical intervention.

41.1.5 Contraindications

- Medical factors that would preclude any surgical intervention.
- Any concern for infection.
- Advanced arthritis of the ankle joint, as fresh allograft is unlikely to improve the patient's condition in a significant and lasting manner.
- Correctable alterations that place undue stress on the graft:
  ○ Malalignment: angulation of the tibial plafond in any direction in relationship to axis of tibia greater 10 degrees may require corrective osteotomy.
  ○ Ankle instability.
  ○ Equinus contracture.
- Relative contraindications: peripheral neuropathy and peripheral vascular disease.

41.2 Goals of Surgical Procedure

The goals of fresh allograft for OLTs include pain relief, ability to bear weight comfortably, and return to activity. One specific caveat, however, is, depending on the size of the allograft,

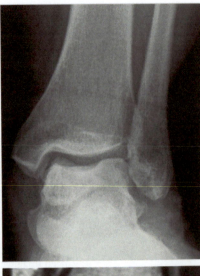
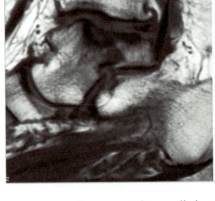
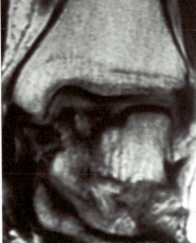

Fig. 41.1 Radiographs and magnetic resonance imaging of a 27-year-old woman with ankle pain and remote history of "ankle sprain" found to have an osteochondral lesion of the talus.

return to running may not be a realistic goal. For example, if a hemitalus or whole talar dome is used, impact sports such as running may no longer be feasible.

41.3 Advantages of Surgical Procedure

Although many procedures are available for the management of OLTs, fresh osteochondral allografting is a powerful procedure in terms of pain relief and improvement in function. Fresh allograft provides viable cells, whereas the cartilage cells are dead in frozen allografts. Additionally, major advantages of fresh allografting over other treatments include avoidance of donor site morbidity and maintenance of ankle motion. The ability to use a whole talar dome allograft also allows for the repair of very large lesions.

41.4 Key Principles

• Judicious preoperative planning including the following:
  ○ Complete imaging of the lesion with size marker for templating.

  ○ Ensuring patient is an appropriate surgical candidate.
  ○ Obtaining the appropriate size-matched allograft.
  ○ Choosing an approach based on lesion location.
• Adequate/appropriate exposure based on location of the defect.
• Preparing the fresh allograft for the lesion.
• Placement and fixation (if needed) of the allograft.
• Prudent soft-tissue handling and closure of the wound.

41.5 Preoperative Preparation and Patient Positioning

41.5.1 Choosing and Obtaining the Allograft

The correct allograft should be chosen based on radiographs performed with a size marker. Measure the talar width 5 mm below the articular surface on AP ankle radiograph. Correct for any magnification based on your radiopaque marker. This width can then be used to calculate the size of your OLT and size of proposed allograft (**Fig. 41.2**). Once the appropriate size is known, it is important to contact the chosen tissue bank to

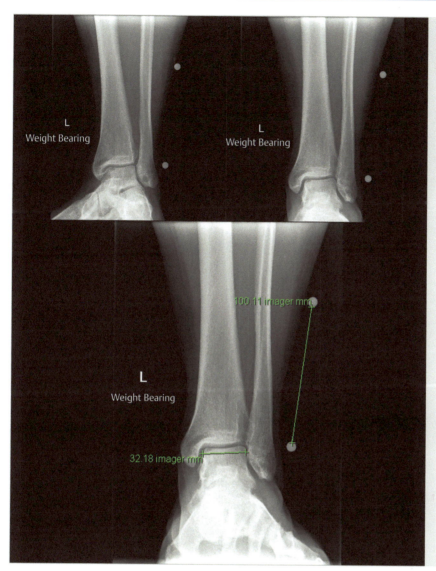

Fig. 41.2 Using X-rays with a radiographic marker for preoperative planning.

obtain the fresh allograft. Developing a relationship with a tissue bank is critical to understand the process for ordering and receiving the allograft. We have used Joint Restoration Foundation (Centennial, CO) in the past with good results. The allograft is procured from the donor within 24 hours of death and must be transplanted within 21 days of harvest. Donors are screened extensively, which requires approximately 2 weeks' time. Grafts should be obtained from a bone bank certified by the American Association of Tissue Banks (AATB).

41.5.2 Positioning

In most cases, the patient should be positioned supine on a radiolucent table with a bump under the hip and a ramp under the extremity. A nonsterile tourniquet is applied. The leg and foot should be prepped in the usual sterile fashion.

41.5.3 Surgical Approach

There are multiple approaches available to the surgeon treating an OLT. The specific approach should be chosen based on the location of the OLT in order to provide the most direct access for preparation of the talus and application of the allograft.

- Medial malleolar osteotomy: First, a skin incision is made from the medial malleolus proximally through skin and subcutaneous tissue to expose the medial malleolus. Care should be taken to protect the saphenous vein. Once the malleolus is adequately exposed, predrill the medial malleolar osteotomy with 3.5-mm cortical screws (**Fig. 41.3a**). Then, under fluoroscopic guidance, perform a medial malleolar osteotomy starting proximally and cutting obliquely down to the corner of the plafond (**Fig. 41.3b**). Once the osteotomy is complete, the bone can be reflected to access the medial talar dome (**Fig. 41.3c, d**). The osteotomy should be fixed at the end of the case, utilizing the predrilled screw holes (**Fig. 41.3e, f**).
- Lateral malleolar osteotomy: A skin incision is made on the lateral ankle overlying the fibula in the standard fashion. Dissection should be carried down to the fibula, elevating anterior and posterior subperiosteal flaps. Care should be taken to protect the superficial peroneal nerve if encountered. A one-third tubular plate can then be chosen prior to osteotomy and contoured to the fibula (**Fig. 41.4a**) and

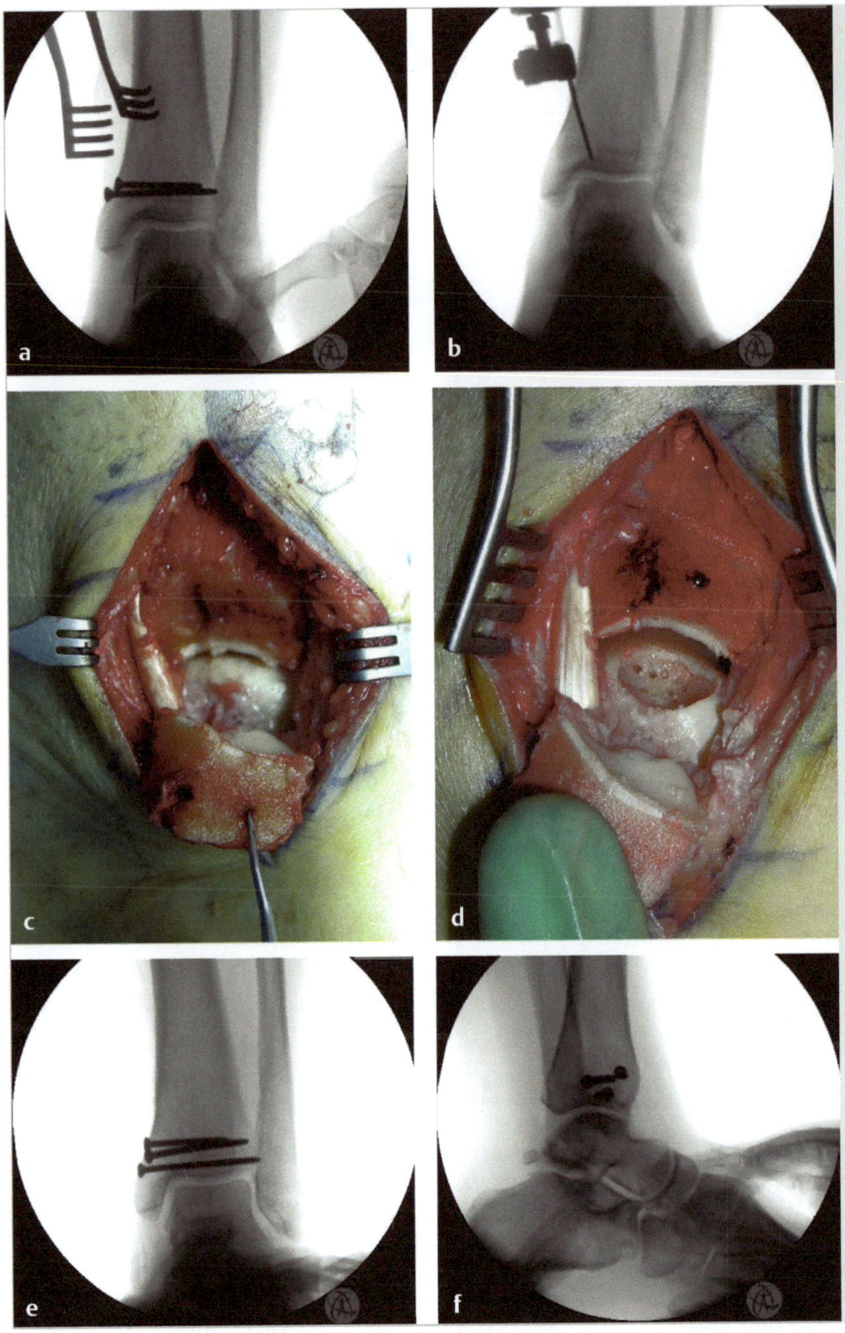

Fig. 41.3 Medial malleolar osteotomy approach demonstrated. Steps include predrilling of medial malleolar osteotomy (a), creation of medial malleolar osteotomy (b), view of the medial talus and defect (c,d), and fixation of the osteotomy (e,f).

osteotomy planned with fluoroscopy. Two cortical screws should then be placed proximally and distally to the site of planned osteotomy and then removed. The osteotomy can then be made using an oscillating saw at approximately a 45-degree angle toward the lateral shoulder of the talus and completed with an osteotome (**Fig. 41.4b**). The fibula can then be reflected posteriorly and inferiorly out of the wound, leaving a small cuff of tissue to allow for ligamentous repair at the end of the procedure (**Fig. 41.4d**). This should then allow for visualization of the lateral talus (**Fig. 41.4c**). The lateral malleolar osteotomy should be fixed at the end of the case, utilizing the precontoured plate and predrilled screw holes (**Fig. 41.4e**).

• Anterior approach: Ankle distraction method: First, an external fixator is placed in order to obtain distraction through the ankle joint that is necessary for visualization. External fixator pins are placed from a medial direction into the talus, calcaneus, and tibia, and then the external fixator assembled (**Fig. 41.5a, b**). The fixator should then be removed in order to make the anterior incision. This incision should be placed near the midline and extend across the joint in the standard fashion. The interval between the tibialis anterior and extensor hallucis longus should be utilized. Once the joint is encountered, an arthrotomy is made, taking care to protect the underlying cartilaginous structures. Subperiosteal dissection can then be taken medially and laterally, exposing the entire talus and tibiotalar joint. The external fixator should then be reapplied, and distraction force applied to further visualize the lesion. With this distraction, excellent visualization should then be possible (**Fig. 41.5c**).

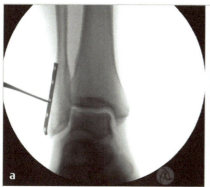
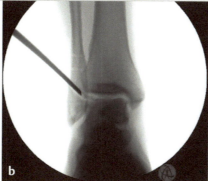

Fig. 41.4 Lateral malleolar osteotomy approach demonstrated. Steps include planning for osteotomy with lateral plate placement (a), creation of the osteotomy under fluoroscopic guidance (b), visualization of the lateral talus (c) after peeling down the osteotomy (d), and fixation of the osteotomy with lateral plate and screws (e).

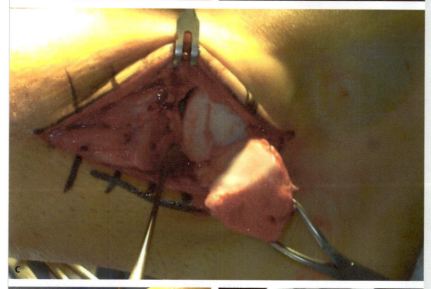

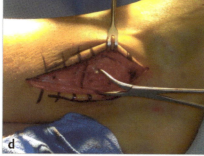
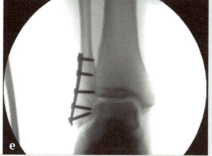

• Anterolateral approach: Tillaux osteotomy: The Tillaux osteotomy allows a window of visualization to the anterolateral talus. An anterolateral approach to the ankle should be utilized. The skin incision is made over the anterolateral ankle joint and is in line with the fourth metatarsal distally. Protect the superficial peroneal nerve, which is likely to run directly across the course of the incision. Sharply incise the fascia over the anterior compartment and retract the extensor tendons of the anterior compartment medially. An arthrotomy can then be made in line with the incision. Next, the anterolateral tibia (Tillaux portion) is predrilled with two 3.5 cortical screws. With the screws removed, the anterolateral tibia is cut with saw and retracted laterally on an intact periosteal hinge. The talus can be visualized and the lesion addressed.

• Posterior malleolar osteotomy: This approach allows access to the posterior talus. In the prone position, a posterolateral approach is utilized. Skin incision is made along the posteromedial border of the fibula and dissection is made with close attention to protecting the sural nerve. Develop the interval between the peroneal tendons laterally and the flexor hallucis longus (FHL) medially, and make an arthrotomy. Osteotomy should be planned as vertical as possible. Predrill screws for eventual fixation of the osteotomy, then complete the osteotomy, and retract it out of the incision. Visualization of the posterior talus is then possible (**Fig. 41.6a, b**). After placement of the graft, the osteotomy should be fixed screws (**Fig. 41.6c, d**).

41.6 Operative Technique

• Debridement of the lesion: After obtaining adequate exposure, the lesion should be debrided in a manner that

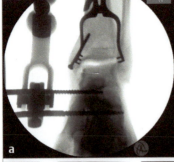
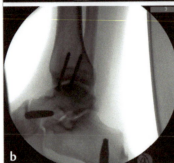
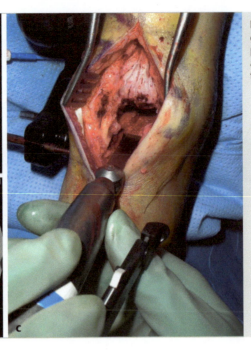

Fig. 41.5 Anterior approach with ankle distraction demonstrated. External fixator is placed (a) and distraction applied across the ankle (b) to allow for anterior access to the talus (c).

facilitates graft placement. The lesion should be removed in one piece as a template if possible. If preparing for an osteochondral plug, preparation should be performed in accordance with the kit being used for preparation of the plug allograft (**Fig. 41.6b**). In general, the cartilage should be debrided until there is a stable rim. After debridement, the bony bed should be fenestrated to facilitate healing.

- Preparation of the allograft: Once the lesion is adequately debrided, the allograft should be prepared. For smaller defects approximately 10 mm or smaller, an osteochondral plug should be created from the allograft. A single plug is preferable over multiple. The plug can be created using a kit such as the Arthrex mosaic plasty kit. Using this kit will allow for creation of an appropriately sized allograft plug that fits the prepared defect site. For larger defects not amenable to use of an osteochondral plug, a custom graft must be made. The excised portion of the talus from the prior debridement can be used as a template to create a custom-sized allograft for implantation (**Fig. 41.7a, b**).
- Placement of the graft and fixation: After preparation of the allograft, it should be placed in the prepared defect. The goal should be exact alignment of the cartilage surface, avoiding leaving the graft proud or sunken. For the osteochondral plugs, fixation will be achieved with a press fit. If it appears the graft remains loose after implantation, fixation should be augmented with screws as needed. For the larger grafts, fixation should be achieved with compression screws with fluoroscopic guidance (**Fig. 41.7c–e**).
- Osteotomy fixation and closure: Once the allograft is in place, the wound should be thoroughly irrigated and attention turned toward closure. If an approach with an osteotomy was chosen, the osteotomy should be fixed with restoration of anatomic alignment and application of adequate fixation across the osteotomy site to prevent nonunion at the osteotomy site to the best of the surgeon's ability (**Figs. 41.3e–f, 41.4e, 41.6c–d**). Wounds should be closed in the standard fashion. After application of a sterile dressing, a well-padded splint in neutral dorsiflexion should be placed.

41.7 Tips and Pearls

- Preparation is key. This includes choosing the appropriate patient, having a thoroughly completed workup, and ensuring availability of the allograft.
- There are several approaches available. Visualization of the lesion is vital; thus, the approach most suitable for the location of the defect should be used.
- Postoperative care involves weight-bearing and activity restriction. Beware of noncompliance. Perform imaging studies early if concerns arise in the early period.
- Long-term follow-up is critical to ensure union of osteotomy and condition of the graft.
- No bridges are burned if the procedure is not effective in providing pain relief.

41.8 Hazards and Pitfalls

- Poor visualization leads to poor ability to reconstruct the anatomy.
- Cost and logistics of obtaining the graft can be burdensome.
- Failure to identify and correct instability, malalignment, or equinus contracture is likely to cause abnormal loading of the graft and ultimate failure.
- Radiographic follow-up is key to ensure union and no graft resorption.

41.9 Complications/Bailout/ Salvage

Complications of any ankle or talus surgery, which have also been observed for this treatment, include symptomatic hardware, iatrogenic injury to surrounding structures, wound healing complications, and deep infection. Specific to certain approaches is a risk for nonunion of the osteotomy site. It is

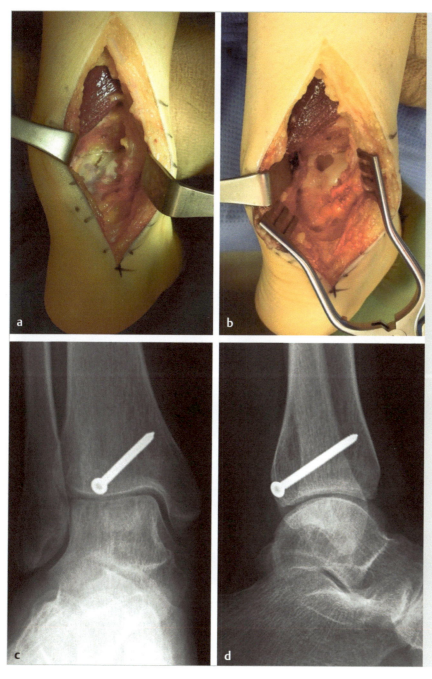

Fig. 41.6 Posterior approach with osteotomy demonstrated. Visualization before (a) and after (b) osteochondral lesions of the talus debridement, (c) anteroposterior, and (d) lateral radiographs after fixation of the osteotomy.

critical to have excellent visualization of the talar lesion before debridement and application of the graft. This often comes at the cost of making an osteotomy, which introduces a risk for nonunion. One clinical example of a fibular nonunion is pictured in **Fig. 41.8**. This patient ultimately underwent allografting to the osteotomy site with subsequent union.

In addition to complications associated with the approach, complications from the allograft itself cannot be overlooked. Disease transmission is rare, but there is a known risk of bone allograft. Risk of human immunodeficiency virus (HIV) transmission is estimated to be 1 in 1.6 million.[4] Another feared complication is graft resorption. Gross's 2001 study, the first on patients treated with fresh allograft for OLTs, reported that three of nine cases had radiographic evidence of graft fragmentation and resorption of greater than 50% of the graft.[5] These

three patients went on to require an ankle fusion. In terms of bailout or salvage, if a patient remains symptomatic, options for ankle arthroplasty or arthrodesis remain available.

41.10 Postoperative Care

Early active range of motion can be initiated after wound is sealed.

Weight-bearing on the other hand should be delayed. For a graft involving the whole talar dome or hemitalus, we recommend restriction to non-weight-bearing for 3 months. With smaller size grafts, 6 weeks of non-weight-bearing is adequate. Formal physical therapy can begin at 6 weeks postoperatively. By 6 months postoperatively, full activity can be allowed.

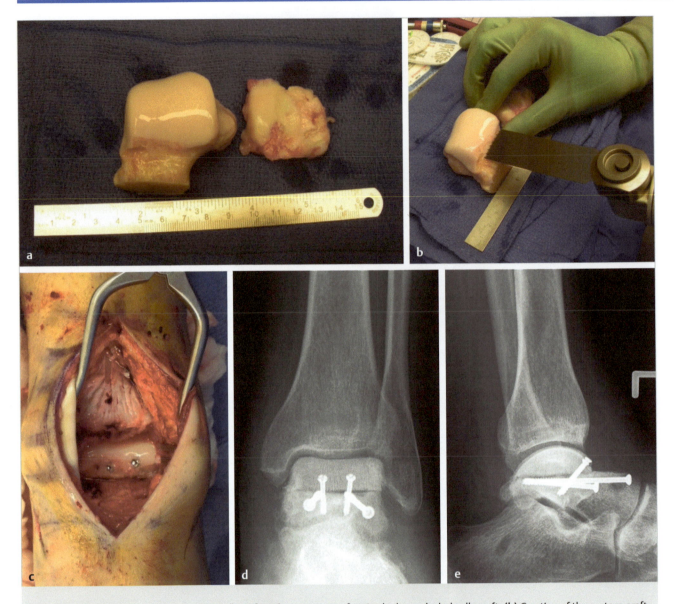

Fig. 41.7 **(a)** Preparation of a large custom allograft with comparison of excised talus and whole allograft. **(b)** Creation of the custom graft on the back table. **(c)** Implantation of the graft. **(d,e)** Postoperative radiographs.

41.11 Outcomes

Fresh allografting for OLT is a powerful tool for treating symptomatic lesions. These fresh allografts can be used to reconstruct the talus and cartilage surface and preserve ankle motion. The goals of treatment as mentioned earlier are an improvement in pain levels and an improvement in function without the addition of donor site morbidity. Multiple studies in the literature indicate that patients experience an improvement in visual analog scale (VAS) pain levels and functional measures after allograft.[5-8] Some patients, however, may have continued pain and dissatisfaction after the procedure.[6] Some reasons for further surgery include removal of hardware and graft resorption resulting in arthritis requiring fusion. In Gross's initial report on OLTs treated with fresh allograft, four of nine patients (44%) required removal of symptomatic hardware and three of nine (33%) required subsequent fusion. In all three of these cases, the graft showed signs of resorption and the ankle showed signs of secondary arthritic changes.[5] Most patients can expect to return to employment and activity after surgery. Gross's study noted that all six patients who had their graft in place (those who had not proceeded to fusion) returned to work and were employed full time. Five of these patients noted no limitation in activity level.[5] The patient's presurgical activity level and line of work may need to be taken into consideration, however. Patients who are quite active at baseline may require a different discussion of goals and outcomes of treatment. A small cohort of highly active U.S. army members was recently studied after allograft. This population showed improved outcomes overall as expected, but the improvement in VAS and functional scores was not as substantial as in civilian populations and national averages.[8] This again reinforces the need to counsel patients appropriately regarding expectations after surgery.

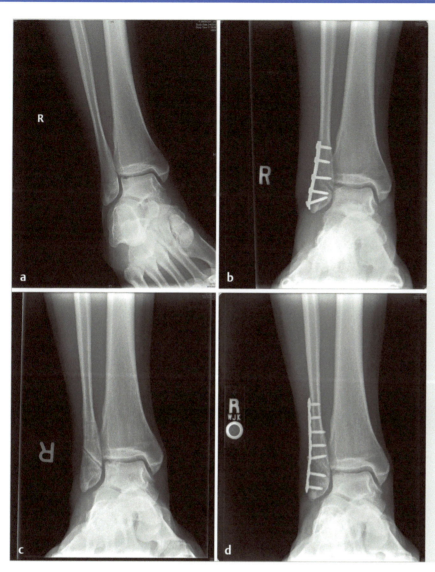

Fig. 41.8 Representative anteroposterior radiographs of a patient with a lateral talar osteochondral lesions of the talus (a) who underwent allografting (b) with subsequent painful nonunion of the fibular osteotomy (c). He had repair of the nonunion with allograft and subsequent clinical and radiographic union (d).

In summary, fresh allografting for OLTs is a powerful tool to improve pain and function in patients with symptomatic lesions. These procedures can be technically challenging depending on the size and location of the lesion. With a combination of thorough preoperative planning, careful intraoperative exposure, appropriate counseling of patients regarding expectations, and routine postoperative care, patients can return to a productive and less painful life.

References

1. Schachter AK, Chen AL, Reddy PD, Tejwani NC. Osteochondral lesions of the talus. J Am Acad Orthop Surg 2005;13(3):152–158
2. McGahan PJ, Pinney SJ. Current concept review: osteochondral lesions of the talus. Foot Ankle Int 2010;31(1):90–101
3. O'Loughlin PF, Heyworth BE, Kennedy JG. Current concepts in the diagnosis and treatment of osteochondral lesions of the ankle. Am J Sports Med 2010;38(2):392–404
4. Buck BE, Malinin TI. Human bone and tissue allografts. Preparation and safety. Clin Orthop Relat Res 1994(303): 8–17
5. Gross AE, Agnidis Z, Hutchison CR. Osteochondral defects of the talus treated with fresh osteochondral allograft transplantation. Foot Ankle Int 2001;22(5):385–391
6. El-Rashidy H, Villacis D, Omar I, Kelikian AS. Fresh osteochondral allograft for the treatment of cartilage defects of the talus: a retrospective review. J Bone Joint Surg Am 2011;93(17):1634–1640
7. Hahn DB, Aanstoos ME, Wilkins RM. Osteochondral lesions of the talus treated with fresh talar allografts. Foot Ankle Int 2010;31(4):277–282
8. Orr JD, Dunn JC, Heida KA Jr, Kusnezov NA, Waterman BR, Belmont PJ Jr. Results and functional outcomes of structural fresh osteochondral allograft transfer for treatment of osteochondral lesions of the talus in a highly active population. Foot Ankle Spec 2017;10(2):125–132

42 Open Lateral Ankle Ligament Reconstruction: Modified Broström Procedure

Jefferson Sabatini and Robert B. Anderson

Abstract

Anatomic repair of the lateral ankle ligament complex of the ankle for chronic recalcitrant ankle instability was first described by Broström in 1966. Since then, there have been numerous modifications and improvements to this technique including augmentation utilizing the inferior extensor retinaculum (Gould's modification), or a split portion of the peroneus brevis tendon (Evans' procedure), as well as utilizing suture anchors to assist the reattachment into the fibular and newer arthroscopic-assisted techniques. This chapter outlines the indications and technique of performing the Broström–Evans procedure, including tricks to optimize results and avoid complications.

Keywords: *ankle instability, ankle ligament reconstruction, Broström, Evans, split peroneus brevis, technique*

42.1 Indications and Pathology

- Chronic lateral ankle instability:
  - Functional: subjective feeling of instability or recurrent symptomatic ankle sprains.
  - Mechanical: ankle motion/laxity beyond the physiologic range.
- Patients that fail 3 to 6 months of conservative management and continue to have symptoms of functional or mechanical ankle instability are candidates for lateral ligament reconstruction.

42.1.1 Clinical Evaluation

- The patient's clinical history and physical examination are key to the diagnosis of lateral ankle instability. Patients usually present with a subjective history of the ankle giving away or the feeling that it might. Occasionally there is pain associated with instability but that may be due to concomitant intra-articular issues. Upon questioning, the patient will often report a history of an ankle sprain or inversion injury at some point in the past. It is not uncommon for this event to have occurred a long time before presentation. The duration of symptoms, frequency of sprains, and previous physical therapy or bracing are important determinants for future treatment.
- The physical exam for lateral ankle instability begins with inspection of the patient's standing alignment. A varus hindfoot or ankle alignment can place the patient at increased risk for inversion injuries. A plantarflexed first ray may also precipitate this varus tendency.
- Palpate the anterior talofibular ligament (ATFL), calcaneofibular ligament (CFL), and syndesmotic ligaments. One should also palpate the peroneal tendons, medial and lateral malleoli, anterolateral dome of the talus, sinus tarsi, lateral process of the talus, and anterior process of the calcaneus to rule out other potential pathologies of lateral ankle pain.
- Anterior drawer and talar tilt testing are the main provocative physical exam maneuvers for lateral ankle instability. The anterior drawer test is when the talus is translated anteriorly in respect to a stabilized tibia. It is aided with the addition of internal rotation. With the deltoid intact, this becomes a rotational movement about the medial malleolus center of rotation. As the ATFL is the primary restraint to anterior translation when the ankle is in planter flexion and the CFL is the primary restraint in neutral, anterior drawer testing in these positions can give information as to which structures may be incompetent. Greater than 10 mm of translation, or 5-mm translation greater than the contralateral side, is considered to be positive. Talar tilt testing is performed by inverting the heel with respect to a stabilized tibia with the ankle and subtalar joint in a neutral position. Any gross difference compared to the contralateral side or soft end point would be suspicious for CFL laxity.

42.1.2 Radiographic Evaluation

- Imaging is important for ruling out other sources of lateral ankle pain, and should be used as an adjunctive to the history and physical examination.
- Obtain weight-bearing anteroposterior (AP), mortise, and lateral images of the affected ankle to look for signs of osteochondral lesions or tibiotalar arthrosis, as well as the overall alignment of the ankle and hindfoot.
- Anterior drawer and talar tilt tests can be quantified using stress radiography. Anterior translation of the talus in a lateral radiograph 10 mm, or 5 mm greater than the contralateral side, is considered positive. Talar tilt stress testing 10 or 5 degrees greater than the contralateral is considered significant. Stress fluoroscopy can also be performed and may be helpful in identifying asymmetries, assuming the patient is relaxed.
- Ultrasound examination can be useful in the setting of potential peroneal pathology as a dynamic examination can reveal tendon subluxation.
- Computed tomography (CT) can provide accurate information about osteochondral lesions of the talus, as well as underlying tarsal coalitions and nonunion of the lateral process of the talus and anterior process of the calcaneus. Weight-bearing CT can also show subtle syndesmotic widening compared to the contralateral side.
- Magnetic resonance imaging (MRI) of the ankle may show attenuation or absence of the lateral ankle ligaments in chronic instability. In addition, it is beneficial to further investigate peroneal tendon pathology, osteochondral lesions, and fibular stress fractures.

42.1.3 Nonoperative Options

- Physical therapy for proprioception and peroneal strength-ening is the mainstay of nonoperative treatment for chronic ankle instability. At least 6 weeks of physical therapy should be completed before surgical intervention is indicated.
- Ankle braces, such as the "lace-up" variety, provide external ankle stability and can be worn inside of shoes. An ankle–foot orthosis (AFO) or double upright brace can also be used to stabilize the ankle.

42.1.4 Contraindications

- Low-demand patients or those with significant medical co-morbidities should be treated nonoperatively with bracing.
- Generalized ligamentous laxity as seen in conditions such as Ehlers–Danlos syndrome is a contraindication to isolated anatomic ligamentous repair, and typically requires a recon-struction enhanced with autograft, allograft, or suture tape.
- Patients with a varus hindfoot alignment should under-go correction of their alignment with a lateralizing (or Dwyer-type) calcaneal osteotomy and/or dorsiflexion first metatarsal osteotomy with reconstruction of their lateral ligaments to prevent recurrence of ankle instability.
- Athletes who require extensive plantar flexion and preserva-tion of inversion such as en pointe in ballet dancers should not undergo the split Evans augmentation to the Broström procedure.

42.2 Goals of Surgical Procedure

- Repair and reconstruct the major static stabilizers of the lateral ankle (AFTL and CFL).
- Re-create a stable ankle mortise during physical activity.
- Prevent future lateral ankle sprains.
- Diminish the risk of degenerative arthritis associated with recurrent ankle sprains.

42.3 Advantages of Surgical Procedure

- Ability to visualize, evaluate, and manage concomitant pero-neal tendon pathology.
- Direct visualization of the ATFL, CFL, and inferior extensor retinaculum.
- Direct exposure of the ATFL into the fibular allowing bony preparation for the reattachment of the ligament.
- Allows utilization of a portion of the peroneus brevis tendon to augment the reconstruction.

42.4 Key Principles

- Initial arthroscopic evaluation of the ankle to exclude or manage any intra-articular pathology.
- Advancing the ATFL back into a decorticated bony bed at the fibular insertion.
- Plicating the CFL with "box" sutures to tighten the ligament.

- Augmentation of the repair utilizing the anterior one-third of the peroneus brevis tendon, secured with an interference screw in a fibular tunnel between the insertional points of the ATFL and CFL.
- Addition/optional augmentation of the repair utilizing the proximal aspect of the inferior extensor retinaculum (Gould's modification).

42.5 Operative Technique

It is the preferred technique of the author to add the split Evans procedure (tenodesis of the anterior 30% of the peroneus brevis tendon to the fibula) to most Broström procedures for added restraint to ankle inversion.

42.5.1 Positioning

- If ankle arthroscopy is going to be performed concomitantly, the patient will need to be supine with the leg in an arthros-copy leg holder.
- Lateral ankle ligament reconstruction can be performed supine with a bump under the ipsilateral hip, overly bumped to produce the so-called sloppy lateral position.
- It is the author's preference to perform the procedure supine with a bump, especially if any concomitant procedures are being performed.

42.5.2 Surgical Approach

- The incision is curvilinear from the posterior aspect fibula proximally, curving around the distal fibula along the course of the peroneal tendons and heading toward the base of the fourth metatarsal (**Fig. 42.1**).

42.5.3 Surgical Procedure

- Any intra-articular pathology in the ankle is first addressed ar-throscopically. If not, then the approach is as outlined earlier.

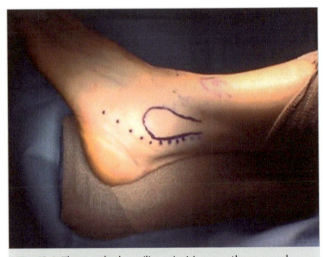

Fig. 42.1 The standard curvilinear incision over the peroneal tendons just posterior to the fibula is marked.

- After incising the skin sharply, use dissecting scissors to dissect through subcutaneous fat distal to the fibula to expose the peroneal tendon sheath. Beware of sural nerve branches along the inferior aspect.
- Sharply incise the more superior of the two peroneal tendon sheaths to expose the peroneus brevis tendon. Carry the sheath incision proximally to the distal aspect of the superficial peroneal retinaculum (SPR) and distally toward the tendon's insertion at the base of the fifth metatarsal (**Fig. 42.2**).
- Expose the sheath over the peroneal tendons proximal to the SPR and incise just off the posterior aspect of the fibula over a distance of 2 cm.
- Carefully inspect the peroneal tendons for pathology and repair as indicated. Excise any tenosynovitis or excessive low-lying muscle belly.
- Use a no. 15 blade to create a longitudinal split in the superior one-third of the peroneus brevis tendon distal to the SPR.
- Cut the needle off a no. 2 nylon suture and feed it through the split in the tendon.
- Using a Gigli saw motion with the suture and continue to split in the tendon distally toward its insertion at the base of the fifth metatarsal (**Fig. 42.3**).
- Next feed a hemostat beneath the SPR from proximal to distal and bring the sutures proximal through the SPR.
- Continue the Gigli saw motion to propagate the tendon split proximally through the SPR and up the posterior aspect of the fibula.
- Sharply cut the one-third width tendon flap at the proximal extent of its split to create a distally attached tendon graft. Wrap the tendon in a wet laparotomy sponge.
- Next sharply incise the periosteum of the distal fibula in a near-vertical manner just posterior to its anterior edge (**Fig. 42.4**).
- Sharply raise a 1-cm periosteal flap proximally off the distal fibula.
- Next, sharply raise the periosteum and attachment of the ATFL and capsule as a single periosteal sleeve. You should be able to easily see into the tibiotalar joint at this time. Inspect the lateral talus for cartilage wear and lesions.

- Using a rongeur, decorticate the anterior distal fibula exposed by reflection of the periosteal flap and ATFL sleeve.
- At this point, identify the CFL deep to the peroneal tendons travelling distal and posterior from the distal tip of the fibula to the calcaneus. Note that it will often appear as two discrete bands.
- Place a "box" stitch (horizontal mattress) with nonabsorbable 2–0 suture in both bands if present but do not secure.
- Now place another "box" stitch as proximal and distal in the ligament as possible and again leave untied. This suture should encase the first one (**Fig. 42.5**).
- Next, drill the guidewire for an interference screw from the anterior edge of the distal fibula (attachment site approximates the halfway point between the CFL and ATFL) proximal and posteriorly exiting out the posterior fibula. It is the author's preference to use the Wright Medical G-Force Interference Screw System (Wright Medical Inc., Memphis, TN).
- Size the tendon using the tendon sizer that accompanies the interference screw system being used and drill the corresponding drill size. This is typically 4 mm.
- Using the guidewire as a Beath needle, bring the end of the peroneus brevis tendon flap through the fibula making sure it easily glides through the tunnel. If it does not fit through, sharply debride the end of the tendon to a smaller diameter (**Fig. 42.6**).
- Next, place a 2–0 nonabsorbable suture in a horizontal mattress manner through the proximal periosteal flap of the distal fibula to the ATFL sleeve, being careful not to take too big a bite on the sleeve to prevent over advancement. Place at least one suture on either side of the tendon graft, likely more than one proximal to the graft will be needed (**Fig. 42.7**).
- Alternatively, and in the case of poor cuff tissue remaining on the fibula, one can place one or more suture anchors into the anterior edge of the distal fibula to attach the ATFL sleeve. In this case, one would want to take bigger bites of the ATFL sleeve in order to advance it, and then suture the sleeve proximal to the bite to the distal fibular periosteal sleeve created earlier.

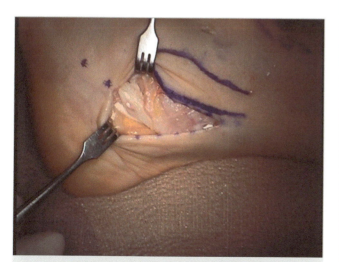

Fig. 42.2 After blunt dissection of the subcutaneous tissues, the peroneus brevis sheath distal to the fibula is opened. In this case, a longitudinal split tear of the tendon was present.

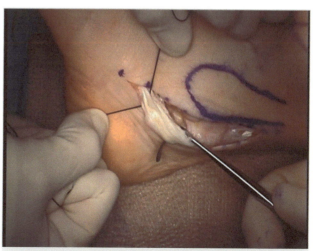

Fig. 42.3 A no. 15 blade is used to make a longitudinal split in the superior one-third of the peroneus brevis tendon distal to the superficial peroneal retinaculum (SPR). A number 2 nylon suture is then passed through and worked back and forth distally toward the tendon insertion to separate the graft.

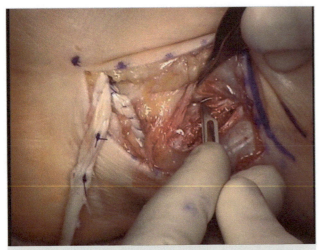

Fig. 42.4 After the modified Evans peroneus brevis flap is created, an oblique incision (anterior–proximal to posterior distal) through the periosteum of the distal fibula is made, and then a full-thickness subperiosteal flap is raised anteriorly off the fibula. The talus should be clearly visible under the flap.

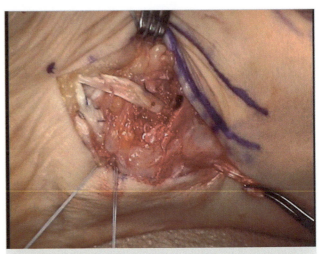

Fig. 42.6 After drilling the graft tunnel from the footprint of the anterior talofibular ligament (ATFL) on the distal fibula aimed proximal and posteriorly, the graft is passed through using a Beath needle.

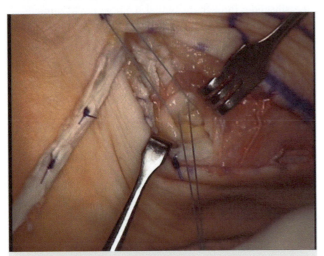

Fig. 42.5 With the peroneal tendons retracted posteriorly, box sutures are placed in the calcaneofibular ligament with nonabsorbable suture.

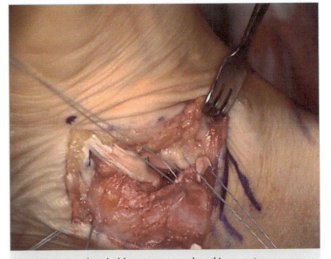

Fig. 42.7 Nonabsorbable sutures are placed in a pants-over-vest fashion through the periosteal sleeve created on the distal fibula and the anterior talofibular ligament (ATFL) to advance the ligament.

- At this point, holding the foot in eversion, mild external rotation, and plantar flexion, secure the sutures in the CFL. Maintain eversion while adding dorsiflexion and posterior translation to secure the sutures in the ATFL.
- Tension the graft and reduce the talus with a posteriorly directed force and hold in neutral varus/valgus position. This is important as securing the tendon in an overly everted position will cause stiffness and possible subtalar joint arthritis.
- Place the interference screw until it is flush with the anterior cortex of the distal fibula to secure the graft. This creates a checkrein against inversion of the talus (**Fig. 42.8**).
- Suture the extra tendon graft exiting posteriorly to the periosteum and fascia on the posterior aspect of the fibula. Trim any excess tendon.
- If one wishes for additional stability, the inferior extensor retinaculum can be sutured to the periosteum of the distal fibula posterior to the ATFL advancement using an absorb-

able 0 suture (Gould modification of the Broström procedure).
- Close the fascia over the peroneal tendons proximal to the SPR with simple interrupted 2–0 absorbable sutures.
- Close the peroneal tendon sheath just distal to the SPR with a single figure-of-eight suture.
- Ensure final ankle stability with anterior drawer and talar tilt tests.
- Closure.

42.6 Tips and Pearls/Hazards and Pitfalls

- A longitudinal incision over the peroneal tendons is preferred over the anterolateral incision originally described for the

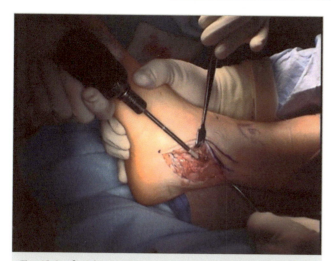

Fig. 42.8 After the Broström lateral ligament advancement has been completed, tension the peroneus brevis graft and reduce the talus with a posterior-directed force and hold it in neutral inversion/eversion. The interference screw is then placed flush with the anterior cortex of the distal fibula.

Broström repair as it allows for management of associated pathology.
- Always consider the possibility of associated peroneal subluxation and longitudinal tears.
- Preserve the superior peroneal reticulum if there is no tendon instability.
- As stated, avoid securing the split Evans transfer in eversion.
- Protect the repair in a potentially noncompliant patient with cast immobilization.

42.7 Complications/Bailout/Salvage

- If the ATFL and lateral capsular tissue are attenuated and will not provide a stout repair, one can use an allograft or autograft hamstring (i.e., gracilis) tendon to re-create the ATFL and CFL (Colville or Chrisman–Snook type procedure). If the patient's peroneus brevis tendon is degenerated and a tendon graft cannot be taken, then one can perform a Broström–Gould procedure alone, or place a suture tape for reinforcement.
- The superficial peroneal nerve runs anterior to the ATFL and can be injured with excessive dorsal dissection; and the sural nerve runs superficial to the peroneal tendons distal to the fibula and can be injured during graft harvesting.
- Incising the ATFL anterior to the fibula instead of over the bone can leave insufficient tissue to advance in the Broström procedure.
- Tensioning the split peroneus brevis graft with the talus everted past neutral can severely restrict hindfoot motion, and can lead to subtalar pain and arthrosis.

42.8 Postoperative Care

- The procedure is performed on an outpatient basis and patients go home the same day.

- Patient returns for first follow-up at 2 weeks where sutures/staples are removed and splint is converted to a walking cast.
- At 4 to 5 weeks, the patient begins walking in a tall CAM walker. Physical therapy may be ordered if it is felt that the patient will need assistance with range of motion (ROM), desensitization, or swelling reduction.
- At 10 weeks, the patient is transitioned out of boot and into a regular shoe. Peroneal strengthening and proprioceptive re-education is initiated.
- At 3 months, patients may begin running in a straight line on a treadmill or even ground.
- At 4 months, patients are allowed to begin to perform cutting activities in the ankle brace. They will begin to feel that the surgery is "behind them," but swelling and atrophy are the last issues to resolve and can take 6 to 12 months.

42.9 Outcomes

- Patients can expect good results with minimal chance of failure.
- Brodsky et al reviewed 73 patients who underwent modified Broström–Gould lateral ligament reconstruction without split Evans modification:
  ○ Average AOFAS (American Orthopaedic Foot and Ankle Society) score at mean 5.3-year follow-up was 95, but only mean physical component score of 84% on the SF-36 (36-Item Short Form Survey).
- A 2015 retrospective study of 19 patients who underwent modified Broström–Evans procedure demonstrated minimal loss of peroneal strength and no recurrent instability or progressive symptomatic subtalar arthritis requiring reoperation at mean 8.7-year follow-up.
- Ankle ROM symmetric in all planes except a 41% decrease in ankle inversion compared to the nonoperative side.

References

1. Brodsky AR, O'Malley MJ, Bohne WH, Deland JA, Kennedy JG. An analysis of outcome measures following the Broström-Gould procedure for chronic lateral ankle instability. Foot Ankle Int 2005;26(10):816–819
2. Colville MR. Surgical treatment of the unstable ankle. J Am Acad Orthop Surg 1998;6(6):368–377
3. Colville MR, Marder RA, Zarins B. Reconstruction of the lateral ankle ligaments. A biomechanical analysis. Am J Sports Med 1992;20(5):594–600
4. Girard P, Anderson RB, Davis WH, Isear JA, Kiebzak GM. Clinical evaluation of the modified Brostrom-Evans procedure to restore ankle stability. Foot Ankle Int 1999;20(4):246–252
5. Hect PJ, Cummins JS, Taylor DC, Easley ME. Modified Broström and Broström-Evans procedures. In Operative Techniques in Orthopaedic Surgery.2nded. Philadelphia, PA: Wolters Kluwer;2016:4899–4911/bok
6. Hsu AR, Ardoin GT, Davis WH, Anderson RB. Intermediate and long-term outcomes of the modified Brostrom-Evans procedure for lateral ankle ligament reconstruction. Foot Ankle Spec 2016;9(2):131–139

43 Broström: Arthroscopic Repair

Jorge I. Acevedo and Peter G. Mangone

Abstract

Current biomechanical and clinical results indicate that arthroscopic lateral ankle ligament reconstruction is becoming an increasingly acceptable method for the surgical management of chronic lateral ankle instability. Traditional methods to stabilize the lateral ankle rely on open approaches for repair or reconstruction. The anatomy of the ATFL and capsular components of the lateral ligament complex is easily visualized during arthroscopic examination and allows for arthroscopic reconstruction techniques. We describe the indications, advantages, and key principles of an arthroscopic Broström repair technique as well as tips and pearls in order to avoid potential pitfalls. The authors have used this technique since 2007 and have published anatomic, biomechanical, and clinical data supporting the outcomes equal to traditional open techniques.

Keywords: *Arthroscopy, Brostrom, lateral ankle ligament repair, ankle instability, ankle sprain*

43.1 Indications

• Symptomatic chronic lateral ankle ligament instability in patients who have failed appropriate nonoperative management.

43.1.1 Pathology

• Chronic attenuation or tears of the lateral ankle ligaments resulting in recurrent inversion ankle sprains or recurrent feelings of lateral ankle instability.

43.1.2 Clinical Evaluation

• Perform complete physical examination of the ankle and hindfoot.
• Important physical examination elements:
  ○ Alignment: cavovarus foot must be corrected with lateral ankle ligament reconstruction to decrease chance of recurrence:
    ❖ "Peek-a-boo" heel.
    ❖ Externally rotated fibula.
    ❖ Rigid plantarflexed first ray.
  ○ Motor strength/tendon assessment:
    ❖ Peroneal muscle strength testing.
    ❖ Tenderness possibly indicates tendon tear.
    ❖ Assess for peroneal subluxation/dislocation.
  ○ Instability:
    ❖ Anterior drawer test.
    ❖ Talar tilt test.
    ❖ Assess for subtalar instability versus ankle instability.
  ○ Palpation:
    ❖ Tenderness over anterolateral ankle.
    ❖ Tenderness over sinus tarsi.

43.1.3 Radiographic Evaluation

• AP (anteroposterior), mortise, and lateral ankle weight-bearing plain radiographs:
  ○ Assess for congruent versus incongruent tibiotalar alignment.
  ○ Assess for osteochondral lesions.
  ○ Assess for degenerative joint space narrowing:
  ○ If severe enough, patient may not be candidate for lateral ligament reconstruction.
  ○ Assess for exostosis:
  ○ Distal tibia—often anterolateral > anteromedial.
  ○ Talus neck—often dorsal and medial.
• Stress radiographs (as needed):
  ○ Anterior drawer.
  ○ Talar tilt.
  ○ Manual versus Telos.
• CT (computed tomography) scan:
  ○ Assess for osteochondral lesions.
  ○ Assess for intra-articular loose bodies.
  ○ Assess for degenerative changes.
  ○ Assess the anatomy of exostoses of the distal tibia and dorsomedial talus.
• MRI:
  ○ Assess for intra-articular pathology such as osteochondral lesions and loose bodies.
  ○ Assess for extra-articular pathology such as peroneal tendon tear.

43.1.4 Nonoperative Options

  ○ Physical therapy focused on proprioception, balance, and peroneal muscle strengthening.
  ○ Ankle gauntlet brace.
  ○ AFO (ankle–foot orthosis) brace (in more severe cases of ankle instability).

43.1.5 Contraindications

• Connective tissue elasticity disorder:
  ○ Ehlers–Danlos syndrome.
  ○ Marfan's syndrome.
• Morbid obesity.
• Heavy-demand patient (relative contraindications).
• Failed previous Broström-type procedure (relative contraindication).
• History of previous failed ligament/capsular reconstruction procedures in other joints (e.g., shoulder).
• Uncorrectable varus heel deformity.

43.2 Goals of Surgical Procedure

- Reconstruct the lateral ankle ligament complex to increase stability and decrease pain.
- Return to premorbid level of activity (including sports activities) as desired.

43.3 Advantages of Surgical Procedure

- Smaller minimally invasive incision technique that has resulted in postoperative clinical course with:
  - Shorter operative time than current open techniques.
  - Decreased pain (anecdotal findings).
  - Decreased swelling.
  - Improved cosmetic appearance.
  - Success rate equivalent to, if not better than, published results with traditional open procedures.[1]

43.4 Key Principles

- Draw out the key landmarks and safe zone prior to starting the initial arthroscopy.
- Perform an extensive debridement/clean out of lateral gutter to remove scar tissue and allow for full visualization of the anterior face of the lateral malleolus and distal tip of the fibula prior to placing the first anchor.
- After placing the first anchor, pass the sutures from that anchor prior to placing the second anchor to avoid suture entanglement.
- Pass the sutures through the skin at least 15 mm inferior to the distal tip of fibula to capture the inferior extensor retinaculum (IER) in the repair.
- Remove distraction prior to tying sutures and hold ankle/foot in neutral to slight eversion, neutral dorsiflexion, and posterior drawer force applied to the ankle.

43.5 Preoperative Preparation and Patient Positioning

Stress radiographs (either manual or with a mechanical stress device) can play a role in the decision making of whether to perform an arthroscopic repair or an open tendon augmentation type of lateral ankle ligament stabilization. MRI or CT scan may be needed to assess for additional intra-articular or extra-articular pathology such as osteochondral lesion, exostosis, and peroneal tendon tear.

A preoperative drawing of anatomic landmarks identifying the "safe zones" in the lateral ankle region is created.[2] The superior margins of the peroneal tendons, distal fibula tip, and intermediate branch of the superficial peroneal nerve (SPN) are outlined on the skin. The lateral calcaneal tubercle is used to identify the IER, which is located 15 mm from the fibula tip with the ankle in neutral dorsiflexion (**Fig. 43.1a,b**).

The patient is positioned supine on the operating room table with a well-padded tourniquet on the proximal thigh. A towel bump is placed under the ankle for distraction. Alternatively, the surgeon may elect to use a noninvasive distractor along with a thigh holder applied during positioning to keep the hip flexed 60 degrees.

43.6 Operative Technique

The arthroscopic Broström repair is typically performed under a regional popliteal block along with monitored anesthesia care (MAC). An additional block of the saphenous nerve is necessary to complete the sensory block over the anteromedial portal. General anesthesia can be used as well if the patient or surgeon prefers.

Prior to the ligament repair, standard anteromedial and anterolateral ankle arthroscopy portals are used to perform the initial diagnostic arthroscopy and treat any concomitant intra-articular pathology. A thorough debridement of the lateral gutter is also necessary in order to clearly visualize the anterior face of the fibula and avoid impingement of anterolateral tissues. All borders of the distal fibular tip should be probed and the anterior fibular face should be denuded in order to improve tissue adherence.

Using the standard anteromedial portal for viewing the lateral ankle joint, the first bone anchor is drilled and inserted, through the standard anterolateral portal, 1 cm superior to the distal tip of the fibula (**Fig. 43.2**). This location corresponds with the inferior origin point of the ATFL on the anterolateral malleolus. The sutures are brought out through the anterolateral portal and then shuttled with a sharp-tipped suture passer (using either an "inside-out" or outside-in" technique) through the lateral ligament complex exiting the skin within the safe zone. The first suture limb is passed just superior to the peroneal tendon margin, while the second suture limb is passed 1 cm dorsal/anterior to the first suture following the arc of the IER (**Fig. 43.3**).

Once the first set of sutures is passed, the second anchor is drilled and inserted 1 cm above the first anchor (usually just

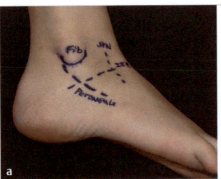
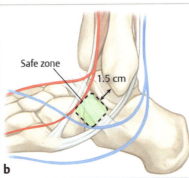

Fig. 43.1 (a) Preoperative drawing and (b) schematic representation of anatomic landmarks and "safe zone."

Safe zone

1.5 cm

below the level of the talar dome) on the anterior face of fibula (**Fig. 43.4a,b**). The second set of sutures is brought out through the anterolateral portal and shuttled, similar to the first suture set (using either an "inside-out" or "outside-in" technique), along the arc of the IER with both suture limbs spaced 1 cm apart (**Fig. 43.5**). Care is taken to assure the exit points are inferior to the intermediate branch of the SPN and within the safe zone.

At this point a 3- to 4-mm incision is made between the two sets of sutures in order to pass the sutures out subcutaneously and then exit the skin (**Fig. 43.6a,b**). A small arthroscopic hook/probe is used to facilitate subcutaneous passage of the sutures. If there is concern of nerve entrapment, a small retractor can be used to elevate the tissue and assure sutures are deep to the SPN.

If peroneal tendon pathology is suspected, the sutures are tagged for tying after this is addressed. Instead of large open incisions, the authors prefer to perform a peroneal tendoscopy or an ancillary mini-incision to evaluate and repair the tendons. The ankle is then held in neutral dorsiflexion and slight eversion while applying a posterior drawer stress for suture tying. The two sets of sutures are individually tied with either a standard surgeon's knot or an arthroscopic slip knot.

Once the sutures are tied, the ankle is tested with a manual anterior drawer and talar tilt to determine whether there is any residual laxity. If additional tightening of the repair is needed, a second suture row (suture bridge) is added proximal to the main anchors. At any point during the repair, the surgeon may revert to an open technique without compromising the final result.

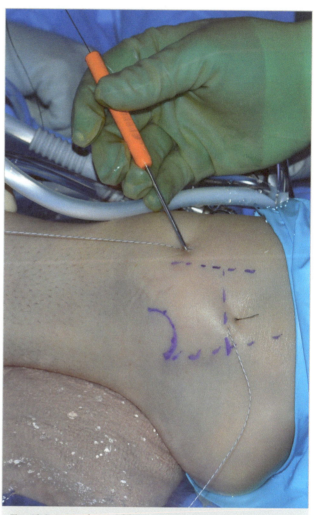

Fig. 43.3 External view of first suture limb exiting superior to the peroneal tendon margin and second suture limb shuttled with suture passer (inside-out technique).

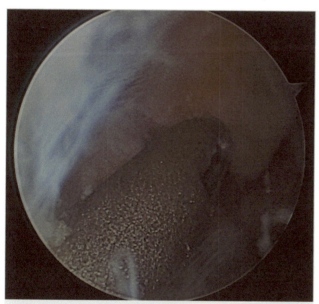

Fig. 43.2 View from anteromedial portal showing placement of cannula for drilling/insertion of first suture anchor.

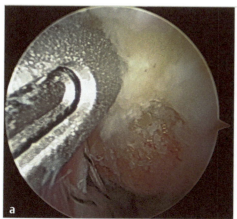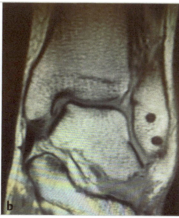

Fig. 43.4 (a) View from anteromedial portal showing placement of cannula for drilling/insertion of second suture anchor. Sutures from first anchor are seen inferiorly after passage through lateral ligament complex. (b) Postoperative magnetic resonance imaging (MRI) showing placement of suture anchors into distal fibula.

43.6.1 Inside-Out Suture Passing Technique

The inside-out technique is based upon the placement of the suture passer from the anterolateral portal out through the lateral ligamentous complex, while the remainder of the general technique is unchanged. Using the anteromedial portal for viewing with the scope, the sharp-tipped suture passer follows a path between the lateral surface of the talus and the suture limbs that were brought out of the anterolateral portal. The suture passer pierces through the lateral ligamentous complex and exits at least 1.5 cm distal to the fibula and within the "safe zone" (between the superior margin of the peroneal tendons and the SPN). If using the Micro Suture-Lasso (Arthrex, Inc.), the internal looped wire is left in place while removing the SutureLasso handle. This wire is then used to shuttle the individual suture limbs. Each suture limb requires a separate passage of the SutureLasso. After passage of the two suture limbs from the first anchor, a second anchor is

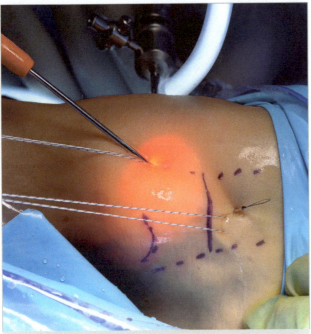

Fig. 43.5 External view of first set of suture limbs exiting superior to the peroneal tendon margin after piercing the lateral ligament complex and second anchor sutures exiting the anterolateral portal prior to shuttling with suture passer (inside-out technique).

inserted as previously described and these sutures are passed in a similar fashion.

43.6.2 Outside-In Suture Passing Technique

The outside-in technique is predicated on placement of the suture passer through the same exit points on the skin as for the inside-out technique while following the same path back into the joint. The suture passer therefore traverses through the skin, subcutaneous tissue, IER, and lateral ligamentous complex under direct arthroscopic view. If using the SutureLasso, the looped wire is advanced within the joint and brought out of the anterolateral portal with an arthroscopic grasper. The looped wire is then used to shuttle each suture limbs back through the soft tissues and exit the skin. Subsequent steps follow the overview of the technique.

43.7 Tips and Pearls

- Obtain MRI before surgery to assess for peroneal tendon pathology. If suspected peroneal tendon pathology is present on MRI, then the surgeon can either proceed with an open technique or the arthroscopic Broström can be performed with a much smaller focused incision used for peroneal tendon exploration and repair.
- Perform an extensive debridement/clean out of lateral gutter to remove scar tissue and allow for full visualization of the anterior face of the lateral malleolus and distal tip of the fibula prior to placing the first anchor.
- After placing the first anchor, pass the sutures from that anchor prior to placing the second anchor to avoid suture entanglement.
- Use an arthroscopic probe with a small hook to pass sutures through the small central incision on the lateral foot.

43.8 Hazards and Pitfalls

Several guidelines can help avoid potential pitfalls.
- If a distractor is used during the procedure, care should be taken to ensure its release prior to tying sutures down.
- Strict adherence to drawing the safe zone may avoid entrapment of the intermediate branch of the SPN and peroneal tendons.

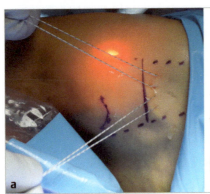
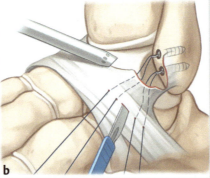

Fig. 43.6 (a) External view of all four suture limbs exiting skin along the arc of the inferior extensor retinaculum. (b) Illustration of both sets of sutures after shuttling through lateral ligament complex and 3-mm incision made between the suture sets before subcutaneous passage.

- The surgeon should identify the medial and lateral margins of the distal fibula prior to anchor placement to avoid intra-articular or lateral skiving.
- Avoid angling the drill guide (superior/inferior) and maintain a horizontal trajectory to avoid inferior placement of the distal anchor.
- It is helpful to use fluoroscopy during initial anchor placement to identify inferior anchor position.
- Once sutures are tied, puckering of the overlying skin may be avoided by spreading the underlying subcutaneous tissues with a hemostat to release them from the deeper tissues.

43.9 Complications/Bailout/Salvage

Potential complications of the arthroscopic Broström repair are mainly related to temporary perturbations or entrapment of anatomic structures. During placement of the standard lateral portal or with shuttling of sutures through the lateral ligament complex, the intermediate branch of the SPN is the primary structure at risk. This can be avoided by elevating the soft tissues with a small retractor placed within the accessory incision in order to confirm sutures are deep to the nerve. Tendon entrapment has not been observed when using the safe zone as a topographical guide. If at any point during the procedure the surgeon is uncomfortable or unable to proceed with the arthroscopic repair, the surgeon may proceed with either a mini-open or a standard open ligament repair without losing recourse. However, if the procedure is completed but the repair is not adequately tight, a "second row" of anchors can be placed 3 cm proximal to the distal fibular tip. The first row sutures may be passed subcutaneously and exit through a 1-cm incision made at the level where the proximal anchor row is planned. Alternatively, a suture tape or allograft tendon is used to augment the repair. In the authors' experience, this is rarely necessary unless compromised tissue or severe laxity is not anticipated preoperatively.

43.10 Postoperative Care

The postoperative care is similar to that of the open procedure. However, the authors have found a trend toward patients accelerating early range of motion and protected weight-bearing due to the decreased swelling and pain using the arthroscopic Broström versus traditional open techniques.

During the first 2 weeks, postoperative dressing and short leg splint remain in place and no weight-bearing is allowed. Sutures are removed at 10 to 14 days. From weeks 2 to 4, patients are allowed 50% weight-bearing as tolerated in a boot walker. Gentle range of motion exercises are encourage while avoiding inversion. During weeks 4 to 6, transition is made to a lace-up style gauntlet ankle brace and the patient is progressed to full weight-bearing. Dorsiflexion/plantar flexion exercises are continued. After 6 weeks, formal physical therapy is initiated emphasizing peroneal muscle strengthening and range of motion. The ankle brace is continued up to 12 weeks and thereafter is used for any sports and higher impact activities until 6 months after surgery.

43.11 Outcomes

Consistent with the stated goals, the patient and surgeon can expect arthroscopic lateral ankle ligament reconstruction to produce a stable, painless ankle that allows for return to premorbid activity, including competitive sports, which is equal to or better than traditional open techniques. Published studies support these expectations with the initial report by Corte-Real et al in 2009.[3]

Since this initial report, multiple additional studies that have been published in peer-reviewed literature demonstrating the results from arthroscopic lateral ankle ligament techniques are at least equal to, if not better than, results from traditional open techniques.[1, 4-6] Most recently, Yeo et al published the first prospective randomized trial comparing an all-inside arthroscopic lateral ligament reconstruction versus an open technique.[1] The authors determined no difference between the two procedures at 1 year after surgery.

The authors have published multiple studies since 2011 detailing patient outcomes after a specific two-anchor arthroscopic lateral ligament technique.[4] To date, this procedure is the only published technique with anatomic, biomechanical, and clinical data supporting the outcomes equal to traditional open techniques.[2,4,5,7]

References

1. Yeo ED, Lee KT, Sung IH, Lee SG, Lee YK. Comparison of all-inside arthroscopic and open techniques for the modified Broström procedure for ankle instability. Foot Ankle Int 2016;37(10):1037–1045
2. Acevedo JI, Ortiz C, Golano P, Nery C. ArthroBroström lateral ankle stabilization technique: an anatomic study. Am J Sports Med 2015;43(10):2564–2571
3. Corte-Real NM, Moreira RM. Arthroscopic repair of chronic lateral ankle instability. Foot Ankle Int 2009;30(3):213–217
4. Acevedo J, Mangone P. Arthroscopic lateral ankle ligament reconstruction. Tech Foot Ankle Surg 2011;10(3):111–116
5. Acevedo JI, Mangone P. Arthroscopic Brostrom technique. Foot Ankle Int 2015;36(4):465–473
6. Nery C, Raduan F, Del Buono A, Asaumi ID, Cohen M, Maffulli N. Arthroscopic-assisted Broström-Gould for chronic ankle instability: a long-term follow-up. Am J Sports Med 2011;39(11):2381–2388
7. Giza E, Shin EC, Wong SE, et al. Arthroscopic suture anchor repair of the lateral ligament ankle complex: a cadaveric study. Am J Sports Med 2013;41(11):2567–2572

44 Ligament Augmentation with the Internal Brace

Gordon M. Mackay and William J. Ribbans

Abstract

The surgical decision making and considerations when preparing to undertake an anatomic ligament repair with augmentation using the Internal Brace are described in this chapter. The Internal Brace supports early mobilization of the repaired ligament and allows the natural tissues to progressively strengthen. The principle established by this experience has resulted in its successful application to other foot and ankle ligaments including the deltoid, spring and syndesmosis complexes as well as other locations including the knee, shoulder, elbow, and hand. The key benefits relate to reduced surgical morbidity and the avoidance of the detrimental effects of immobilization. This has transformed the patient experience. For over 30 years, the accepted orthopaedic approach to joint instability secondary to ligament injury has been reconstruction with allograft or autograft in both the acute and chronic situation. With the Internal Bracing principles and the evolution of technology, we have been able to successfully return to ligament repair.

Keywords: *ankle instability, anterior talar fibular ligament, augmentation, Internal Brace, FiberTape*

44.1 Indications

Broström discounted nonanatomical repairs in favor of an anatomical repair and recognized crucially that, even in chronic situations, it is possible to utilize the damaged ligament in the repair (**Fig. 44.1**). Concerns regarding the potential weakness of direct soft-tissue repair were in part addressed by the Gould modification incorporating the free edge of the inferior extensor retinaculum (IER) to reinforce the repair.

A spectrum of different approaches and techniques has been described to achieve the goal of tightening the lateral restraining tissues of the ankle joint.

Repair of the lateral ligaments utilizing a Broström technique results in a construct initially much weaker than the native ligament. Conversely a high proportion of subjects fail to return to their pre-injury level of sport with more traditional nonanatomical approaches—up to 50% in some papers.

Our technique for Internal Bracing has reflected this understanding, focusing on augmenting anatomically the anterior talofibular ligament (ATFL; **Fig. 44.2**). The detrimental effects of immobilization itself may have been underestimated. Only by restoring equivalent natural strength of the ATFL at time zero can immediate mobilization be encouraged with confidence.

It is recommended that surgeons use their preferred Broström technique in conjunction with the Internal Brace to optimize results. The biomechanical strength of the Broström alone is insufficient to confidently support early mobilization. The load to failure was 68 N for anatomical sutures and 79 N for fibula suture anchors; both were significantly weaker than the intact ATFL (161 N) in one recent biomechanical study.

The **need to augment the repair is clearly recognized** by surgeons with a multitude of techniques described. The Broström procedure describes a surgical continuum.

The use of the **fibula periosteum, IER, or a portion of the peroneus brevis tendon** to augment lateral ligament reconstruction has been described by several authors. This may be associated with additional morbidity and still requires postoperative protection.

Augmentation of a Broström repair, or its replacement, with an **allograft** tendon has been advocated in certain situations, for example, failed previous repairs, hyperlaxity, and long-standing instability. A recent paper has compared the strength of a semitendinosus allograft with an intact ATFL and reported similar ultimate load to failure—170 N (allograft) compared to 154 N (intact ATFL). Unfortunately, this dead tissue can attenuate during early remodeling.

The **Internal Brace** augments the Broström repair, ensuring sufficient initial strength of reconstruction to safely mobilize as tolerated.

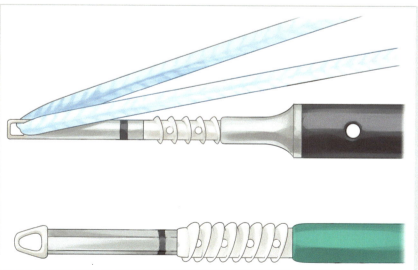

Fig. 44.1 FiberTape attached to a 3.5-mm BioComposite SwiveLock (above) for fibula attachment. 4.75-mm BioComposite SwiveLock (below) to which the FiberTape is attached for talus attachment.

44.1.1 The Internal Brace

The Internal Brace was conceived by one of the authors (GMM) and has been used to augment ligament and tendon repair following injury.

The Internal Brace construct comprises the FiberTape and two BioComposite SwiveLock screws.

The anatomy and biomechanical properties of the lateral ligament complex and the principles of various associated surgical procedures to restore stability have been validated by Dr. Tom Clanton's expert research. Clanton and coworkers comprehensively reviewed and published a series of papers from the Steadman Philippon Research Laboratory in Vail, Colorado. These papers concluded that direct soft-tissue fixation to ana-tomical sutures or bone anchors was not of sufficient strength to support early mobilization (**Fig. 44.3**). This essential appreciation has helped determine the biomechanical advantages derived from using an augmentation technique to support early mobilization.

The mean ultimate load to failure of the Internal Brace–Broström combination (251 N) was significantly higher than the native ATFL (154 N) and concluded that the "ATFL with suture tape augmentation is at least as strong and stiff as the native ATFL at time zero in a fresh-frozen cadaveric model" and that "adding strength to the Broström repair, through the addition of suture tape, may be valuable in patients with generalized ligamentous laxity, in large patients or elite athletes, or when graft reconstruction is not feasible."

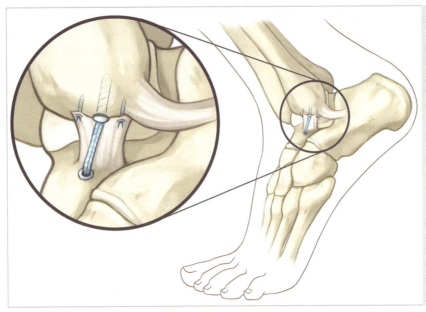

Fig. 44.2 Internal Brace mimics anterior talofibular ligament (ATFL) anatomy.

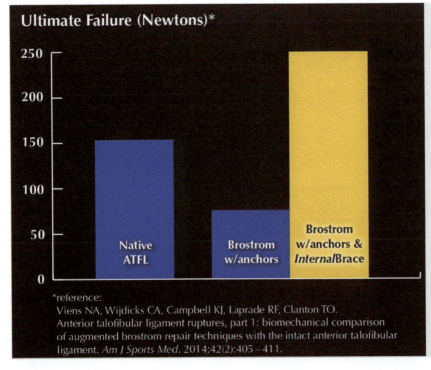

Fig. 44.3 Suture anchors alone insufficient to restore native strength of anterior talofibular ligament (ATFL), but the Internal Brace restores native strength at time zero.

*reference:
Viens NA, Wijdicks CA, Campbell KJ, Laprade RF, Clanton TO. Anterior talofibular ligament ruptures, part 1: biomechanical comparison of augmented brostrom repair techniques with the intact anterior talofibular ligament. *Am J Sports Med*. 2014;42(2):405–411.

44.1.2 Expert Opinion

From a patient's perspective, we can see few reasons why a patient should be subjected to an unnecessary and potentially dangerous period of immobilization after ligament repair.

Initially it was assumed that the benefits of the Internal Brace would be limited to the subgroups listed earlier, but the benefits are even greater for patients with significant comorbidities, for example, the diabetic, the obese, those unable to use crutches safely, or even the acute trauma case.

44.1.3 Clinical Evaluation

- Most patients present with a history of chronic or recurrent lateral ankle ligament instability and sprains.
- Pain usually accompanies the acute sprain, but is not a frequent symptom of ankle instability.
- Patients may have tenderness over their ATFL anterior to the distal fibular.
- Clinical instability of the ankle should be able to be reproduced through an anterior drawer test and varus mechanical stress test clinically.
- Patients should be evaluated for associated conditions such as peroneal tendon dysfunction, cavovarus foot alignment, or osteochondral lesions of the talus (OLT).

44.1.4 Radiographic Evaluation

- Standard weight-bearing radiographs should be evaluated for hindfoot alignment, loose bodies or OLTs in the ankle, old allusion fractures off the fibular, or talar insertions of the ATFL.
- Magnetic resonance imaging (MRI) is rarely indicated, except in equivocal cases of functional (nonmechanical) instability, or to evaluate for associated pathologies, particularly when pain is the predominant presenting symptom (more than instability).

44.1.5 Nonoperative Options

- Physical therapy for peroneal strengthening and proprioceptive training.
- Brace immobilization.
- Activity modification.

44.1.6 Contraindications

- Any patient undergoing a lateral ankle ligament reconstruction is a candidate for Internal Brace augmentation unless
  ○ Active infection at the surgical site.
  ○ Allergy or history of reaction to FiberWire or FiberTape material.

44.2 Goals of Surgical Procedure

- Restore physiologic strength (load to failure) to the ATFL/lateral ankle ligament.
- Allow early weight-bearing and ankle motion.
- Allow rapid return to function and minimize muscle disuse atrophy.

- Limit immobilization time to diminish risks of DVT (deep vein thrombosis)/pulmonary embolism (**Fig. 44.4**).

44.3 Advantages of Surgical Procedure

The use of the Internal Brace should not been seen as a substitute for an anatomical repair or for less exacting surgical standards in performing a Broström procedure. However, the superior strength of the combined construct allows for earlier mobilization postoperatively. The principle of Internal Bracing to facilitate early mobilization, ligament healing, and restoration of optimal function should and can be applied to all ligaments.

The FiberTape has an impressive safety record. It is known to have excellent biocompatibility with over 750,000 inserted over 9 years with 0.0001% reported synovial reactions.

44.4 Key Principles

- Standard Broström lateral ankle ligament reconstruction.
- Initial talar footprint Internal Brace fixation.
- Appropriate tensioning of the FiberTape prior to fibular fixation.
- Final fibular Internal Brace fixation.

44.5 Preoperative Preparation and Patient Positioning

44.5.1 Anesthetic Preparation

Surgery can be performed under general, spinal, or regional anesthetic utilizing either a thigh or calf tourniquet according to surgeon and patient preference. Antibiotics are routinely administered prior to tourniquet inflation.

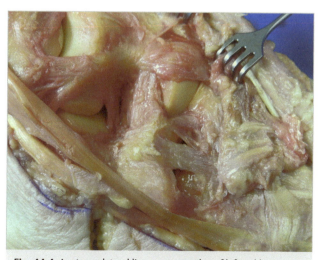

Fig. 44.4 Anatomy-lateral ligament complex of left ankle.

44.5.2 Arthroscopy and Operative Planning

An ankle arthroscopy is undertaken if the preoperative clinical and imaging evaluation identifies potential intra-articular pathology. A skin marker is used to mark the outline of the fibula and courses of the superficial peroneal nerves (SPN) and sural nerves.

44.6 Operative Technique

44.6.1 Surgical Incision

A curved longitudinal (**Fig. 44.5b**) or curved transverse incision (**Fig. 44.5a**) can be utilized. If the surgery is to be combined with a peroneal tendon procedure, the longitudinal incision should be sited more posteriorly and inferiorly.

44.6.2 Soft-Tissue Preparation

Following careful dissection of the subcutaneous fat and control of any vessels, the free edge of the IER is identified and mobilized carefully. It is carefully separated from the underlying talocrural capsule and ATFL and calcaneofibular ligament (CFL). The authors choose to mobilize this separately to ensure a distinct laminar repair, provide a repairable layer in the event of inadequate capsular tissue, for example, in the presence of a sizable avulsion fragment, and to provide a tissue plane between the IER and capsule for later passage of the Internal Brace if desired.

The capsule and ATFL are separated from the fibula by sharp dissection in a curvilinear fashion. Care must be taken not to make this incision too distal, especially if there is an underlying loose ossicle, to allow adequate tissue length for later repair. Care must be taken to avoid straying too far anteriorly to prevent injury to the SPN. The authors' posterior landmark is the peroneal sheath and this allows inspection of the tendons if pathology is suspected.

If additional tissue is required, the fibula periosteum is elevated from distal to proximal starting at the cut edge of the capsule and reflected.

Any loose ossicle is carefully excised taking care to preserve the capsule and as much of the integrity of the ATFL as possible for later reconstruction. The distal fibula is prepared with a rasp and bone rongeurs to enhance healing following ligament fixation. The CFL is inspected and its integrity ascertained.

44.6.3 Internal Brace Positioning at the Talar Neck

The insertion point for the Internal Brace is located on the nonarticulating surface of the lateral border of the talus at the point of insertion of the ATFL. With the ankle in **neutral**, a drill guide is used in a direction of 45 degrees medial and parallel to the floor with the foot in neutral to avoid entering the sinus tarsi or ankle joint.

The talus is drilled at 45 degrees to the sagittal plane. If there is initial unfamiliarity with the position of the ATFL insertion, a more extensive dissection at the level of the talar neck can allow direct visualization of this landmark. The drill hole is fully tapped with a 4.75-mm tap.

The 4.75-mm BioComposite SwiveLock is inserted into the talar hole preloaded with the FiberTape through the eyelet and secured in the tunnel. The Internal Brace is passed deep to the IER but superficial to the capsule and ligaments and emerges proximally ready for later fibular fixation.

The authors advise talar fixation first.

Alternatively, leave the tap in situ to facilitate location and orientation of the talar hole later. In these circumstances, the proximal fixation steps are completed first, including Internal Brace fixation to the fibula. The talar fixation is completed as the last step and ensuring correct tensioning of the FiberTape.

It is theoretically mechanically weaker to fix the open end of the FiberTape to the softer fibular bone, but it is still strong enough either way and depends upon the surgeon's preference. The fixation points for the Internal Brace should be drilled under direct vision prior to standard Broström repair.

Initial talar fixation can simplify fibular fixation at the end of the procedure.

It minimizes the impact of soft-tissue swelling and facilitates the tensioning process. The FiberTape can then be used as a convenient retractor for the ligament repair.

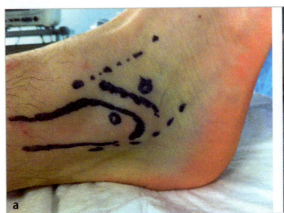 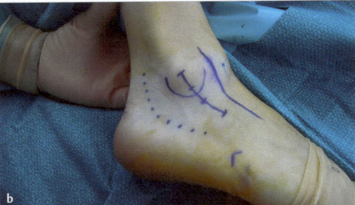

Fig. 44.5 (a) Anterolateral incision made 1 cm distal to fibula. (b) Incision from lateral malleolus to sinus tarsi.

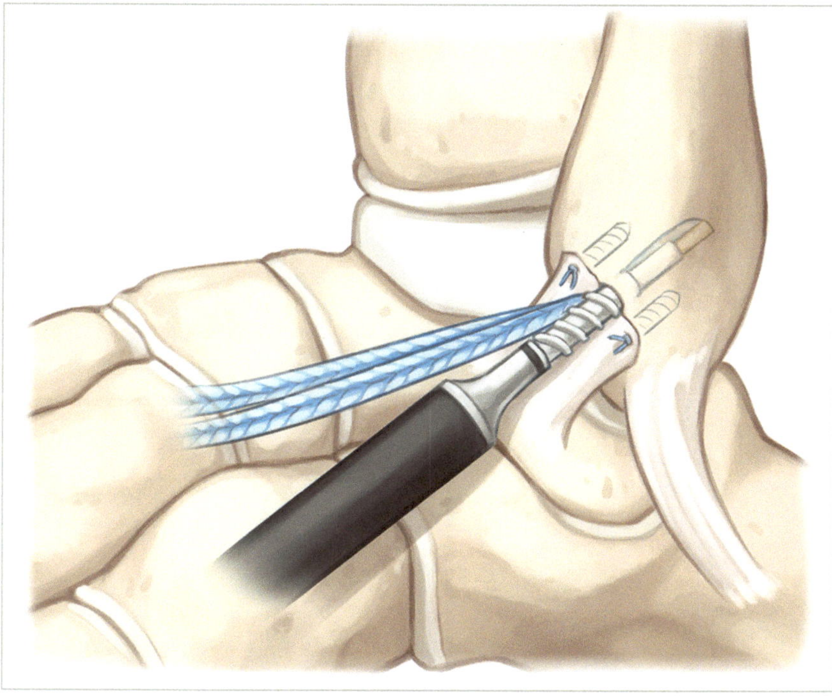

Fig. 44.6 Attachment of Internal Brace to fibula.

44.6.4 Internal Brace Positioning at the Fibula

A 2.7-mm drill hole at the fibula origin of ATFL approximately 14 mm from the tip of the fibula is made (**Fig. 44.6**). The drill hole is tapped with a 3.5-mm tap to assist screw placement.

44.6.5 Standard Broström

Prior to securing the Internal Brace, the authors perform the stages of the Broström utilizing the FiberWires attached to the distal fibula by bone anchors.

The number and siting of osseous anchors are decided next. If the CFL is to be repaired, an Arthrex FASTak 2.4-mm bone anchor loaded with 2–0 FiberWire is placed at its origin 5 mm from the tip of the fibula. A further one or two anchors are placed anterior to the Internal Brace position in the distal fibula for attachment of the capsule and ATFL. The ligaments and capsule are reattached to the fibula under tension by the FiberWire sutures.

The Internal Brace can be laid over the ATFL and anchored to the fibula initially or as a final step, whichever the surgeon finds easier.

44.6.6 Internal Bracing Fixation at the Fibula

A 3.5-mm BioComposite SwiveLock is loaded with the Fiber-Tape. It is inserted into the prepared fibula tunnel with the foot held in neutral.

The length of the FiberTape between the fibula and talus is calculated to allow for the correct length of insertion with the SwiveLock.

The tension in the Internal Brace at the point of tightening and attached of the FiberTape is important and creates considerable confusion as surgeons are familiar with the concept of soft-tissue tensioning often with the ankle in eversion.

Overtightening of the construct could restrict postoperative normal talocrural movement and, theoretically, stress shield the underlying Broström repair, resulting in poorer healing. Conversely, undertightening of the FiberTape will negate the biomechanical advantages of the Internal Brace. Measuring of the anatomical length of ATFL allows consistent and appropriate length to be established. This importantly allows the Internal Brace to act as a seat belt rather than a synthetic ligament. This can be assessed by checking that the tip of a hemostat can be placed between the FiberTape and underlying tissue prior to anchor tightening. This allows minimal laxity in the stabilized construct reflecting normal anatomy. This is the key to its success.

44.6.7 Final Suturing

The redundant FiberTape is cut flush with the fixation. The free proximal edge of the IER can be sutured to the capsule, and, if utilized, the mobilized periosteum overlapped and sutured over the IER.

Finally, the ankle is placed through a full range of movement and ankle stability confirmed with confidence. The wounds are irrigated and closed.

44.7 Tips and Pearls

• If there is any confusion about the insertion point of the ATFL, with the foot in neutral, its point equates with a horizontal line drawn from the tip of the fibula. This is just off the articular surface and equates with midpoint of the vertical talar height as illustrated by Clanton (**Fig. 44.7**).

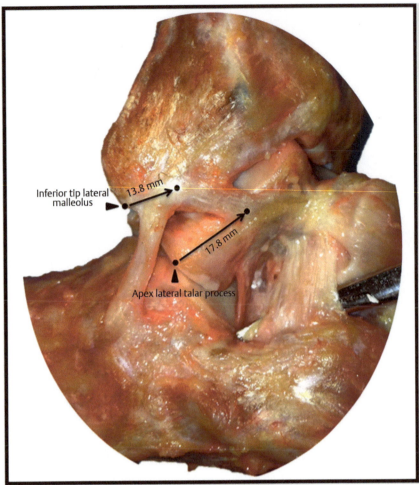

Inferior tip lateral malleolus

13.8 mm

17.8 mm

Apex lateral talar process

Fig. 44.7 Anatomy of anterior talofibular ligament (ATFL) as illustrated by Clanton.

- When completing the talar neck bone tunnel, **a sinus probe** is used to ensure the tunnel is both blind ending and has not inadvertently encroached upon the superior wall of the sinus tarsi.
- Fully tap talus to avoid screw breakage.
- The surgeon can confirm that the correct tension has been established if the tip of a hemostat can be placed between the FiberTape and underlying tissue prior to anchor tightening. This allows minimal laxity in the stabilized construct reflecting normal anatomy.
- The ankle is placed in neutral during tightening of the anchor into the fibular.

44.8 Hazards and Pitfalls

- Do not overtighten the Internal Brace. The Internal Brace is designed as a checkrein to the Broström, not as the ligament reconstruction itself.
- If overtightened, the Internal Brace will not stretch out with time as is usually seen with overtightened ligament and tendon repairs.
- Ensure that the bone tunnels do not cut out of the fibular or talar bone by being eccentrically placed. This will result in failure of the SwiveLock anchor fixation, and as such of the Internal Brace itself. If this occurs, the bone tunnel should be redrilled and a new swivel lock anchor inserted.

- Placement of the fibular bone tunnel should be in between the anchors used for the Broström procedure, ensuring that the anchors are not compromised during drilling.

44.9 Complications/Bailout/Salvage

- Infection.
- Neural irritation.
- Overtensioning.
- Nonanatomical placement.

44.10 Postoperative Care

The procedure is performed either as day-case or overnight surgery. The ankle is dressed. The senior author (GMM) uses no postoperative cast and allows immediate partial weight-bearing as in a removable boot according to comfort. This is to ensure satisfactory wound healing rather than to protect repair. The surgeon's normal postoperative antithromboembolic regime should be utilized. Sutures are removed at 2 weeks and the patient referred to physical therapy.

44.10.1 Rehabilitation Protocol

It is now normal for patients to walk with a normal gait 2 weeks after surgery. Patients are expected to be able to return to water-based activities after satisfactory wound healing, cycling at 2 weeks, and straight line running from 8 weeks. Some patients can tolerate antigravity treadmill running at 50% body weight from the third or fourth week. Return to contact sports needs to be individually assessed between 8 and 12 weeks postoperatively. Patients are advised to wear a supportive ankle brace or strap when initially returning to play. Time to return to sport and work has been reduced by half.

44.11 Outcomes

Early results have been very promising for all patients even if nonsporting. Early mobilization, reduced pain, and early restoration of function were the shared experience.

The Surgical Outcome System (Arthrex, Naples, FL) is being used to capture independently validated outcome data on patients being managed with an Internal Brace and Broström procedures. These have demonstrated significant improvement in FFI (Foot Function Index) and FAAM (Foot and Ankle Activity Measure) from presurgery out to 2 years postsurgery. The earliest return to professional sport was a premiership rugby player who played a full match 8 weeks post-op. There were no reports of synovitis.

All sports-oriented patients were back running at 12 weeks. A range of different sports were represented and the only complication reported involved one superficial wound infection.

These data are currently unpublished.

44.12 Conclusion

This chapter points to a profound change in orthopaedic practice. For over 30 years, the accepted orthopaedic approach to instability secondary to ligament injury has been reconstruction in both the acute and chronic situation. The Internal Brace has allowed us to refocus on the restoration of normal anatomy and in turn function. It supports early mobilization of the repaired ligament and allows the natural tissues to progressively strengthen and heal with minimal surgical morbidity. Reconstruction should be indicated only if the tissues fail to heal adequately after augmentation and repair.

References

1. Mackay GM, Blyth MJ, Anthony I, Hopper GP, Ribbans WJ. A review of ligament augmentation with the Internal-Brace™: the surgical principle is described for the lateral ankle ligament and ACL repair in particular, and a comprehensive review of other surgical applications and techniques is presented. Surg Technol Int 2015;26:239–255
2. Waldrop NE III, Wijdicks CA, Jansson KS, LaPrade RF, Clanton TO. Anatomic suture anchor versus the Broström technique for anterior talofibular ligament repair: a biomechanical comparison. Am J Sports Med 2012;40(11):2590–2596
3. Viens NA, Wijdicks CA, Campbell KJ, Laprade RF, Clanton TO. Anterior talofibular ligament ruptures, part 1: biomechanical comparison of augmented Broström repair techniques with the intact anterior talofibular ligament. Am J Sports Med 2014;42(2):405–411
4. Acevedo J, Vora A. Anatomical reconstruction of the spring ligament complex: "internal brace" augmentation. Foot Ankle Spec 2013;6(6):441–445
5. Gilmer BB, Crall T, DeLong J, Kubo T, Mackay G, Jani SS. Biomechanical analysis of Internal Bracing for treatment of medial knee injuries. Orthopedics 2016;39(3):e532–e537
6. Lubowitz JH, MacKay G, Gilmer B. Knee medial collateral ligament and posteromedial corner anatomic repair with internal bracing. Arthrosc Tech 2014;3(4):e505–e508
7. Smith JO, Yasen SK, Palmer HC, Lord BR, Britton EM, Wilson AJ. Paediatric ACL repair reinforced with temporary internal bracing. Knee Surg Sports Traumatol Arthrosc 2016;24(6):1845–1851
8. Heitmann M, Dratzidis A, Jagodzinski M, et al. Ligament bracing--augmented cruciate ligament sutures: biomechanical studies of a new treatment concept [in German]. Unfallchirurg 2014;117(7):650–657
9. McWilliam JR, Mackay G. The Internal Brace for midsubstance Achilles ruptures. Foot Ankle Int 2016;37(7):794–800
10. Mackay GM, Ribbans WJ. The addition of an "Internal Brace" to augment the Broström technique for lateral ankle ligament instability. Tech Foot Ankle Surg 2016;15(1):47–56
11. Broström L. Sprained ankles. VI. Surgical treatment of "chronic" ligament ruptures. Acta Chir Scand 1966;132(5):551–565

45 Semitendinosus Allograft Augmentation of Lateral Ankle Ligament Reconstruction

Steven M. Raikin

Abstract

Failure of rehabilitation for chronic lateral ankle ligament instability often requires surgical reconstruction. Direct anatomic surgical techniques (Broström–Gould) have been described with good long-term outcomes. There are certain situations where direct repair cannot be achieved or where the patient's available tissue quality or underlying deformity would lead to high failure rates. In these situations, local repair can be augmented with near anatomic reconstruction utilizing allograft semitendinosus tendon. This avoids risking injury to the previously described utilization of the patient's peroneus brevis tendon (Chrisman–Snook type procedures), which will weaken the dynamic stabilizers of the lateral ankle. An additional advantage is utilizing biologic tissue to enhance local tissue deficiency, positioned isometrically to optimize function and stability.

Keywords: *ankle instability, semitendinosus, allograft, augmentation, cavovarus, ligament laxity*

45.1 Indications

- Recurrent deformity from failed modified Broström type anatomic reconstruction.
- Recurrent deformity from nonanatomic split peroneus brevis reconstruction.
- Poor local tissue quality due to generalized ligamentous instability (Ehlers–Danlos syndrome).
- Severe varus ankle deformity (varus talar tilt >30 degrees based on weight-bearing radiographs) with complete loss of locally usable tissue.
- Severe hindfoot varus deformity with concomitant lateral ankle ligament instability.
- Associated high-grade tears of their peroneus brevis tendons requiring reconstruction with concern that the dynamic stabilizer of the ankle would be suboptimal and augmentation utilizing an allograft would be beneficial.

45.1.1 Pathology

- Lateral ankle ligament instability.
- Recurrent sprains of the ankle.
- Associated pathology (described earlier) precluding direct anatomic repair.

45.1.2 Clinical Evaluation

History

- Recurrent ankle sprains.
- History of failed physical therapy.
- History/family history of generalized ligamentous instability:
  - Ehlers–Danlos syndrome.
  - Marfan's syndrome.
  - Recurrent joint instability (shoulder, patella, etc.).
- History of prior surgical reconstruction.

Examination

- Lateral ankle ligament instability:
  - Positive anterior drawer test.
  - Positive varus stress test.
- Scars from previous surgical repairs may be present.
- Peroneus brevis dysfunction/pain/weakness despite adequate therapy.
- Evaluate for associated cavovarus deformity.
- Evaluate for generalized ligamentous instability:
  - Beighton score >6/9.

45.1.3 Radiographic Evaluation

- Weight-bearing ankle and foot radiographs should be obtained:
  - May be normal in many cases.
  - Evaluate for cavovarus deformity (hindfoot or forefoot driven).
  - Varus talar tilt >30 degrees (without additional varus stressing of the ankle).
- Magnetic resonance imaging (MRI):
  - Assess for associated pathology:
    - ❖ Peroneal tendon pathology.
    - ❖ Osteochondral lesions talus.
    - ❖ Ankle/hindfoot arthritis.

45.1.4 Nonoperative Options

- Physical therapy with focus on peroneal strengthening and proprioception training.
- Brace immobilization:
  - Semi-rigid ASO (Ankle Stabilizing Orthosis) brace usually insufficient for these severe instability cases.
  - Rigid ankle–foot orthosis (AFO; Arizona brace or molded ankle–foot orthosis [MAFO] brace) usually required.
- Activity modification.

45.1.5 Contraindications

- Immune compromise (high risk for allograft transplantation).
- History of or active perioperative site infection.
- Inadequate bone stock for required bone tunnels (usually fibular).
- Severe ankle arthritis requiring arthrodesis (in patient who is not a candidate for ankle arthroplasty that can be performed concomitantly with this procedure).

45.2 Goals of Surgical Procedure

- Lasting stability of the lateral ankle ligamentous complex.
- Maintenance of ankle function and range of motion.
- Prevention of recurrent ankle instability.

45.3 Advantages of Surgical Procedure

- Fresh frozen allograft can be utilized.
- This is freely available in most institutions.
- No immune typing or cross-matching is required.
- No donor site morbidity.
- Allows anatomic positioning of bone tunnels for ligament reconstruction.

45.4 Key Principles

- Anatomic positioning of bone tunnels:
  - Anterior talofibular ligament (ATFL) footprint in talus.
  - ATFL insertion into fibular.
  - Common flexor tendon (CFT) insertion into fibular.
  - CFT attachment into calcaneus.
- Adequate length on semitendinosus allograft.
- Interference fixation into bone tunnels.
- Fixation in ankle eversion with maximal tightness of allograft.
- Procedure can be performed in isolation, or combined with anatomic ligament repair.

45.5 Preoperative Preparation and Patient Positioning

- Lateral or sloppy lateral position with a wedge or beanbag under the ipsilateral hip.
- Calf or thigh tourniquet can be used.
- Concomitant procedures are carried out as needed.

45.6 Operative Technique

- The exposure for the reconstruction is dependent on associated procedures.
  - If this is the primary procedure, as with cases of Ehlers–Danlos syndrome where the local tissue quality is known to be deficient, a more percutaneous approach can be used. Four small incisions are utilized, one over the ATFL insertion footprint into the talus, a second at the ATFL insertion into the anterior distal fibular, one posterior to the distal fibula, and a final incision over the lateral calcaneus at the calcaneofibular ligament (CFL) insertion (**Fig. 45.1a**).
  - If peroneal or lateral ankle joint exposure is required, the procedure is performed through a curvilinear incision along the path of the peroneal tendons, posterior to the fibula. The flap is elevated in order to gain access to ATFL and CFL (**Fig. 45.1b**).

45.6.1 Graft Preparation

- Different tendon allograft can be used. The semitendinosus tendon is optimal due to the length of the tendon, which should be at least 20 cm long.
- The allograft is thawed and soaked in antibiotic solution prior to use.
- On the back table, a whipstitch is run through each end of the tendon, tubularizing the tendon (**Fig. 45.2**).
- A "Chinese finger trap" wrapping suture can be placed around the tendon end with absorbable suture to bullet-tip the end of the tendon and prevent fraying and jamming of the tendon during passage through the bone tunnels.
- Suture ends are left long to pull and tension the tendon through the bone tunnels.
- We usually manually pre-tension the tendon prior to implantation, but the necessity for this remains controversial.
- The thickness of each end of the tendon is measured utilizing a known diameter measuring system (**Fig. 45.3**).

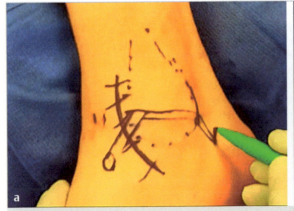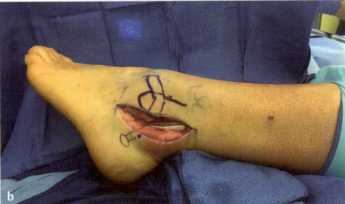

Fig. 45.1 (a) Incision planning for primary procedure with small incision anterior to fibular over anterior talofibular ligament (ATFL) insertion. (b) More extensive lateral incision is made when repair of the peroneal tendons is required.

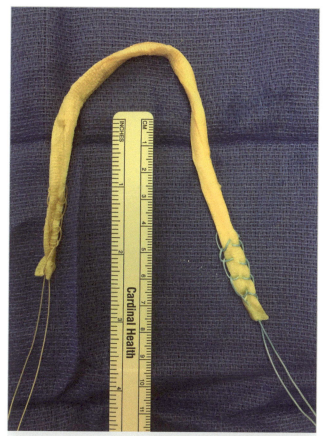

Fig. 45.2 Semitendinosus allograft of adequate length with locking stitches at each end.

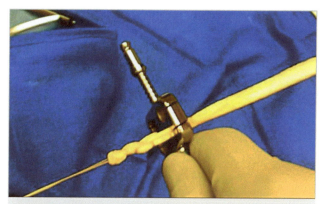

Fig. 45.3 Measuring the thinner end of the tendon's diameter.

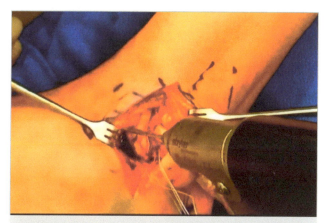

Fig. 45.4 Talar bone tunnel is planned by placing a Beath pin into the anterior talofibular ligament (ATFL) footprint.

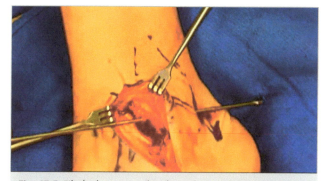

Fig. 45.5 Fibular bone tunnel is planned using the Beath pin from the anterior talofibular ligament (ATFL) insertion into the fibular.

45.6.2 Tunnel Placement

- Whether done open or percutaneously, three bone tunnels are created through which the allograft tendon is passed.
- Initially a Beath pin is drilled from lateral to medial across the talar neck at the footprint of the ATFL insertion point (**Fig. 45.4**).
  - This can be located by direct visualization or under image intensification guidance.
  - This is just anterior to the anterior end of the cartilage of the talar dome, close to the true footprint of the ATFL attachment.
- Based on the tendon diameter, the Beath pin is then over-drilled with a matching sized reamer.
  - The tendon must be able to freely slide through the chosen diameter bone tunnel.
  - In most cases, there is a thinner and thicker end to the tendon. The thinner end will usually slide through a 5-mm tunnel or should be trimmed to allow easy passage through this diameter tunnel.
  - A 5-mm tunnel is then drilled across the talus over the Beath pin at the isometric point of the insertion of the ATFL into the talus.
- A second bone tunnel is made in the distal fibular, again drilled over a Beath Pin (**Fig. 45.5**).
  - This is usually also a 5-mm-diameter tunnel.
  - The tunnel starts anteriorly at the insertion of the ATFL on the anterior distal fibula and exits the fibula posteriorly between the insertion points of the CFL and posterior

talofibular ligament (PTFL). This is a relative bare spot of the distal fibula and can be confirmed with pin placement prior to drilling.
  - This allows a single tunnel to be used in the fibular limiting the risk of bone tunnel fracture and loss of fixation, but care must be taken not to fracture the cortex of the fibular while making the bone tunnel (**Fig. 45.6a,b**).
  - The path of the reconstructed ATFL is oriented approximately 130 degrees with respect to the CFL, corresponding to the normal anatomy. While this does not truly replicate the CFL insertion into the fibular, it allows a single straight bone tunnel to be created in the fibular.

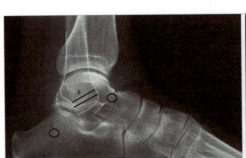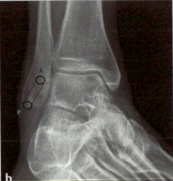

Fig. 45.6 Lateral radiograph (a) demonstrating the anterior talofibular ligament (ATFL) footprint in the talus (A); the fibular bone tunnel directed posteriorly and inferiorly (B), and the calcaneofibular ligament (CFL) insertion point in the calcaneus (C). On the mortise view (b), the fibular bone tunnel is seen within the fibular bone to prevent cutout. The tunnel extends from anterior superior (A) to posterior inferior (P) to the CFL insertion.

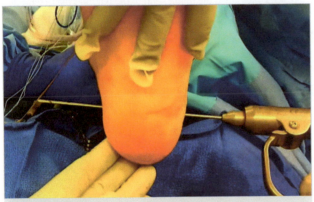

Fig. 45.7 Planning the calcaneal tunnel for attachment of the calcaneofibular ligament (CFL) portion of the graft.

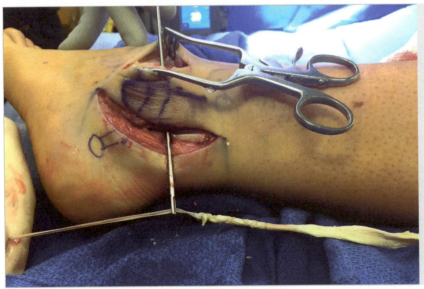

Fig. 45.8 The Beath pin is used to pull the graft through the fibular bone tunnel.

- The third bone tunnel is made across the calcaneus at the insertion point of the CFL (**Fig. 45.7**).
  - This is for the thicker end of the tendon graft, and is sized according to the tendon allograft diameter.
  - Care must be taken to assure that the pin used to guide this hole does not penetrate the subtalar joint.
  - The calcaneus can usually accommodate up to an 8-mm bone tunnel.

45.6.3 Allograft Passage and Fixation

- The allograft is initially passed from the posterior fibular through the fibular bone tunnel anteriorly (**Figs. 45.8, 45.9**).
  - No fixation in the fibular tunnel is utilized.
- The narrow end of the allograft is then pulled through the talar neck into the talar bone tunnel from lateral to medial.
- The graft is fixated into the talar bone tunnel with an interference screw (**Fig. 45.10**).

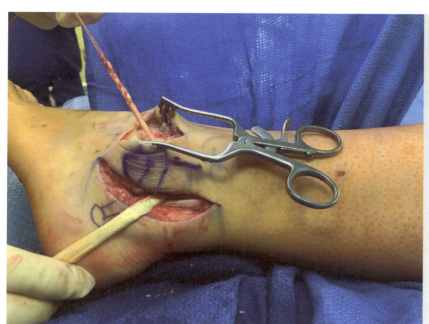

Fig. 45.9 The graft is freely mobile within the fibular tunnel and planned for attachment into the talus (reconstructs the anterior talofibular ligament [ATFL]), and the calcaneus (reconstructs the calcaneofibular ligament [CFL]).

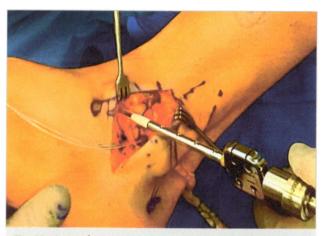

Fig. 45.10 Interference screw fixation into the talar tunnel.

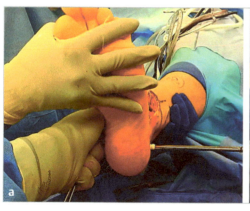
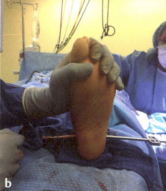

Fig. 45.11 The ankle is held in neutral dorsiflexion and eversion (**a**), while the graft is tensioned and fixed with an interference screw (**b**).

○ The interference screw is sized 0.5 mm larger than the bone tunnel.
• The allograft is the passed under the peroneal tendons, replicating the CFL.
  ○ If there is associated peroneal tendon subluxation, the graft can be placed over the peroneal tendons to act as a restraint against dysmotility of the peroneals.

○ The allograft is then passed through the calcaneal bone tunnel exiting through a small medial incision to allow free tensioning of the graft.
• The ankle is brought into a position of slight dorsiflexion and eversion (**Fig. 45.11a**).

o The talus must be neutrally reduced within the mortise given that it is frequently anterior subluxed in cases of instability or cavovarus.
o The graft is maximally tensioned by pulling through the calcaneal tunnel medially.
o Fixation into the calcaneus is obtained with a second inter-ference screw placed from the lateral side (**Fig. 45.11b**).
o Excess tendon graft medially is trimmed deep to the skin.
o Following wound closure, the limb is splinted in slight eversion and neutral flexion, and maintained in this position in a cast for a total of 6 weeks, with the patient non-weight-bearing on the extremity.

45.7 Tips and Pearls

• Check the allograft before surgery to ensure adequate length and quality is available.
• A slither of allograft is sent for culture to ensure that there is no contamination of the graft.
  o The graft is thawed by soaking in antibiotic impregnated solution.
• Perform any associated procedures before final calcaneal tunnel fixation.
• Ensure adequate strength suture is used in the tensioning end (thicker end) of the allograft.
  o absorbable suture is adequate for the talar end of the graft.
  o No. 2 or thicker suture is required for the calcaneal/tension end.
    ❖ Inadequate strength suture may rupture when being tensioned.
• An anatomic (Broström-type) repair can be performed in conjunction with an allograft augmentation.
  o The bone tunnel within the fibular should be positioned anteriorly just superior to the ATFL insertion in this case.
  o Ideally, suture anchors should not be used, but when used, ensure the tunnel can be created without disrupting the anchors, or risking damage to the allograft by the anchors.

45.8 Hazards and Pitfalls

• The true ATFL and CFL ligaments are flat broad structures, which cannot be truly reproduced utilizing an allograft ten-don. The round and bulky structure of the tendon was felt to be needed to ensure adequate strength of the reconstruction construct.
• Care must be taken in creating the bone tunnels:
  o Talar tunnel must be within the center of the talus to pre-vent cutout and loss of fixation.
  o Fibular tunnel must be within the center of the fibular with enough surrounding bone to prevent fracture while allowing the tendon to easily pass through the tunnel.
    ❖ If the fibular is small and a 5-mm tunnel will result in fracture, the graft should be thinned out to allow pas-sage through a smaller bone tunnel.
    ❖ This can lead to graft failure and should be reserved for limited cases.
• Graft should be obtained from a reliable American Associ-ation of Tissue Banks (AATB) facility and should be appro-priately tested for communicable diseases and bacterial contamination.

45.9 Complications/Bailout/Salvage

• Complications with this procedure are rare and include the following:
  o Wound healing complications.
  o Infections:
    ❖ Allograft related infections are very rare.
  o Graft cutout of the bone tunnels or tunnel fracture leading to failed fixation and stabilization.
  o Delayed graft stretching and failure may be seen:
    ❖ Particularly if associated cavovarus deformities are not corrected.
  o Sural or superficial peroneal nerve injury:
    ❖ Usually temporary numbness.
    ❖ No motor weakness effect.
    ❖ May result in chronic numbness or hypersensitivity.

45.10 Postoperative Care

• Patients are kept non-weight-bearing in a short leg cast for 6 weeks:
  o Allograft tissue requires longer stabilization than local anatomic tissue.
• Weight-bearing as tolerated in a boot is initiated at 6 weeks:
  o This may be delayed if required by the associated bony procedures.
• Physical therapy is initiated at 6 weeks:
  o Peroneal strengthening and proprioceptive training fo-cused.
  o Avoid inversion beyond neutral until 12 weeks postsur-gery.
• At 12 weeks, patients are weaned to a stirrup brace in a sneaker:
  o Physical therapy is allowed to start gentle inversion, with continued strengthening.
• Brace is weaned at 18 weeks.
• Sports participation is progressed as tolerated, but side-to-side cutting is avoided for 6 months.

45.11 Outcomes

• Dierckman and Ferkel[1] reviewed 33 ankles stabilized with an isolated semitendinosus allograft reconstruction:
  o One hundred percent of patients were completely satisfied with the procedure at an average 38 months.
  o AOFAS-AH (American Orthopaedic Foot and Ankle Society Ankle–Hindfoot) score significantly improved from a mean of 60.3 to 87.5 ($p < 0.0001$).
  o VAS (visual analog scale) pain scores significantly de-creased from 7.3 to 1.9 ($p < 0.0001$).
  o Twenty-two of 31 patients (71%) either returned to or were one level below their preinjury Tegner activity level.
  o On stress radiographs, the mean talar tilt decreased from 14.3 to 3.1 degrees.
• Jung et al[2] evaluated 66 ankles at an average 22-month follow-up.
  o Mean AOFAS-AH score improved from 71.0 to 90.9 ($p < 0.05$).

- The mean VAS pain score decreased from 5.5 to 1.3 ($p < 0.05$).
- The mean Karlsson–Peterson score improved from 55.1 to 90.3.
- Talar tilt decreased from 14.8 to 3.9 degrees.
- There was no significant difference in clinical outcomes between the pre-tensioned and non–pre-tensioned groups.
- Wang and Xu[3] and Xu et al[4] independently reviewed patients undergoing percutaneous semitendinosus allograft lateral ligament reconstruction:
  - The mean AOFAS score increased on average from 71.1 to 95.1 ($p < 0.001$).
  - Significant improvement in stress radiographic parameters was noted for the talar tilt angle, with reduction from a mean of 14.0 to 3.8 degrees ($p < 0.001$).
  - No difference was seen in outcome whether a semitendinosus allograft or autograft was used.
- Miller et al[5] reviewed 29 patients undergoing semitendinosus allograft reconstruction for failed prior anatomic ligament repairs, generalized ligamentous laxity, or severe associated talar tilt and/or cavovarus deformity.
  - Median FAAM (Foot and Ankle Ability Measure) sports score increased from 41.7 to 95.2 after surgery ($p < 0.001$).
  - Median VAS of pain decreased from 8 before surgery to 1 after surgery ($p < 0.001$).
  - Radiographs demonstrated correction of preoperative varus malalignment in all but 1 patient.

- No patients developed subsequent arthritis.
- Three patients had mild persistent instability, all of which was managed nonoperatively.
- At final follow-up, 25 of 28 patients rated their satisfaction as good or excellent and 3 as fair.
- No patients required revision surgery.

References

1. Dierckman BD, Ferkel RD. Anatomic reconstruction with a semitendinosus allograft for chronic lateral ankle instability. Am J Sports Med 2015;43(8):1941–1950
2. Jung HG, Shin MH, Park JT, Eom JS, Lee DO, Lee SH. Anatomical reconstruction of lateral ankle ligaments using free tendon allografts and biotenodesis screws. Foot Ankle Int 2015;36(9):1064–1071
3. Wang B, Xu XY. Minimally invasive reconstruction of lateral ligaments of the ankle using semitendinosus autograft. Foot Ankle Int 2013;34(5):711–715
4. Xu X, Hu M, Liu J, Zhu Y, Wang B. Minimally invasive reconstruction of the lateral ankle ligaments using semitendinosus autograft or tendon allograft. Foot Ankle Int 2014;35(10):1015–1021
5. Miller AG, Raikin SM, Ahmad J. Near-anatomic allograft tenodesis of chronic lateral ankle instability. Foot Ankle Int 2013;34(11):1501–1507

46 Tibiotalar Fusion: Open

Meshal Alhadhoud and Mark Glazebrook

Abstract

The open tibiotalar fusion with fibular sparing Z-osteotomy (FSZO) technique increases stability of the ankle fusion to maintain alignment when compared with fibular-sacrificing ankle arthrodesis due to preservation of the fibula acting as lateral strut. Excellent surgical exposure of the weight-bearing surfaces of ankle joint may help the surgeon to perform a more thorough joint debridement and allow for better correction of any preexisting deformities, potentially decreasing malunion and nonunion rates. Preservation of the anatomy of the fibula allows for the option of future revision to a total ankle arthroplasty, which is a familiar lateral approach to an orthopaedic surgeon that is easy and safe. These potential benefits suggest that FSZO ankle arthrodesis may prove to be a superior or at least an equally effective technique for ankle arthrodesis in treatment of end-stage ankle arthritis.

Keywords: *fibular sparing, Z-osteotomy, ankle arthrodesis*

46.1 Indications

• Ankle arthritis:
  ○ Most commonly posttraumatic.

46.1.1 Clinical Evaluation

• In order to formulate an appropriate differential diagnosis and successful treatment, a careful initial history must be obtained, then a systematic physical examination in order to identify the major joint dysfunction. Typically, patients complain of anterior ankle joint pain that increases with walking for short period or prolonged standing, and decreases with rest. A careful history taking should include review of ankle fracture, tibia plafond fracture, ankle dislocation, ankle sprain, and osteochondral lesion of the talus.[1] Systemic diseases include rheumatoid arthritis; systemic lupus can cause ankle arthritis, but it is not common as posttraumatic arthritis.[2]
• Inspect the ankle joint for any previous surgical scars, swelling, and deformities.
• Palpation at the medial and lateral joint space induces pain; periarticular osteophytes can be palpated.
• There is decrease of range of motion in a sagittal plane, usually forced motion associated with a pain.
• In long-standing arthritis, varus or valgus deformity forms and gait abnormality will occur.
• Neurovascular examination is required.

46.1.2 Radiographic Evaluation

• Weight-bearing radiographs include a true anteroposterior, lateral, and mortise views of the ankle. Hindfoot alignment view can be helpful to measure the severity of the deformity.[3] Decrease of joint space, periarticular osteophytes, subchondral sclerosis, cyst formation, and ankle malalignment can be seen in the anteroposterior view, and anterior and posterior impingement seen in the lateral view. Always obtain a long film to evaluate the lower limb for any deformity.
• There is no role of MRI (magnetic resonance imaging) and CT (computed tomography) scan in ankle arthritis diagnosis. SPECT-CT (single-photon emission computed tomography and CT) scan has 94% sensitivity and 95.45% specificity in detecting joint arthritis, around the foot and ankle.[4]

46.1.3 Nonoperative Options

• Activity modification.
• Bracing.
• Injections (corticosteroids and viscosupplementation).
• Medications (analgesia and anti-inflammatory) and nutritional supplements (chondroitin and glucosamine).
• Patient education.
• Physical therapy.
• Shoe wear modification (rocker-bottom shoe wear) and shoe orthotics.
• Weight reduction.[5]

46.1.4 Contraindications

• Active infection.
• Charcot neuropathic process.
• Generally sick patient or those with poor circulation.

46.2 Goals of Surgical Procedure

Recently, there has been increase of periarticular arthritis in the midfoot and hindfoot joints in the long-term follow-up of patients with prior ankle arthrodesis. This has led some surgeons to convert ankle arthrodesis to total ankle arthroplasty, which is contraindicated if the lateral malleoli are scarified. This chapter describes a fibular sparing Z-osteotomy (FSZO) surgical technique that is designed to preserve the anatomy of the ankle joint while providing excellent exposure to correct preexisting deformity and allowing rigid stable fixation.

46.3 Advantages of Surgical Procedure

The lateral approach is familiar to all surgeons who fix ankle fractures. It provides excellent exposure for correction of deformity and stable fixation while avoiding neurovascular structures located anteriorly and medially. The lateral approach spares the anterior soft tissue that will need to be used if conversion to a total ankle arthroplasty is necessary.

46.4 Key Principles

- Extensile lateral approach of the ankle.
- Z-osteotomy of the fibula.
- Taking medial third of the fibula to use as bone graft.
- Clear visualization of all articular surfaces.
- Using osteotome in joint preparation.
- Insert the talus screw first to achieve good compression at the fusion site.

46.5 Preoperative Preparation and Patient Positioning

- Open discussion with the patient on the risks, benefits, and limitations of ankle arthrodesis.
- Patient history and physical examination should be taken to determine medical fitness for surgery.
- Patient should also be examined for ipsilateral lower extremity deformities above the ankle that may need to be corrected first.
- Patient should have standing lateral and anteroposterior radiographs of the foot and ankle to determine if there is preexisting deformity or fracture that may need concurrent treatment.

46.6 Operative Technique

- The patient is positioned on the operating table in the lateral decubitus position with the operative limb up. This facilitates easy approach to the ankle joint and avoids interference from the operating table that the surgeon may experience in the supine position.
- Further, the lateral position also provides an excellent view of the coronal and sagittal hindfoot alignment, which is essential for successful positioning of ankle arthrodesis.

- A tourniquet is applied to the thigh and inflated to 350 mm Hg. The leg is prepared, draped, and then sterilized using a soap scrub before betadine painting.
- The incision is made on the lateral aspect of the ankle directly over the fibula starting distal in the sinus tarsi region, then carried in a curved fashion proximally to a point approximately 10 cm from the initiation of the incision (**Fig. 46.1**).
- The skin and subcutaneous soft tissue are then incised down to the fibula with care taken not to cut neural vascular structures.
- Soft tissue is then gently dissected off the anterior and posterior border of the fibula to allow placement of retractors to visualize the site of the FSZO (**Fig. 46.2**).
- A mini-sagittal saw with a long thin blade is used to make the initial 2-cm cut (**Fig. 46.3**) along the longitudinal axis of the fibula in the sagittal plane, beginning approximately 2 to 3 cm proximal to the ankle joint. The second cut is made in the axial plane beginning at the fibula (**Fig. 46.4**), thus separating the fibula into distal and proximal portions.
- The distal portion of the fibula may then be rotated externally, using a posterior soft-tissue hinge, thus providing excellent exposure (**Fig. 46.5**) to the weight-bearing surface of the ankle joint, allowing distraction of the joint using a laminar spreader (**Fig. 46.6**).

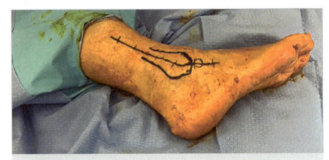

Fig. 46.1 Extensile lateral ankle incision of the right ankle.

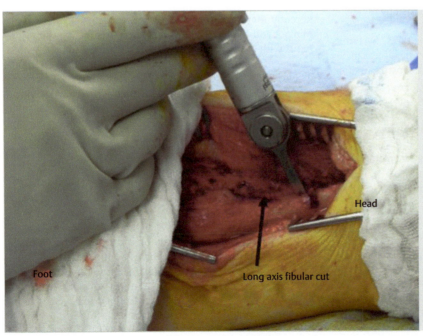

Fig. 46.2 Long axis cut of the Z-osteotomy of the fibula in the sagittal plane for the left ankle.

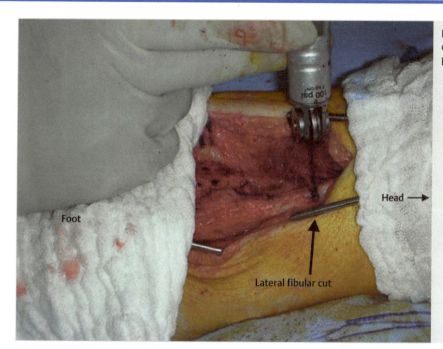

Fig. 46.3 Lateral aspect cut of the Z-osteotomy of the fibula in the transverse plane proximally for the left ankle.

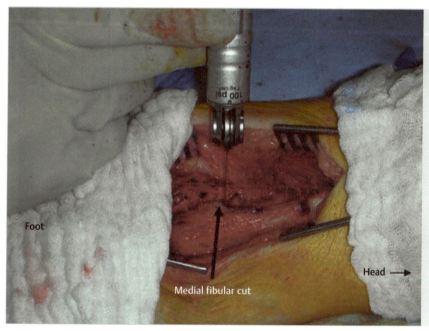

Fig. 46.4 Medial aspect cut of the Z-osteotomy of the fibula in the transverse plane distally for the left ankle.

- The arthrodesis site is prepared by decorticating any remaining arthritic cartilage from the talar dome and the tibial plafond using a combination of osteotomes, rongeurs, and curettes.
- The decorticated surfaces of the ankle joint are then foraged using a 2-mm drill bit on high-speed drill, while all bones removed during the decortication process are stripped of all soft tissues and cartilages (**Fig. 46.7a,b**).
- These bones are then morselized and if necessary mixed with a bone graft substitute and grafted into the arthrodesis site.
- Stable fixation of the FSZO ankle arthrodesis in the appropriate position (90-degree dorsiflexion, 5-degree valgus, and slight external rotation) is then achieved using cannulated 7.3-mm half-threaded cancellous screws.
- The first screw is placed obliquely across the fusion site entering the talus at the superior portion of the sinus tarsi and directed to the medial border of the tibia. The second screw is also placed obliquely across the fusion site entering the lateral border of the tibia approximately 3 cm proximal to the fusion site and directed toward the medial wall of the talar body, taking great care not to enter the subtalar joint (**Fig. 46.8a,b**).
- Once adequate fixation is achieved, an intraoperative fluoroscopy is used to confirm adequate hardware placement and fusion positioning.
- The fibula osteotomy is then reduced and fixed with a small fragment plate, using a combination of cortical and cancellous screws.
- Wounds are then irrigated and closed using a no. 1 Vicryl suture for deep layer and 2.0 Vicryl suture for subcutaneous layer with staples in the skin.

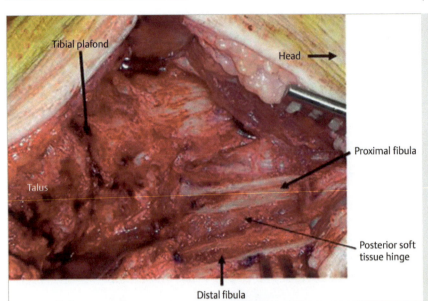

Fig. 46.5 Completed opening of the Z-osteotomy of the fibula laterally exposing lateral aspect of the left ankle joint.

Tibial plafond

Head

Talus

Proximal fibula

Posterior soft tissue hinge

Distal fibula

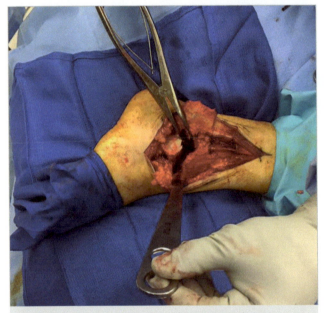

Fig. 46.6 Distraction of the right ankle joint using laminar spreader.

- A compression dressing is then applied, tourniquet deflated, and plaster of Paris posterior and "U" slabs are applied that are converted to a circumferential cast at 10 to 14 days postoperatively with stich removal and wound inspection.

46.7 Tips and Pearls

- Extensile lateral ankle approach with fibular Z-osteotomy facilitates visualization of all ankle joints.
- Resect the medial third of the fibula and morselize it to use it as a graft.
- Dismantle cartilage from the medial malleolus by using the osteotome to allow a slight medial translation of the talus to be perfectly positioned under the tibia plafond.
- Forage the sclerotic subchondral bone with a 2.5-mm drill bit to enhance revascularization.

- The aim position is neutral position in sagittal plane, 5-degree valgus, and 5- to 10-degree external rotation. The external rotation must be symmetrical to the contralateral physiological normal ankle.
- Valgus ankle deformity is cut more from the lateral side of the joint to correct the deformity, while varus deformity is cut more from medial side of the joint to correct the deformity.
- Start with talar screw first to achieve more compression at the fusion site.

46.8 Hazards and Pitfalls

- Avoid breaking the fibula during Z-osteotomy and make sure that the sagittal osteotomy level is in the middle of the fibula.
- Avoid injury of the peroneal artery specially when dissecting syndesmosis posteriorly to open the Z-osteotomy of the fibula.
- Avoid using high-speed burr to prepare the articular surface; it causes localized osteonecrosis that may delay healing.
- Avoid taking too much of the subchondral bone; the bone surface should be uniformly leveled to avoid malposition.
- Avoid varus or excessive valgus ankle.
- Avoid equinus especially in cavus or forefoot plantar flexion.
- Avoid penetrating subtalar joint with the screw directed anterolateral of the tibia to posteromedial of the talus; fluoroscopy image is recommended at this stage.

46.9 Complications/Bailout/Salvage

46.9.1 Early Complications

- Risk of anesthesia and risk related to patient health.
- Malposition.
- Superficial wound infection or wound dehiscence.
- Neurovascular injury especially the superficial peroneal nerve.

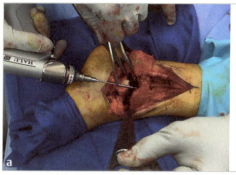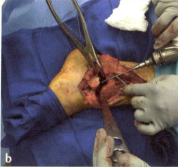

Fig. 46.7 (a) Forage the tibial articular surface for the right ankle using a 2-mm drill bit. **(b)** Forage the talar articular surface for the right ankle using a 2-mm drill bit.

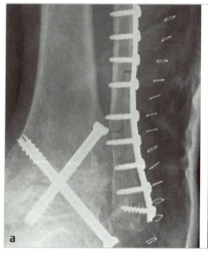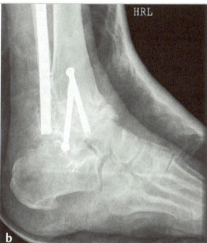

Fig. 46.8 (a,b) AP (anteroposterior) and lateral radiographs of FSZO (fibular sparing Z-osteotomy) immediately postoperative with crossing cannulated screws securing the ankle arthrodesis and small fragment plate and screws securing the Z-osteotomy.

46.9.2 Late Complications

- Nonunion, especially in smoker patients.
- Malunion.
- Failure of fixations.
- Late infection.
- Adjacent segment arthritis:
  - Subtalar joint.
  - Midfoot.

46.10 Postoperative Care

- Hospital stay of 1 to 3 days with a return clinic visit at 10 to 14 days for cast change and suture removal.
- The patient should be instructed to remain non-weight-bearing for 6 weeks, then be allowed to progressively increase weight-bearing at the rate of 25% of body weight per week in a removable cast boot, which subsequently weans after full weight-bearing is achieved.
- The patient is then informed to modify weight-bearing activities according to the pain and swelling experience over the next 6 months.

46.11 Outcomes

- The clinical data of patients who underwent an FSZO ankle arthrodesis were studied preoperatively and at 6 months postoperatively. There were no records of cases of complications in the Canadian Orthopaedic Foot and Ankle Society Surgical Treatment of Ankle Arthritis Outcome Study.

- The initial mean total ankle osteoarthritis score was significantly improved when compared with the 6-month follow-up ankle osteoarthritis score ($p < 0.001$).[5]
- The American Orthopaedic Foot and Ankle Society showed significant improvements from preoperative measurement to the 6-month postoperative measurement ($p = 0.01$).[5]
- The foot function index failed to show an initial statistically significant improvement from preoperative measurements to 6-month postoperative measurement ($p = 0.06$).[5]
- No significant difference was found in the SF-36 (36-Item Short Form Survey) physical or mental health subscales between preoperative and postoperative values.[5]

References

1. Daniels T, Thomas R. Etiology and biomechanics of ankle arthritis. Foot Ankle Clin 2008;13(3):341–352, vii
2. Thomas RH, Daniels TR. Ankle arthritis. J Bone Joint Surg Am 2003;85-A(5):923–936
3. Lee W-C, Moon J-S, Lee HS, Lee K. Alignment of ankle and hindfoot in early stage ankle osteoarthritis. Foot Ankle Int 2011;32(7):693–699
4. Singh VK, Javed S, Parthipun A, Sott AH. The diagnostic value of single photon-emission computed tomography bone scans combined with CT (SPECT-CT) in diseases of the foot and ankle. Foot Ankle Surg 2013;19(2):80–83
5. Glazebrook MA, Holden D, Mayich J, Mitchell M, Boyd G. Fibular sparing Z-osteotomy technique for ankle arthrodesis. Tech Foot Ankle Surg 2009;8(1):34–37

47 Salto Talaris Total Ankle Replacement

Mark E. Easley, Matthew Stewart, and Andrew Harston

Abstract

The Salto Talaris total ankle replacement is a fixed-bearing implant used to treat end-stage ankle arthritis with the goals of providing pain relief, restoring mechanical alignment, and allowing motion of the ankle joint. This chapter aims to describe the operative technique of the Salto Talaris total ankle replacement with step-by-step instructions for the procedure, as well as pearls for implantation and tips to optimize outcomes and limit complications. This chapter also highlights preoperative preparation, hazards and pitfalls of the operation, salvage options, and postoperative care.

Keywords: *Salto Talaris, total ankle replacement, total ankle arthroplasty, ankle arthritis, posttraumatic ankle arthritis, ankle osteoarthritis, fixed bearing, technique guide*

47.1 Indications and Pathology

• This procedure is reserved for end-stage tibiotalar degeneration secondary to osteoarthritis, posttraumatic arthritis, or inflammatory arthritis.

47.1.1 Clinical Evaluation

• A thorough preoperative assessment is performed to include a history of prior trauma to the ankle or other less common etiologies such as inflammatory arthropathy, gout, or infection. A detailed physical examination is performed that includes gait analysis, range of motion of the ankle and hindfoot, and a neurovascular examination. It is especially important to take note of previous ankle operations, the quality of the soft tissues, and overall alignment of the ankle and foot. This is critical for planning of potential adjunctive procedures such as hardware removal, ligament balancing, equinus correction, or reconstructive procedures (osteotomies and tendon transfers).[1-3]

47.1.2 Radiographic Evaluation

• Patients are evaluated with a complete series of weight-bearing ankle and foot radiographs to evaluate the extent of their arthrosis, predict component sizing, check talar dome shape, and plan for potential adjunctive procedures, particularly hardware removal or reconstructive procedures requiring deformity correction.[1]
• Advanced imaging with computed tomography (CT) can be useful to evaluate patients with questionable bone stock or to evaluate cystic lesions.

47.1.3 Nonoperative Options

• Activity modification.
• Physical therapy.
• Nonsteroidal anti-inflammatory drugs (NSAIDs).

• Shoe wear modification with a rocker-bottom.
• Bracing with an ankle–foot orthosis for mechanical unloading.
• Cortisone injections.

47.1.4 Contraindications[1-3]

• Active ankle joint infection or osteomyelitis of the surrounding bone.
• Inadequate soft-tissue envelope.
• Morbid obesity.
• Inadequate bone stock.
• Severe deformity.
• Patient preference for ankle arthrodesis.
• Loss of protective sensation/neuro-arthropathy.
• Osteonecrosis.
• Severe vascular disease.

47.2 Goals of Surgical Procedure

• To provide pain relief with restoration of the mechanical alignment and soft-tissue stability of the ankle joint.

47.3 Advantages of Surgical Procedure

• Potential to maintain or restore ankle joint motion.
• Avoidance of nonunion risk with ankle arthrodesis.
• Improved gait kinematics compared to arthrodesis.
• Avoidance or reduction of adjacent joint disease.

47.4 Key Principles

• Diligent preoperative planning to identify and avoid potential pitfalls. This involves being prepared for potential adjunctive procedures to correct alignment and provide stability to the ankle.
• Meticulous soft-tissue handling.
• Minimal bone resections to provide compact bone for impaction of implants and to conserve bone stock.
• Be familiar with the instrumentation to ensure efficient and reproducible results.

47.5 Preoperative Preparation and Patient Positioning

47.5.1 Templating

We do not routinely template preoperatively, and this is why: We tend to intentionally undersize the initial tibial cut (using a size 1 or 0 cutting block) in order to not cut too much malleoli at the outset. The final determination of tibial implant size will ultimately be determined during implant trialing using a lateral fluoroscopic image to verify coverage in the anterior to posterior dimension. We feel it is critical to ensure adequate implant coverage in this plane so that the tibial baseplate has adequate support on the posterior cortex. If upsizing is necessary at this point, it is then easy to gradually increase the medial to lateral width with the reciprocating saw as needed. For the talus, it is the same initial cutting guides for the 1, 2, and 3 talar prostheses. This means that typically the final decision for implant size does not need to be made until after the initial cuts. Additionally, it is imperative to take into account whether an ankle is "tight" or "loose," which will be in intraoperative finding. A looser ankle demands less bony resection (in the superior-to-inferior plane) and thus often results in a smaller talar component. This protocol allows us to make intraoperative decisions that best fit the patient, for both the tibia and the talus.

47.5.2 Anesthesia

- This procedure is performed under a regional take-home anesthetic block and/or general anesthesia with preoperative antibiotics. The regional anesthetic is typically an indwelling popliteal catheter with a single-shot saphenous block.

47.5.3 Positioning

- Supine, foot positioned at the end of a radiolucent table.
- Bump under the operative hip to place the foot in a neutral position and prevent external rotation.

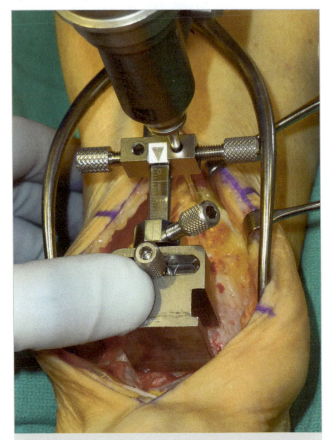

Fig. 47.1 Placement of the external alignment guide. Note how to control resection level (set screw A), mediolateral orientation (set screw B), and rotation (set screw C) with guide.

- Thigh tourniquet recommended.
- Large C-arm fluoroscopy used, brought in perpendicular to the table from the operative side.
- Stack of towels or custom bone foam under the operative ankle is optional. This elevates the operative extremity above the contralateral extremity to aid with imaging.

47.6 Operative Technique

47.6.1 Exposure: Anterior Approach to the Ankle Joint

- A 10- to 12-cm longitudinal, midline incision is marked out. It starts a fingerbreadth lateral to the tibial crest and extends longitudinally toward the second web space.
- Incise through skin. Find and protect the superficial peroneal nerve, resting just above the fascia. Retract the nerve laterally.
- Incise the extensor retinaculum and divide longitudinally over the extensor hallucis longus (EHL) sheath. The EHL is retracted lateral and the tibialis anterior is kept within its sheath and retracted medially. The neurovascular bundle will be seen laterally under the EHL. Once the bundle is safely identified and protected, incise straight down to bone on the medial side of the bundle. There are always crossing veins, which should be cauterized. Raise medial and lateral subperiosteal flaps proximally and distally.
- Incise the anterior ankle joint capsule longitudinally and reflect the capsule and subperiosteal flaps up until both the medial and lateral gutters are accessible. Place a deep self-retaining retractor at the level of the ankle joint.

47.6.2 Placement of Tibial Alignment Guide

- This guide (**Fig. 47.1**) should be placed parallel to the tibia's mechanical axis and in neutral rotation to the ankle joint.[4] A pin is placed in the tibial tubercle to secure the guide proximally. Make a small incision over the tubercle. Predrill and place the pin.
- Place the alignment guide over the tubercle pin in the neutral hole with about two fingers between the guide and tibial tubercle. Distally the guide should rest flush to the tibia at the level of the plafond. The guide should also be roughly aligned centrally within the plafond in the medial to lateral plane. Have the height adjustment set initially at 15 mm (position zero) to allow for translation proximally in a few steps.
- Stabilize the guide distally with a pin through the distal, medial hole (the guide should be positioned in the center of the metaphysis).

47.6.3 Adjustments of the Alignment Guide

- Use intraoperative fluoroscopy and direct inspection to determine the appropriate alignment, tibial component size, and resection level as guided by the external tibial alignment and cutting guides (**Fig. 47.2**).
- Varus/valgus alignment: With the distal end of the guide at the level of the plafond, check an anteroposterior (AP) image

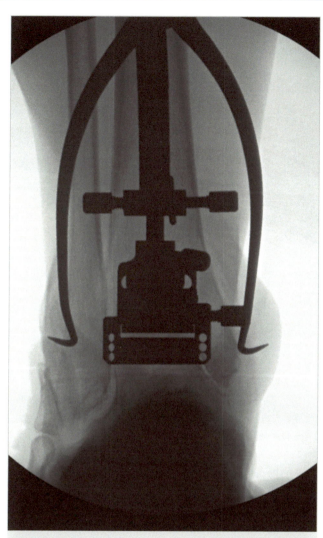

Fig. 47.2 Fluoroscopic image used for sizing confirmation of the cutting block.

to confirm that the resection will be perpendicular to the mechanical axis of the tibia. If a change needs to be made, move the guide on its proximal pinholes.
- Resection level: The minimal recommended resection level is 9 mm (accounts for the composite thickness of the tibial plate and the lowest thickness of polyethylene [PE]). Use set screw A to translate the guide proximally from the level of the plafond to the desired resection level (if the guide was set at position zero, this will allow for up to 15 mm of translation). Tighten screw A to lock in the height of your cut.
- Rotation: The goal is to have the alignment guide set at the bisection of the malleoli. Place the rotational jig on the distal end of the alignment guide and place a pin through the articulating arm. With the ankle in neutral position, check that the pin is aligned with the second ray. Confirm that set screw C is tightened to lock in rotation.
- Medial to lateral alignment: Translate the alignment guide so that it aligns over the axilla of the medial malleolus. The rotational jig also has a series of medial and lateral holes that correspond to the available implant sizes (0, 1, 2, and 3). Tighten set screw B to lock in the mediolateral position once satisfied with position.

- Place the cutting block on the alignment guide. The cutting block size should correspond to preoperative planning and the size confirmed by the last step.
- Lateral slope: The alignment guide should be parallel to the anterior tibial slope on a lateral image. If a change in the slope needs to be made, raise or lower the guide on its proximal pin.

47.6.4 Cutting the Tibia

- Once satisfactory position of the cutting guide is obtained, drill and fill the top medial and lateral holes in the cutting guide and mallet pins down to level of guide (protects malleoli from the sweep of the saw). Drill the remaining four distal holes bicortically to prepare the vertical cuts (drill holes but do not place pins).
- Confirm that all set screws are tightened and perform the horizontal tibial cut with an oscillating saw, carefully avoiding penetration deep to the posterior tibial cortex. Slide the cutting block off. Complete the vertical cuts with a small osteotome or reciprocating saw. Remove the distal tibial segment.

47.6.5 Talar Pin Placement

- The talar pin setting guide is placed on the distal end of the alignment guide. Maintain the ankle in neutral dorsiflexion and the foot in neutral rotation during pin placement. Predrill and place a pin in the hole (**Fig. 47.3**).

47.6.6 Posterior Talus Resection

- Place the appropriately sized talar dome resection guide over the talar pin. There is a guide for size 0 and one for sizes 1, 2, and 3. Use the largest size that will not impinge on either malleolus (**Fig. 47.4**).
  ○ Remember that the final talar component MUST be the same size as the tibial component or one size less.
- The paddles on the resection guide must be flush with the dome of the talus. Confirm with a lateral fluoroscopic image. Drill and place four pins through the resection guide. Each pin should exit at the posterior articular surface of the talar dome.
- The four pins define the upper plane of the talar cut. Remove the talar dome resection guide from the pins. Place ribbon retractors next to each malleoli to protect from the sweep of the saw blade. Make the talar dome resection with an oscillating saw, cutting flush on the top of the four pins (**Fig. 47.5**).

47.6.7 Anterior Talar Chamfer Resection

- Remove all osteophytes from the talar neck with a rongeur. Place the anterior talar chamfer guide (with the talar position spacer inserted in the chamfer guide's oblong window) on to the cut surface of the talar dome. The foot and ankle should be positioned at neutral dorsiflexion and neutral rotation, and the handle to the guide should be appropriately aligned

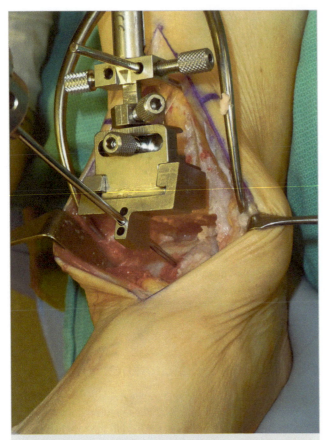

Fig. 47.3 Placement of talar pin setting guide. Emphasizes the importance of this step as final position of talus based off this and demonstrates maintaining the ankle in neutral dorsiflexion and the foot in neutral rotation during pin placement.

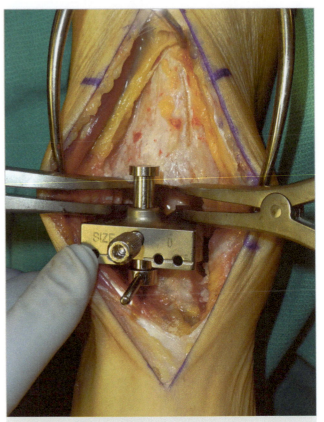

Fig. 47.4 Placement of talar dome resection guide.

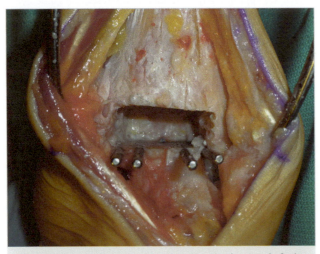

Fig. 47.5 Picture after talar dome resection (and removal of talar dome resection guide). Shows how the four pins define the upper level of the talar cut.

down the second ray for correct rotation. Confirm positioning with a lateral fluoroscopic image. The anterior tibial cortex should be co-linear with the calibration line on the talar position spacer and the chamfer guide should rest flush on the cut surface of the talar dome. Once appropriately positioned, drill and pin the chamfer guide in place.

- Remove the talar position spacer from the chamfer guide and insert the reaming guide in its place. Ream the anterior chamfer through the guide, then flip the reaming guide 180 degrees and ream again to complete the anterior chamfer surface. Remove the reaming guide and the anterior chamfer guide and use a rongeur to clean up any areas of the anterior chamfer surface that need trimming (typically the medial and lateral margins).

47.6.8 Lateral Talar Resection and Talar Plug Preparation

- Place the correct-sided lateral resection guide on the cut surface of the talus. The guide has a mediolateral position gauge on it. The winged component of the gauge should face laterally such that the tip of the wing sits flush with the lateral talus to establish mediolateral orientation. The wing should also be positioned at the apex of the anterior and posterior chamfer surfaces of the talus to establish AP orientation. Secure the guide with pins and joint distractors. Remove the mediolateral position gauge and drill for the talar plug with the bell saw. The bell saw will advance to a hard stop. Remove the bell saw and place the fixation plug to further stabilize the guide (**Fig. 47.6**).

- Complete the lateral talar resection through the guide with an oscillating saw. Remove the fixation plug and the lateral resection guide. Thoroughly irrigate to remove any debris from the joint (**Fig. 47.7**).

47.6.9 Trialing Implants

- Impact the talar trial component in place (**Figs. 47.8**, **47.9**).
- The trial tibial baseplate is secured to a trial poly component to form a monoblock. Thickness of this monoblock can vary from 8 to 11 mm. The monoblock trial is inserted. There is an engraved line on the superior surface of the trial tibial component that should align with the anterior tibial cortex in the correct position. Confirm position on lateral fluoroscopic image to ensure the trial tibial baseplate is resting flush with the distal tibial cut surface prior to keel preparation.

47.6.10 Keel Preparation and Placement of Final Implants

- Drill the most inferior hole in the anterior phalange of the tibial tray and place a pin in the hole to secure the trial (slightly drop hand toward the toes while drilling to prevent posterior liftoff). Drill the second hole, then drill the keel hole with the 7.9-mm drill bit. Remove all trial components. Finish up the keel fin by connecting the drill holes with small osteotome or reciprocating saw. Check the appropriate keel thickness and depth with a graduated osteotome. Lastly, bevel the distal portion of anterior groove with the guide rasp to allow the tibial implant to rest flush on the distal tibial resection.
- Impact the final talar implant in place using direct inspection and a lateral fluoroscopic image.
  The final tibial baseplate and PE component are assembled as a monoblock with an assembly clamp on the back table. Impact the tibial PE component into its final position using direction inspection and a lateral fluoroscopic image (**Fig. 47.10**).

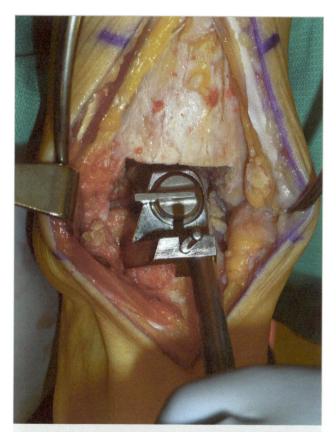

Fig. 47.6 Determining how to place the lateral talar resection guide and using the winged portion of the mediolateral gauge to establish the correct mediolateral orientation on the talus.

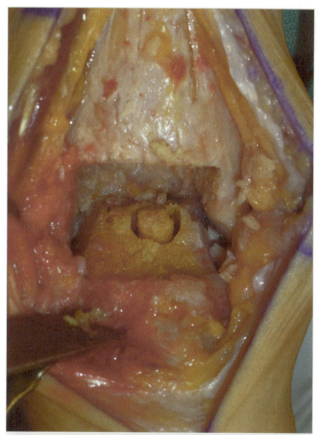

Fig. 47.7 Showing final bony resection. Note the lateral chamfer and talar plug relief preparations.

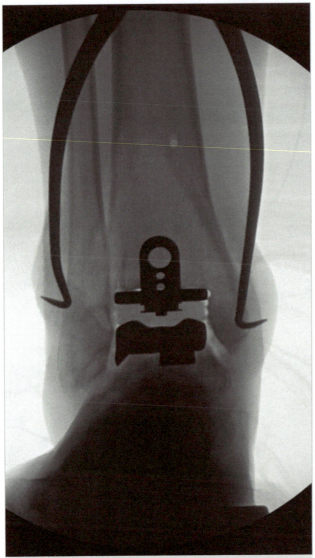

Fig. 47.8 AP (anteroposterior) fluoroscopy of trial components. Note adequate distance from the implants to the medial tibial cortex (protecting from medial malleolar stress fracture).

47.6.11 Wound Closure and Postoperative Care

- Perform a layered closure of joint capsule, extensor retinaculum, subcutaneous tissues, and skin. We routinely will leave a closed suction drain above the retinaculum closure. Apply a well-padded short leg cast with the ankle in the neutral position.

47.7 Tips and Pearls

47.7.1 2015 Instrumentation Update

- Tibial cutting block: Instead of using drill holes to make the vertical resection, this cutting block has slots on the medial and lateral aspect of the guide so that an oscillating saw can be used.
- Posterior talar dome resection guide: Instead of drilling four pins that are used to guide the resection, this guide has a

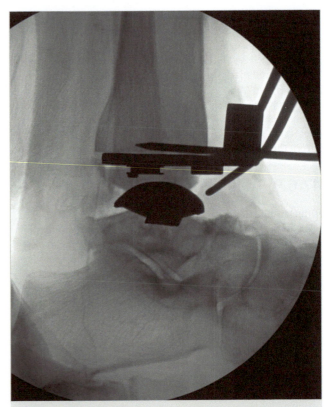

Fig. 47.9 Lateral fluoroscopy of trial components. Note pin aimed-up, helping prevent posterior "lift-off" of final components.

horizontal slot to guide the resection. There are two pinholes on either side of the horizontal slot to stabilize the guide and protect from the sweep of the oscillating saw.
- Anterior chamfer resection guide: The updated guide has additional pinholes for stabilization.
- Lateral talar resection and talar plug resection: The lateral chamfer resection and talar plug are completed through the preliminary talar trial. The correct size trial should extend to but not past the lateral and medial margins of the talus. The trial has a laser mark that corresponds to the apex of the anterior and posterior chamfer cuts to ensure proper positioning in the AP orientation. Confirm proper positioning of the trial using direct inspection and a lateral fluoroscopic image and stabilize with a pin. A joint distractor can be used for further stabilization. The bell saw cut is now performed through this trial. The trial has a lateral cutting slot that allows for a narrow oscillating saw or reciprocating saw to be used for the lateral chamfer resection.

47.7.2 Exposure: Anterior Approach to the Ankle Joint

- Length of the incision should be adequate to insert a distal tibia pin in the metaphyseal region and extend to the neck of the talus distally.
- Meticulous soft-tissue handling and avoidance of aggressive retraction of the skin is essential to avoid damage to neurovascular structures and cause skin necrosis.

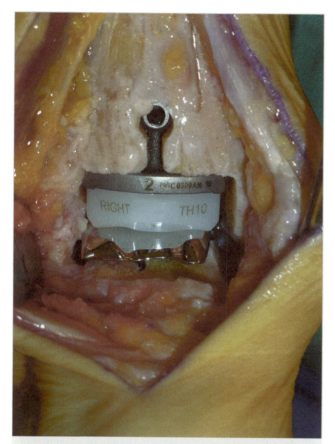

Fig. 47.10 Final implants pictured. Note size 2 tibial component, size 1 talar component, and polyethylene (10-mm thick).

- Highlight the superficial peroneal nerve with a skin marker to facilitate identification during the operation.
- We prefer to use the EHL tendon sheath for our deep exposure. The tibialis anterior tendon sheath is acceptable, but in our experience the EHL tendon sheath allows for improved wound closure and avoidance of postoperative tendon adhesions.
- Once the plane of the subperiosteal flaps has been started, the use of a medium-sized key elevator can be helpful.
- Varus malalignment oftentimes requires a medial release of the deltoid ligament to realign the talus within the plafond. This can be done sharply with a no. 15 blade or with a small osteotome or Cobb.
- Resect any large osteophytes on the anterior surface of tibia or neck of talus with a rongeur or a 0.5-inch osteotome. Use a combination of reciprocating or oscillating saws to expose the tibial plafond, as this is the point from which the tibial resection is measured.

47.7.3 Placement of Tibial Alignment Guide

- Place a small osteotome in the medial gutter to use as a reference for the orientation of the tubercle pin. Have an assistant check that the drill aligns with this osteotome prior to drilling.
- When placing the distal end of the guide at the level of the plafond, it is oftentimes easier to place an osteotome in the

joint and bring the guide down to rest on the osteotome. Leaving the distal end of the guide 1 to 2 mm off the distal tibia allows for easier translation as you set the rotation, alignment, and resection level.

47.7.4 Adjustments of the Alignment Guide

- Resection level: We will cut 8 mm in patients with ligamentous laxity.
- Rotation: It can be helpful to place pins within the medial and latter gutters to use as a reference to make sure the rotation jig is placed at the malleolar bisector.
- Sizing and medial and lateral position: Place a pin in the sizing hole 1 both medially and laterally and evaluate the coverage. Repeat with next size (up or down) until you are satisfied with estimation of implant size.
- Sizing confirmation: Use the largest size that does not threaten malleolus as assessed with direct inspection and fluoroscopy. There are several ways to do this:
  ○ Simply place a pin in the top medial hole of the cutting block for direct inspection to confirm that you are not cutting too much medial malleolus.
  ○ Check an AP image at this point. You should see all six holes of the cutting block that correspond to the width of the tibial cut. This will also confirm the frontal plane alignment (varus/valgus) of the cutting block.
  ○ Pin the cutting block in place through the proximal medial and lateral hole, remove the cutting block, and take an AP image and visually inspect. The two pins will confirm the width of the cut.
- Confirming amount of bone resection: Place a saw blade in the cutting block slot to check the amount of resection and the slope of the resection on a lateral image.
  ○ This system has 3 degrees of anterior slope built in. We typically aim for a cut that is neutral to the mechanical axis, so we take out this built-in slope. This requires moving the alignment guide up a few millimeters on its proximal pin.

47.7.5 Cutting the Tibia

- To avoid damage to the posterior neurovascular structures, cut posteriorly, stop the saw, and check that bone is still remaining. Cut an additional couple of millimeters and check for bone again. Repeat until you cut through the posterior cortex.
  ○ If desired, use a small malleable retractor for additional protection of the posterior neurovascular structures. Make a small incision just behind the medial malleolus and dissect through the posterior tibial tendon sheath to place the retractor.
- Insert a 0.75-inch, curved osteotome and carefully try to remove the distal tibial bone block in whole. If not possible, then we will remove the block piecemeal with the combination of the reciprocating saw, rongeur, and 90-degree curved curettes.
  ○ Oftentimes, it is easier to remove the anterior two-thirds of the tibial block at this step and remove the posterior one-third of bone after the talar dome resection. Additionally, use a joint distractor to provide a larger space to work during bone removal.

47.7.6 Talar Pin Placement

- This is a very important step, as the final position of the talus depends on placement of this pin. Confirm pin placement and angle with lateral image.

47.7.7 Posterior Talus Resection

- For a talus that has uneven wear, use an osteotome or key elevator to remove remaining articular cartilage from the least worn side. This will ensure that the paddles of the talus resection guide rest flush on the medial and lateral sides of the dome. For large talar defects on the dome, there are 1-, 2-, and 3-mm paddle augments that can be used to compensate.
- Two joint distractors, such as lamina spreaders, can be helpful to stabilize the guide's paddles on the talar dome. Each distractor is leveraged with one side on a paddle and the other side against the tibial cut.

47.7.8 Trialing Implants

- This is the time to assess ankle stability and range of motion to determine if alteration of PE thickness is necessary or if additional soft-tissue releases are necessary (deltoid release, lateral ankle ligament reconstruction, Achilles lengthening, or gastrocnemius recession).

47.7.9 Keel Preparation and Placement of Final Implants

- Ensure complete congruity between the tibial baseplate and the tibial resection surface by using the insertion handle to drive the component up against the bone during insertion. Do this by slightly lowering your hand toward the foot and maintaining good contact between the bone and implant as you impact.
- Graft the keel plug with morselized bone from the previous bone resections.

47.8 Hazards and Pitfalls

- Avoid a tibial cut that is too wide and will put you at risk for a medial malleolus fracture.
- Ensure adequate retraction during all saw cuts to avoid tendon lacerations or cutting into the malleoli.
- When removing the distal tibial bone block, do not lever on the medial malleolus with instruments, as this could cause an iatrogenic fracture.
- When trialing, ensure that there is no gutter impingement. If present, then judiciously perform a gutter debridement with a rongeur or reciprocating saw.
- Bone graft any cysts if present, typically on the talar side.
- For patients with a flattened talus on their preoperative

X-rays where talar bone stock may be an issue, we recommend using the Salto XT system, which utilizes a single flat cut across the talus.

47.9 Complications/Bailout/ Salvage

- Iatrogenic medial malleolar fractures can be fixed with parallel screws in a similar fashion to a traumatic fracture. Screws should project in a path outside of the implant so as to be able to continue with the standard operation.
- If there exists a remote possibility of preexisting infection within the joint, obtain intraoperative frozen specimens. Err on the side of caution and place an antibiotic spacer when necessary.
- We recommend including ankle arthrodesis as part of the informed consent in the rare occurrence of intraoperative findings that wound contraindicate a replacement. These could include massive talar cysts or bone loss that would provide inadequate bony support to prosthesis.

47.10 Postoperative Care

- Patients are placed in a well-padded short-leg cast and allowed to weight-bear to tolerance on postoperative day 2 with a cast shoe.
- Patients return to clinic at 3 weeks post-op to have their sutures removed. They are converted to a CAM walking boot to start gentle range-of-motion exercises.
- At 6 weeks post-op, they return to clinic for a return surveillance X-ray.

47.11 Outcomes

- Patients are counseled preoperatively that they can expect significant improvements in pain and quality of life with this operation. They are able to return to low-impact sporting activities (such as swimming, hiking, golf, and skiing) but are cautioned to avoid high-impact activities (jogging or sports that involve running or jumping). Many studies over the last 15 years have supported ankle replacement with good results as it pertains to implant survivorship, patient satisfaction, and clinical outcomes.[5-8] Our institution showed a 96% survivorship in short-term follow-up with significant improvement in their American Orthopaedic Foot and Ankle Society (AOFAS) hindfoot scores, pain scores, and functional scores (**Figs. 47.11**, **47.12**).[7] At midterm follow-up, Bonnin et. al showed survivorship ranging from 92 to 98% with similar trends in improvement of pain and functional outcomes.[5] While this operation is still relatively immature as compared to hip and knee arthroplasty, the results are promising and should continue to improve with surgeon experience and continued innovation.

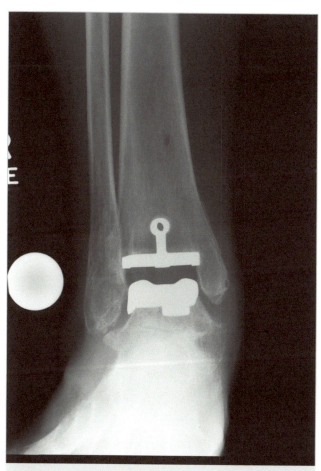

Fig. 47.11 AP (anteroposterior) radiograph at 1-year follow-up.

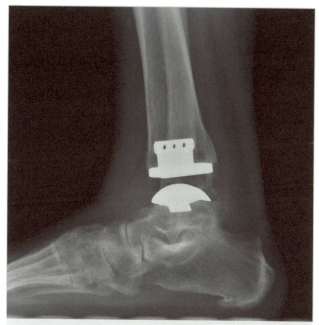

Fig. 47.12 Lateral radiograph at 1-year follow-up.

References

1. Colombier JA, Judet T, Bonnin M, Gaudot F. Techniques and pitfalls with the Salto prosthesis: our experience of the first 15 years. Foot Ankle Clin 2012;17(4):587–605
2. Halloran JP, Parekh SG. Salto-Talaris Total Ankle Arthroplasty: features, surgical technique, and results. In:DeOrio JK, Parekh SG, eds. Total Ankle Replacement: An Operative Manual. Philadelphia, PA: Lippincott Williams & Wilkins; 2014
3. Schweitzer KM, Adams SB, Easley ME, DeOrio JK, Nunley JA II. Total ankle arthroplasty with a modern fixed-bearing system: the Salto Talaris Prosthesis. JBJS Essential Surg Tech 2013;3(3):e18
4. Salto Talaris Surgical Technique Guide. Edina, MN: Tornier, Inc
5. Bonnin M, Judet T, Colombier JA, Buscayret F, Graveleau N, Piriou P. Midterm results of the Salto Total Ankle Prosthesis. Clin Orthop Relat Res 2004(424):6–18
6. Piriou P, Culpan P, Mullins M, Cardon JN, Pozzi D, Judet T. Ankle replacement versus arthrodesis: a comparative gait analysis study. Foot Ankle Int 2008;29(1):3–9
7. Schweitzer KM, Adams SB, Viens NA, et al. Early prospective clinical results of a modern fixed-bearing total ankle arthroplasty. J Bone Joint Surg Am 2013;95(11):1002–1011
8. Singer S, Klejman S, Pinsker E, Houck J, Daniels T. Ankle arthroplasty and ankle arthrodesis: gait analysis compared with normal controls. J Bone Joint Surg Am 2013;95(24):e191–(1–10)

48 Scandinavian Total Ankle Replacement (STAR)

David I. Pedowitz

Abstract

The Scandinavian Total Ankle Replacement (STAR) system is a mobile bearing total ankle replacement designed to achieve physiologic ankle motion and minimize stresses at the bone–implant interface. It is the only implant approved by the Food and Drug Administration (FDA) for use in the United States without cement and therefore relies on bony ingrowth into its porous surfaces. Long-term results suggest that the STAR is reliable in achieving pain relief and good function for the treatment of end-stage tibiotalar arthritis.

Keywords: *total ankle replacement, arthroplasty, tibiotalar arthritis, posttraumatic arthritis*

48.1 Indications and Pathology

- End-stage degenerative, posttraumatic, or inflammatory tibiotalar arthritis.

48.1.1 Clinical Evaluation

- Tenderness over tibiotalar joint line.
- Patients should have pain with weight-bearing activity.
- May present with or without significant ankle, midfoot, or hindfoot deformity.
- May have some decreased sagittal arc of motion at ankle joint.

48.1.2 Radiographic Evaluation

- Plain weight-bearing X-rays of the foot and ankle looking for the following:
  - Tibiotalar congruence.
  - Intra versus extra-articular deformity at the ankle.
  - Hindfoot deformity and how, if at all, it effects ankle joint.
  - Bone loss.
  - Collapse or signs of avascular necrosis (AVN) of the talus.
  - Location of preexisting hardware as it affects placement of implant and impacts the need for removal at the time of arthroplasty.
  - Anterior or posterior subluxation of the talus.
  - Adjacent segment (subtalar and talonavicular) arthritic change.
- Magnetic resonance imaging (MRI):
  - Used in the setting of suspected AVN of the talus that may be a contraindication for arthroplasty.
- Computed tomography (CT) scan:
  - Used to assess bone stock when cysts or osteochondral lesions can be seen with plain radiography.
  - Used to assess talar morphology in the setting of collapse or prior fracture that may affect choice of talus implant or helping to anticipate the need for bone grafting.

48.1.3 Nonoperative Options

- Brace immobilization.
- Activity modification.
- Rocker-bottom sole and cushioned heel to shoe; orthotic inserts.
- Medications: cortisone injection, hyaluronic acid injections, anti-inflammatory medications.

48.1.4 Contraindications

- Insufficient bone stock to support the implant, particularly on the talar side.
- Extensive AVN of the talus. The authors' recommendation is that arthroplasty should be highly cautioned when greater than 30% of talar AVN exists.
- Severe neuropathy.
- Active infection.
- Prior infection remains a relative contraindication and ankle replacement may be performed under select circumstances in which latent infection can largely be ruled out.
- Psychiatric or psychosocial conditions that may make a patient unable to follow the postoperative protocol.
- Smoking remains relative contraindication. The authors do not perform total ankle arthroplasty in smokers.
- Uncontrolled diabetes with an HgA1c greater than 6.5 brings with it an unusually high complication rate and those patients who have an elevated HbA1c should be cautioned about elective surgery.
- BMI (body mass index) greater than 40. This has been shown to lead to an increased rate of complications in hip and knee arthroplasty. To date, no hard recommendations have been set forth for the ankle. Some surgeons use this as a relative contraindication.

48.2 Goals of Surgical Procedure

- Pain- and brace-free ambulation.
- Plantigrade, balanced ankle with correction of any coronal plane deformity.
- Functional range of motion of the tibiotalar joint.
- Protection of the adjacent joints from increased biomechanical stress and potential degeneration.

48.3 Advantages of Surgical Procedure

- It is the only three-piece design available for use in the United States (**Figs. 48.1, 48.2**).
- It is the only FDA-approved ankle implant in the United States for use without cement.

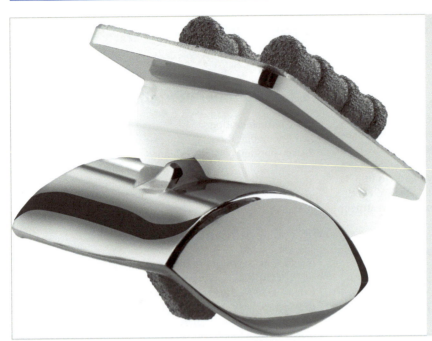

Fig. 48.1 Scandinavian Total Ankle Replacement (STAR) total ankle prosthesis.

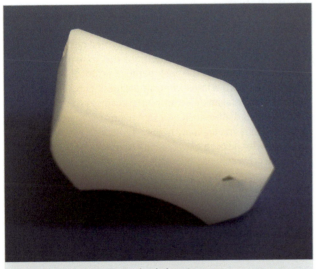

Fig. 48.2 Mobile bearing polyethylene insert.

- Medial and lateral talar resurfacing allows the implant to address some degree of gutter arthrosis without the need for aggressive gutter debridement.
- Minimal tibial resurfacing leaves ample bone stock for potential revision procedures.
- Total resection as small as 12 mm.
- Mobile bearing allows ankle to
  - Establish its own axis of motion.
  - Minimize stress transfer to implant/bone interface as shear and torque and translational forces are dissipated through the bearing surface.
- Window trial for the talar component allows one to confirm and ensure bony contact of talar component with talus prior to implantation.

48.4 Key Principles

- Care must be taken to make sure that the distal tibial and proximal talar cuts are parallel to the ground/plantar aspect of the foot so that the implant is loaded evenly.
- Extra-articular deformities may be compensated for through supramalleolar osteotomies or the bony cuts themselves.
- Effort is made to choose implants that cover as much exposed bony surface as possible.
- Determining the best marriage of stability and range of motion is assessed by trailing polyethylene inserts of various sizes.
- Achilles tendon lengthening or gastrocnemius recession should be assessed for and employed at the end of the procedure as needed.

48.5 Preoperative Preparation and Patient Positioning

- Preoperative weight-bearing X-ray images should be visible in the operating room.
- Patient is placed supine with a bump under the ipsilateral hip to achieve neutral rotation of the lower extremity such that the patella and ankle are facing the ceiling.
- The patient is positioned within 2 inches of the foot of the operating room table.
- Regular (not mini) C-arm image intensifier should come in from the contralateral side with the image view screen near the head of the bed for unobstructed visualization while operating.
- General or spinal anesthesia with a popliteal block or catheter placed for postoperative pain relief.
- Thigh tourniquet.

- When not contraindicated, 2 g of a second-generation cephalosporin and an aminoglycoside antibiotic should be administered.
- Chlorhexidine-based scrub followed by an alcohol-based paint for prep.

48.6 Operative Technique

- A 15-cm anterior incision exposes interval between tibialis anterior and flexor hallucis longus, protecting the superficial peroneal nerve and the deep anterior neurovascular bundle (**Fig. 48.3**).
- A shorter incision will not allow placement of the distal tibial alignment jig adjacent to the tibia.

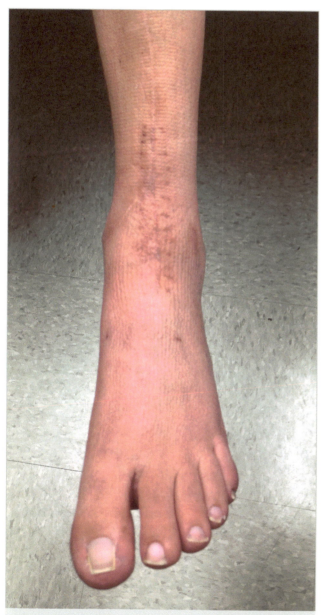

Fig. 48.3 Healed anterior incision for total ankle arthroplasty.

- The extramedullary alignment guide is placed parallel to the mechanical and anatomic axis of the tibia in the coronal and sagittal plane and is pinned to the tibial tubercle.
- The rotational axis of the implant should be in line with the second ray.
- In a tibia without any deformity, the distal tibial cut should be perpendicular to the mechanical and anatomic axis.
- Tibial resection is performed to ensure adequate bone removal and preservation of an ample medial malleolar bridge.
- Talar sizing is accomplished with a talar cut template that is the exact size of the implant itself. It is important to make sure maximum bony contact is achieved, but that the implant does not overhang over the bone.
- Talar cuts are then based on a "datum," an engineering term referring to a point of reference. It is imperative that the datum do not move when the various cutting jigs are applied and removed given this will change the plane in which the talus is prepared.
- Care is taken to use the proper depth and angle with the reciprocating blade when performing the lateral chamfer cut. This will avoid cutting the lateral process of the talus.
- Once proper implant sizes are chosen, care must be taken to drop one's hand while inserting the tibial component to prevent posterior lift-off (**Fig. 48.4**).
- Anterior overhang of the tibial implant is common and acceptable.

48.7 Tips and Pearls

- Once tibial resection height is chosen on a lateral X-ray, always recheck the resection level on an anteroposterior (AP) X-ray to ensure enough medial malleolus has been preserved to prevent fracture.
- Place medial malleolar screws if there is concern that the medial malleolar bone bridge is narrow.
- Treating deformity:
  - Make sure tibial and talar cuts are parallel to the plantar aspect of the foot.
  - Balance ankle accordingly with subperiosteal deltoid release, lateral ankle ligament imbrication, and/or the use of larger polyethylene spacers.
  - Once the components are implanted balanced and parallel to the weight-bearing surface, the decision can then be made to correct any residual hindfoot deformity or gastrocnemius recession as needed.
  - In some cases, once an incongruent deformity has been corrected, there is no longer an associated hindfoot deformity requiring correction.
- When deciding on a size for the tibial implant, we tend to favor better coverage than undersizing. So a larger implant may be chosen when a patient is in between sizes.
  - If one suspects gapping on any area where bony contact should occur on the talar side, morselized bone graft from the anterior chamfer reaming may be applied to the undersurface of the implant.
  - Barrel holes should be grafted anteriorly so that full ingrowth occurs and the implant is "sealed" into the tibia anteriorly.

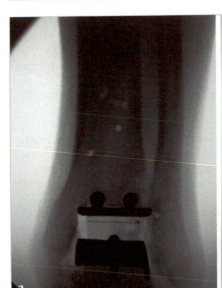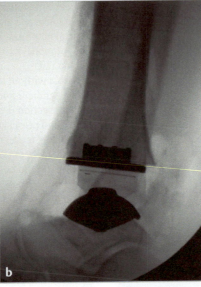

Fig. 48.4 Scandinavian Total Ankle Replacement (STAR) total ankle replacement following implantation on anteroposterior (a) and lateral (b) radiographs.

48.8 Hazards and Pitfalls

- If the medial malleolus is fractured, perform open reduction though the anterior incision and percutaneous screw fixation through small medial incisions.
- *Do not* test intraoperative range of motion without trial implants in place. Without a bearing surface, abnormal impingement of the medial talar neck and medial malleolus can result in a fracture of medial malleolus in dorsiflexion.

48.9 Complications/Bailout/ Salvage

- Sutures are preferred to staples for skin closure. In cases of wound breakdown, local care and prompt evaluation by plastic surgery is recommended.
- In cases of implant failure, revision should be contemplated. When revision is not advisable secondary to infection or poor bone stock, tibiotalocalcaneal (TTC) arthrodesis should be considered.
- Complications:
  - Medial malleolar fracture—use fixation as needed (**Fig. 48.5**).
  - Bearing dislocation—since the tibial tray and polyethylene liner are de-coupled and move independently, there is the possibility of the polyethylene liner dislocating anteriorly or posteriorly. While the authors are not aware of any posterior dislocations, under rare circumstances, particularly if the polyethylene has fractured, it can subluxate anteriorly. Fortunately, the polyethylene liner has two wires in it, which allow it to be visualized on an X-ray. In cases of dislocation, polyethylene liner revision is mandatory and should be considered urgent.
  - Lack of tibial and talar bony ingrowth can lead to loosening, subsidence, and implant failure. Poor bony contact, AVN of the underlying bone and smoking all contribute to this complication. Salvage is either with revision total ankle arthroplasty or tibiotalar arthrodesis. TTC arthrodesis may also be considered when the remaining talar bone

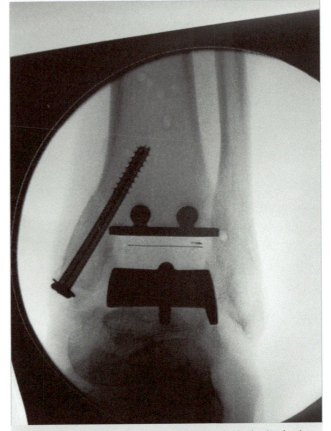

Fig. 48.5 In this patient, a narrow medial malleolar bridge lead to an intraoperative hairline fracture. This was fixed with two 4.0 cannulated screws.

would fail to support either a revision arthroplasty or an isolated ankle arthrodesis.
  - Periprosthetic joint infection is a known, devastating complication in all joints in which arthroplasty is performed. To date, there are no specific recommendations for the delineation of early and late fixation or their respective treatments. Nonetheless, as in the hip and knee, early

infections may be washed out with a concomitant polyethylene exchange, while chronic or delayed infections should be managed with staged re-implantation after a cement spacer and appropriate course of intravenous antibiotics have been administered.

48.10 Postoperative Care

- Hemovac drain is placed and removed at 24 hours to decompress hematoma, which forms underneath the retinacular closure.
- Patients are maintained in a splint in the plantigrade position non-weight-bearing for 2 weeks postoperatively.
- Sutures are removed at 2 weeks.
- Weight-bearing is allowed as tolerated in a controlled ankle motion (CAM) boot at 2 weeks.
- Formal physiotherapy commences at 6 weeks post-op.

48.11 Outcomes

- Recent studies have reported a 78 to 90% midterm survival rate for the STAR prosthesis (ranging from 7.5 to 10 years post-op).[1-3]

- Revision rates range significantly, but appear to be more common at later time periods and appear to be largely related to loosening of the metallic components.
- Data are scant on the relative long-term benefit of a mobile bearing but does not appear to be a detriment to the success of the system.

References

1. Mann JA, Mann RA, Horton E. STAR™ ankle: long-term results. Foot Ankle Int 2011;32(5):S473–S484
2. Kerkhoff YR, Kosse NM, Metsaars WP, Louwerens JW. Long-term functional and radiographic outcome of a mobile bearing ankle prosthesis. Foot Ankle Int 2016;37(12):1292–1302
3. Jastifer JR, Coughlin MJ. Long-term follow-up of mobile bearing total ankle arthroplasty in the United States. Foot Ankle Int 2015;36(2):143–150

49 Cadence Total Ankle Replacement

David I. Pedowitz, Selene G. Parekh, and Timothy R. Daniels

Abstract

The cadence total ankle replacement system is a fixed bearing condylar ankle replacement designed to take minimal talar bone and prevent fibular impingement. Inserted through a standard anterior approach, the system also allows for the correction of talar subluxation in the sagittal plane using anteriorly and posteriorly biased polyethylene inserts.

Keywords: *total ankle replacement, arthroplasty, tibiotalar arthritis, posttraumatic arthritis*

49.1 Indications and Pathology

- End-stage degenerative, posttraumatic, or inflammatory tibiotalar arthritis.

49.1.1 Clinical Evaluation

- Tenderness over tibiotalar joint line.
- Patients should have pain with weight-bearing activity.
- May present with, or without, significant ankle, midfoot, or hindfoot deformity.
- May have some decreased sagittal arc of motion at ankle joint.

49.1.2 Radiographic Evaluation

- Plain weight-bearing X-rays of the foot and ankle looking for the following:
  - Tibiotalar congruence.
  - Intra versus extra-articular deformity at the ankle.
  - Hindfoot deformity and how, if at all, it affects ankle joint.
  - Bone loss.
  - Collapse or signs of avascular necrosis of the talus.
  - Location of preexisting hardware as it affects placement of implant and impacts the need for removal at the time of arthroplasty.
  - Anterior or posterior subluxation of the talus.
  - Adjacent segment (subtalar and talonavicular) arthritic change.
  - Talar dome anatomy.
- Magnetic resonance imaging (MRI):
  - Used in the setting of suspected avascular necrosis of the talus that may be a contraindication for arthroplasty.
- Computed tomography (CT) scan:
  - Used to assess bone stock when cysts or osteochondral lesions can be seen with plain radiography.
  - Used to assess talar morphology in the setting of collapse or prior fracture that may affect choice of talus implant or helping to anticipate the need for bone grafting.
  - Used to evaluate the presence of adjacent joint arthritis.

49.1.3 Nonoperative Options

- Brace immobilization.
- Activity modification.
- Rocker-bottom sole and cushioned heel to shoe; orthotic inserts.
- Medications: cortisone injection, hyaluronic acid injections, anti-inflammatory medications.

49.1.4 Contraindications

- Insufficient bone stock to support the implant, particularly on the talar side.
- Extensive avascular necrosis (AVN) of the talus. The authors' recommendation is that arthroplasty should be highly cautioned when greater than 30% of talar AVN exists.
- Severe neuropathy.
- Active infection.
- Prior infection remains a relative contraindication and ankle replacement may be performed under select circumstances in which latent infection can largely be ruled out.
- Psychiatric or psychosocial conditions that may make a patient unable to follow the postoperative protocol.
- Smoking remains relative contraindication. The authors do not perform total ankle arthroplasty in smokers.
- Uncontrolled diabetes with an HgA1c greater than 6.5 brings with it an unusually high complication rate and those patients who have an elevated HbA1c should be cautioned about elective surgery.
- BMI (body mass index) greater than 40. This has been shown to lead to an increased rate of complications in hip and knee arthroplasty. To date, no hard recommendations have been set forth for the ankle. Some surgeons use this as a relative contraindication.

49.2 Goals of Surgical Procedure

- Pain- and brace-free ambulation.
- Plantigrade, balanced ankle with correction of any coronal plane deformity.

49.3 Advantages of Surgical Procedure

- Cutout in the tibial implant to match the natural incisura prevents fibular impingement (**Fig. 49.1**).
- Minimal talar resection preserves bone stock needed in case of revision.
- Anteriorly and posteriorly biased polyethylene inserts allow for restoration of sagittal alignment.
- Joint space evaluator allows one to estimate tibial resection and ensure cuts have taken enough bone for implantation of the components.
- Minimal violation of talus with pins in order to reduce vascular insult.

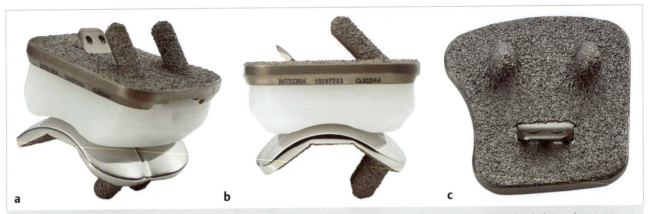

Fig. 49.1   (a-c) Assembled cadence implants. Note cutout in lateral tibial implant to match the anatomy of the distal tibia and prevent fibular impingement.

49.4 Key Principles

- Anterior incision exposes interval between tibialis anterior and extensor hallucis longus, protecting the superficial peroneal nerve and the deep anterior neurovascular bundle.
- The extramedullary alignment guide is placed parallel to the mechanical and anatomic axis of the tibia in the coronal and sagittal planes.
- The rotational axis of the implant should be in line with the second and third rays.
- Care must be taken to make sure that the distal tibial and proximal talar cuts are parallel to the ground/plantar aspect of the foot so that the implant is loaded evenly.
- Extra-articular deformities may be compensated for through supramalleolar osteotomies or the bony cuts themselves.
- Effort is made to choose implants that cover as much exposed bony surface as possible.
- Determining the best marriage of stability and range of motion is assessed by trailing polyethylene inserts of various sizes.
- Sagittal alignment may be adjusted using anteriorly or posteriorly biased polyethylene inserts.
- Achilles tendon lengthening or gastrocnemius recession should be assessed for and employed at the end of the procedure as needed.

49.5 Preoperative Preparation and Patient Positioning

- Preoperative weight-bearing X-ray images should be visible in the operating room.
- Patient is placed supine with a bump under the ipsilateral hip to achieve neutral rotation of the lower extremity such that the patella and ankle are facing the ceiling.
- The patient is positioned within 2 inches of the foot of the operating room table.
- Regular (not mini) C-arm image intensifier should come in from the contralateral side with the image view screen near the head of the bed for unobstructed visualization while operating.
- General or spinal anesthesia with a popliteal block or catheter placed for postoperative pain relief.
- Thigh tourniquet.

- When not contraindicated, antibiotic prophylaxis with 2 to 3 g of a second-generation cephalosporin and 1 g of vancomycin should be administered.
- Chlorhexidine-based scrub followed by an alcohol-based paint for prep.

49.6 Operative Technique

- Balance the ankle prior to placing the external medullary guide.
- Use joint spacer to estimate resection on tibia.
- Place the medial gutter tibial resection jig initially to grossly estimate correct position of the jig.
- Place the "angel wing" such that it is at the level of the subchondral bone, not the ankle joint (**Fig. 49.2**).
- Note the initial size of the tibia from the tibial resection jig.
- Use a reciprocating saw to "connect the dots" on the medial tibial resection.
- If in between sizes on talus, downsize to avoid impingement.
- At times, depending on patient anatomy, the anterior tibial slope may cause the lateral side of the tibial tray to be more prominent. In these cases, consider using a burr to remove 2 to 3 mm of anterior medial tibia to allow for further posterior placement of the tibial tray.
- When implanting on the final tibial component, ensure that the tray is being placed parallel to the cut tibial surface (**Fig. 49.3**).
- If anterior or posterior talar subluxation is present, use biased poly to provide improved talar alignment (**Fig. 49.4**).

49.7 Tips and Pearls

49.7.1 Treating Deformity

- Congruent deformity:
  ○ Make tibial and talar cuts parallel to the plantar aspect of the foot.
  ○ Balance ankle accordingly with subperiosteal deltoid release, lateral ankle ligament imbrication, and/or the use of larger polyethylene spacers.
- Incongruent deformity.

49.7.2 Varus Ankle

• Once dissection is performed to the joint, place a laminar spreader into the medial joint.
• If the talar surface can be made parallel to the tibial surface, then no further adjunctive procedures should be undertaken at this time.
• If the talar surface does not correct, consider the following:
  ○ Medial deltoid release versus medial malleolar osteotomy.
  ○ Modified Broström procedure.

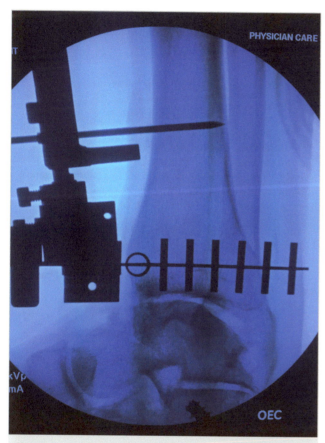

Fig. 49.2 Intraoperative fluoroscopic view assessing tibial bone resection.

• Once corrected, proceed with total ankle.
• If cavovarus foot, consider bony, soft-tissue, and tendon transfer procedures as required.

49.7.3 Valgus Ankle

• Once dissection is performed to the joint, place a laminar spread into the lateral joint.
• If the talar surface can be made parallel to the tibial surface, then no further adjunctive procedures should be undertaken at this time.
• If the talar surface does not correct, consider the following:
  ○ Lateral ligament release.
  ○ Deltoid reconstruction.
• Once corrected, proceed with total ankle.
• If pes planus foot, consider bony, soft-tissue, and tendon transfer procedures as required.

49.8 Hazards and Pitfalls

• When placing talar cutting jig, ensure ankle is plantigrade; otherwise, component will be flexed or extended.
• Once tibial resection height is chosen on a lateral X-ray, always recheck the resection level on an AP (anteroposterior) X-ray to ensure enough medial malleolus has been preserved to prevent fracture.
• Place medial malleolar screws if there is concern that the medial malleolar bone bridge is narrow.

49.9 Complications/Bailout/Salvage

• Medial malleolar fracture: use fixation as needed.
• Lack of tibial and talar bony ingrowth can lead to loosening, subsidence, and implant failure. Poor bony contact, avascular necrosis of the underlying bone, and smoking all contribute to this complication.

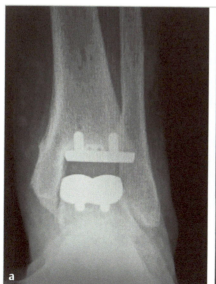
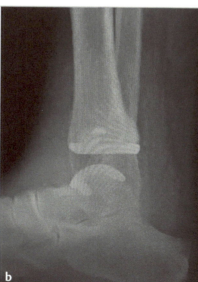

Fig. 49.3 (a,b) Final implants impacted. Note posterior fin has engaged posterior tibia. On an anteroposterior radiograph, a well-sized tibial implant will appear as if the implant impinges on the fibula because it is wider anteriorly to match tibial anatomy.

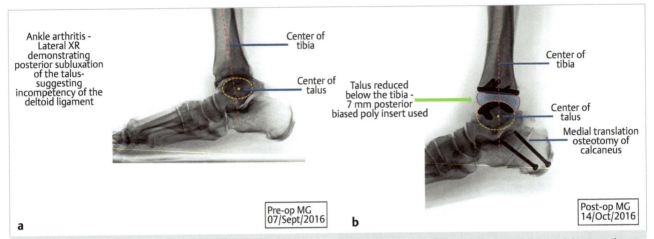

Fig. 49.4 Anteriorly and posteriorly biased polyethylene inserts can reestablish sagittal alignment as seen in the following **(a)** pre- and **(b)** postoperative X-rays.

- Periprosthetic joint infection is a known, devastating complication in all joints in which arthroplasty is performed. To date, there are no specific recommendations for the delineation of early and late fixation or their respective treatments. Nonetheless, as in the hip and knee, early infections may be washed out with a concomitant polyethylene exchange, while chronic or delayed infections should be managed with staged re-implantation after a cement spacer and appropriate course of intravenous antibiotics have been administered.

49.10 Postoperative Care

- Hemovac drain is placed and removed at 24 hours to decompress hematoma that forms underneath the retinacular closure.

- Patients are maintained in a splint in the plantigrade position non-weight-bearing for 2 weeks postoperatively.
- Sutures are removed at 2 to 3 weeks.
- Weight-bearing is allowed as tolerated in a controlled ankle motion (CAM) boot at 2 to 3 weeks.
- Formal physiotherapy commences at 6 weeks post-op.

49.11 Outcomes

No long-term data exist on this implant system given that it is new to the global market.

50 INFINITY/Prophecy Total Ankle Arthroplasty

Steven L. Haddad

Abstract

Total ankle arthroplasty is an accepted and validated technique to treat end-stage ankle arthritis. Experience through the 1990s and early 2000s with longer-term follow-up of second-generation prostheses allowed surgeons to recognize failure through osteolysis and over-resection of the native bone leading to progressive implant subsidence. Lower-profile prostheses (especially the talus component) were then advocated to maximize residual talar bone at the time of implant revision. The INFINITY implant performs minimal resection of talar bone while allowing excellent implant stability (minimizing shear) through component interface with the native talus, and increased radius of curvature for coronal plane stability. Accuracy of implantation is enhanced through the Prophecy system, and it allows the surgeon to carefully plan the surgery prior to entering the operating room (decreasing operative time), minimizing the need for fluoroscopic assistance. Choosing implant size prior to surgery prevents over-resection of bone (and subsequent malleolar fracture) while allowing appropriate sagittal plane coverage to minimize the risk of subsidence. This chapter outlines the methodical approach to advance total ankle implantation through the INFINITY Prophecy system. Tips and pearls will assist the surgeon in maximizing operative efficiency, and hazards and bailouts are linked to prevent the surgeon from defaulting to ankle arthrodesis should intraoperative difficulties arise. Postoperative protocols are described to educate the surgeon on methodology to allow early range of motion without compromising the anterior surgical incision, ultimately creating fluid ankle movement without secondary scar contracture.

Keywords: *ankle arthritis, total ankle arthroplasty, INFINITY implant, Prophecy system*

50.1 Indications

- End-stage ankle arthritis.
- Ankle fusion on opposite extremity.
- Hindfoot fusion/significant adjacent joint arthritis.
- Adequate bone stock (nonneuropathic/Charcot's bone destruction).
- Prior ankle fusion with symptomatic adjacent joint arthritis.

50.2 Pathology

- Ankle arthritis from one of three sources: primary osteoarthritis, posttraumatic arthritis, and systemic arthritis (e.g., rheumatoid, psoriatic).
- There was a time in the history of replacing ankles when one would avoid significant preoperative deformity, ligament instability, or bone loss. It is now clear that all of these pathologic states can be managed with ankle replacement through a structured plan (either single-stage or two-stage correction).

50.2.1 Clinical Evaluation

- The patient is observed standing for malalignment of the ankle and hindfoot, and the full limb is assessed for tibia vara or genu valgum (**Fig. 50.1**).
- Any malalignment must be assessed and measured prior to surgical procedure to assist with planning. Structural alignment of the foot is also assessed weight-bearing for either cavovarus foot or pes planovalgus.
- Weight-bearing stretch (dorsiflexion and plantar flexion) is measured with the examiner on the floor to increase accuracy.
- When viewed from behind, heel alignment is measured, and the patient is asked to rise onto tiptoes to assess both Achilles tendon strength and posterior tibial tendon strength (and ankle stability).
- Seated, the physician performs a neurologic examination to assess for neuropathy and assesses anterior and posterior pulses (and capillary refill) to evaluate vascular status. If either of these assessments creates concern, advanced testing is mandatory.
- The examiner documents prior incision placement, especially in posttraumatic cases, given that this may dictate safety and location of the anterior ankle incision approach. Quality of the skin is assessed for healing potential, and swelling documented to consider compression wraps to minimize this pathology prior to surgery (and lower tension on surgical incisions).
- Documentation of forefoot deformity assists with foot alignment assessment.
- Finally, gait is assessed to look for external rotation, antalgic pattern, and the potential for ankle replacement to have value in improving the patient's gait.

50.2.2 Radiographic Evaluation

Weight-bearing radiographs of the foot and ankle are mandatory to understand not only the arthritis (and deformity) at the ankle, but also the alignment of the foot (**Fig. 50.2**). I also obtain a weight-bearing hindfoot alignment view to assist with deformity correction.

- I prefer a computed tomography (CT) scan over a magnetic resonance imaging (MRI) for assessment of ankle (and adjacent joint) arthritis because this gives a better interpretation not only of the arthritic condition, but also of the quality of bone within the ankle joint (location of cysts, and need for bone grafting following resection for prosthesis implantation).
- I prefer a diagnostic ultrasound for soft-tissue assessment (over an MRI) because this test is dynamic and can discern soft-tissue contracture that may require release or repair at the time of the replacement.
- In addition, for Prophecy cutting block guide design, a CT scan formatted per protocol including both the ipsilateral knee and ankle is necessary to determine the mechanical and anatomic axis of the extremity.

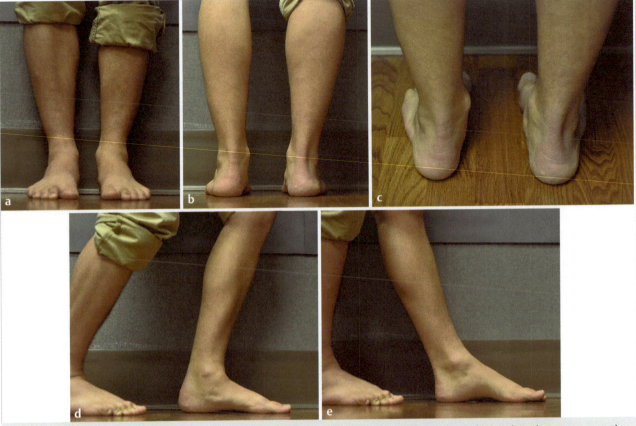

Fig. 50.1 Assessment of clinical alignment of the involved patient with left hemophilic ankle arthritis. **(a,b)** Standing alignment assessed and compared to opposite (right) side. **(c)** Hindfoot alignment assessed for varus/valgus heel. **(d,e)** Flexion/extension measured for comparative purposes.

50.2.3 Nonoperative Options

- Brace management ("Arizona" brace, or more commonly solid nonarticulated ankle foot orthosis).
- Injection of cortisone (preferably under fluoroscopy) for both diagnostic and potentially therapeutic information. These injections should be given no sooner than every 4 months.
- Physical therapy has a limited role, and in fact can aggravate symptoms in an arthritic ankle.

50.2.4 Contraindications

- Prior deep infection/osteomyelitis, though the temporal nature of prior infection should be assessed, and under certain circumstances bone biopsies done in advance of ankle replacement might determine lack of residual infectious process.
- Charcot's or neuropathic bone destruction creates risk for component subsidence and failure (diabetes is not a contraindication, even with mild peripheral neuropathy).
- Severe bone loss (with the INFINITY implant). The INFINITY is a low-profile prosthesis and needs sufficient bone stock for structural support.

50.3 Goals of Surgical Procedure

- Pain relief, not only with ambulatory pain, but also with deep ache that wakes patient up at night.

- Improve motion at the ankle joint, which is now an achievable goal with ankle replacement.
- Lower risk of progressive arthritis developing at adjacent joints surrounding the ankle joint.
- Increase cadence and stride length from preoperative arthritic condition.
- Resume nonimpact activities such as hiking, skiing, and golf in a pain-free (or pain-improved) participant.

50.4 Advantages of Surgical Procedure

- The INFINITY implant is a low-profile prosthesis with the goal of preservation of sufficient bone stock to facilitate revision ankle replacement surgery in the future (and avoid defaulting to often unsuccessful ankle fusion using intercalary bone blocks).
- The INFINITY implant is fixed bearing, allowing multiplanar stability from the implant itself, helpful in grossly unstable patients.
- The INFINITY implant has coronal plane stability through the sulcus geometry of the polyethylene–talus component interface. This allows more aggressive gutter debridement, which improves motion and lessens tricompartmental ankle pain.
- The Prophecy system allows critical preoperative planning, determining the placement of the prosthesis prior to surgery, helping avoid surgeon misjudgment in both extramedullary and intramedullary alignment systems. Also, the surgeon

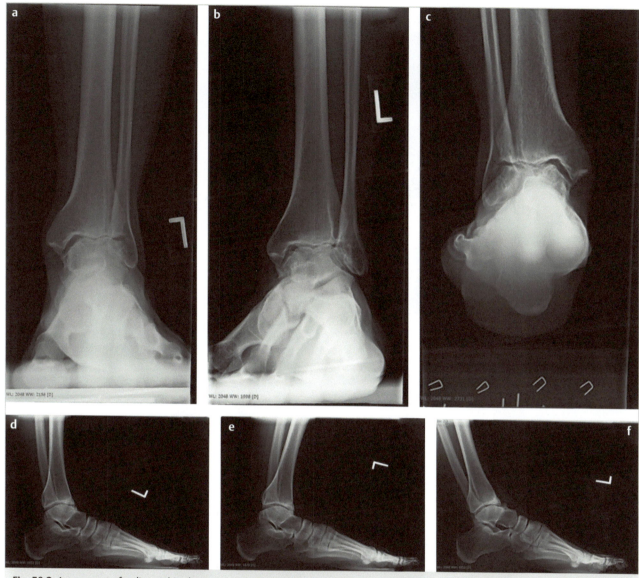

Fig. 50.2 Assessment of radiographic alignment in the same patient. **(a,b)** Anteroposterior and mortise views to assess ankle alignment. **(c)** Standing axial calcaneus view to assess heel position with respect to the tibia and talus. **(d)** Standing lateral ankle/foot view to assess cavus or planus foot and apex of deformity to allow complete plantigrade correction. **(e,f)** Flexion/extension weight-bearing to accurately measure preoperative motion.

can study the ability of the prosthesis to correct deformity without making the incision, and locate bone cysts that might cause late-term subsidence of the prosthesis. Finally, decisions on the need to remove preexisting hardware can be made in advance of the surgery.

50.5 Key Principles

- Central incision placement.
- Limited exposure due to bone sparing implant.
- Prophecy system.
- Reduced reliance on fluoroscopy.
- Reduced operative time spent on component positioning.
- Simplified tibial tray preparation, single cut, and single broach system for fixation.

- Simplified talus preparation, one guide for chamfer cuts incorporates both anterior reaming and posterior cut under direct visualization of posterior structures.
- Mismatch tibia/talar implant size capability allows gutter resections to enhance motion.

50.6 Preoperative Preparation and Patient Positioning

- Standard weight-bearing radiographs of the ankle. This author also always obtains weight-bearing ankle flexion/extension views, three weight-bearing radiographs of the foot (to study alignment and need for supplementary osteotomies/arthrodesis), and a weight-bearing hindfoot alignment view (axial calcaneus).

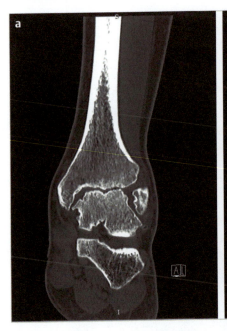
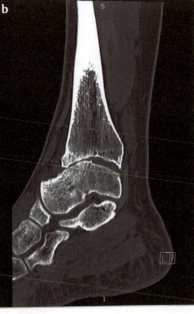

Fig. 50.3 (a,b) CT (computed tomography) obtained with Prophecy protocol includes full ankle scan and knee scan.

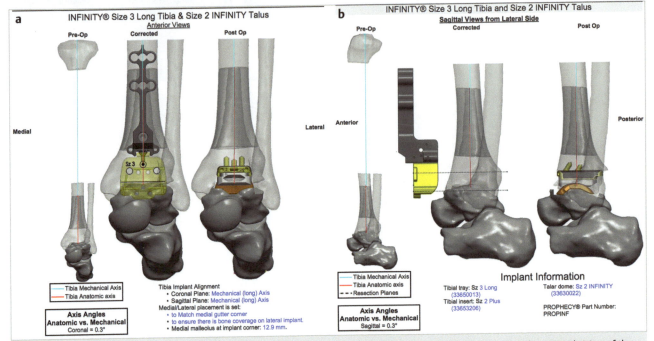

Fig. 50.4 Example of preoperative Prophecy report, manufactured for the involved patient. This report illustrates the coronal sizing of the implant (**a**) and the sagittal sizing (**b**), allowing the surgeon to make preoperative adjustments in size and position of the prosthesis.

- Preoperative testing includes a Prophecy protocol CT scan (**Fig. 50.3**), which incorporates the knee and ankle joints to determine simulated mechanical and anatomic axes of the extremity, and is used to develop and manufacture Prophecy cutting block guides for the tibia and talus. The surgeon is responsible for reviewing the plan (**Fig. 50.4**) and approving it, and should study it carefully because it gives all information about proposed implant sizing, alignment, bone resection, and obstacles (i.e., hardware) that must be removed. This author also provides the company with weight-bearing radiographs to increase the knowledge base on alignment.

- If vascular insufficiency is suspected, preoperative venous and arterial Doppler exams are appropriate. If concern is present, an arteriogram is appropriate (especially in post-traumatic arthritis).
- Patient positioning is done with the ipsilateral hip bumped to bring the ankle to neutral (not internally or externally rotated), the heel at the end of the operating table, and the ipsilateral side as close to the border of the operating table as possible.
- Fluoroscopy is positioned on the ipsilateral side and the scrub tech/nurse is on the opposite side of the involved extremity.

50.7 Operative Technique

- Standard anterior surgical approach, normally 8 to 10 cm in length. The superficial peroneal nerve is defined and retracted. Though most state that the surgeon should not expose either the anterior tibial tendon or the extensor hallucis longus tendon, it is difficult not to do this. Thus, it is more important to preserve the overlying retinaculum for later repair.
- Retract deep peroneal nerve and anterior tibial artery on the lateral side. Elevate directly off bone to minimize injury to these structures.
- The surgeon must remove all periosteum, scar, fibrous tissue overlying the distal tibia bone to allow appropriate fitting of the cutting block guide (**Fig. 50.5**).
- Place the cutting block guide in the position determined by the report, and place one pin in the tibial portion of the guide. Place the longitudinal axis wire into the guide to check guide position under fluoroscopy (**Fig. 50.6**). Check central position of the guide and varus/valgus alignment. If confirmed, place the other three pins in the guide, and check one last time.

- Remove the cutting block guide, and place the Coronal Sizing Guide/Prophecy Conversion Instrument over these wires (**Fig. 50.7**). Use fluoroscopy to center the bull's-eye on the guide, and again use the report as a reference to make sure the implant positioning is correct. Check to be sure the holes within the guide (which represent the corners of the tibial tray) do not violate the malleoli, confirming appropriate size. If you are "coupling" the tibia/talus cuts, bring the ankle to neutral and place two talus pins through the guide. Then, drill the two corner holes in the guide.
- Remove the Coronal Sizing Guide and place the actual cutting block over the wires (**Fig. 50.8**). Place gutter pins in the guide and cut all pins flush. Then, make saw cuts (tibia/medial/lateral, or with a coupled cut, tibia/medial/lateral/talus). Remove cutting block guides and all pins except the most proximal two tibial pins.
- For uncoupled cuts, denude the talus of any residual cartilage and/or fibrous tissue/scar tissue. Place the talar alignment guide (cutting block guide) over the talar neck, and pin in place with the oblique pin, followed by a single parallel pin. Check under sagittal fluoroscopy that the resection margin

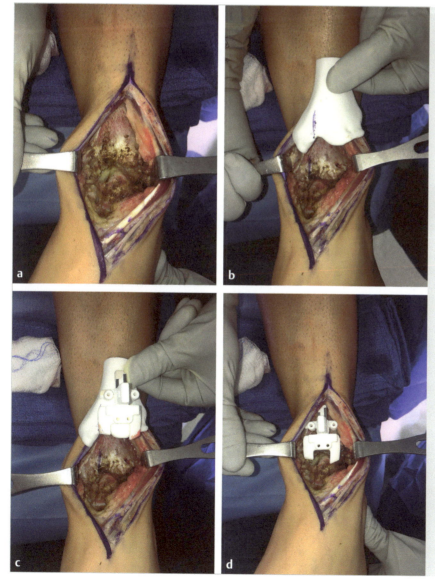

Fig. 50.5 All periosteum has been removed (**a**) from the distal tibia to allow appropriate fitting of the cutting block guide. The model of the distal tibia (**b**) is used to compare placement of the cutting block guide upon it (**c**) improving accuracy of final placement (**d**).

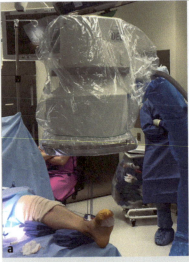
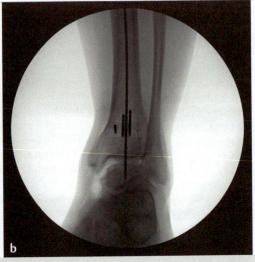
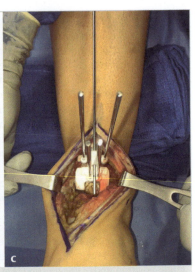

Fig. 50.6 Fluoroscopy is used to check cutting block guide position **(a)**, and, once confirmed that it matched the preoperative report **(b)**, the guide is pinned in position with all four pins **(c)**.

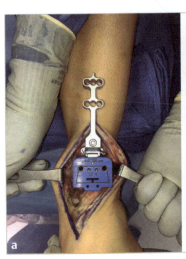
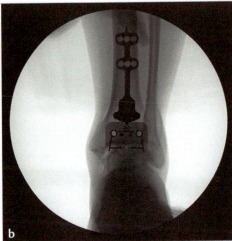

Fig. 50.7 The Coronal Sizing Guide is set in place **(a)** and checked under fluoroscopy **(b)** for accurate positioning (bull's-eye must be centered in the guide to increase accuracy).

off the dome of the talus is correct. Then place the second parallel pin, remove the oblique pin, and place the cutting block back through the two remaining pins. Replace gutter pins and cut the talus. Remove the cutting block guide and remove as much talus bone as is accessible.

- Place the tibial tray trialing (anteroposterior [AP] sizing) guide over the two proximal pins in the tibia, and secure the guide into the prior saw cut. Check sagittal imaging to ensure the guide sits flush with the tibia, and check the sizing (long vs. standard) by evaluating the "notch" in the guide and determining its location with respect to the patient's posterior tibia at the cut line (**Fig. 50.9**). Broach the three tibial pegs (first posterior, then the anterior two pegs).
- Leave the tibial alignment guide in position, and place the talar component sizing guide onto the dome of the talus (now cut flush), and check sagittal imaging to ensure the two triangles cut into the guide are visible symmetrically (**Fig. 50.10**). Place the two anterior oblique pins into this guide. Then remove all components (trial polyethylene first, then tibial tray, and then talus trial).
- Place the talar resection guide base over these pins, and cut the pins short (**Fig. 50.11**). Under direct visualization, cut the

posterior chamfer for the talus. Place the vertical pin into this guide, and remove the two oblique pins. Cut the vertical pin short, and ream the anterior chamfer by first using the scalloped guide, followed by the smooth guide. Remove the pins and talus guide, and clean up any residual talar bone with a reciprocating saw and/or a rongeur.

- Place all trial components into the joint, and place the ankle through a range of motion (**Fig. 50.12**). Use the talus trial to determine appropriate gutter resection margins. Make sure the components are centered, then place the oblique pin through the talus guide, followed by drilling for the two anterior talar pegs. Remove all components.
- Begin with insertion of the tibial tray using the insertion handle and the Offset Tibial Tray Impactor. Start posterior with the impactor to avoid translating the tibial tray posteriorly (use pure axial impaction), followed by anterior impaction. Check sagittal fluoroscopic imaging to ensure seating of the tibial tray.
- Manually place the talus component in the appropriate positioning, and impact with the Talar Dome Impactor (**Fig. 50.13**). Again, ensure appropriate seating in the sagittal place.

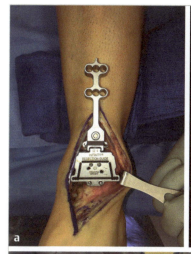
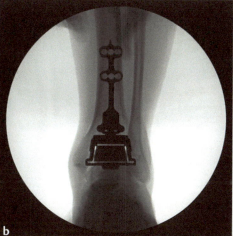
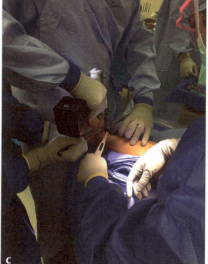
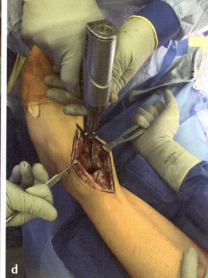

Fig. 50.8 The cutting block is placed over the previously drilled wires (a), and may be checked again under fluoroscopy for accuracy of placement and appropriate resection margin (b). Once gutter pins are in place, the saw cuts are safely made (c). Gutters should be debrided (bone impingement removed) at this time (d) to ensure true talar motion.

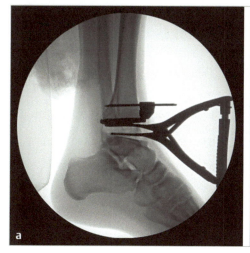
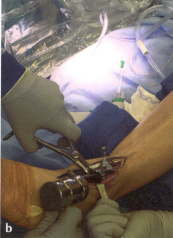

Fig. 50.9 Sagittal imaging is used to confirm the tibial tray is flush with the cut surface of the distal tibia (a), followed by broaching for the tibial pegs (b).

- Trial polyethylene at different thicknesses, and choose the thickness that provides appropriate ligament tension to balance the ankle joint (**Fig. 50.14**). Use the Poly Inserter Assembly over the Attachment Screws to first push the poly to engage the lock detail, followed by the screw-home mechanism to insert the poly into the tibial tray (until the lock detail is engaged). Rarely the poly is not fully seated and the Straight Tibial Tray Impactor is used to complete engagement of the lock detail (**Fig. 50.15**).
- Perform supplementary procedures (Achilles tendon surgery, osteotomies, ligament reconstruction).

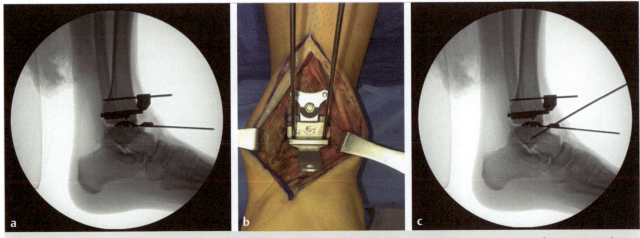

Fig. 50.10 Sagittal imaging is again used to confirm proposed sagittal positioning of the talus component **(a)**. Range of motion is used to determine the "sweet spot" of the talus. Once confirmed (assessed by the perfect "triangles" in the fluoroscopic talar trial), the guide is pinned in place **(b,c)**.

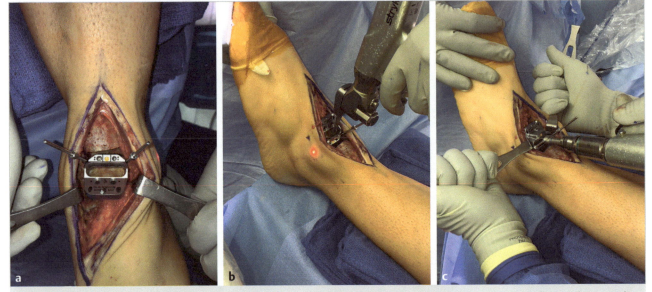

Fig. 50.11 Talar resection guide base in place and pinned securely **(a)**. Posterior chamfer cut made under direct visualization **(b)** to avoid posterior structures. Anterior chamfer is reamed to ensure accuracy in more dense cortical bone **(c)**.

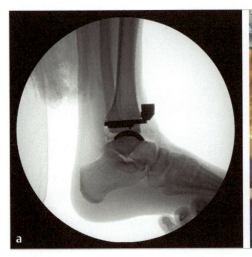

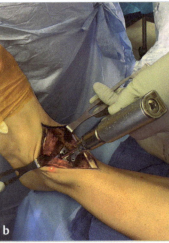

Fig. 50.12 Sagittal imaging showing all trial components in place **(a)**. Ankle is placed through range of motion to ensure accuracy prior to drilling talar peg holes **(b)**.

• Close the deep soft tissue over the prosthesis, followed by the retinaculum over the anterior tibial tendon and extensor hallucis longus tendon, with braided absorbable suture. Use monofilament absorbable suture in the subcutaneous tissue (liberally to take the tension off the incision line) followed by a 3–0 nylon suture in a modified vertical mattress closure.

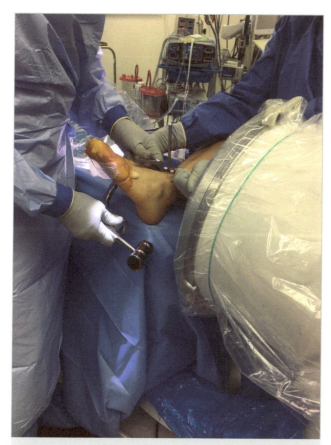

Fig. 50.13 Impaction of final components is performed with Offset Tibial Tray Impactor first.

50.8 Tips and Pearls

• Use a Bovie to remove all scar and fibrous tissue overlying the distal tibia. A fishtail elevator can be used to supplement this removal. It is critical to remove all soft tissues to ensure the cutting block guide fits as proposed.

• Use the provided models of the distal tibia and talus along with the cutting block guides to determine appropriate positioning on the native tibia/talus. Mark the medial and lateral borders of the guide as it fits on the models, and hold the models up to the native bone to reproduce those marks on that native bone. This helps in positioning of the guide on the native tibia.

• With the Coronal Sizing Guide in place and the bull's-eye centered, slightly rotate the ankle medial until the drill hole is perfectly symmetrical. This will give the surgeon an accurate interpretation of the medial corner of the prosthesis. Rotate the same laterally to confirm.

• Be sure not to plunge with the tibia and talus saw cuts. The neurovascular complex can be within 5 mm of the posterior tibial cortex. Gently cut through the posterior bone. In addition, make all talar saw cuts under direct visualization with the ankle plantarflexed (except coupled cuts). This is especially true with the posterior talar chamfer cut. With maximal ankle plantar flexion, the surgeon can watch the saw blade penetrate the posterior talar cortex (this avoids sectioning the flexor hallucis longus tendon, which is directly posterior).

• Perform gutter resection before determining the "sweet spot" with the talar dome trial. This will allow increased range of motion while determining the "sweet spot," making that assessment more accurate. This is particularly important given the limited radius of curvature of this trial.

• Be sure to impact the tibial tray axially (with respect to the distal tibia). Posterior translation of the final tibial tray (due to orientation of the pegs) will create uncovering of the anterior tibial cortex by the prosthesis, enhancing the risk of tibial component subsidence.

• Place on osteotome between the native talus bone anteriorly and the anterior border of the talar component during

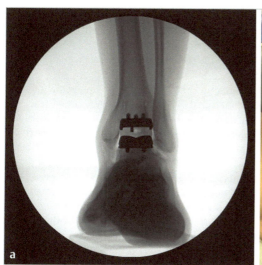
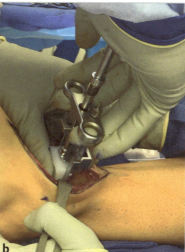
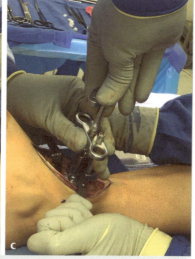

Fig. 50.14 Following talus component impaction, ligament tension is checked with varying polyethylene thicknesses **(a)**. The chosen polyethylene is first engaged via the "syringe" mechanism **(b)**, followed by the "screw home" mechanism to engage the lock detail **(c)**.

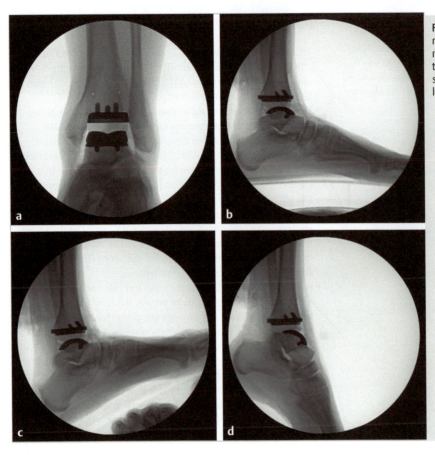

Fig. 50.15 Final implant position in the coronal plane (a) and sagittal plane (b). Range of motion must be assessed (c,d) to determine the need for either a gastroc-soleus recession or Hoke triple step cut Achilles tendon lengthening.

impaction. Lever the osteotome superiorly to prevent the anterior portion of the talar component from being driven into the talar neck, plantar flexing the prosthesis. Once the component is in the correct orientation on sagittal plane imaging, use the impactor without the osteotome to drive it squarely into the talar bone.

- Carefully check ligament tension (particularly the deltoid ligament) during polyethylene trialing. One can lengthen the gastrocnemius or Achilles tendon if required; tensioning creates more limited motion.

50.9 Hazards and Pitfalls

- Be certain that the initial tibial cutting block guide is perfectly positioned. Even slight deviation can create angular malalignment of the final prosthesis or create partial resection of the malleolus/malleoli.
- Implant sizing is critical in both planes, but it is most critical to be sure sagittal plane coverage of the implant reaches the anterior cortex of the tibia. This generally results in the use of the "long" implant.
- Poorer quality tibial bone can create difficult fixation of the tibial component. The tibial component does, however, get excellent stability from its medial/lateral limbs.
- Resecting too much talar bone with the initial talus cut will then create notching of the talar neck during anterior chamfer reaming. This then creates the potential for stress fractures within the talar neck.
- Overstuffing the talus implant (too much coronal plane width) will lead to gutter impingement and ankle joint stiffness/pain.

50.10 Complications/Bailout/ Salvage

- If the initial tibial cutting block guide is pinned incorrectly, remove that pin, and use one different pin site to place the pin into the block after realignment. It is critical to not put more than one pin in at a time, given that block adjustment must be precise to the millimeter, and if one tries to use a hole where a pin was already placed, the guide will invariably be driven to that prior poor position.
- Use the screw home mechanism within the Tibial Tray Trial to give 1-mm overhang of the trial on the native tibia. Then, when broaching (and with impaction) slight posterior translation will still provide complete anterior coverage of the tibial component.
- During gutter resection, do not resect into the medial/lateral portions of the proximal part of the tibial resection (near the transverse limb). That bone must maintain the width provided by the initial saw cuts to allow an interference fit of the tibial tray. Also, you may use cement around the tibial tray pegs to assist with implant stability, and still allow bone ingrowth in anterior and posterior locations.
- If too significant bone resection of the talus is performed during the initial saw cut, do not use the INFINITY talus. Rather, use the INBONE II talus upon the INFINITY tibia (they are compatible due to identical radius of curvature and configuration of the polyethylene). If that decision has been made, you may convert with a formal INBONE II Adjustment Block cut guide to complete implant height positioning, or free-hand the cut with the required bone removal to avoid

placing the implant under too much tension (too much resection for the INFINITY, but too little resection for INBONE II).

- On most occasions, the talus component is one size less (mismatched) from the tibial tray to facilitate an aggressive gutter resection. This not only allows enhanced range of motion, but also eliminates gutter pain. This does not compromise stability, but if preexisting instability is present (usually lateral ligaments), then ligament repair (usually modified Broström) is necessary to balance the ankle joint prosthesis.

50.11 Postoperative Care

- Day 2: Begin compression wrap protocol (**Fig. 50.16**). In our facility, it is performed by the physical therapists, in conjunction with range of motion of the ankle (passive) at each visit. This limits scar contracture around ankle.
- Day 14: Sutures out if incisions are acceptable and continue physical therapy for aggressive passive range of motion.
- Week 4: Begin weight-bearing stretch exercises if osteotomies/arthrodesis were NOT performed at the time of the replacement. If ligament reconstruction(s) were done at the time of the index replacement, use a stirrup brace while performing weight-bearing stretch.
- Week 6: If osteotomies/arthrodesis done at the time of replacement, get CT scan to check healing, then commence weight-bearing stretch. The patient may stand on extremity as much as desired and transfer steps 10 to 20 with immobilization.
- Week 10: Advance to a shoe (if no osteotomies/arthrodesis performed).
- Week 12: If osteotomies/arthrodesis is done at time of replacement, get CT scan to check bone healing, then advance to a shoe. If ligament reconstruction(s) is done at the time of index replacement, use a stirrup brace or lace-up brace until 4 to 6 months postsurgery depending on the level of preexisting instability.

- Six months, 9 months, 1 year, and every year thereafter. Radiographs with flexion/extension views (with three views weight-bearing foot, three views weight-bearing ankle) to confirm well-aligned prosthesis and absence of osteolysis. Any suspicion of osteolysis warrants a CT scan to confirm size and location of lesion. Early bone grafting may be required for lesions in regions that compromise implant stability (medial malleolus, anterior cortical break through tibia, and/or talus). Otherwise they may be monitored with second CT scan 6 months later.

50.12 Outcomes

- This prosthesis was launched for surgeon use 2.5 years ago. There are no short-, mid-, or long-term outcome studies in the literature on the INFINITY prosthesis. At the time of this writing, the author's personal use involves implantation of 88 INFINITY implants over a 3.4-year period (implant was available to designers before national and international launch as a part of a premarket trial). This author's "lower" numbers are due to initial reserved use only in limited deformity or single-stage total ankle arthroplasty procedures. Indications have now been expanded based on durability and success of implant during this initial phase. Forty-two INFINITY implants were performed in 2016 as indications continue to expand.
- During this time, one implant has required early revision at 4 months postsurgery for tibia tray subsidence and one implant required bone grafting for early osteolysis at 3.2 years postsurgery. Four patients required posterior capsule release with medial and lateral gutter debridement to enhance range of motion due to scar tissue and bone overgrowth postsurgery (all four were posttraumatic arthritic presurgical patients).
- The Prophecy implantation system has been reviewed by a variety of authors. Hamid et al compared patient-specif-

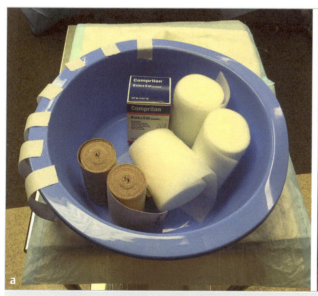 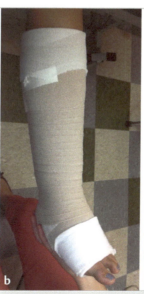 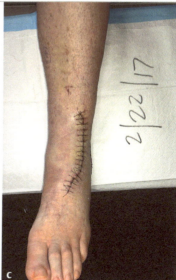

Fig. 50.16 Materials required for compression wrap **(a)**. The wrap is applied every 2 to 3 days **(b)** to eliminate postoperative edema surrounding the incision and lessen incisional wound complications **(c)**. This patient had a prior anterolateral incision from two previous failed total ankle arthroplasties. This photo is at 8 days post revision (×2) surgery with compression wraps removed. Note use of old incision, and note lack of edema (promoting early range of motion).

ic instrumentation (PSI) versus standard (extramedullary guidance) instrumentation for accuracy and cost savings.[1] The prosthesis in this study was the INFINITY implant. These authors found both implantation systems equivalent with respect to postsurgical alignment, but the PSI provided a US $863.00 net savings per case over standard instrumentation. This cost savings was based on an average of 38 minutes operative time saved through PSI, and must be weighed against the cost of corporate development of the report and cutting block guides. Thus, this study must be considered institution specific, given that operative pricing is variable as is that of creating the instrumentation.

- A cadaveric study[2] evaluated the ability to place the implant guides (cutting block guides for INBONE II) in the position expected by the preoperative report. This study found that, after four separate trials per implant guide, the average deviation between preoperative plan and intraoperative guide placement was less than 2 degrees in all planes.
- A more recent study[3] evaluated 29 INBONE II and 13 INFINITY prostheses evaluated pre- and postoperative alignment along with accuracy of PSI to place the implant in the proposed location based on the preoperative report. This study found that this technology allowed the surgeon to place the ankle in a neutral angular position regardless of preoperative deformity. Postoperative weight-bearing alignment views documented ± 3 degrees from the predicted coronal and sagittal plane alignment based on the preoperative report. Predictive implant sizing on the preoperative report was more accurate for the tibial tray (100% INBONE II, 92% INFINITY) versus the talus (76% INBONE II, 46% INFINITY). In all cases, the report was one implant size larger than actually used. This makes sense, as we commonly downsize the talus in order to allow more aggressive gutter resection, and the engineers who design the reports are not clinicians, and do not account for ankle range of motion in arthritic circumstances as a physician would. This emphasizes the fact that the clinician makes the ultimate decision on the accuracy and utility of the preoperative report, and must communicate his or her wishes to the engineers in order to place the perfect implant.

References

1. Hamid KS, Matson AP, Nwachukwu BU, Scott DJ, Mather RC III, DeOrio JK. Determining the cost-savings threshold and alignment accuracy of patient-specific instrumentation in total ankle replacements. Foot Ankle Int 2017;38(1):49–57
2. Berlet GC, Penner MJ, Lancianese S, Stemniski PM, Obert RM. Total ankle arthroplasty accuracy and reproducibility using preoperative CT scan-derived, patient-specific guides. Foot Ankle Int 2014;35(7):665–676
3. Hsu AR, Davis WH, Cohen BE, Jones CP, Ellington JK, Anderson RB. Radiographic outcomes of preoperative CT scan-derived patient-specific total ankle arthroplasty. Foot Ankle Int 2015;36(10):1163–1169
4. Daigre J, Berlet G, Van Dyke B, Peterson KS, Santrock R. Accuracy and reproducibility using patient-specific instrumentation in total ankle arthroplasty. Foot Ankle Int 2017;38(4):412–418

51 Hintegra Total Ankle System

Beat Hintermann and Roxa Ruiz

Abstract

The Hintegra ankle is a three-component ankle that uses a flat, 4-mm-thick loading plate with six pyramidal peaks for full coverage of resection surface of tibia. The talar component is anatomically shaped with a conical form with a smaller radius medially rather than laterally. It has two 2.5-mm rims on the medial and lateral sides which ensure stable position of the polyethylene insert. The insert is available with the thickness of 5 to 9 mm. Given the parallelism of the two interfaces, the Hintegra ankle does provide, in contrast to other current ankles, intrinsic stability in the frontal plane. Its unique design permits to use the Hintegra ankle as a part of hindfoot reconstruction, which may also include correcting osteotomies above and below the ankle, fusion of periarticular joints, ligament reconstructions, and tendon transfers. It also allows to revise a failed ankle arthrodesis to total ankle replacement. With the available revision components with thicker tibial platform and flat talar undersurface, respectively, the Hintegra ankle also enables the surgeon to manage bone defects, as typically encountered in revision of failed component. Conceptor and nonconceptor studies have proven effectiveness of the Hintegra ankle in the clinical use with a survivor-ship of 86 to 93% at 10 years.

Keywords: *total ankle replacement, Hintegra ankle, surgical technique, indication, contraindication, design, revision arthroplasty*

51.1 Introduction

- In the past decade, total ankle replacement has evolved to a valuable alternative to arthrodesis for end-stage osteoarthritis of the ankle.
- The Hintegra ankle is composed of three components and was introduced in 2000 to the market (not yet approved by the Food and Drug Administration for U.S. market).
- Numerous studies have reported very satisfactory outcomes with a survivorship of 86 to 93% at 1 year.

51.2 Indications

- Primary and secondary end-stage osteoarthritis of the ankle.
- Salvage of failed ankles.
- Salvage for failed ankle fusions.
- Low and moderate demands for sports.
- Associated hindfoot or midfoot arthritis, bilateral ankle arthritis.
- Patient not wanting an ankle fusion.

51.2.1 Clinical Evaluation

While the patient is standing, perform a thorough clinical investigation of both lower extremities to assess
- Alignment.
- Deformities.
- Foot position.
- Muscular atrophy.

While the patient is sitting with free-hanging feet, perform an assessment of
- Extent to which a present deformity is correctable.
- Preserved joint motion at the ankle and subtalar joints.
- Ligament stability of the ankle and subtalar joints with anterior drawer and tilt tests.
- Supination and eversion power (e.g., function of posterior tibial and peroneus brevis muscles).

51.2.2 Radiographic Evaluation

- Standard weight-bearing X-rays including alignment view (**Fig. 51.1**).
- CT scan to assess bone stock.
- SPECT-CT to assess neighboring joints.
- MRI to assess vascularity.

51.2.3 Nonoperative Options

- Brace immobilization.
- Activity modification.
- Rocker bottom sole and cushioned heel to shoe; orthotic inserts.
- Medications: cortisone injection, hyaluronic acid injections, anti-inflammatory medications.

51.2.4 Contraindications

Relative

- Severe osteoporosis.
- Immunosuppressive therapy.
- Increased demands for physical activities (e.g., jogging, tennis, downhill skiing).

Absolute

- Infection.
- Avascular necrosis of more than one-third of surface at either talar or tibial side.
- Nonmanageable instability/misalignment.
- Neuromuscular disorders.
- Charcot neuroarthropathy.
- Metal allergy or intolerance.
- Highest demands for sports.

51.3 Goals of Surgical Procedure

- To replace the worn-out articular surfaces of tibia and talus with minimal bone resection.
- To restore mechanics of the ankle as closely as possible.
- To mimic physiologic load transfer at bone–implant interface and thus ensure for long-term stability of components.

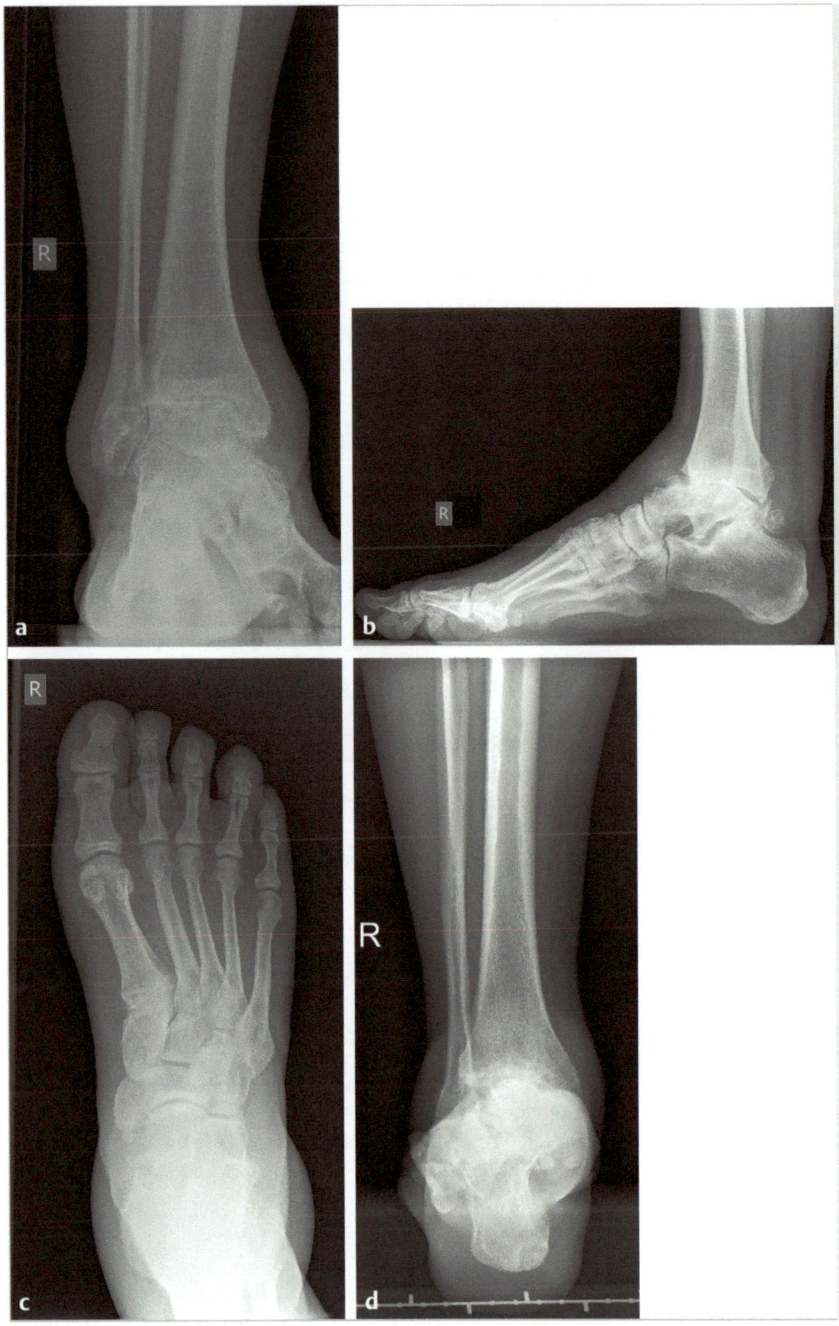

Fig. 51.1 Standard weight-bearing radiographs including **(a)** AP view of the ankle, **(b)** lateral view of the foot and ankle, **(c)** AP view of the foot, and **(d)** Saltzman hindfoot alignment view.

51.4 Advantages of Surgical Procedure

- Simple and reliable instrumentation.
- Nonconstrained three-component device.
- Includes revision implants.

51.5 Key Principles

- Anterior approach to the ankle.
- Mounting and adjusting tibial resection bloc, tibial cut.
- Step-by-step talar resection.
- Debridement of medial, lateral, and posterior gutters.
- Insertion of implants:
  - Talar component.
  - Tibial component.
  - Polyethylene insert.
- Additional procedures, if necessary:
  - To align the ankle joint complex.
  - To stabilize the ankle joint complex.
- Wound closure.

51.6 Preoperative Preparation and Patient Positioning

51.6.1 The Device (Fig. 51.2)

- Design of tibial component:
  - Maximal contact area.
  - Physiological load transfer.

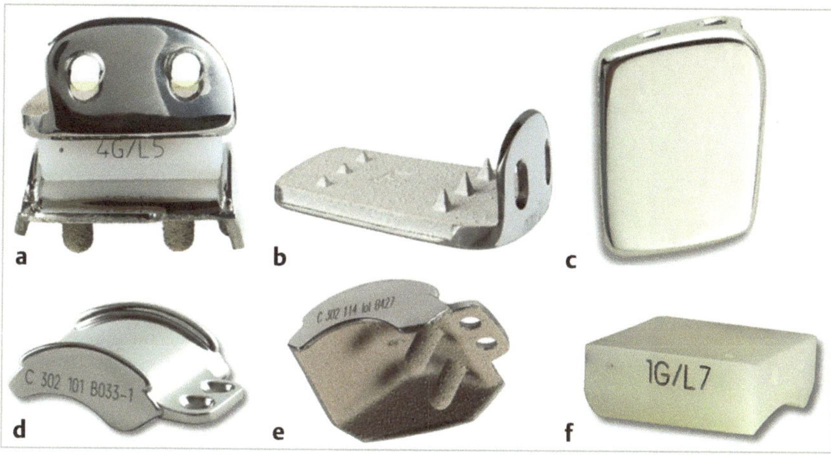

Fig. 51.2 (a) The Hintegra ankle (anterior view): the tibial component— **(b)** medial view and **(c)** plantar view—has an anatomic shape to fit to fully cover the resection surface and to get support on circumferential cortex; the talar component— **(d)** dorsomedial view and **(e)** dorsoplantar view—has a conical form with medially a smaller curvature; and the polyethylene insert— **(f)** anterior view.

- Design of talar component:
  - Anatomically shaped
  - Guides the polyethylene insert
- Design of polyethylene insert:
  - Covers talus completely.
  - Optimal force distribution.
  - Minimal deformation forces.
- Resurfacing alone:
  - Minimal bone resection.
  - Minimal disturbance of vascularity.
  - No stress shielding.
- Minimal thickness:
  - Minimal stress forces.
  - Minimal dislocation.

51.6.2 Anatomy

- The superior extensor retinaculum is a thickening of the deep fascia above the ankle, running from the tibia to the fibula including the tendons of the tibialis anterior, extensor hallucis longus, and extensor digitorum longus.
- The anterior neurovascular bundle lies consistently between the extensor hallucis longus and extensor digitorum longus tendons.
- The neurovascular bundle contains the tibialis anterior and the deep peroneal nerve.

51.6.3 Positioning

- The patient is positioned with the feet on the edge of the table.
- The ipsilateral back is lifted until a strictly upward position of the foot is obtained.
- The tourniquet is mounted at the ipsilateral thigh.

51.7 Operative Technique

51.7.1 Exposure

- An anterior longitudinal incision of 10 to 12 cm in length is made to expose the retinaculum.
- The retinaculum is incised along the lateral border of the anterior tibial tendon.
- The distal tibia is exposed, and arthrotomy is made.

- Loose bodies and osteophytes are removed.
- The Hintermann distractor is mounted on anteromedial side to distract the ankle joint (**Fig. 51.3a**).

51.7.2 Tibial Resection (Fig. 51.3b, c)

- The tibial cutting block with its alignment rod is positioned using the tibial tuberosity as the proximal reference, and the anterolateral border of the ankle as the distal reference.
- The final adjustment is made as follows:
  - Sagittal plane: The rod is moved until a position parallel to the anterior border of the tibia has been achieved.
  - Frontal (coronal) plane: After preliminary fixation of the block with a long pin, the tibial resection block is rotated until proper varus/valgus alignment and ligament tension have been achieved.
  - Vertical adjustment: The tibial resection block is moved proximally until the desired resection height is achieved. Usually, resection of approximately 2 mm on the apex of the tibial plafond is desired.
- The tibial cutting guide is slid into the cutting block, creating a slot in which the saw blade will be guided. The width of the slot limits the excursion of the saw blade, thereby protecting the malleoli from being hit and fractured.
- Tibial cut is done with an oscillating saw.

51.7.3 Talar Resection

- The talar resection block is inserted into the tibial cutting block.
- The resection block is moved distally as much as possible to properly tension the collateral ligaments.
- While the foot is held in neutral position, the resection block is fixed by two pins.
- Talar cut is done with an oscillating saw.
- The 12-mm-thick spacer, representing the thickness of the tibial and talar components and the thinnest 5-mm inlay, is inserted into the created joint space. While the foot is held in neutral flexion position, the surgeon should check (**Fig. 51.3d**):
  - If an appropriate amount of bone has been resected.
  - If the achieved alignment is appropriate (**Fig. 51.3e**).
  - If the medial stability and lateral stability are appropriate.
- The spacer is removed and the Hintermann distractor mounted using the same pins.

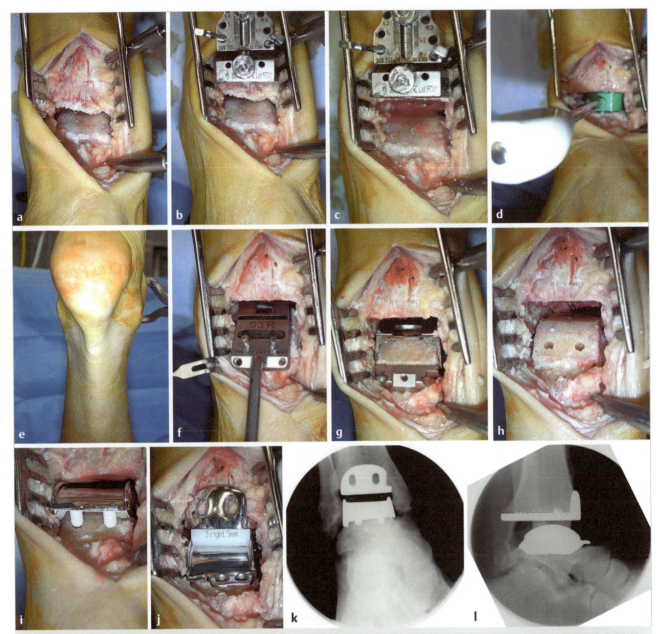

Fig. 51.3 Surgical technique; for details, see text. **(a)** Exposure of the ankle with the Hintermann distractor mounted on anteromedial side; **(b)** tibial resection bloc mounted and aligned before and **(c)** after tibial resection cut; **(d)** the 12-mm-thick spacer is inserted to check the amount of resection cut, the stability, and **(e)** alignment of the foot; **(f)** the talar resection bloc is mounted; **(g)** after having done the resection cuts and cleaned all gutters, talar trial is placed in a press-fit manner, and the anterior bony surface is prepared; **(h)** final talar cuts after having drilled the two holes for the pegs; **(i)** talar component is inserted; **(j)** prosthesis in place; final fluoroscopic check in the **(k)** AP-view and **(l)** lateral view.

- The size of the talar resection block is determined so as not to oversize the previously determined size of tibial component by more than one size.
- The talar resection bloc is first adjusted to the posterior surface of talus regarding the two hooks at its posterior aspect, and second aligned along the medial border of the talus such that 1 to 2 mm of bone will be removed from the medial side of the talus (**Fig. 51.3f**).
- Fixation of the talar resection bloc with two to three pins.
- Posterior resection is made with the oscillating saw through the slot.

- Medial and lateral resections of the talus are made with the reciprocating saw that is guided along the talar cutting block.
- The medial and lateral gutters are cleaned using a chisel and rongeur.
- After resection of the anterior surface, the drill-bit is mounted and the holes for the pegs are made (**Fig. 51.3g,h**).
- The remaining bone and capsule of the posterior compartment are removed.

51.7.4 Insertion of Components

- The bony surfaces are carefully checked. If there are cysts, they are removed with a curette, and then filled with bone.
- The talar component is such that the pegs can glide into the two drilled holes; a hammer and an impactor are used to get a proper fit of the component to the bone (**Fig. 51.3i**).
- The tibial component is inserted along the medial malleolus until proper fit to the anterior border of the tibia is achieved; hammer and impactor may be used for appropriate fit to the bone.
- After having determined the appropriate thickness of insert using the trial components, the polyethylene insert (same size as the talar component) is inserted (**Fig. 51.3j**).
- It is also highly recommended to check the position of the implants by fluoroscopy (**Fig. 51.3k, l**).

51.7.5 Additional Procedures

- Before total ankle replacement:
  - Correcting osteotomy of distal tibia (for malunited tibia with angular deviation > 6 degrees.
  - Arthrodesis of peritalar joints (for osteoarthritis, instability, and fixed deformities).
- After total ankle replacement:
  - Heel cord lengthening (if dorsiflexion < 10 degrees can be achieved after maximal mobilization into dorsiflexion of the foot).
  - Lateral ankle ligament reconstruction (for persistent lateral instability).
  - Peroneus longus to peroneus brevis transfer (for incompetent peroneus brevis).
  - Correcting calcaneal osteotomy (for persistent inframalleolar deformity).
  - Arthrodesis of syndesmosis (for unstable syndesmosis).
  - Correcting osteotomy of first ray (for dorsi- or plantar-flexion deformity).

51.7.6 Wound Closure

- Wound closure over a drain (without suction) is obtained by suture of the tendon sheath and retinaculum and of the skin.
- A careful dressing is made to avoid any pressure to the skin.
- A splint is used to keep the foot in neutral position.

51.8 Tips and Pearls

- The soft tissue beneath the anterior tibial tendon is always free from the neurovascular bundle and thus is called the "safe spot" while approaching the anterior ankle joint.
- Proper frontal (coronal) plane alignment may best be achieved while pulling the talus distally with a rasp (placed in the center of the tibiotalar joint), thereby tightening the medial and lateral ligaments.
- In varus ankles, there is usually need for more tibial resection, whereas in valgus ankles, and/or in the presence of high joint laxity, less bone resection is advised.

- If in doubt (e.g., if the anterior border of the tibia is projected onto the gauge between two markers), the bigger size for tibial component might be selected.
- If in doubt, the smaller size for talar component might be selected.
- The posterior capsule should be removed completely until fat tissue and tendon structures are visible to get full dorsiflexion.
- If the foot is moved in dorsiflexion with the surgeon's maximal power, settling of the implant may be improved, and remaining soft-tissue contracture on the posterior aspect of the ankle may be released; if, with this, 10 degrees of dorsiflexion cannot be achieved, heel cord lengthening is considered.
- Fluoroscopy allows detecting any remaining bony fragments or osteophytes that could be a potential source of pain or motion restriction.

51.9 Hazards and Pitfalls

- Attention should be paid so as not to insert the saw blade too deeply into the joint given the tibial nerve might be at risk.
- If old scars from previous surgeries or injuries are not respected, breakdown of critical areas may occur.
- Positioning of the resection block too posterior will lead to insufficient bony support of the talar component, thus creating sagittal plane instability.

51.10 Complications/Bailout/Salvage

- Too-aggressive motion during the first postoperative days may lead to breakdown of soft tissues.
- Primary or secondary infection.
- Loosening of component.
- Mechanical failure due to insufficient balancing of the ankle:
  - Instability with polyethylene insert dislocation.
  - Misalignment with asymmetric wear of polyethylene insert.

51.11 Postoperative Care

- The dressing and splint are removed and changed after 2 days.
- When the wound condition is dry and proper, typically 2 to 4 days after surgery, the foot is placed in a stabilizing cast or walker that protects the ankle against eversion, inversion, and plantar flexion movements for 6 weeks.
- Weight bearing is allowed as tolerated. Usually, full weight bearing is achieved after 1 week.
- A rehabilitation program should be started for the foot and ankle after cast or walker removal, including stretching and strengthening of the triceps surae.
- The first clinical and radiologic follow-up is made at 6 weeks, to check wound situs and osteointegration and position of the implants (**Fig. 51.4**).
- The patient should be advised to wear a compression stocking for further 4 to 6 months to avoid swelling.

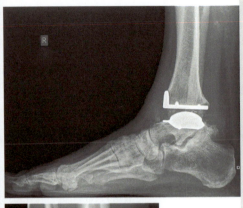

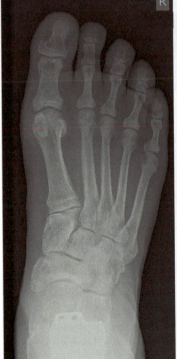

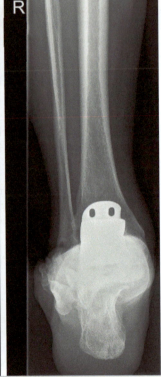

Fig. 51.4 Standard weight-bearing radiographs including after 1 year showing a balanced ankle and stable implants.

51.12 Outcomes

- Out of 779 consecutive TARs with HINTEGRA, 722 ankles were available for follow-up control after 6.3 ± 2.9 years (range, 2.0–12.2 years).
- The average VAS pain score decreased from 7.2 ± 2.4 (range, 5–10) to 1.7 ± 1.5 (range, 0–3) ($p < 0.001$).
- The average AOFAS hindfoot score increased significantly from 39 ± 20 (range, 15–78) to 76 ± 18 (range, 52–97) ($p < 0.001$).

- The average range of motion increased significantly from 22.5 ± 10.6 degrees (range, 11–52 degrees) to 34.3 ± 9.4 degrees (range, 28–56 degrees) ($p < 0.01$).
- Thirty-five ankles (8.4%) had to be revised at a mean of 3.2 years (range, 0.5–7.9 years) after the index surgery; 27 revision total ankle arthroplasties (6.5%; using HINTEGRA total ankle prosthesis) and 8 ankle arthrodeses (1.9%; using anterior double plating system) were performed: most likely the revision was performed in patients with first-generation prosthesis with single coating with hydroxyapatite ($n = 17$),

rather than in patients with second- (n = 10) or third- (n = 8) generation prosthesis.

- The reasons for revision were aseptic loosening of one or both components (n = 23), subsidence of talar component (n = 5), cyst formation (n = 2), deep infection (n = 1), unmanageable instability (n = 1), and painful arthrofibrosis (n = 3).
- In 16 of the remaining 380 ankles (4.1%), radiolucency around the prosthesis components was seen; however, in none of the ankle, progression of radiolucency was observed over the time.
- Overall survival rate for the series was 94 and 84% after 5 and 10 years, respectively.

References

Conceptor studies

1. Barg A, Knupp M, Henninger HB, Zwicky L, Hintermann B. Total ankle replacement using HINTEGRA, an unconstrained, three-component system: surgical technique and pitfalls. Foot Ankle Clin 2012;17(4):607–635
2. Barg A, Zwicky L, Knupp M, Henninger HB, Hintermann B. HINTEGRA total ankle replacement: survivorship analysis in 684 patients. J Bone Joint Surg Am 2013;95(13):1175–1183
3. Choi GW, Kim HJ, Yeo ED, Song SY. Comparison of the HINTEGRA and Mobility total ankle replacements. Short- to intermediate-term outcomes. Bone Joint J 2013;95-B(8):1075–1082
4. Daniels TR, Younger AS, Penner M, et al. Intermediate-term results of total ankle replacement and ankle arthrodesis: a COFAS multicenter study. J Bone Joint Surg Am 2014;96(2):135–142
5. Gougoulias N, Khanna A, Maffulli N. How successful are current ankle replacements?: a systematic review of the literature. Clin Orthop Relat Res 2010;468(1):199–208– Review
6. Hintermann B, ed. Total Ankle Arthroplasty: Historical Overview, Current Concepts and Future PerspectivesBerlin: Springer;2004
7. Hintermann B, Barg A. The Hintegra prosthesis: why I designed it this way. In: Haddad S, ed. Total Ankle Replacement. AAOS Monograph Series;2015:117–133
8. Hintermann B, Barg A, Knupp M, Valderrabano V. Conversion of painful ankle arthrodesis to total ankle arthroplasty. J Bone Joint Surg Am 2009;91(4):850–858
9. Hintermann B, Valderrabano V, Dereymaeker G, Dick W. The HINTEGRA ankle: rationale and short-term results of 122 consecutive ankles. Clin Orthop Relat Res 2004(424):57–68
10. Hintermann B, Zwicky L, Knupp M, Henninger HB, Barg A. HINTEGRA revision arthroplasty for failed total ankle prostheses. J Bone Joint Surg Am 2013;95(13):1166–1174
11. Jung HG, Shin MH, Lee SH, Eom JS, Lee DO. Comparison of the outcomes between two 3-component total ankle implants. Foot Ankle Int 2015;36(6):656–663
12. Lefrancois T, Younger A, Wing K, et al. A prospective study of four total ankle arthroplasty implants by non-designer investigators. J Bone Joint Surg Am 2017;99(4):342–348
13. Nery C, Fernandes TD, Réssio C, Fuchs ML, Godoy Santos AL, Ortiz RT. Total ankle arthroplasty: Brazilian experience with the HINTEGRA prosthesis. Rev Bras Ortop 2015;45(1):92–100
14. Nigg BM, von Tscharner V, Stefanyshyn DJ, Goepfert B, Hintermann B. Gait analysis in ankle osteoarthritis and total ankle replacement. Clin Biomech (Bristol, Avon) 2007;22(8):894–904

52 The Zimmer Trabecular Metal Total Ankle System

Alireza Mousavian and Lew C. Schon

Abstract

The Zimmer Trabecular Metal Total Ankle represents a paradigm shift from existing systems. A utilitarian lateral approach through a fibula osteotomy permits sparing of the deltoid ligament and correction of deformities. A frame is used to achieve alignment and stability. The bone-sparing curved shape implant follows the contours of the natural joint. The implant materials are unique including porous tantalum trabecular metal and highly crossed-linked polyethylene. The technique will cover exposure, fibular osteotomy, release of contracture, alignment, bony stabilization, routing of the surfaces, rail guide drilling, trial reduction, implantation of the prosthesis, fixation of the fibula, restoration of the lateral ligaments, closure, and postoperative management.[1-5]

Keywords: *lateral approach, fibular osteotomy, highly cross-linked polyethylene, tantalum trabecular metal, curved implant, alignment, frame*

52.1 Indications

- Symptomatic arthritis of the ankle.
- A contralateral ankle fusion.
- Symptomatic arthritis of the ankle with adjacent joint arthritis.
- Ankle deformity that involves a malunion or deformity of the fibula.
- Sagittal plane deformity (anterior or posterior translation) of the ankle.
- Valgus deformity with shortened or valgus fibula.
- Varus deformity with varus fibula and contracted deltoid.
- Rotational deformity of the ankle.
- Prior ankle fusion with intact fibula.
- A lateral approach may be the best option for a patient with compromised anterior tissue.
- Prior lateral scar from fracture fixation, lateral ligament reconstruction, or peroneal tendon surgery.
- Flat top talus or low domed talus with ankle arthritis.[6-8]

52.1.1 Clinical Evaluation

- Evaluate the range of motion of the ankle, subtalar, and transverse tarsal joints.
- Test muscle strength and look for atrophy.
- Evaluate the neurovascular status.
- With the patient standing, evaluate overall alignment of the lower extremity, and especially the foot.
- Watch the patient walk to check for dynamic deformities and mechanical contributions from other lower extremity pathology.
- Determine if there is a deformity. If yes, is it passively correctable?
- Carefully assess the etiology of ankle malalignment: instability of medial or lateral ligaments, arthritis, contracture, and/or weakness due to a neurologic situation. Is there bony deformity from joint erosion: tibial, fibular, and talar malunion?

- Evaluate for pes planovalgus from posterior tibial tendinopathy.
- Check for cavovarus from peroneal tendon pathology.
- Document previous incisions and the quality of the lateral tissues. Make sure adequate skin bridges will be present with the lateral approach.
- Medically optimize the patient by vitamin D replacement to midrange level using 50,000 IU weekly for 12 weeks in patients with low or deficient levels.
- For patients with rheumatologic diseases, altering their use of disease-modifying antirheumatic drugs and biologics to increase the drug-free time before and after surgery may decrease infection and wound complications.[7,9-11]

52.1.2 Radiographic Evaluation

- Standing anteroposterior (AP) and lateral views of the ankle, including the lower two-thirds of the tibia. An AP view of the foot to identify occult deformities. In cases of significant malalignment of the ankle or leg, include more proximal leg and comparative views of the opposite side.
- A standing AP view that includes the hip, knee, and foot is helpful in difficult cases of malalignment.
- Dorsiflexion and plantarflexion standing lateral views.
- A Saltzman view for hindfoot and ankle alignment.
- An MRI will demonstrate arthritis of the ankle and/or subtalar joint that may not be detected on plain radiographs. Tendon damage should be assessed.
- A CAT scan will demonstrate bony voids, cysts, or fracture nonunions that may need to be addressed.
- Technetium- and indium-labeled WBC scan to assess for infection.[9-13]

52.1.3 Nonoperative Options

- Brace immobilization.
- Ambulatory aids: cane, crutches, walker.
- Activity modification.
- Shoe modifications with rocker bottom sole and cushioned heel: orthotic inserts.
- Medications: cortisone injections, hyaluronic acid injections, anti-inflammatory medications.

52.1.4 Contraindications

- Acute avascular necrosis of the talus.
- Charcot arthropathy.
- Local/systemic infection.
- Severe neurologic or vascular disease affecting the extremity.
- Poor lateral skin quality.

Relative Contraindications

- Severe osteoporosis or compromised bone stock.
- Immunosuppressive therapy.

- Previous joint infection.
- Severe non-reconstructable deltoid insufficiency.
- A non-reconstructable nonplantigrade foot.
- An absent fibula or medial malleolus.

52.1.5 Indication Controversies

- Body mass index of the patient must be taken into consideration.
- The size 1 (smallest) implant is rated for 250 lb.
- Age less than 50 years.

52.2 Goals of Surgical Procedure

The goals are to achieve reduced pain, improved range of motion, and better function in patients suffering from ankle arthritis. The implant surfaces are milled after accurately aligning the joint to follow the natural ankle contours. All variables that contribute to malalignment are addressed with this system. Early range of motion and weight bearing at 10 days permit improved motion and less atrophy.

52.3 Advantages of Surgical Procedure

The Zimmer Trabecular Metal Total Ankle represents a paradigm shift from existing systems. A utilitarian lateral approach through a fibula osteotomy allows for correction of fibula deformity and clear access to the anterior, posterior, and lateral aspects of the joint.[10]

Typically, this permits sparing of the deltoid ligament and correction of deformities in all planes: coronal, sagittal, axial, and rotational. A frame is used to achieve an accurate algorithm-driven correction of the alignment. The system uses a coupled resection for optimal positioning and intrinsic stability. The external fixation provides stabilization for an accurate guide-driven milling of the surfaces. The bone-sparing curved

shape implant follows the contours of the natural joint and has coronally oriented rails for bone to metal purchase. The implant materials are unique. The bone interface is porous tantalum trabecular metal. The polyethylene insert is bicondylar and is highly crossed linked for maximum durability (FN highly cross-linked poly FAI). The talar dome is cobalt chrome with a bicondylar matching contour (**Fig. 52.1**).[1-5, 14]

52.4 Key Principles

Key principles are to preserve bone stock and restore anatomic alignment and integrity of bone and soft tissues. The fibular osteotomy permits correction of contributory deformities. Rail orientation in the coronal plane and curve-to-curve stability maintain positioning of the implants. The correction of the deformity is accurately achieved sequentially beginning with soft-tissue release and positioning of the calcaneus, the talus, and finally the tibia in all planes. Coupled bony resections permit geometry precision milling for implant to bone apposition.

52.5 Preoperative Preparation and Patient Positioning

- The heel should be 6 inches from the end of the table, to allow room for the frame.
- Ensure that there is sufficient space to allow the frame to be near the center of the table (**Fig. 52.2**).
- If the leg-rests of the table are not firm, a stiff board is used to prevent the frame from shifting.
- A bump or bean bag under the ipsilateral hip to lift up the hemipelvis 15 to 20 degrees which places the femoral bicondylar axis 15 to 20 degrees of internal rotation and the fibular–medial malleolus axis parallel to the floor.
- An arm rest placed at the side of the end of the table allows the contralateral leg to be stable on the table while providing more room for the affected ankle.
- Secure the opposite leg so that it is not inadvertently pushed off the operating room (OR) table during the case.

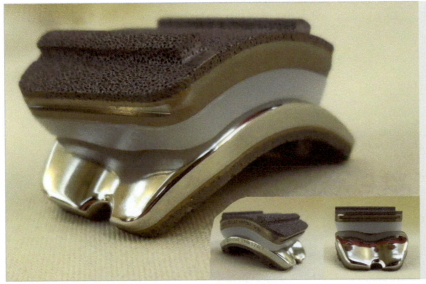

Fig. 52.1 Trabecular Metal components— note the semiconstraint bicondylar shape and porous tantalum–bone interface.

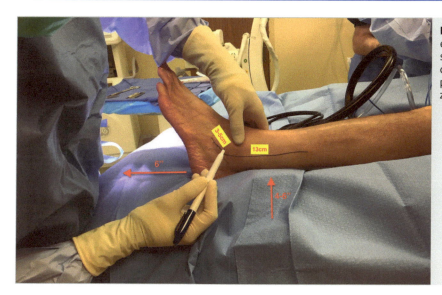

Fig. 52.2 Positioning and incision: The leg is elevated 4 to 6 inches off the table and the sole of the foot is 6 inches distance to the end of table. 13-cm-long lateral incision along the posterior border of the fibula with 3-cm horizontal distal extension over the sinus tarsi.

- A pile of folded blankets 4 to 6 inches thick and large enough in length and width to support the frame is placed from the end of the table to the level of the knee. Secure it with circumferential tape to the table. This elevates the operative leg to facilitate the lateral C arm images without the obstruction from the contralateral limb (**Fig. 52.2**).
- A thigh tourniquet is placed and secured. Typically, it is not inflated.
- Set up the large C-arm. Multiple AP and lateral images will be required during the case.
- Lead gowns must be worn before scrubbing as the large C-arm is used.

52.6 Operative Technique

The leg is not yet in the alignment stand:
- Along the posterior border of the fibula, make the incision approximately 13 cm proximal to the ankle joint. Extend it distally, just distal to the tip of the fibula over the sinus tarsi for 3 to 5 cm (**Fig. 52.2**). This permits more anterior exposure of the ankle joint and allows for less aggressive soft-tissue retraction anteriorly.
- Open the peroneal sheath along the fibula just over the posterior edge of the bone and elevate the periosteal flap to the anterior aspect of the fibula (**Fig. 52.3a, b**).
- Distally, at the tip of the fibula, leave the superior retinaculum intact by preserving the inferior and posterior aspect of the periosteum on the bone (**Fig. 52.3a**).
- Elevate the anterior periosteum and then in the same flap transect the anterior talofibular ligament off the fibula.
- Elevate the anterior capsule and periosteum off the distal 3-4 cm of the tibia, staying below the peroneal artery.
- Continuing the periosteal flap anterior to the ankle joint to allow exposure to the medial joint line.
- Place a suture tag on the edge of the anterior talofibular ligament and the capsular periosteal flap to facilitate identification and closure.
- If there is no fibula deformity, a five-hole fibular reconstruction plate is applied. A screw is placed proximally above the

level of the osteotomy to anticipate the contour of the bone. Three holes are predrilled and measured distally (**Fig. 52.3e**). *Note*: If the tissues laterally are thin, a semi tubular or lower profile plate should be used.
- An oblique osteotomy in the sagittal plane or coronal plane will be made in the fibula.
- The distal-most aspect of the cut should be 1.5 to 2 cm proximal to the ankle joint, to allow adequate room for milling and placement of the tibial implant.
- Place a 0.45 K-wire obliquely across the fibula first, and evaluate under C-arm to plan the position of the osteotomy (**Fig. 52.3d**).
- If there is sagittal malalignment or in cases of no deformity, make an oblique cut with a thin micro-sagittal saw from proximal–lateral to distal medially, angled about 45 degrees to the long axis, under cool water irrigation (**Fig. 52.3f**).
- An alternative osteotomy is made obliquely in the coronal plane like a Weber B fracture. This osteotomy allows for lengthening or shortening of the fibula as well as correction of varus or valgus deformity.
- Incise the lower syndesmotic ligaments sharply anteriorly and posteriorly to mobilize the fibula.
- Use a medium-size elevator to free up the fibula from the syndesmosis, so that it can be hinged distally (**Fig. 52.3f, g**). If there is a partial synostosis of the syndesmosis, use a chisel to take it down.
- Leave intact the calcaneofibular and posterior talofibular ligaments.
- Pin the fibula against the foot into the calcaneus under oscillation mode with a 1.6-mm K-wire so that it does not obstruct the sweep of the router along the posterior talus. Bend, cut, and cover the wire with a pin cap.
- Place a periosteal elevator in the joint and twist it between the tibia and talus to release contractures (**Fig. 52.3h**). The elevator should be used to release the posterior capsule by placing it deeply between the tibia and talus and sliding and turning it as it moves from the inside to the outside of the joint posteriorly. Later during the milling, this permits placement of the posterior retractor and protection of the posterior medial structures.

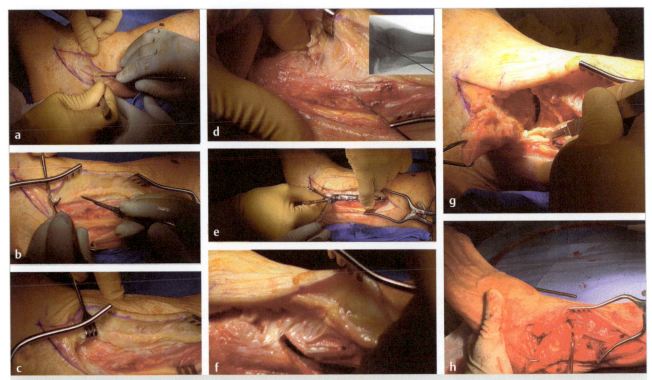

Fig. 52.3 Lateral approach: **(a)** Incise the periosteum along with skin and subcutaneous incision along the posterior edge of fibula preserving 1 cm most distal attachment of superior peroneal retinaculum. **(b)** Peel off the periosteum anteriorly. **(c)** Cut the anterior talo fibular and anterior inferior tibi fibular ligaments. **(d)** Place a K-wire in line with proposed osteotomy and check with fluoroscopy to determine that the cut will be 1.5 cm above the joint line. **(e)** Apply and (if needed) contour the fibular plate before osteotomy. Drill one hole above the osteotomy and insert a screw to finalize the apposition to the bone. Then drill and measure three distal hole sizes. **(f)** Fibular osteotomy. **(g)** Turning down the distal fragment with gradual cutting of connecting ligaments of syndesmosis. Preserve the calcaneofibular ligament and posterior talofibular ligament. **(h)** Freeing the posterior and anterior capsule off the tibia using a periosteal elevator.

- An arthrotomy of the medial ankle may be required to remove bony impingement, especially in the medial gutter along the anterior or distal aspect of the medial malleolus or medial neck of the talus.
- A severe varus deformity can be more readily corrected with a medial arthrotomy. This releases the superficial deltoid and allows for placement of a medial laminar spreader or pin distraction spreader (Hintermann's distractor; **Fig. 52.4**).
- The deep deltoid is rarely, if ever, released in this system.

52.6.1 Implant Sizing

- With the leg still out of the frame, measure the width of the talus with the Zimmer depth gauge. Go all the way to the medial border of the talus. Confirm proper placement with fluoroscopy (**Fig. 52.9**). Determine the largest implant that can be used, without any medial-lateral overhang. Use the smaller measurement in between sizes to preserve more medial malleolar bone stock.
- Confirm the size with the AP sizer or silhouette, although this rarely effects the decision.
- Once the size is determined, remove any large anterior spurs with a rongeur, and assess the need for a percutaneous Achilles lengthening or Gastrocnemius recession.
- If there is still a contracture, the foot can be placed in the frame in 5, 10, or 15 degrees.

52.6.2 Guide Frame Application

- Place the leg in the frame, as outlined in the Zimmer instruction manual in the middle and parallel to the long bars of the frame (**Fig. 52.5a, b**).
- Make sure the proper internal rotation is set with the medial edge of the foot parallel to the oblique medial border of the foot plate (**Fig. 52.5c**).
- To check that the talar internal rotation is correct, place the wide and flat end of the probe inside the router guide and against the anterior half of the lateral body of the talus. It should be flush to the surface. Make sure the milling tower is tight to maximize accuracy of this step.
- Use Coban to hold the forefoot to the plate. Ensure that the foot posts are not pressing into the foot.
- Make sure the leg is positioned high enough (superiorly) in the frame so that a clear lateral fluoroscopic image can be obtained without the other leg being in the way. The folded blankets should have facilitated this (**Fig. 52.5d**).
- The heel should be in the heel rest, but 1 to 2 cm off the foot plate to facilitate distraction of the joint with the calcaneal pins (**Fig. 52.5a**).
- The surgeon can place the calcaneal pin, parallel to the talar joint surface, prior to placement in the frame or once in the frame (**Fig. 52.6a, b**).
- As the calcaneal pin is tightened, take a few C-arm images. Eccentric tightening of the pin may be needed to bring the talus into a neutral positon. The heel now should be resting against the foot plate.

- Rotational malalignment can be adjusted using the calcaneal pin holders in different holes.
- Images to check for overall talar and tibial alignment via horizontal and vertical reference bars should be performed (**Fig. 52.6**).
- The talar pin is placed through the pin to post clamp that is on the talar post. The starting point should be 1 cm distal and 1 cm anterior to the tip of the medial malleolus.
- The talar pin is started at the junction of the middle and lower third of the talus neck. It is angled from distal to proximal and from posterior to anterior avoiding the dome of the talus laterally (**Fig. 52.6c, d**).
- Check an AP and lateral image to be sure that the placement is correct.
- The talar pin can be used as a "joystick" to make further corrections in talar alignment.[15]

52.6.3 Cutting Guide

- Attach the cutting guide of appropriate size onto the lateral cut guide assembly. Place the Center Probe, flat side first, into the Tibial 2 hold. Place it across the front of the ankle. The cutting guide may have to be raised anteriorly to accomplish this (**Fig. 52.5e**).
- The tibial alignment rod should be in line with the long axis of the tibia. Parallax created by fluoroscopy can make this determination challenging. Use the lateral border of the tibia as a reference.
- The Center Probe should be parallel to the planned talar joint surface of the prosthesis. The alignment rod will be 90 degrees to the Center Probe (**Fig. 52.6a**).

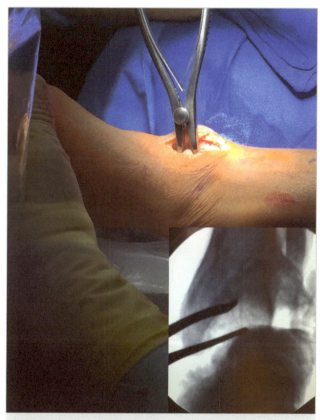

Fig. 52.4 Medial incision for severe rigid varus cases and to remove osteophytes and insert a distractor or laminar spreader to release the deltoid ligament.

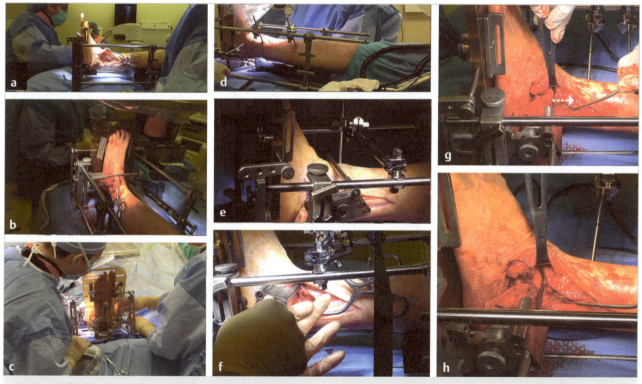

Fig. 52.5 (a,b) Place the leg frame, middle to the long bars in anteroposterior and lateral view. (c) Medial side of foot is parallel to medial side of foot plate. (d) Proximal pins are inserted medially. (e) In case of sagittal imbalance, insert first proximal pin anterior to posterior and (f–h) fasten it to a transverse accessory carbon bar.

- Make final adjustments to achieve fluoroscopic confirmation that the talus joint line is horizontal to the longitudinal bar or parallel to the horizontal bar. This may require adjustment/tensioning of the calcaneal pin or joy sticking the talar pin.
- Lock the talar pin to the talar pin post.
- Now check the AP and sagittal images.
- If there is any sagittal malalignment of the ankle, it is best to place the most distal tibial pin from anterior to posterior, approximately 5 cm from the joint (**Fig. 52.5e**). It may

not be possible to hold the corrected position without it. This pin is placed off a carbon bar secured anteriorly to the frame. During this correction in the sagittal plane, the tibia is elevated, depressed, or rotated manually to help achieve the correction. Pulling the pin anteriorly or pushing it posteriorly with the T-handled chuck will fine tune the correction.

- Before inserting the tibial pins, residual varus or valgus alignment of the tibia can be corrected by angling the proximal frame medial or lateral in relation to the leg.

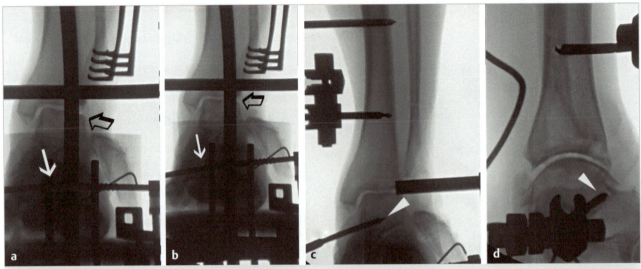

Fig. 52.6 **(a–d)** Calcaneal pin adjustment can manipulate talar surface coronal orientation **(a,b)** The calcaneal pin (*solid white arrow*) is tensioned medially to coronally correct the talus from varus (*open arrow*) to neutral. **(c)** The talar pin (*solid arrowhead*) can be used to finely adjust the talus so it is parallel to the horizontal bar, and then to adjust the tibial alignment and insert the tibial pins. **(d)** The anterior to posterior tibial pin is used to correct the sagittal alignment.

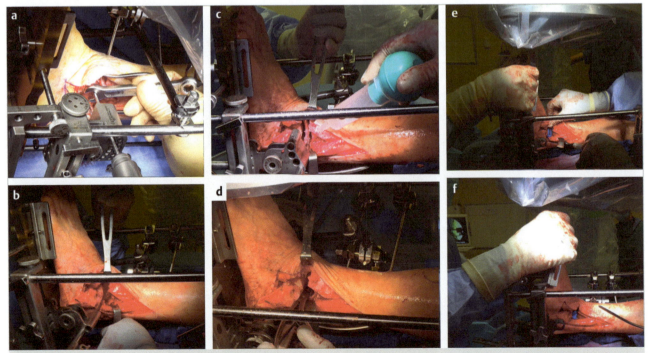

Fig. 52.7 Bone surface preparation: **(a)** Place drill guide and drill talar and tibial holes. **(b)** Using cutting guide, cut 7/8th middle talar surface. **(c)** Then cut tibia 1. **(d)** Remove the tibial shelf first with rongeur and finalize through tibial 2 routing. Then with better visualization and retraction, complete the more anterior and posterior routing of the talus and tibia medially. **(e,f)** Put trial components and control test range of motion.

- When inserting the lower tibial pin, the assistant should provide a counter force on the tibia to avoid inadvertent posterior translation.
- Place the tibial pins through the frame to pin clamp with the clamp relatively tightened close to its final position. This avoids some rotation of the tibia during tightening of the nuts.
- The most proximal tibial pin is always inserted from medial to lateral (**Fig. 52.5d**).

52.6.4   Setting the AP Positioning

- The Center Probe is used to determine the appropriate joint line, as discussed in the Zimmer technique guide.
- Start with the probe in the position hole of the router guide locked in position and find the apex or high point of the dome of the talus (**Fig. 52.5g**).
- Unlock the router guide and trace along the joint line. The path should follow the joint line or be symmetrically coursing along it (e.g., it may touch the apex centrally but trace an arc that is off a symmetric amount anteriorly and posteriorly).
- Next, translate the cutting jig proximally 1.5 to 2 mm proximal to the anatomic joint line (**Fig. 52.5g, h**). With the probe in the position hole, this typically corresponds to the lower tibial margin. Elevating the joint line to restore the normal mechanics may require translation proximally of 3 to 4 mm above the joint line sulcus when a flat top talus is present. This position minimizes the amount of talar bone resected.
- As the probe is swung anterior and posterior, make sure to examine where the burr will excise the talar neck. Too much notching (more than 3 mm) means that the guide is probably set too inferior on the talus.
- The appropriate anteroposterior position is set.

52.6.5   Bone Resection/Burring

- Once the guide is locked into position, the drilling and burring can begin. First place the drilling block on the cutting jig

and, using the drill in the central talar hole, drill from lateral to medial (**Fig. 52.7a**).
- Check the depth of the drill on image and set the chuck for further drilling (**Fig. 52.8a**).
- Sometimes, the drill bit will be deflected from the hard talar surface. Use the open end of the wrench to counteract this force (**Fig. 52.7a**).
- Once the talar holes are drilled, drill the tibial holes.
- Then place the burr cutting guide (**Fig. 52.7b, c**).
- Place the router in the talar hole resting against the talus and use the contralateral plastic talar trial to set the burr depth guide.
- The burring process can generate a lot of heat, and should be done under continuous irrigation (**Fig. 52.7c**). Two bulb syringes may be used. The use of an IV bag, tubing, and continuous irrigation may also be helpful.
- An army navy retractor must be used anteriorly (**Fig. 52.7d**).
- A malleable or "Z" retractor posteriorly to protect the soft tissue, tendons, and neurovascular structures (**Fig. 52.7c, d**). The posterior retractor must be carefully placed hugging the posterior tibia and talus across the medial aspect to protect the tendons and neurovascular structures.
- The depth of the router must be checked under fluoroscopic image before progressing medially.
- Use more of a pecking than a sweeping technique with the burr, to help minimize skiving, especially on the hard talar bone.
- Initially burr the central 7/8th of the talus and tibia, leaving the most anterior and posterior medial aspects to the end. This is the best way to protect the anterior and posterior tissues.
- The medial-most aspect of the talus should be excised with the burr, to assure proper fit of the prosthesis.
- When milling the tibia side, check the depth again to ensure that the medial malleolus is not being compromised (**Fig. 52.8b**).
- Once finishing the talus and tibial 1 milling except for the anterior and posterior 1/8th, use a rongeur to remove the tibial 2 shelf of bone (**Fig. 52.7d**).
- Then mill the remaining portion of the tibial 2 shelf with the router.

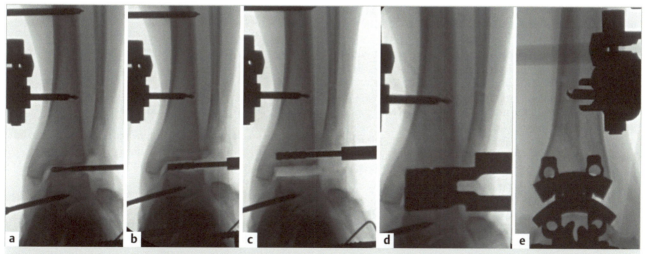

Fig. 52.8 (a) Measure the correct length of first drill and (b) first talar burr. (c) Measure the length of burr in tibia 2 cut again to ensure enough space for medial malleoli. (d,e) Place rail guides and insert the largest possible "U-shaped" spreader pin in between. Make sure that rail guides are resting on the bone by wiggling the rail guides into final survey on curve resting position. Center the guides so that they do not overhang anteriorly or posteriorly.

- Now with clear direct vision and optimal retraction, the posterior- and anterior-most aspects of the tibia and talus are milled.
- Once the bone is removed, go over the surfaces with your finger. They should be smooth, and the far medial side decompressed with no bone spicules that can prevent the prosthesis from seating fully.

52.6.6 Cutting the Rail Slots

- Insert the rail guides.
- If there is difficulty placing them, some bone may need to be resected.
- Wiggle the guides to achieve final apposition of curve against curve.
- Each guide should be independently set. The tibial guide should be flush with the anterior tibia, without posterior overhang. The talar guide should be set at 90 degrees to the tibia, under the weight-bearing axis.
- AP and lateral images are obtained to see that the rail holes will be in bone and to check the anterior and posterior positioning (**Fig. 52.8c, d**).
- Place the spreader pin between the guides to compress them against the surfaces (**Fig. 52.8d**).
- With fluoroscopy assure that the rail holes are perfectly aligned (see the Zimmer technique guide). The rail guides should ideally be completely flush on the tibia and talus, although there is often a 1-mm acceptable gap visible between the talus and the talar rail guide (**Fig. 52.8e**).
- Place the pins to secure the rail guide to the tibia and talus and drill the rail holes. Save the bone graft from the drill for later use at the fibular osteotomy site.

52.6.7 Trial and Final Components

- Remove the rail holes and irrigate out the space. Detach the footplate from the frame and place the trials (**Fig. 52.7d, e**). Evaluate valgus laxity and appropriate tension on the deltoid ligament. If there is valgus stress induced laxity, insert a larger poly trial until stable. Place the ankle through a range of motion (**Fig. 52.7d, e**). DO NOT PERFORM A VARUS STRESS BECAUSE THE MEDIAL MALLEOULUS MAY BE COMPROMISED.
- With the tibial trial in place, reattach the footplate but without the foot plate stabilizing pins in place, to allow dorsiflexion of the ankle.
- For permanent component insertion, start with removing the talar trial first. Secure the final talar component (with control of size, side, and direction) to the holder.
- Adjust the medial side of talar component to the insertion site.
- Make sure the talar component is set into the rail holes by pushing and slightly adjusting so that the rail slides along its path without resistance. It must be flush against the surface. Once it is well seated in the rail hole and advances 3 to 4 mm, then begin insertion. The assistant should apply dorsiflexion of the footplate to create compression on the component during insertion (**Fig. 52.9a, b, Fig. 52.10a**). If the implant is going in at an angle, start over. If the fibula is in the way of the inserter, detach the implant and finish with the hand-held impactor.

- The tibial component is inserted next, with dorsiflexion of the footplate implant after the implant is seated 3 to 4 mm (**Figs. 52.9c, 52.10b**). Check final images.

52.6.8 Fibular Reduction and Closure

- Reduce the fibula and apply the lateral plate. Repair the ATFL with several slowly absorbable sutures, such as 2-0 PDS or nonabsorbable 0 Ethibond (**Fig. 52.9d, e**). Advance and reef the extensor retinaculum over the knots onto the lateral distal fibula (**Fig. 52.9f**). The retinaculum both covers the bulky knots and reinforces the repair.
- This can be done in the frame with the anterior lateral bar removed.
- Place bone graft from the rail hole drilling around the fibular osteotomy site.
- Check final images (**Fig. 52.11**).
- A syndesmotic screw or suture button device may be needed in rare cases of syndesmotic instability.
- The periosteal sleeve is now closed.
- The soft tissues and skin are closed.
- Concentrated bone marrow obtained from the iliac crest is injected percutaneously at the end of the case.

52.7 Tips and Pearls[15]

52.7.1 Surgical Approach

- Follow old incisions if present even if they are more anterior or posterior.
- Make the distal end of the fibular cut sufficiently proximal so that there is sufficient room to insert the prosthesis.
- The fibula will not flip down if the posterior tibiofibular ligament is left intact. It needs to be cut along the posterior lateral aspect of the tibia.
- An alternative to turning the fibula distally is to hinge it posteriorly. A wire fixed to the fibula or to the calcaneus can secure its position. This is an option when the CF is not present. When doing this, the posterior talus exposure during milling is facilitated by securing the ankle in the frame in 10 to 15 degrees of equinus.
- Make sure there is access to about 1 cm of the posterior tibia and the anterior neck of the talus, permitting effective soft-tissue retraction.

52.7.2 Frame Application

- There are no clear guidelines of how much deformity can be corrected in the frame, without a tibial osteotomy.
- Thirty-five degrees of bony or ligamentous valgus or varus correction can be achieved routinely.
- When correcting a severe bony varus, it may be necessary to use a chisel to resect a wedge of the distal lateral plafond to coronally correct the talus out of varus.
- Sagittal translation of 2 cm is readily correctable. Resected lip of the tibia anteriorly or posteriorly may help with this correction.
- A more proximal tibial deformity may require a tibial osteotomy.

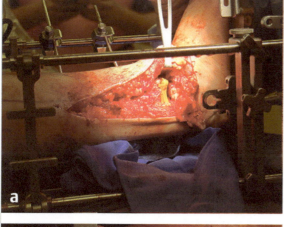
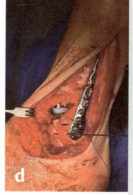
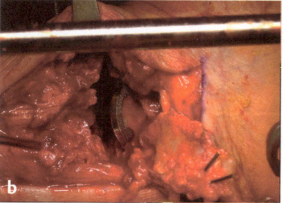
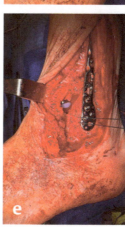
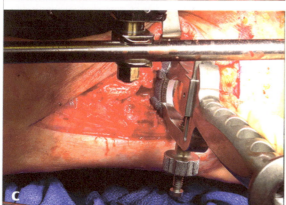
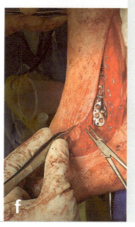

Fig. 52.9 (a) The talus trial is removed and the ankle is lavaged. **(b)** The talus prosthesis is inserted with the tibial trial in place and then the tibial trial is removed for tibial lavage. **(c)** The tibial prosthesis with its poly tray is inserted. **(d)** The fibula is reduced and plated. Drill holes are made to reattach the ligamentous tissues and capsule. **(e)** The ligaments are sutured to the fibula. **(f)** The periosteal sleeve is now placed over the plate and reattached to the posterior retinaculum.

52.7.3 Cutting Guide Application

- Visualize the knee joint with the C-arm. Scan down to the ankle. The knee joint should be 90 degrees to the alignment rod, and parallel to the ankle joint.
- Accurate placement of the leg in the frame, with correction of any ankle malalignment, is critical. This is the time to be meticulous and make it as perfect as possible.
- Distraction of the ankle joint with a lamina spreader will allow for less bone to be removed from the tibial and talus, but may only be needed for more severe rigid deformities.
- A medial arthrotomy is probably not needed if careful visualization of the medial joint is done from the lateral side.
- Placing a carbon bar from the talar pin to the lower tibial pin will secure the correction of deformity and make the construct more rigid for accurate milling. REMEMBER TO REMOVE IT BEFORE DOING TRIAL PLACEMENT AND RANGE OF MOTION.

- Always check the final leg position in both planes. Varus–valgus angulation and sagittal subluxation of the ankle joint must be corrected at this stage.
- An arthrotomy of the medial ankle may be required to remove bony impingement, especially in the medial gutter or tip of the medial malleolus.

52.7.4 Setting the AP Positioning

- One of the best ways to determine appropriate position of the cutting guide is to assure that not more than two times the burr width, or 11 mm is taken off of the tibia. Once the guide is set, place the burr into the tibia 1 hole, which should be one burr width above the joint line.
- Place the burr in the talar hole. Approximately two-thirds of the burr width of talar bone should be removed if the

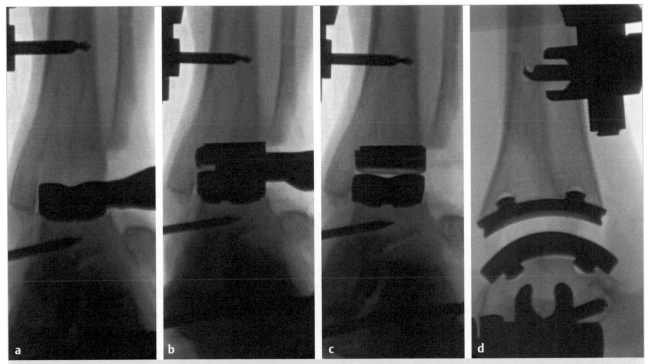

Fig. 52.10 (a) Insert talar component while leaving tibial trial in place. (b) Insert tibial component next. (c,d) Final fluoroscopic images in the coronal and sagittal planes before fibular reduction and plating.

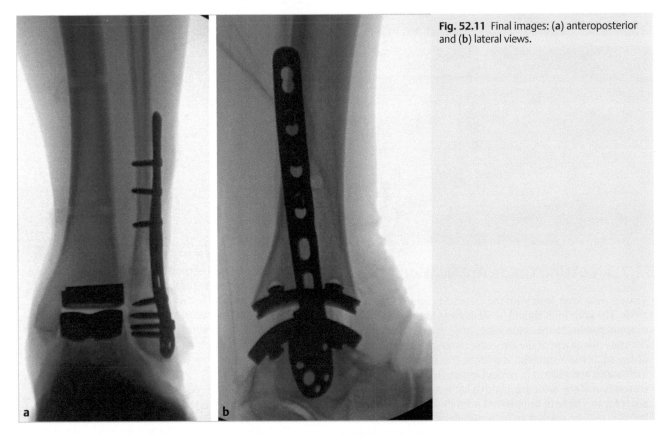

Fig. 52.11 Final images: (a) anteroposterior and (b) lateral views.

position is correct. The burr is 5.5 mm, and approximately 4 mm of bone should be removed. If too much bone will be resected, raise the guide 1 to 2 mm.

- Sweep with the probe in the tibial hole and see that the resection of the tibia will be relatively perpendicular to the tibia. If there is anterior sloping, the jig can be moved more posteriorly. Check the effect of this move on the talar cut.
- When performing the sweeps, tighten the three cutting guide screws (two that secure the proximal to distal transla-

tion and one that secures the anterior posterior adjustments) to maximize accuracy and minimize wiggling.
- There is no evidence that notching of the talar neck is deleterious.

52.7.5 Bone Resection and Burring

- Advance the drill under fluoroscopic guidance. When the proper depth is reached, reset the drill in the chuck. This creates a positive depth stop, rather than eyeballing the laser etched lines on the drill. Drill all of the talar holes. Downward pressure on the drill with a small wrench will prevent it from skiving on the hard talar bone.
- Advance the burr under fluoroscopic guidance.
- Be careful not to remove too much of the medial malleolus. If there is a concern, place a medial malleolar screw at the end of the case.
- Remember that the tibia narrows proximally. The depth of tibia 1 will therefore be a few millimeters shorter than the depth of talar and tibia 2. Always check the burr advancement with the C-arm, to avoid excessive resection of the medial malleolus.
- Check the position of the malleable retractor under the C-arm to ensure it is sufficiently medial to protect the neurovascular bundle during burring.
- Always evaluate the final resection with both AP and lateral images.

52.7.6 Cutting the Rail Slots

- Make sure there is no overhang of the rail guides laterally, or the fibula will not be able to reduce properly. If there is too much potential compromise of the tibia medially, a small concavity can be created in the fibula to accommodate the lateral overhang.
- Measure the distance between the lateral guide and the edge of the bone. This is the same distance that should be present when the final implant is inserted.
- The notch in the tibial rail hole should be centered in the tibia. Do not insert the guides too far medially.
- The rail holes are not designed to extend to the medial edge of the resected tibia and talus.

52.7.7 Trial and Final Components Implantation

- Be cautious not to insert the implant too far medially. Follow the insertion process by C-arm if there is any question.
- Place pressure on the medial malleolus while inserting the implant, both to apply counter pressure and avoid an inadvertent fracture.
- When testing for stability, remember that it is all off the deltoid, and there is no lateral stability with the fibular cut. NO VARUS STRESSING.

52.7.8 Fibular Reduction and Closure

- The fibular osteotomy may need to be trimmed to gain perfect apposition. Place a lag screw through the plate and across the osteotomy, if possible.

- There may be a benefit to predrilling the distal fibular plate holes before the osteotomy is made at the start of the case. This approach may interfere with the correct final position of the plate if there is fibular deformity that requires varus, valgus, rotation, lengthening, or shortening of the fibula.

52.8 Hazards and Pitfalls

- Use prior incisions to minimize wound complications.
- Conserve the peroneal artery by not dissecting anterior to the fibula beyond 3 to 4 cm above the joint line.
- Protect the peroneal tendons from harm when doing the exposure and osteotomy.
- Release the posterior capsule to allow for retractor placement posteriorly to avoid the neurovascular bundle and the posterior tibial tendon.
- Irrigate during routing.
- Use the army navy retractor anteriorly.
- Check the depth of the router at the talus and tibial levels.
- Do not do a varus ankle stress because it may fracture the medial malleolus.
- Do not over impact the prosthesis into the media malleolus.

52.9 Complications[8,10,11,16-18]

- Schon's series:
  ○ Malalignment, 3%.
  ○ Loss of correction, 0%.
  ○ Medial malleolar fracture: 2% intraoperative; 3% postoperative.
  ○ Delayed fibular union, 2%.
  ○ Nonunion, 0%.
  ○ Lucency, 2%.
  ○ Neurovascular compromise, 0%.
  ○ Delayed superficial wound healing: 10%,-treated with local wound care.
  ○ Infection, 4%.
- Of 100 patients, 16 returned to the OR:
  ○ Three medial ankle bone resection.
  ○ One calcaneal and cuneiform osteotomy.
  ○ Four hardware removal.
  ○ One Strayer.
  ○ Three medial malleolar fractures.
  ○ Two infections with I&D beads poly swap.
  ○ One infection with I&D removal of fibular plate and no poly swap.
  ○ One below knee amputation (eight prior complicated surgeries with prior infection).

52.10 Postoperative Care

- A bulky dressing is applied with the ankle in neutral.
- The patient is seen 2 weeks after the surgery, at which time the sutures are removed and a boot brace is applied.
- Deep knee bending protocol beginning at 10 to 14 days out of the brace five times a day for 20 minutes.
- A night splint to protect the lateral ligament reconstruction and to avoid pressure of the brace against the lateral incision.
- At 6 weeks, a WB set of X-rays is obtained and walking in the boot can be started.

- The brace can be discontinued by 6 to 8 weeks after surgery, and physical therapy started, if appropriate.
- Patients are advised not to do standing internal or external rotational movements to avoid stressing the malleoli.
- Most of the time, the night splint is discontinued at 3 months.
- The healing is roughly 75% complete at 3 months and 90% complete at 6 months.
- It is important to remind patients that it can take up to 1 year to be 99% healed and for the total ankle to become "a forgotten joint," and reach maximal improvement.[1]

52.11 Outcomes[18]

Senior author's (Dr. Schon's) first 100 patients:
- 80% had deformity correction.
- 6- to 52-month follow-up.
- During OR:
  o 11 Tendo Achilles lengthening or gastrocnemius recession.
  o 4 Peroneal tendons reconstruction, groove deepening.
  o 5 Osteotomies (calcaneal, cuneiform, first metatarsal).
  o 3 Hindfoot fusions.
  o 36 Hardware removal.
  o 11 Medial malleolar screws for thin or at risk for fracture. Two nondisplaced fractures.
- Results:
  o 92/100 Improved pain and function.
  o 81/100 Improved ROM.
  o No loss of deformity correction.
  o No nonunions, two delayed unions which resolved without surgery.
  o 4 Infections: 3 successfully treated with implant retention, 1 BKA (clubfoot with 8 prior complicated surgeries with infection).
  o One asymptomatic tibial lucency.
  o One symptomatic tibial and talar lucency.

References

1. Barg A, Lyman M, Gililland J. Trabecular metal total ankle using transfibular approach. Foot Ankle Orthop 2016;1(1):2473011416S00024

2. Bischoff JE, Fryman JC, Parcel J, Orozco Villaseñor DA. Influence of crosslinking on the wear performance of polyethylene within total ankle arthroplasty. Foot Ankle Int 2015;36(4):369-76. doi: 10.1177/1071100714558507. Epub 2014 Nov 4.

3. Bischoff JE, Fryman JC, Parcell J, Villaseñor DAO. Influence of crosslinking on the wear performance of polyethylene within total ankle arthroplasty. Foot Ankle Int 2015;36(4):369–376

4. Giannini S, Mazzotti A, Romagnoli M. A new ankle prosthesis model implanted with a lateral surgical approach: preliminary results at 18 months. Foot Ankle Surg 2016;22(2, Suppl 1):96

5. Wentorf FA, Steven Herbst MD, Gillard D, Parduhn C, Smyth S. Kinematic evaluation of the Zimmer® Trabecular Metal™ Ankle using robotic technology

6. Pedowitz DI, Kane JM, Smith GM, Saffel HL, Comer C, Raikin SM. Total ankle arthroplasty versus ankle arthrodesis: a comparative analysis of arc of movement and functional outcomes. Bone Joint J 2016;98-B(5):634–640

7. Sagherian BH, Claridge RJ. Salvage of failed total ankle replacement using tantalum trabecular metal: case series. Foot Ankle Int 2015;36(3):318–324

8. Usuelli FG, Maccario C, Pantalone A, Serra N, Tan EW. Identifying the learning curve for total ankle replacement using a mobile bearing prosthesis. Foot Ankle Surg 2017;23(2):76–83

9. Usuelli FG, Maccario C, Manzi L, Tan EW. Posterior talar shifting in mobile-bearing total ankle replacement. Foot Ankle Int 2016;37(3):281–287

10. Usuelli FG, Manzi L, Brusaferri G, Neher RE, Guelfi M, Maccario C. Sagittal tibiotalar translation and clinical outcomes in mobile and fixed-bearing total ankle replacement. Foot Ankle Surg 2017;23(2):95–101

11. Usuelli FG, Mason L, Grassi M, Maccario C, Ballal M, Molloy A. Lateral ankle and hindfoot instability: a new clinical based classification. Foot Ankle Surg 2014;20(4):231–236

12. Kumar NM, de Cesar Netto C, Schon LC, Fritz J. Metal artifact reduction magnetic resonance imaging around arthroplasty implants: the negative effect of long echo trains on the implant-related artifact. Invest Radiol 2017;52(5):310–316

13. Usuelli FG, Maccario C, Indino C, Manzi L, Gross CE. Tibial slope in total ankle arthroplasty: anterior or lateral approach. Foot Ankle Surg 2017;23(2):84–88

14. Goetz JE, Rungprai C, Tennant JN, et al. Variable volumes of resected bone resulting from different total ankle arthroplasty systems. Foot Ankle Int 2016;37(8):898–904

15. Usuelli FG, Indino C, Maccario C, Manzi L, Salini V. Total ankle replacement through a lateral approach: surgical tips. SICOT J 2016;2:38

16. Netto CC, Maccario C, Tan E, et al. Early outcomes of a novel transfibular total ankle replacement system. Foot Ankle Surg 2016;22(2, Suppl 1):87

17. Tan EW, Maccario C, Talusan PG, Schon LC. Early complications and secondary procedures in transfibular total ankle replacement. Foot Ankle Int 2016;37(8):835–841

18. Usuelli FG, Maccario C, Manzi L, Gross CE. Clinical outcome and fusion rate following simultaneous subtalar fusion and total ankle arthroplasty. Foot Ankle Int 2016;37(7):696–702

53 Tibiotalocalcaneal Fusion: Intramedullary Nail

Jacob R. Zide and James W. Brodsky

Abstract

Combined ankle and subtalar joint arthritis, failed ankle arthroplasty, neuroarthropathic Charcot's ankle collapse, talar osteonecrosis, and ankle and hindfoot deformity with bone loss are difficult problems to manage surgically. Combined tibiotalocalcaneal arthrodesis utilizing a compressing, retrograde, intramedullary (IM) nail fixation is a powerful technique for difficult reconstructions, even and especially when associated with significant bone loss. The IM nail device is a load-sharing device, and offers excellent bending stiffness and improved fusion rates, attributable to power of compression across both ankle and subtalar joints. This chapter outlines the technique for implantation and tips to obtain optimal results.

Keywords: *ankle joint, subtalar joint, arthritis, tibiotalocalcaneal, ankle arthrodesis, subtalar arthrodesis, bone loss, avascular necrosis*

53.1 Indications

- Concomitant ankle and subtalar arthritis (degenerative, post-traumatic, or inflammatory).
- Severe concomitant ankle and hindfoot deformity (**Fig. 53.1a–d**).
- Extensive bone loss of ankle and hindfoot with arthritis or deformity.
- Failed total ankle arthroplasty.
- Avascular necrosis of the talus with collapse (**Fig. 53.2a–d**).
- Failed previous ankle arthrodesis.
- Ankle arthritis after prior subtalar or triple arthrodesis.

53.1.1 Clinical Evaluation

- *Alignment*: careful standing evaluation of lower extremity alignment including the knee, ankle, and hindfoot is critical

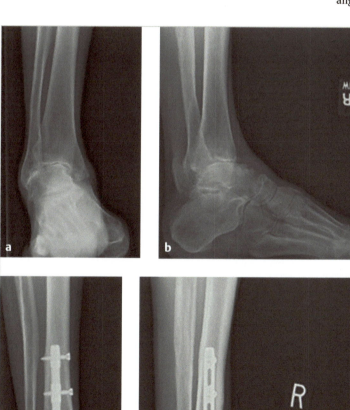

Fig. 53.1 (a,b) AP and lateral views of a patient with severe varus ankle arthritis. (c,d) AP and lateral views after successful tibiotalocalcaneal fusion.

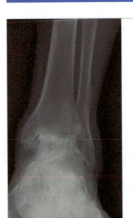
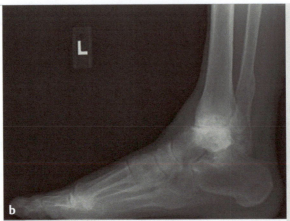
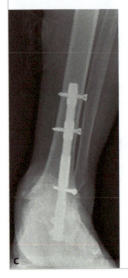
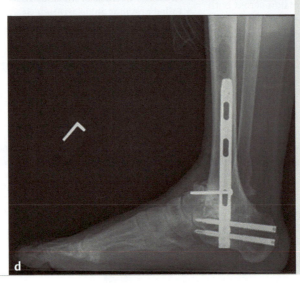

Fig. 53.2 **(a,b)** AP and lateral X-rays demonstrating posttraumatic talar osteonecrosis with collapse of the talar body. **(c,d)** AP and lateral X-rays demonstrating successful union of the tibiocalcaneal fusion. In this case, the talar neck has been fused to the anterior face of the tibia.

to plan for deformity correction. Associated forefoot varus/valgus should also be assessed.

- *Skin*: previous incisions are noted so that they can either be incorporated into the surgical approach or be avoided altogether.
- *Vascular*: examination of pedal pulses is crucial. Weak or impalpable pulses should prompt further work-up with arterial studies (ABI and toe pressures) and/or vascular surgery consultation.
- *Neurological*: sensory examination with light touch is evaluated. It is important to be on the lookout for peripheral neuropathy (whether diabetic, idiopathic, or from another cause). If neuropathy is suspected, Semmes-Weinstein testing with a 5.07 monofilament should be performed along with consideration of neurology consultation.
- *Motor*: assessment of power about the ankle, especially as it pertains to the posterior tibialis and peroneals, is valuable since soft-tissue balancing may be required in order to correct varus/valgus deformity.

53.1.2 Radiographic Evaluation

- Standing X-ray evaluation with anteroposterior (AP), oblique, and lateral views of the foot and ankle should be performed.
- If there is an associated malalignment of the knee or tibia,

consider longstanding radiograph of the lower extremities to assess.
- Computed tomography (CT) scan is obtained to fully evaluate the intra-articular deformity and any associated bone loss which may require bone grafting.
- A hindfoot alignment view may be helpful.

53.1.3 Nonoperative Options

- Bracing with an over-the-counter lace-up ankle brace, custom ankle-foot orthosis (AFO), or Arizona brace may provide symptomatic pain relief.

53.1.4 Contraindications

- Peripheral vascular disease.
- Active infection, remote osteomyelitis.
- Uncontrolled diabetes.
- Poor soft-tissue envelope.
- Malnutrition.
- Inability to comply with postoperative non-weight-bearing.
- Tobacco use (relative).
- Neuropathic arthropathy has higher risk of nonunion or breakage than patients who have normal sensation.

53.2 Goals of Surgical Procedure

- Pain relief.
- Solid union of the tibiotalar and subtalar joint arthrodesis.
- Deformity correction with restoration of plantigrade alignment of foot.
- Maximize reconstruction of limb length after bone loss.
- Maximize restoration of activity.

53.3 Advantages of Surgical Procedure

The primary advantages of using an intramedullary nail (IMN) for tibiotalocalcaneal (TTC) fusion are mechanical. The nail is a load-sharing device that demonstrates higher bending stiffness, increased rotational stability, and the capability for dynamic compression in comparison to other forms of internal fixation. It can achieve distal fixation to the calcaneus, better than with plates or screws alone.

The TTC nail is a powerful tool in cases with loss of the talar body, working well with bulk allograft to fill the bony defect; it also extends the indications for tibiocalcaneal arthrodesis because of the strong fixation in the calcaneus.

53.4 Key Principles

- Use of the nail is simply a form of fixation.
- The key to and challenge of the procedure is the surgical skill to do the following, which can be difficult, especially with bone loss and large deformity:
  ○ Prepare good bone surfaces with excellent contact and apposition.
  ○ Fashion the bony construct in proper alignment in three planes.
- Bone grafting to fill defects and augment healing.
- Satisfactory alignment in hindfoot valgus (coronal plane), ankle dorsiflexion (sagittal plane), external rotation (axial plane), and translation of the foot relative to tibial axis.
- Some degree of medialization of the foot relative to the tibia to aid nail placement.

53.5 Preoperative Preparation and Patient Positioning

53.5.1 Surgical Approach

A variety of surgical approaches are possible, according to surgeon preference, locations and type of deformity, previous incisions and implants, and soft-tissue issues.

- An anterior approach to the ankle with a lateral approach to the subtalar joint is commonly utilized. It provides a familiar view of both joints for most orthopaedic surgeons. It is best used for patients without severe varus/valgus deformity.
- An extensile lateral approach is useful with large deformities, especially in valgus. The fibula may be harvested and used as autograft.

- Combined limited anterior ankle and lateral subtalar incisions can be used when there is minimal deformity.
- A posterior, Achilles-splitting approach with the patient prone is valuable in cases of poor anterior soft-tissue envelope or large talar defect. In the latter situation, grafting from the posterior tibial to the calcaneal tuberosity mechanically augments the salvage. The malleoli can be resected and used as autograft. Intraoperative evaluation of hindfoot alignment is easier with patient prone.
- While uncommon, a medial approach to both the ankle and subtalar joints can be done with careful dissection of the neurovascular structures and a medial malleolar osteotomy.

53.5.2 Patient Positioning

- As above, the patient may be positioned in the supine, lateral, or prone position.
- A thigh tourniquet is utilized.
- The knee should be prepped into the sterile field to assist assessment of alignment.
- The patient should be positioned so that the foot is just at the end of the table to facilitate nail placement and imaging.

53.6 Operative Technique

53.6.1 Joint Preparation

- In a patient with good alignment and adequate bone stock, preparation for arthrodesis saves the shape of the joints, removing only the remaining cartilage and sclerotic bone, with sharp curettes and osteotomes. The subchondral bone can be either carefully removed to expose the cancellous surface, while preserving bone contour, or thoroughly perforated with a drill bit and/or "fish-scaled" with a sharp, narrow osteotome.
- Significant bony defects require more surgical creativity, in order to make a structurally sound construct. It is helpful to expose cancellous bone and create surfaces with wide contact, especially if structural bone graft is required.
- Hindfoot valgus is corrected first and foremost by external rotation of the calcaneus relative to the talus. The talus must be seated beneath the center of the tibial plafond, with simultaneous attention to rotation and coronal plane tilting.
- Shortening of the limb is often necessary, and has been shown to be consistent with good clinical results in patients with bone loss due to avascular necrosis of the talus.
- If the bone loss is very large, bony defects can be filled with use of a femoral head allograft, and augmented with malleable bone preparations that contain stem cell lines for bone growth, which help to fill defects.

53.6.2 Fixation

- Once the construct is complete and voids have been filled with bone graft, provisional fixation with a Steinmann pin holds the alignment during preparation for the nail. The pin must be peripheral, away from the central path of the nail.

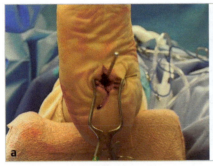 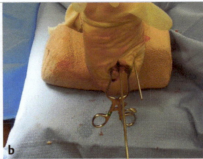

Fig. 53.3 (a,b) These photos show the patient's right foot. The eccentric provisional 2-mm Steinmann pin holding the construct during preparation for definitive arthrodesis (smaller, medial pin) as well as the long guidewire (larger, lateral pin) in place for reaming for the nail, after positioning under fluoroscopy in the AP and lateral planes.

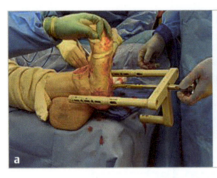 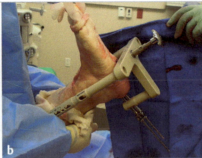

Fig. 53.4 (a) Insertion of the PANTA nail mounted on a radiolucent guide, for placement of calcaneal locking/transfixion screws. (b) Drill bits in place in the calcaneus and through the nail, just prior to insertion of posterior to anterior calcaneal locking screws.

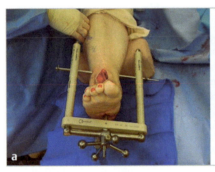 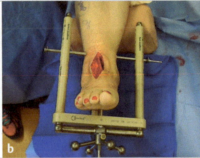

Fig. 53.5 (a,b) The metal "goal post" jig mounted inside a radiolucent jig, from different perspectives. The compression rod is passing through the jig and the slotted portion of the nail just prior to activation of the compression mechanism.

- Next, a 3- to 4-cm longitudinal plantar incision is centered on the axis of the ankle/tibia, about 2 to 3 cm proximal to the calcaneocuboid joint. Dissection of the soft tissues over the calcaneus is done to protect the lateral plantar nerve.
- The most important point in nail placement is the position of the starting guidewire. The insertion point will usually need to be as medial as possible in order to achieve a central position within the tibia in both the coronal and sagittal planes (**Fig. 53.3a,b**).
- Medialization of the talus within the ankle mortise by either narrowing or resection of the medial bone from malleolus or talus can be required if the guidewire is too lateral in the tibia.
- Once the guidewire is positioned, it is drilled and then over-reamed to a diameter of 0.5 mm over the selected width of the IMN.
- The guidewire is removed and the nail is inserted. Our preference is to use a nail with direct bone compression. The distal fixation is placed first, with two screws inserted longitudinally in the calcaneus (**Fig. 53.4a,b**).

- The construct is manually compressed before activating the compression jig.
- Then one or two compression rods are placed through the jig and through the slotted portion of the nail. The compression mechanism pulls the calcaneus and tibia together through the bone fixation of screws and rods, respectively (**Fig. 53.5a,b**).
- The compression rods typically bend once maximum compression is achieved.
- Then, the proximal locking screws are inserted into the tibia.
- While most nails have holes or slots for fixation in the talus, we almost never use them. The most common complication of any arthrodesis that aims to achieve fusion on two sides of a bone segment is nonunion on one side. In the last century, Charnley showed that arthrodesis is improved by compression. By using direct bone compression between tibia and calcaneus, the talus or bulk allograft is compressed in a "sandwich" on both the proximal and distal surfaces. Screws in the intercalary talar segment increase the risk of distraction or uneven compression, and so may increase the risk of nonunion.

53.7 Tips and Pearls

- Medialize the talus by debridement of the medial gutter and/or bone resection from malleolus or talus to align the foot with the tibia axis.
- Forego fixation of the talus to achieve simultaneous compression across both the ankle and subtalar joints, and to prevent distraction.
- Use an eccentric long Steinmann pin to provisionally hold alignment, then check with fluoroscopy in multiple planes; leave in place to insert guidewire.
- Consider a posterior approach in cases with multiple anterior surgeries, poor soft-tissue envelope, and severe talar loss.
- Check and augment bone graft after fixation of calcaneus, but before compression and placement of tibial screws.
- Calcaneal screws often exit the medial cortex of anterior process of calcaneus. This is not a problem and augments the strength of the distal fixation.

53.8 Hazards and Pitfalls

- Failures most often arise from creation of an inadequate surgical construct, with gaps in bone contact or poor alignment.
- Failure to adequately medialize the foot on the tibia makes fixation more difficult.
- Late stress reactions or stress fractures proximally at the tip of the nail are not uncommon and not predictable, but usually resolve easily by immobilization or removal of nail, after healing is complete.

53.9 Complications/Bailout/Salvage

53.9.1 Nonunion

- In the setting of a delayed union with intact hardware, an external bone stimulator may be utilized.
- If union is not present by 6 months postoperatively and the patient is symptomatic, we recommend revision arthrodesis with bone grafting of the nonunion. The IMN can be exchanged or dynamized, or a different type of fixation construct can be attempted for increased compression if necessary.
- In the setting of a symptomatic nonunion with avascular necrosis of the talus or a failed femoral head allograft, talectomy with direct tibiocalcaneal arthrodesis should be considered.

53.9.2 Infection

- If there is an acute deep infection of the device, the treatment is with thorough surgical debridement and a course of intravenous antibiotics managed by an infectious diseases specialist. The patient is kept on antibiotics until fusion is achieved and the IMN can be removed.

- In the setting of recurrent deep infection despite debridement and antibiotics, the internal fixation is removed and the patient can be converted to an Ilizarov's ring external fixator construct for TTC arthrodesis.

53.9.3 Failure

- If attempts at fusion fail multiple times, the patient has intractable pain, or if there is uncontrollable infection, below-knee amputation serves as the final salvage procedure.
- Proximal stress fracture:
  - Rarely, and most often in patients with impaired sensation, the proximal stress fracture becomes a nonunion. This usually resolves with fixation using a tibial IMN from proximal.

53.10 Postoperative Care

Postoperatively, the patient is non-weight-bearing and placed into a well-padded splint. The first follow-up visit is 2 weeks after surgery. Sutures are removed between 2 and 4 weeks. The patient is in a series of short leg, non-weight-bearing casts for another 6 weeks, after which she or he is allowed progressive weight-bearing in a walking cast for another 4 to 6 weeks. Subsequent advancement to a removable boot is then followed by physical therapy for gait training and proximal limb strengthening. Patients with neuropathy are instructed to remain non-weight-bearing for 12 weeks and sometimes more.

53.11 Outcomes

Kile et al popularized the IMN for TTC, publishing results of 30 patients, of whom 26 reported high level of satisfaction. Visual analogue scale (VAS) pain scores declined from 8.3 to 1.7.

In 2013, a multicenter study by Rammelt et al demonstrated an 84% rate of union and a 5.3% overall rate of infection in 38 patients.

Brodsky et al demonstrated good outcomes and deformity correction of 30 patients with severe deformity using the IMN. In their study, mean varus/valgus deformity correction was 13.2 degrees, and they achieved final deformities of less than 5 degrees of coronal plane deformity in 76% of their patients postoperatively. Outcome measures demonstrated significant improvements in VAS pain scale (6.5 pre-op, 1.3 post-op), AOFAS scores (29.7 pre-op, 74.3 post-op), and SF-36 scores (85.7 pre-op, 98.8 post-op). Complications included one nonunion, three tibial stress reactions at the proximal end of the nail, three infections (one deep, two superficial), and three transient plantar paresthesias.

Significant improvements in gait parameters after TTC arthrodesis have been reported as well. Tenenbaum et al compared gait characteristics of 21 patients before and after TTC arthrodesis. Their study demonstrated significant increases in cadence and walking speed as well as decreased total support time postoperatively. They also showed a significant improvement in gait symmetry.

References

1. Asomugha EU, Den Hartog BD, Junko JT, Alexander IJ. Tibi-otalocalcaneal fusion for severe deformity and bone loss. J Am Acad Orthop Surg 2016;24(3):125–134

2. Brodsky JW, Verschae G, Tenenbaum S. Surgical correction of severe deformity of the ankle and hindfoot by arthrod-esis using a compressing retrograde intramedullary nail. Foot Ankle Int 2014;35(4):360–367

3. Charnley J. Compression arthrodesis of the ankle and shoulder. J Bone Joint Surg Br 1951;33B(2):180–191

4. Jeng CL, Campbell JT, Tang EY, Cerrato RA, Myerson MS. Tibiotalocalcaneal arthrodesis with bulk femoral head al-lograft for salvage of large defects in the ankle. Foot Ankle Int 2013;34(9):1256–1266

5. Kile TA, Donnelly RE, Gehrke JC, Werner ME, Johnson KA. Tibiotalocalcaneal arthrodesis with an intramedullary de-vice. Foot Ankle Int 1994;15(12):669–673

6. McGarvey WC, Trevino SG, Baxter DE, Noble PC, Schon LC. Tibiotalocalcaneal arthrodesis: anatomic and technical considerations. Foot Ankle Int 1998;19(6):363–369

7. Rammelt S, Pyrc J, Agren PH, et al. Tibiotalocalcaneal fusion using the hindfoot arthrodesis nail: a multicenter study. Foot Ankle Int 2013;34(9):1245–1255

8. Shah KS, Younger AS. Primary tibiotalocalcaneal arthrode-sis. Foot Ankle Clin 2011;16(1):115–136

9. Tenenbaum S, Coleman SC, Brodsky JW. Improvement in gait following combined ankle and subtalar arthrodesis. J Bone Joint Surg Am 2014;96(22):1863–1869

10. Tenenbaum S, Stockton KG, Bariteau JT, Brodsky JW. Salvage of avascular necrosis of the talus by combined ankle and hindfoot arthrodesis without structural bone graft. Foot Ankle Int 2015;36(3):282–287

11. Thomas RL, Sathe V, Habib SI. The use of intramedullary nails in tibiotalocalcaneal arthrodesis. J Am Acad Orthop Surg 2012;20(1):1–7

54 Tibiotalocalcaneal Fusion with a Plate

Clifford L. Jeng

Abstract

Arthrodesis of the tibiotalar and subtalar joints is a procedure to alleviate arthritis pain, correct deformity, or provide stability. The procedure is done through a transfibular approach, which provides excellent visualization of the two joints for preparation. Excellent correction of even severe deformities can be accomplished with this approach. Multiple dedicated tibiotalocalcaneal fusion plate systems are available, but alternative fixation can be achieved with a pediatric blade plate or proximal humeral locking plate inserted "upside-down" as well.

Keywords: *tibiotalocalcaneal, ankle, subtalar, arthritis, arthrodesis*

54.1 Indications

- Ankle and hindfoot arthritis.
- Ankle deformity.
- Avascular necrosis of the talus.
- Charcot arthropathy.
- Failed total ankle replacement.
- Failed arthrodesis.
- Flaccid paralysis.
- Trauma.
- Rheumatoid arthritis.
- Reconstruction after tumor resection.
- Osteomyelitis.

54.1.1 Clinical Evaluation

- Standing alignment of both the operative leg and normal contralateral leg to determine desired limb alignment and any limb length inequality.
- Evaluation of the ankle joint, subtalar joint, and transverse tarsal joints to determine arthritic involvement and which joints need to be included in the fusion procedure.
- Vascular evaluation to determine circulation with noninvasive arterial ultrasound studies if there are no palpable pedal pulses.

54.1.2 Radiographic Evaluation

- Weight-bearing plain radiographs of the foot and ankle, including a heel alignment view.
- Computed tomography (CT) scan and magnetic resonance imaging (MRI) as needed to assess alignment, quality of bone, and presence of avascular necrosis.
- White cell–labeled nuclear scintigraphy to assess for potential infection if there is a clinical concern.

54.1.3 Contraindications

- Active infection.
- Poor soft-tissue envelope.
- Inadequate bone stock to hold fixation.
- Medical comorbidities.
- Inability to remain non-weight-bearing or to comply with postoperative protocols.
- Metal allergy.
- Relative contraindications include peripheral vascular disease, uncontrolled diabetes, and smoking.

54.1.4 Nonoperative Options

- Brace immobilization.
- Activity modification.
- Rocker bottom sole and cushioned heel to shoe; orthotic inserts.
- Medications: cortisone injection; hyaluronic acid injections; anti-inflammatory medications.

54.2 Goals of Surgical Procedure

- The goal of a tibiotalocalcaneal arthrodesis is a stable, plantigrade, painless limb.

54.3 Advantages of Surgical Procedure

- The biggest advantage of plate fixation is that there are more points of fixation available in the calcaneus compared to an intramedullary rod.
- There is also less risk of injury to the plantar nerves because no incision or reaming is required on the plantar aspect of the heel.

Disadvantages: The main downside to lateral plate fixation is that the plate is not load-sharing, and if a nonunion occurs, the screws will eventually break. An additional disadvantage is that if a wound-healing problem occurs, the lateral plate is more likely to get infected and require removal.

54.4 Key Principles

- Appropriate debridement and preparation of the joint surfaces of the ankle and subtalar joints for fusion.
- Reestablish anatomic alignment of the ankle and subtalar joints in neutral (0 degrees) dorsiflexion and 5 to 10 degrees of valgus and 10 degrees of external rotation.

- Compression of the ankle and subtalar joints through a separate screw from the calcaneus into the distal tibia anteriorly.
- Rigid fixation of the ankle and hindfoot with the plate.

54.5 Preoperative Preparation and Patient Positioning

It is easiest to do this procedure in the lateral decubitus position as long as no additional medial-sided work needs to be done. Assessing alignment can be slightly more difficult in this lateral position, especially rotational alignment. Supine or "sloppy lateral" positions are also acceptable positions that make it easier to approach the medial ankle gutter through a separate arthrotomy or to include a talonavicular fusion to the procedure. Make sure that the patient is well padded with axillary roll if necessary and egg crate/sponge under the down side. A thigh tourniquet is helpful given this procedure can be fairly bloody. A popliteal block or other regional anesthesia prior to the induction of general anesthesia can be helpful for postoperative pain relief. The operative limb should be prepped and draped above the knee so that alignment of the fusion can be accurately assessed and proximal tibial bone graft can be harvested if necessary. TED hose and a sequential compression device on the down leg during surgery may be helpful in preventing deep venous thrombosis. Preoperative intravenous antibiotics must be given. A Foley catheter may be helpful to avoid excessive bladder distension during what can often be a lengthy anesthetic.[1-5]

54.5.1 Anatomic Issues to Consider

The sural and superficial peroneal nerves are vulnerable in this approach. The sural nerve is found distally over the calcaneal tuberosity and the superficial peroneal nerve proximally near where the fibula is transected. The fibula is difficult to remove due to the strong interosseous membrane and syndesmotic ligaments. Once the fibula is removed, it is important to find and cauterize the peroneal artery, which will be cut from incising the interosseous membrane. The peroneal tendons at the distal end of the incision can be either retained or excised. There are no long-term negative effects from excising the peroneal tendons. Two large bony prominences, the lateral process of the talus and the Chaput tubercle of the tibia, interfere with laying the plate flat against the bone. These must be removed in order to position the plate flush, which is important because if the plate is elevated off the bone, it can be difficult to obtain a good closure distally. The posterior facet of the subtalar joint is surprisingly vertical. The middle facet of the subtalar joint is visualized distal and medial to the posterior facet and should be prepared as well to maximize fusion surface area. The medial gutter of the ankle joint can be prepared either across the ankle using a lamina spreader and angled curettes or through a separate anteromedial arthrotomy. Throughout the procedure, be careful not to injure the neurovascular bundles lying anteriorly and posteromedially.[6]

54.6 Operative Technique

54.6.1 Surgical Approach

Make a 15-cm longitudinal incision centered over the middle of the fibula. It is helpful to use the planned internal fixation plate to measure how proximal the fibula will need to be transected. Dissect through the subcutaneous tissue in order to identify the superficial peroneal and sural nerves. The superficial peroneal nerve will be in the proximal aspect of incision running from posterior to anterior. The sural nerve will be distal in the incision over the calcaneal tuberosity. The sural nerve always runs together with a large vein from posterior to anterior. Protect these nerves and then incise directly down to bone on the fibula, talus, and lateral aspect of the calcaneus. Expose subperiosteally the fibula and lateral malleolus. Identify the syndesmosis anteriorly with a scalpel blade and then use a Cobb elevator or osteotome to release the syndesmosis and interosseous membrane between the tibia and fibula. Use Hohmann retractors anterior and posterior to the fibula as far proximally as your incision will allow and make a fibular osteotomy using a sagittal saw. The osteotomy should be either transverse or beveled slightly distally to avoid a sharp point underneath the skin. Continue to release what is left of the interosseous membrane and syndesmosis until the fibula is free and remove it to the back table to be harvested for bone graft. Find the peroneal artery which is routinely cut in this approach and cauterize it (**Figs. 54.1, 54.2**).

54.6.2 Joint Exposure

Identify the ankle and subtalar joints. The peroneal tendons cover the posterior facet of the subtalar joint and may be either retracted during joint preparation or excised. There are no long-term negative effects of excising the peroneal tendons. Approach the subtalar joint first, using scalpel and rongeur to remove the contents of the sinus tarsi including the interosseous ligament which will interfere with distracting the joint open. An elevator can then be inserted into the subtalar joint and twisted to pry apart the capsular ligaments. Once this is complete, insert a toothed lamina spreader into the sinus tarsi and distract open the posterior facet of the subtalar joint. Further debridement medially is necessary to see the middle facet of the joint (**Fig. 54.4**). Now remove the lamina spreader and insert it in between the tibia and talus to expose the ankle joint. If it is too tight, a Cobb elevator can be passed anterior and posterior to the ankle joint to gently pry off the capsule, and a scalpel can then be used to release subperiosteally around the joint. Be careful not to overstrip the periosteum, which may damage the blood supply to the tibia and talus and impair healing. An elevator can then be inserted between the tibia and talus and twisted to pry open the remaining capsular ligaments. Now a toothed lamina spreader is inserted between the tibia and talus to fully expose the joint for preparation (**Fig. 54.3**).

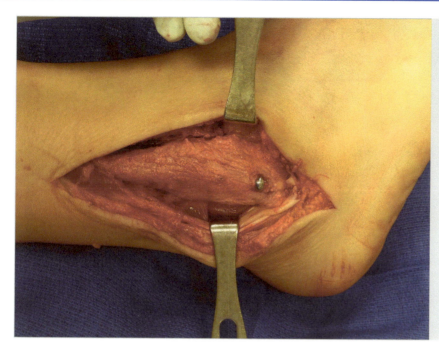

Fig. 54.1 Subperiosteal dissection over the fibula prior to osteotomy and removal of fibula.

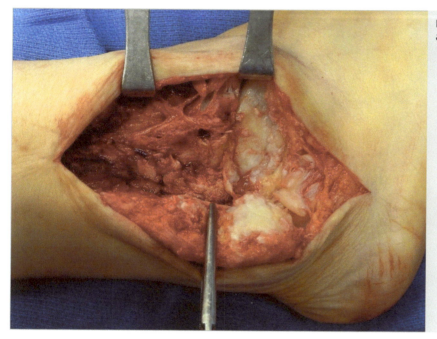

Fig. 54.2 Fibula is removed revealing ankle and subtalar joints.

54.6.3 Joint Preparation for Fusion

Remove articular cartilage from both sides of the ankle and subtalar joints including the medial gutter of ankle joint and the middle facet of subtalar joint. Prepare the underlying subchondral bone surfaces per surgeon preference (drill, scale, feather, burr). An alternative option for preparing the ankle joint is to make flat parallel cuts on the distal tibia and proximal talus while holding the foot and ankle in a plantigrade position. While this is quicker and can be useful to correct severe deformities with contracture, it shortens the limb slightly and is technically more difficult to obtain neutral ankle alignment.

A separate anteromedial ankle arthrotomy can be made to prepare the medial ankle gutter for fusion if desired. In flexible ankles, the medial gutter can sometimes be prepared from the lateral approach using angled curettes.

54.6.4 Bone Grafting

Obtain autogenous bone graft from either the ipsilateral iliac crest or proximal tibia. Other options are to use allograft bone or bone graft substitutes. Insert these into the ankle and subtalar joints after thorough irrigation of the surgical field (**Figs. 54.5, 54.6**).

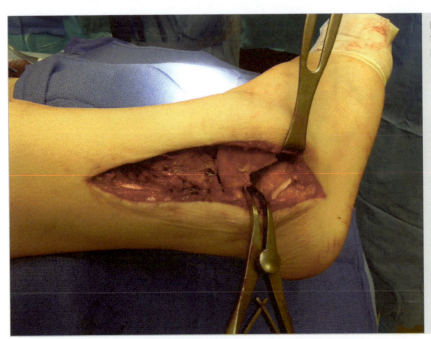

Fig. 54.3 Lamina spreader in the posterior facet of subtalar joint to expose for joint preparation.

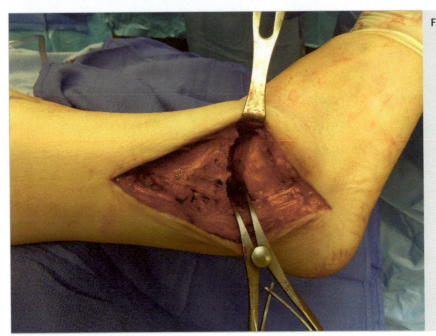

Fig. 54.4 Lamina spreader in the ankle joint.

54.6.5 Joint Alignment

Align the ankle into the optimal position now with 90 degrees of flexion, 5 to 10 degrees of valgus, and rotation of the foot so the tibial crest aligns with the second ray of the foot. Adjustments to this "ideal" alignment should be made based on the contralateral leg alignment assessed preoperatively assuming this is normal. Also, in obese patients, the heel is fused intentionally in slightly more valgus to avoid lateral overload during gait. In patients with anterior or posterior subluxation of the talus beneath the tibia, a Weber reduction clamp can help center the lateral process of the talus below the tibia. Patients with severe varus malalignment may require soft-tissue release of the deltoid ligament and posterior tibial tendon. Pin across the ankle and subtalar joints from the heel up through the tibial cortex to hold this position. Check the final position both clinically and under fluoroscopy (**Fig. 54.7**).

54.6.6 Plate Fixation for Fusion

- A large 7.0-mm axial screw placed from under the calcaneus and directed proximally across both joints and into the hard cortical bone of the tibia is inserted first to compress across the fusion sites. This is usually positioned in the sagittal plane from the posterior inferior calcaneal tuberosity into the anterior tibial cortex. Some lateral tibiotalocalcaneal plate designs allow an axial screw to be inserted through a distal screw hole that wraps under the calcaneus.

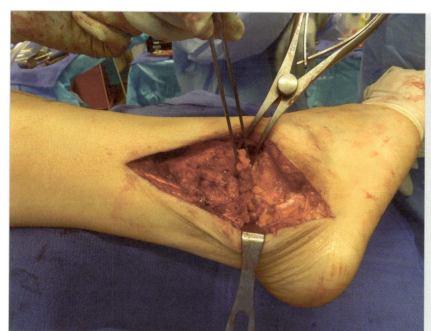

Fig. 54.5 Combination of proximal tibia bone graft and fibula autograft is placed into the ankle joint.

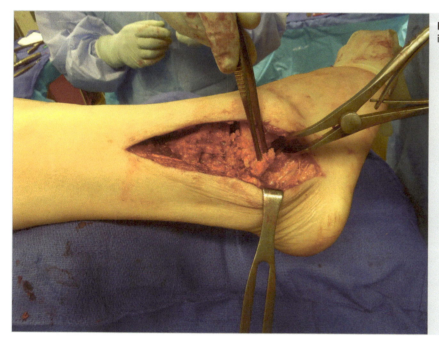

Fig. 54.6 Autogenous bone graft inserted into the subtalar joint.

• The plate is now provisionally placed on the lateral aspect of the bone to identify prominent areas that will prevent the plate from sitting flush along its entire length. A saw is used to brush flat these problem areas until the plate fits flat against the bone. This is critical because if the plate is prominent it can make closure at the end of the case difficult. The plate should be pinned into position and its alignment relative to the tibia and calcaneus checked with fluoroscopy. Calcaneal fixation is achieved first with screws through the distal end of the plate. Locked versus unlocked screw fixation should be determined by the quality of the bone. Further compression is then obtained by inserting screws in dynamic compression mode into the proximal holes of the plate obtaining purchase into the hard cortical bone of the tibial diaphysis. The remaining screw holes are then filled, includ-

ing fixation into the talar body. Intraoperative fluoroscopy is used to check for final alignment and satisfactory positioning of all hardware (**Figs. 54.8, 54.9, 54.10**).

54.6.7 Closure

Insertion of a drain is up to surgeon preference. It is critical to get a deep layer closed over the plate so that if there is a superficial wound dehiscence, the hardware will not automatically be exposed. Anything possible to close dead space between the skin and plate will be beneficial in avoiding a large subcutaneous hematoma. Usually the skin has very little tension during closure due to the removal of the fibula. However, in severe valgus cases when the deformity is corrected, the skin can become very tight. A sterile compressive bandage with plaster splints is applied.

54.7 Tips and Pearls

- There must be a good skin and soft-tissue envelope laterally over the fibula to perform this procedure. In patients with severe valgus deformity, it may become difficult to adequately close the incision once the deformity has been corrected due to the increased tension on the soft tissues.
- Avoid injuring the superficial peroneal and sural nerves during the lateral approach.

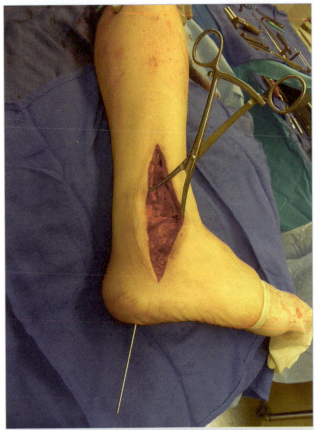

Fig. 54.7 The ankle and subtalar joints are reduced into a neutral/plantigrade position and held in place with a stout guide pin.

- Make sure that the talus is aligned correctly in both the sagittal and coronal planes prior to applying fixation. The most common malalignments are anterior translation or lateral subluxation of the talus beneath the tibia.
- Meticulously prepare joint surfaces for fusion including removal of all articular cartilage and aggressive perforation of the subchondral bone.
- Add autograft or allograft bone and/or bone graft substitutes to help augment the fusion.
- Make sure that the plate fits flat against the bone along its entire length by removing the Chaput tubercle of the tibia and the lateral process of talus. Additional trimming of any prominent areas of bone using a saw or osteotome may be necessary.
- Compress the ankle and subtalar joints with an axial partially threaded screw from the posterior heel to the anterior tibial cortex prior to applying the lateral plate.
- Be certain to meticulously close the deep layer to cover the plate completely. This can protect it from infection if there is a superficial wound dehiscence.

54.8 Hazards and Pitfalls

- Wound-healing problems.
- Infection.
- Nerve injury.
- Nonunion.
- Malunion.
- Painful hardware.

54.9 Complications/Bailout/ Salvage

If plate fixation fails, the surgeon can convert to intramedullary nail fixation or screws alone. If all else fails, a multiplanar external fixator can be applied to hold the fusion. Additionally, in cases where the internal fixation is questionable, an external fixator can be applied to supplement the stability of the construct.

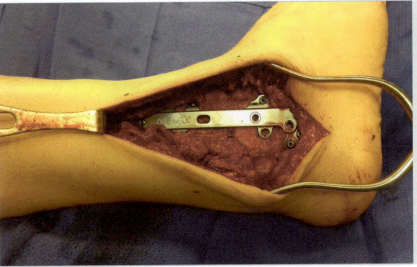

Fig. 54.8 Lateral tibiotalocalcaneal fusion plate is affixed to lateral aspect of ankle after removing bony prominences.

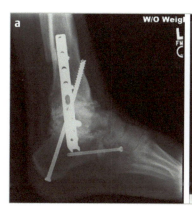 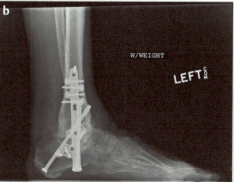

Fig. 54.9 (a) Tibiotalocalcaneal fusion fixed with pediatric blade plate, and (b) fusion fixed with dedicated lateral tibiotalocalcaneal fusion plate.

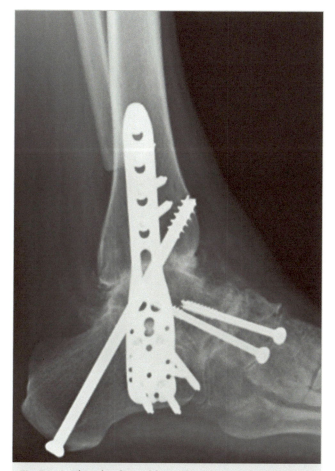

Fig. 54.10 Tibiotalocalcaneal fusion fixed with proximal humeral locking plate applied upside-down.

54.10 Postoperative Care

The postoperative splint is changed and stitches are removed at 2 weeks. Patients are immobilized in a below-the-knee cast and kept non-weight-bearing for 12 weeks. A CT scan is ordered at 12 weeks postoperatively to confirm healing of both arthrodesis sites. If there is only partial healing present, the patient is converted to a removable CAM boot and kept non-weight-bearing for an additional month.

54.11 Outcomes

Several small series have documented satisfactory fusion rates for tibiotalocalcaneal fusion with lateral plate fixation. Özer et al had an 87% fusion rate in 8 patients followed for 32 months with no signs of failure of fixation.[7] Kheir et al used an inverted 90-degree blade plate in a diverse group of 11 patients with a 91% fusion rate.[8] Ahmad et al used an upside-down 3.5-mm proximal humeral locking plate in 18 fusions for Charcot, avascular necrosis of the talus, neuromuscular disease, and arthritis. At 20-month follow-up, 94% of the patients had successfully fused with improved AOFAS outcome scores.[9]

References

1. Chiodo CP, Acevedo JI, Sammarco VJ, et al. Intramedullary rod fixation compared with blade-plate-and-screw fixation for tibiotalocalcaneal arthrodesis: a biomechanical investigation. J Bone Joint Surg Am 2003;85-A(12):2425–2428

2. Alfahd U, Roth SE, Stephen D, Whyne CM. Biomechanical comparison of intramedullary nail and blade plate fixation for tibiotalocalcaneal arthrodesis. J Orthop Trauma 2005;19(10):703–708

3. O'Neill PJ, Logel KJ, Parks BG, Schon LC. Rigidity comparison of locking plate and intramedullary fixation for tibiotalocalcaneal arthrodesis. Foot Ankle Int 2008;29(6):581–586

4. Chodos MD, Parks BG, Schon LC, Guyton GP, Campbell JT. Blade plate compared with locking plate for tibiotalocalcaneal arthrodesis: a cadaver study. Foot Ankle Int 2008;29(2):219–224

5. Ohlson BL, Shatby MW, Parks BG, White KL, Schon LC. Periarticular locking plate vs intramedullary nail for tibiotalocalcaneal arthrodesis: a biomechanical investigation. Am J Orthop 2011;40(2):78–83

6. Rausch S, Loracher C, Fröber R, et al. Anatomical evaluation of different approaches for tibiotalocalcaneal arthrodesis. Foot Ankle Int 2014;35(2):163–167

7. Özer D, Bayhan Aİ, Keskin A, Sarı S, Kaygusuz MA. Tibiotalocalcaneal arthrodesis by using proximal humeral locking plate. Acta Orthop Traumatol Turc 2016;50(4):389–392

8. Kheir E, Borse V, Bryant H, Farndon M. The use of the 4.5 mm 90° titanium cannulated LC-angled blade plate in tibiotalocalcaneal and complex ankle arthrodesis. Foot Ankle Surg 2015;21(4):240–244

9. Ahmad J, Pour AE, Raikin SM. The modified use of a proximal humeral locking plate for tibiotalocalcaneal arthrodesis. Foot Ankle Int 2007;28(9):977–983

55 Ankle Fractures

Trapper A.J. Lalli and Dane K. Wukich

Abstract

Ankle fractures account for approximately 9% of all fractures and are among the most common fractures treated by orthopaedic surgeons, second only to proximal femur fractures as the most common lower extremity fracture.[1] The complexity in treating ankle fractures arises in their variable presentation and mechanism of injury. Due to these factors, every patient with an ankle fracture should be thoroughly evaluated. Each ankle fracture should be assessed for specific characteristics, including bone quality, fracture comminution, marginal impaction, presence of additional fractures, soft-tissue injury, and host factors. Detailed preoperative evaluation, surgical planning, meticulous surgical technique, and management of soft tissues are keys to help obtain good outcomes. This chapter provides surgical tips and pearls to achieve excellent outcomes and maximize patient function.

Keywords: *ankle fracture, bimalleolar, trimalleolar, open reduction, internal fixation*

55.1 Introduction

55.1.1 Pathology/Classification

- **Anatomic**
  - Isolated medial malleolar fracture.
  - Isolated lateral malleolar fracture.
  - Bimalleolar fracture.
  - Trimalleolar fracture.
  - Maisonneuve's injury.
- **Danis–Weber:**
Describes the level of the medial aspect of the fibular fracture:
  - A: infrasyndesmotic:
    - Usually a transverse avulsion-type fracture as a result of an inversion mechanism.
    - Most commonly stable and does not require ORIF.
  - B: transsyndesmotic:
    - Usually an oblique or spiral fracture.
    - May or may not be stable requiring ORIF.
    - Syndesmotic ligaments usually intact.
  - C: suprasyndesmotic:
    - An unstable fracture most commonly requiring ORIF.
    - Syndesmotic ligaments usually disrupted and requires fixation.
- **AO/ATA:**
  - 44A: infrasyndesmotic.
  - 44B: transsyndesmotic.
  - 44C: suprasyndesmotic.
- **Lauge-Hansen:**
The first descriptor describes the position the foot was in at the time of the deforming injury mechanism. The second descriptor describes the direction of force on the ankle at the time of injury. Each type of injury has a subset of sequential progression of injury severity.
  - **Supination-adduction:**
    - **I:** talofibular sprain or distal fibular avulsion.
    - **II:** vertical medial malleolus and impaction of anteromedial distal tibia.
  - **Supination-external rotation (SER):**
    - **I:** anterior tibiofibular ligament sprain.
    - **II:** lateral short oblique fibula fracture (anteroinferior to posterosuperior).
    - **III:** posterior tibiofibular ligament rupture or avulsion of posterior malleolus.
    - **IV:** medial malleolus transverse fracture or disruption of deltoid ligament.
  - **Pronation-abduction:**
    - **I:** medial malleolus transverse fracture or disruption of deltoid ligament.
    - **II:** anterior tibiofibular ligament sprain.
    - **III:** transverse, comminuted fibula fracture above the level of the syndesmosis.
  - **Pronation-external rotation:**
    - **I:** transverse medial malleolus fracture or disruption of deltoid ligament.
    - **II:** anterior tibiofibular ligament disruption.
    - **III:** short oblique/spiral fracture of fibula above the level of the joint.
    - **IV:** posterior tibiofibular ligament rupture or avulsion of posterior malleolus.

55.2 Nonoperative Treatment

55.2.1 Indications

- Isolated fibula fracture with < 3-mm displacement:
  - Negative stress radiograph.
- Isolated, nondisplaced medial malleolus fracture or tip avulsion.
- Posterior malleolus fracture with < 25% joint involvement or < 2-mm displacement.

55.2.2 Treatment

- Short leg cast or controlled ankle motion (CAM) boot.

55.2.3 Clinical Evaluation

- Assess soft-tissue envelope.
- Assess neurovascular status.
- Physical examination is an unreliable indicator of deltoid ligament injury.[2]

55.2.4 Radiographic Evaluation

Standard Radiographs

- Anteroposterior (AP), mortise, lateral.
- Obtain radiographs of joints proximal and distal to injury:
  ○ Evaluate for Maisonneuve's injury and concomitant foot fractures.

Gravity Stress Radiograph[3]

- Equivalent to manual stress radiograph.
- Use for initial screening tool to distinguish SER II from SER IV equivalent.

External Rotation Stress Radiograph

- Intraoperative stress radiograph to assess competency of deltoid ligament:
  ○ Medial clear space of > 5 mm with external rotation stress is predictive of deep deltoid disruption.

Syndesmosis Evaluation

- Decreased tibiofibular overlap:
  ○ Normal > 6 mm on AP view.
  ○ Normal > 1 mm on mortise view.
- Increased medial clear space widening:
  ○ Normal less than or equal to 4 mm.
- Increased tibiofibular clear space:
  ○ Normal < 6 mm on both AP and mortise views.

Radiographic Measurements

- Talocrural angle:
  ○ Measured by bisection of line through tibial anatomical axis and another line through the tips of the malleoli.
  ○ Shortening of lateral malleoli fractures can lead to increased talocrural angle.

55.2.5 Contraindication to Open Reduction and Internal Fixation

- Medical health precluding surgical treatment.
- Poor vascularity to the affected limb.
- Poor soft-tissue envelope at the surgical site.
- Active surgical-site infection.

55.3 Goals of Procedure

- Stable, anatomic reduction of the talus within the ankle mortise.
- Ensure less than 1-mm shift of the talus within the mortise:
  ○ Greater than 1-mm shift causes 42% decreased tibiotalar contact area.[4]
- Allow early range of motion of stable ankle joint.

55.4 Advantages of ORIF

- Anatomic reconstruction of the ankle mortise.
- Reconstruction of tibiotalar congruency.
- Rigid fracture fixation.
- Early range of motion of the ankle joint.
- Prevention of posttraumatic arthritis of the ankle.

55.5 Key Principles of the Surgical Procedure

- Outcomes correlate with anatomic reduction.
- Restore length and rotation of fibula.
- Use "dime sign" (Shenton's line) to determine proper length of fibula.
- Ensure rigid fixation of the ankle bony fractures to allow early ankle motion.

55.6 Operative Technique

- **Indications:**
  ○ Medial clear space widening of > 4 to 5 mm on the ankle mortise radiograph.[5]
  ○ Isolated, displaced medial or lateral malleolus fracture.
  ○ Bimalleolar fracture or bimalleolar equivalent fracture.
  ○ Talar displacement.
  ○ Open fracture.
  ○ Bosworth's fracture/dislocation.
  ○ Associated syndesmosis injury.
  ○ Fibular shortening.
  ○ Dynamic instability on stress views.
  ○ Marginal impaction of the tibial plafond.

55.6.1 Patient Positioning

- Supine on a radiolucent table.
- Operative extremity is placed on a radiolucent bump or stack of blankets.
- Place a bump under the ipsilateral hip to put the extremity in a neutral position:
  ○ If the medial malleolus requires fixation, the bump can be removed to allow external rotation.
- Place 4-5 sterile towels under the distal leg, proximal to the heel:
  ○ Avoids anterior translation of the talus.

55.6.2 Surgical Approach

- The distal fibula is approached through a lateral incision over or just posterior to the fibula, centered over the fracture site (**Fig. 55.1**):
  ○ The superficial peroneal nerve (SPN) crosses the fibular from posterior to anterior at a level 7 cm proximal to the tip of the fibula. This needs to be dissected out, mobilized, and protected for fractures requiring an incision extended down to this level.

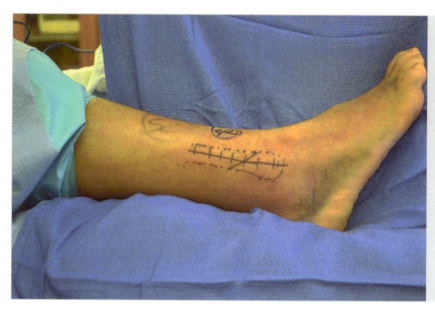

Fig. 55.1 Lateral view of the operative extremity with skin incision drawn out.

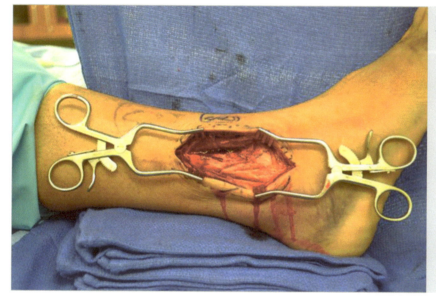

Fig. 55.2 Dissection to fracture site with soft tissues retracted.

55.6.3 Procedure

- **Lateral approach** (**Fig. 55.2**):
  - The skin is sharply incised and hemostasis is achieved with electrocautery.
  - Blunt dissection is carried out with a hemostat to expose the fracture site.
  - Be aware of the SPN, especially in the proximal extent of the incision.
  - With the fracture site exposed, 1 to 2 mm of periosteum is elevated sharply with a scalpel to aid in a cortical read for reduction.
  - A pointed reduction clamp can be placed on the proximal and distal fragments and used to expose the ends of the fracture site (**Fig. 55.3**).
  - The fracture hematoma should then be irrigated from the ends of the bone and the fracture site should be cleared of soft tissue.
  - Avoid damaging the cortical ends because they are critical to aid in reduction.
  - Once the fracture is cleared of hematoma and soft tissue, the reduction maneuver is performed.
  - A pointed reduction clamp can be used to grasp the proximal and distal fragments. A combination of pronation/supination and internal/external rotation can be used to reduce the fracture and regain length. Traction and manipulation of the foot are often helpful in fracture reduction (**Fig. 55.4**).
  - Once the fracture is reduced, a reduction clamp can be placed across the fracture site to hold the reduction while internal fixation is placed (**Fig. 55.5**).
  - In general, oblique fractures are treated with lag screw fixation with a 3.5-mm, fully threaded cortical screw and neutralization plating. Lag screws are placed perpendicular to the fracture site and are done through AO technique (**Fig. 55.6**).

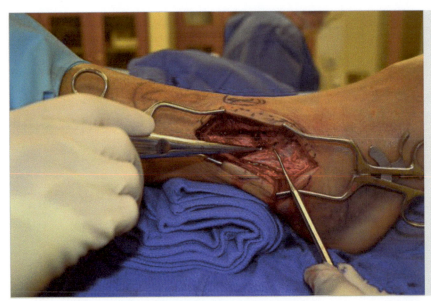

Fig. 55.3 Exposure of fracture site with removal of interposed soft tissue and fracture hematoma.

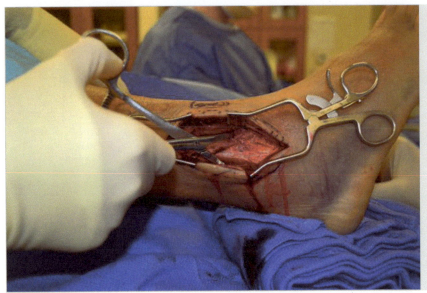

Fig. 55.4 Fracture reduction with reduction clamp.

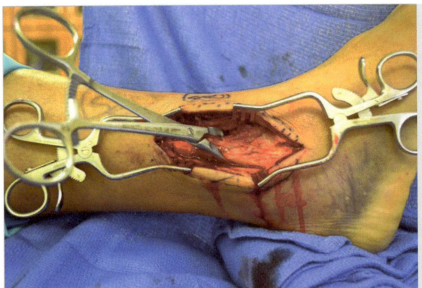

Fig. 55.5 Reduced lateral malleolus fracture with reduction clamp in place.

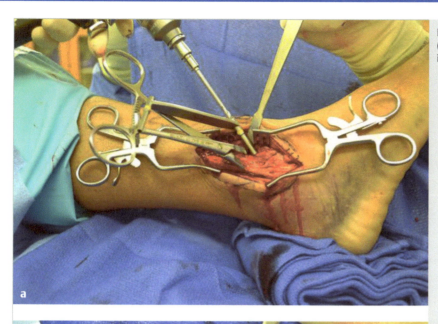
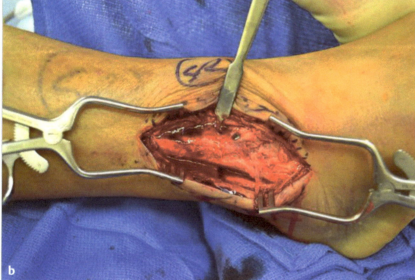

Fig. 55.6 (a) Drilling for lag screw placement. (b) Lateral malleolus fracture with lag screw in place.

- Small oblique fragments may be more amenable to 2.7-mm lag screw fixation.
- If there is not adequate purchase with the initial lag screw, a 4.0 cancellous screw can be used.
- With lateral plating, the distal screws must be unicortical to avoid penetrating the ankle joint.
- 1/3 tubular plates are used, unless the patient has poor bone quality, a distal fracture, or diabetes; then, a distal fibular locking plate is more appropriate (**Fig. 55.7**).
- **Medial approach:**
  - The medial malleolus is approached through a longitudinal incision along the midline of the medial tibia. Carry the incision 1 to 2 cm distal to the end of the bone to allow access to the anterior colliculus.
  - The skin is sharply incised and care is taken to avoid the saphenous neurovascular bundle. Blunt dissection is used to identify, mobilize, and protect the neurovascular bundle.
  - The fracture site can then be identified and 1 to 2 mm of periosteum dissected from the fractured ends to expose the cortical bone and aid in reduction.

- The fracture site must be booked open to allow evacuation of the hematoma and removal of any interposed soft tissue.
- The fracture can then be reduced and held in place with a 0.062 K-wire. Once the fracture is provisionally held in place, use fluoroscopy to confirm the reduction. When reduction is confirmed, internal fixation can be placed.
- The preferred technique for internal fixation is with two 4.0 partially threaded cancellous screws, usually 40 to 50 mm in length, placed across the fracture site and into the tibial metaphysis.
- These screws should be placed parallel to each other on the lateral radiograph. They should be as perpendicular to the fracture as possible. The anterior screw should be at the anterior colliculus and the posterior screw should be no more posterior than the center of the intercollicular groove to avoid damage to the posterior tibial tendon.
- In patients with poor bone quality, or a small fragment, consider using one screw and an antirotational K-wire.
- Other options for patients with poor bone quality is to use long, bicortical screws.
- Vertical shear fractures are treated with antiglide plating.

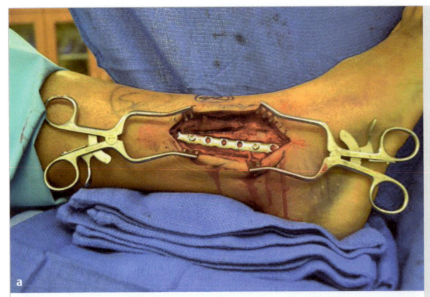

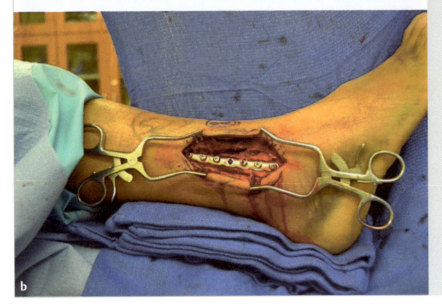

Fig. 55.7 **(a)** Plate placement with initial fixation in place. **(b)** Plate placement with final fixation in place.

- **Syndesmosis fixation:**
  - Syndesmosis stability is assessed after ankle fixation is completed. This is done with the external rotation test under fluoroscopy. If more than 1 to 2 mm of widening is found, syndesmosis fixation is performed.
  - Syndesmosis fixation is done laterally to medially, with either suture button fixation or screw fixation.
  - A pelvic reduction clamp is useful to reduce the syndesmosis. One tine of the reduction clamp is placed in the distal fibula and one tine is placed in the anteromedial aspect of the tibia. Avoid placing the heel on the bed during reduction because this can cause the talus to anteriorly displace and may malreduce the syndesmosis.
  - Choice of syndesmosis fixation is controversial, without clear superiority. Generally, one 3.5-mm, fully threaded cortical screw is placed across four cortices. Screws should be placed 2 cm proximal and parallel to the tibiotalar joint. They should be angled 20 to 30 degrees anteriorly in the tibia.
  - In high-level athletes, we opt for a suture button instead of a screw.

- **Lateral malleolus (Fig. 55.8)**
- Plate placement:
  - Lateral plating:
    - ❖ Straight lateral incision.
    - ❖ Lag screw fixation with neutralization plating.
    - ❖ Bridge plating technique for severe comminution.
  - Posterior plating:
    - ❖ Posterolateral incision.
    - ❖ Antiglide technique:
      – Lag screw fixation with neutralization plating.
      – Biomechanically stronger than lateral plating.
    - ❖ Disadvantage:
      – Peroneal irritation.
    - ❖ Transverse fracture pattern:
      – Intramedullary retrograde 3.5 screw.
      – Requires minimal soft-tissue dissection.[6]
    - ❖ Minimally invasive plate osteosynthesis:
      – Less periosteal stripping.[7]
- **Medial malleolus:**
  - Lag screw fixation:
    - ❖ 4.0 cancellous screws.

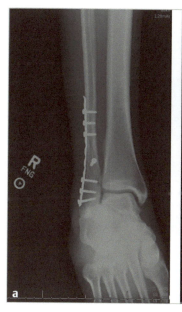 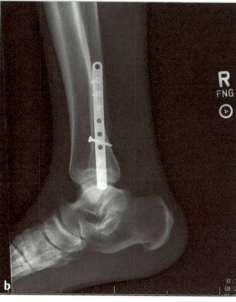

Fig. 55.8 (a) Mortise view of lateral malleolus fracture with internal fixation. **(b)** Lateral view of lateral malleolus fracture with internal fixation.

- Antiglide plate:
  - Best for vertical shear fractures.
  - Tension band fixation.
- **Posterior malleolus[8]:**
  - Posteromedial approach:
    - Best for posteromedial fragment.
    - Allows for concomitant treatment of medial malleolus fractures.
  - Posterolateral approach:
    - Provides good visualization.
    - Allows simultaneous fixation of a fibula fracture.
    - Done in prone position.
  - AP screw fixation:
    - Dental pick can be useful to aid reduction.
  - K-wires can provisionally hold fragment.
- **Syndesmosis injury:**
  - Most common in Weber C fracture patterns.
  - Fixation usually not required when fracture within 4.5 cm of plafond.
  - Length and rotation of fibula must be accurately restored.
  - Outcomes correlated with anatomic reduction:
    - Malreduction is common, can be around 30%.[9]
  - Fixation technique is controversial (**Fig. 55.9**):
    - Screw size, 3.5 or 4.5 mm.
    - Number of screws:
      - One or two cortical screws placed 2 to 4 cm above joint and angled 30 degrees posterior to anterior.
  - Screw fixation versus suture button construct.
  - Number of cortices: 3 or 4.
  - Screw removal versus screw retention:
    - If removing screws, do so at 8 to 12 weeks.
- Outcomes are similar at 1 year.[10]

55.7 Diabetic Ankle Fractures

- **Tips and pearls**
  - Carefully evaluate preoperative neurovascular status.
  - Enhance fixation[11]:
    - Multiple tetracortical syndesmotic screws:
    - Even in the absence of syndesmotic injury.

- More rigid fixation:
  - Small fragment locking plates.
  - Compression plates.
  - Consider temporary tibiotalar Steinmann pins (i.e., Childress pin) (**Fig. 55.10**).
- Sprinkle vancomycin powder in wounds prior to closure.[12]
- Meticulous control of postoperative blood glucose levels.[13]
  - < 200 mg/dL.
- Postoperative care:
  - Double time spent non-weight-bearing (8–12 weeks).
- Complications[14]:
  - Increased risk of malunion, nonunion, hardware failure.
  - Infection.
  - Charcot neuroarthropathy.
  - Increased length of stay and in-hospital mortality.

55.8 Tips and Pearls

- If you are unable to reduce the lateral malleolus, assess the medial and lateral gutters.
- When placing syndesmosis fixation, elevate the leg on towels to allow your hand to drop to the appropriate 30-degree angle.
- If medial clear space widening remains after syndesmosis fixation, assess medial gutter for soft-tissue interposition and need for deltoid ligament repair.
- Small medial malleolus fractures can be fixed with K-wires, if they are too small to be fixed with a screw.
- Use of a washer spreads out compressive forces over medial malleolus and is useful in osteopenic bone.
- CT scan is imperative for evaluation of posterior malleolus fracture fragment size (**Fig. 55.11**).

55.9 Hazards and Pitfalls

- Avoid injury to the SPN laterally and sural nerve medially.
- Avoid fracture comminution with lag screw placement.
- Identify and address marginal impaction of tibia:
  - Bone graft and use internal fixation.

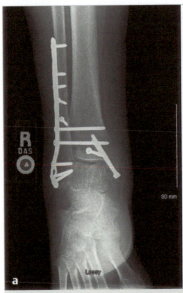
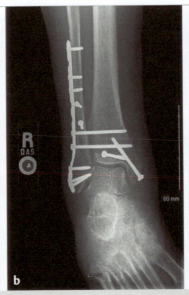
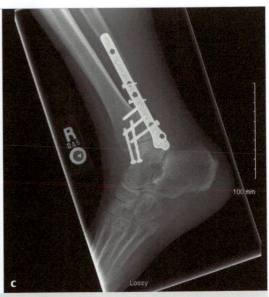

Fig. 55.9 **(a)** Anteroposterior view of trimalleolar ankle fracture with transsyndesmotic fixation in place. **(b)** Mortise view of trimalleolar ankle fracture with transsyndesmotic fixation in place. **(c)** Lateral view of trimalleolar ankle fracture with transsyndesmotic fixation in place.

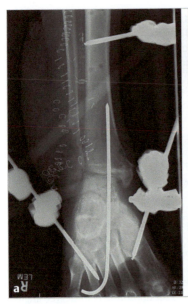
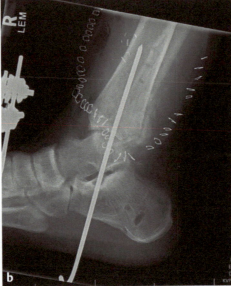

Fig. 55.10 **(a)** Anteroposterior view of a bimalleolar ankle fracture in a patient with diabetes with tibiotalocalcaneal Steinmann pin in place and A-frame external fixation. **(b)** Lateral view of a bimalleolar ankle fracture in a patient with diabetes with tibiotalocalcaneal Steinmann pin in place and A-frame external fixation.

55.10 Complications[15]

- Overall rate of complications after ORIF varies between 5 and 40%:
  - Open injuries, elderly patients, patients with insulin-dependent diabetes, peripheral vascular disease and smokers are at higher risk.[16]
- Wound complications: 1 to 18%.[17-19]

55.11 Postoperative Care

55.11.1 Postprocedure

- All patients are non-weight-bearing and placed in a well-padded splint.

55.11.2 Weeks 0 to 2

- Rest, ice, elevation.
- Sutures removed at 2 week postoperative visit, if no wound problems.
- Remove splint, transition to short leg cast or boot.

55.11.3 Weeks 2 to 6

- Multiplane hip strengthening.
- Core and upper extremity strengthening.
- Continue non-weight-bearing status.

55.11.4 Six Week Postoperative Visit

- Obtain AP, mortise, lateral radiographs to assess healing.

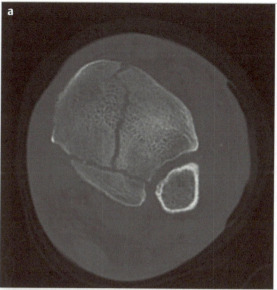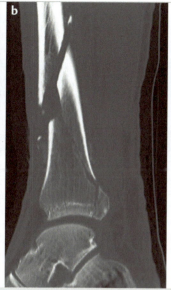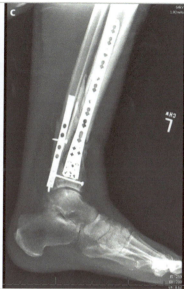

Fig. 55.11 (a) Axial computed tomography view of a pilon fracture with posterior malleolar fragment. (b) Sagittal computed tomography view of a pilon fracture with posterior malleolar fragment. (c) Lateral radiograph of a pilon fracture treated with internal fixation.

• Transition to CAM boot at 6 weeks, if patient has been in a cast.
• Wean off crutches.

Physical Therapy

• Gradual progression to full weight-bearing at 6 to 10 weeks postoperatively in CAM boot.
• Restore normal gait mechanics.
• Full active and passive ROM in all planes.
• Isometric and isotonic ankle strengthening.
• Foot intrinsic strengthening.
• Proprioception training.
• Nonimpact cardiovascular work.
• Edema control.
• Scar massage.

55.11.5 Week 12 Postoperative Visit

• Weight-bearing radiographs.

Physical Therapy

• Transition from CAM boot to ankle brace.
• Restoration of full range of motion in all planes.
• Advance foot and ankle intrinsic strengthening.
• Pool running progressing to dry land.
• Linear progression to lateral and rotational functional movements.
• Bilateral progression to unilateral plyometric activity.
• Continue modalities.

55.11.6 Weeks 12 to 16

Physical Therapy

• Advance impact and functional progressing.
• Sport/job-specific functions with functional brace.
• Functional bracing during sports for first year.
• Continue modalities PRN.

55.11.7 Six Month Postoperative Visit

• Weight-bearing radiographs.
• Continue bracing during competitive activities.

55.11.8 One Year Postoperative Visit

• Weight-bearing radiographs.

55.12 Outcomes

• At 1 year, 90% have no limitations or limitations only in recreational activities[20]:
  ○ Age less than 40 years: more likely to gain greater than 90% recovery at 1 year.
  ○ Men, ASA class 1 or 2, and absence of diabetes are predictors of better functional recovery at 1 year.
• Prolonged recovery expected:
  ○ Up to 2 years to obtain maximum functional improvement.
• Worse outcomes with lower education level, alcohol use, elderly, smokers, medial malleolar fracture.[21]

- Posttraumatic arthritis[22]:
  - Seen in 63% at 10 years.
  - 10% severe arthritis.
  - Fracture dislocation at the time of injury is a significant predictor of long-term posttraumatic radiographic osteoarthritis.

References

1. Court-Brown CM, Caesar B. Epidemiology of adult fractures: a review. Injury 2006;37(8):691–697
2. DeAngelis NA, Eskander MS, French BG. Does medial tenderness predict deep deltoid ligament incompetence in supination-external rotation type ankle fractures? J Orthop Trauma 2007;21(4):244–247
3. Schock HJ, Pinzur M, Manion L, Stover M. The use of gravity or manual-stress radiographs in the assessment of supination-external rotation fractures of the ankle. J Bone Joint Surg Br 2007;89(8):1055–1059
4. Ramsey PL, Hamilton W. Changes in tibiotalar area of contact caused by lateral talar shift. J Bone Joint Surg Am 1976;58(3):356–357
5. Egol KA, Amirtharajah M, Tejwani NC, Capla EL, Koval KJ. Ankle stress test for predicting the need for surgical fixation of isolated fibular fractures. J Bone Joint Surg Am 2004;86-A(11):2393–2398
6. Bankston AB, Anderson LD, Nimityongskul P. Intramedullary screw fixation of lateral malleolus fractures. Foot Ankle Int 1994;15(11):599–607
7. Siegel J, Tornetta P III. Extraperiosteal plating of pronation-abduction ankle fractures. J Bone Joint Surg Am 2007;89(2):276–281
8. Tenenbaum S, Shazar N, Bruck N, Bariteau J. Posterior malleolus fractures. Orthop Clin North Am 2017;48(1):81–89
9. Gardner MJ, Demetrakopoulos D, Briggs SM, Helfet DL, Lorich DG. Malreduction of the tibiofibular syndesmosis in ankle fractures. Foot Ankle Int 2006;27(10):788–792
10. Hamid N, Loeffler BJ, Braddy W, Kellam JF, Cohen BE, Bosse MJ. Outcome after fixation of ankle fractures with an injury to the syndesmosis: the effect of the syndesmosis screw. J Bone Joint Surg Br 2009;91(8):1069–1073
11. Wukich DK, Kline AJ. The management of ankle fractures in patients with diabetes. J Bone Joint Surg Am 2008;90(7):1570–1578
12. Wukich DK, Dikis JW, Monaco SJ, Strannigan K, Suder NC, Rosario BL. Topically applied vancomycin powder reduces the rate of surgical site infection in diabetic patients undergoing foot and ankle surgery. Foot Ankle Int 2015;36(9):1017–1024
13. Sadoskas D, Suder NC, Wukich DK. Perioperative glycemic control and the effect on surgical site infections in diabetic patients undergoing foot and ankle surgery. Foot Ankle Spec 2016;9(1):24–30
14. Chaudhary SB, Liporace FA, Gandhi A, Donley BG, Pinzur MS, Lin SS. Complications of ankle fracture in patients with diabetes. J Am Acad Orthop Surg 2008;16(3):159–170
15. Miller AG, Margules A, Raikin SM. Risk factors for wound complications after ankle fracture surgery. J Bone Joint Surg Am 2012;94(22):2047–2052
16. Belmont PJ Jr, Davey S, Rensing N, Bader JO, Waterman BR, Orr JD. Patient-based and surgical risk factors for 30-day postoperative complications and mortality after ankle fracture fixation. J Orthop Trauma 2015;29(12):e476–e482
17. Basques BA, Miller CP, Golinvaux NS, Bohl DD, Grauer JN. Morbidity and readmission after open reduction and internal fixation of ankle fractures are associated with preoperative patient characteristics. Clin Orthop Relat Res 2015;473(3):1133–1139
18. Mak KH, Chan KM, Leung PC. Ankle fracture treated with the AO principle--an experience with 116 cases. Injury 1985;16(4):265–272
19. Höiness P, Engebretsen L, Strömsöe K. Soft tissue problems in ankle fractures treated surgically. A prospective study of 154 consecutive closed ankle fractures. Injury 2003;34(12):928–931
20. Egol KA, Tejwani NC, Walsh MG, Capla EL, Koval KJ. Predictors of short-term functional outcome following ankle fracture surgery. J Bone Joint Surg Am 2006;88(5):974–979
21. Gougoulias N, Khanna A, Sakellariou A, Maffulli N. Supination-external rotation ankle fractures: stability a key issue. Clin Orthop Relat Res 2010;468(1):243–251
22. Regan DK, Gould S, Manoli A III, Egol KA. Outcomes over a decade after surgery for unstable ankle fracture: functional recovery seen 1 year postoperatively does not decay with time. J Orthop Trauma 2016;30(7):e236–e241

56 Talus Neck Open Reduction Internal Fixation (ORIF)

James C. Krieg

Abstract

The goals of ORIF) of the talar neck are an anatomic reduction and stable internal fixation. This is best achieved through two surgical approaches, anterolateral and medial. Reduction is performed through both approaches, as is fixation. Fixation typically consists of lag screws, positioning screws, minifragment plates, or a combination thereof. Reduction techniques and fixation strategies will be discussed. Examples will be shown.

Keywords: *fracture, neck of talus, surgical approach, reduction, fixation*

56.1 Indications

- Displaced fractures of the talar neck.
- Nondisplaced fractures in order to allow for early motion and to ensure healing without displacement.
- Often occur in conjunction with other injuries, both local and remote. Timing and surgical incisions need to take this into account.

56.1.1 Clinical Evaluation

- Swelling and contusion around the ankle.
- Varus alignment of the hindfoot.
- Beware of tenting of the skin with displaced fractures, which can lead to skin ischemia.
- Neurovascular evaluation must be carefully done as the talar body fragment can displace posteromedially and injure the neurovascular bundle.
- Approximately 15% of injuries are open fractures.
- High vigilance for associated injuries in high-velocity injuries:
  - Thirty percent of displaced fractures have concomitant medial malleolar fractures.
  - Calcaneal or pilon fractures.
  - Pelvic or spinal fractures.

56.1.2 Radiographic Evaluation

- Imaging includes anteroposterior (AP), lateral, oblique of foot, AP and mortise, and lateral of the ankle.
- The Canale view of the foot gives a true AP of the talar neck. This is performed with the foot 15 degrees internally rotated on the X-ray plate, and the beam aimed 15 degrees from vertical, aimed cephalad and centered over the talar neck.
- Computed tomography (CT) scan of the ankle is recommended in most cases to define displacement and comminution.

56.1.3 Mechanism of Injury

- Most commonly high-velocity trauma (motor vehicle injury; fall from height).
- Hyperdorsiflexion of the foot on the leg with axial loading.

56.1.4 Nonoperative Options

- Non-weight-bearing cast immobilization can be used for undisplaced fractures.
- Surgical reduction and fixation is recommended for all displaced fractures unless the patient is not a surgical candidate for medical reasons.

56.1.5 Classification of Talar Neck Fractures

The classification was described by Hawkins into four types and is dependent on the congruency of the peritalar joints. The degree of comminution or displacement is not addressed by this classification.

- Hawkins I: Undisplaced vertical fracture of the talar neck.
- Hawkins II: Displaced fracture of the talar neck with subluxation or dislocation of the subtalar joint (the ankle joint remains well aligned):
  - Vallier et al divided Hawkins II fractures into IIA (where the subtalar joint was subluxated) and IIB (where the subtalar joint was dislocated).[1]
- Hawkins III: Displaced fracture of the talar neck with subluxation or dislocation of the subtalar and ankle joints (the talonavicular joint remains congruent).
- Hawkins IV: Displaced fracture of the talar neck with subluxation or dislocation of the subtalar, ankle, and talonavicular joints.

With each increasing Hawkins type, the risk of talar osteonecrosis and posttraumatic arthritis increases.

56.1.6 Contraindications

- Nonviable limb due to unreconstructable vascular or server soft-tissue/nerve injury.
- Active infection at the surgical site.
- Medically unstable patient.

56.2 Goals of Surgical Procedure

The primary goals of the procedure are to obtain an anatomic reduction of the fracture fragments and achieve stable internal fixation. Additionally, there are often fragments loose in the subtalar joint and occasionally in the tibiotalar joint. These must be removed in order to prevent later symptoms and degenerative arthritis. In the attempt to achieve these goals, it is important to remember the blood supply to the talus and to preserve it as much as possible. This will facilitate healing and help minimize the risk of avascular necrosis (AVN).

56.3 Advantages of Surgical Procedure

Given the tenuous nature of the blood supply to the talus, direct reduction and stable internal fixation will greatly increase the likelihood of union after fracture. The talus is the vital connection between the hindfoot and the midfoot. It is a functional part of the ankle, subtalar, and transverse tarsal joints, all of which are essential to normal foot function. Alteration of the talar morphology, by malunion in particular, will affect foot position and function.

56.4 Key Principles

- Two approaches required.
- Preserve dorsal soft-tissue attachments.
- Reduction with direct control of fragments, using joysticks, clamps, picks.
- Reduction assessment by interdigitating fracture on tension side.
- Canale, mortise, and lateral views to assess reduction on fluoroscopy.
- Fixation must also be bicolumnar, corresponding with the two approaches.
- Screw fixation when the fracture is simple.
- Miniplates can span areas of comminution.

56.5 Preoperative Preparation and Patient Positioning

56.5.1 Timing of Surgery

- Historically, displaced talar neck fractures have been considered surgical emergencies. While we advocate these to be fixed in a timely fashion, it is better and safer to wait for the soft-tissue envelope swelling to resolve prior to surgery than to operate early and risk wound-healing complications.
- No correlation with timing of surgery and incidence of osteonecrosis or posttraumatic arthritis.[2,3]

56.5.2 Preparation and Positioning

Diagnosis and planning will require radiographs of the foot and ankle. Fracture features are often seen well on the plain X-rays. Include mortise and lateral views of the ankle and AP, lateral, and oblique views of the foot. However, the detail of a CT scan is often invaluable (**Fig. 56.1**). The additional information gained in the CT scan is generally worth the extra cost and radiation exposure. It is also important to remember that a significant number of talar neck fractures will have associated injuries, both locally and systemically. For example, many neck fractures of the talus will also have a fracture of the lateral process of the talus, which can be seen much better on a dedicated CT scan.

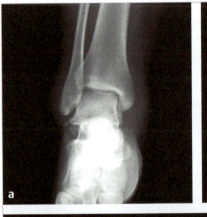
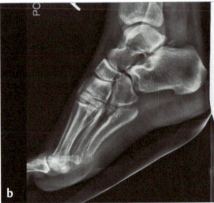
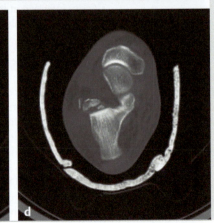

Fig. 56.1 (a,b) Mortise and lateral views of talar neck fracture. (c) CT scan with axial cut showing comminution not seen on plain X-rays. (d) CT scan showing osteochondral fragment in the subtalar joint.

Planning will include anticipating the need for mini-fragment plates, in addition to mini- and small-fragment screws (3.5/2.7/2.4/2.0 mm). A micro-oscillating saw will be needed if a medial malleolar osteotomy is necessary.

Assessment of reduction and proper hardware placement will require use of intraoperative fluoroscopy. A completely radiolucent operating table will facilitate use of fluoroscopy. In order to avoid interference with the operating team, a table with a cantilever radiolucent extension is preferred.

The patient is positioned supine, with a small bump placed under the ipsilateral hip. A completely radiolucent positioning "ramp" can be placed under the lower leg prior to the prep. This will greatly facilitate the ability to obtain lateral images without having to move the operative limb. Additionally, a sterile triangle positioning support can be placed under the knee, which will position the foot in a more plantigrade position relative to the table. This greatly enhances use of fluoroscopy.

56.6 Operative Technique

56.6.1 Surgical Exposure

Two approaches are necessary to adequately reduce and fix the vast majority of talar neck fractures. The approaches are used simultaneously, so it does not matter which is made first. The incision for the medial approach is centered between the anterior tibialis and posterior tibialis tendons. It should reach from the anterior tip of the medial malleolus to the navicular. Prior to making the incision, draw a proximal extension that will curve across the medial malleolus as it proceeds proximally, from the anterior tip of the medial malleolus to the posterior border of the tibial shaft (**Fig. 56.2a**). This proximal extension can be used if the need for a medial malleolar osteotomy arises. Skin flaps are kept full thickness.

Deep dissection involves cutting the capsule of the tibiotalar joint just anterior to the deltoid ligament. Distally, the talonavicular joint capsule is incised and it can be exposed dorsally. The dorsomedial talar neck is exposed subperiosteally. Care is taken, however, to limit the amount of subperiosteal dissection carried out dorsally, in order to preserve the soft-tissue attachments that may provide some blood supply to the fragments. In the proximal part of the dissection, the ankle capsule and dorsal soft tissues can be safely retracted to allow visualization of the articular surface all the way across to the lateral side. Exposure should include the articular dome of the talus, the dorsomedial cortex of the neck, and the medial aspect of the head.

More lateral exposure of the head can be obtained by abducting the foot at the talonavicular joint.

The lateral incision is in line with the distal tibiofibular joint and the medial side of the fourth metatarsal, or the third interspace. The dissection should elevate full-thickness flaps, but care needs to be taken proximally to look for and preserve the superficial peroneal nerve, which is generally encountered. The extensor retinaculum is incised and the long toe extensors are retracted medially. The extensor brevis musculature is generally retracted laterally (**Fig. 56.2b**). The sinus tarsi fat can be excised, and the lateral cortex can be exposed subperiosteally. Proximally, the ankle capsule is incised, and the anterior retraction of the capsule and dorsal soft tissues allows for the visualization of the lateral dome, across to the medial exposure. As with the medial side, the dorsal dissection is limited to the ankle capsule, to avoid stripping the dorsal blood supply from the neck fragments and remainder of the talus.

The lateral dissection of the ankle capsule can be extended distally, along the lateral facet of the talus, to the lateral process. Dissection in the plantar direction beyond the lateral process will expose the posterior facet of the subtalar joint. The capsule of the subtalar joint and the interosseous ligament can be excised, facilitating the visualization. There is often osteochondral debris in the subtalar joint. Excision of these fragments is important in minimizing the effect they can have on the subtalar joint.

56.6.2 Reduction

The majority of talar neck fractures occur because of forced dorsiflexion and some inversion. This means that the anteromedial neck is loaded in compression, leading to comminution of the bone in this part of the neck. The lateral neck and sometimes the inferomedial neck are often loaded in tension and will therefore fail with a simple fracture pattern. Reduction should begin at the zone of the fracture that lacks comminution. The goal is to use the interdigitation of the fracture edges to help guide reduction in these areas. The fracture edges need to be exposed subperiosteally to allow for the use of these edges for a fracture "read." Often, a more vertical fracture will exit through the chondral surface of the talar dome. In these cases, assessment of the reduction is facilitated by using the edge of the chondral surface as a landmark for fracture alignment. After the simple fracture line is reduced, attention can be turned to the areas of comminution. Obviously, cases with more comminution will be harder to accurately reduce.

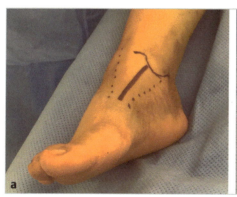
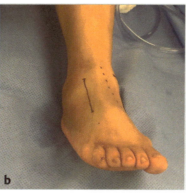

Fig. 56.2 (a) Planned medial incision. (b) The lateral incision is drawn out.

Manipulation of the fragments is often facilitated by placement of 2.5-mm Schanz screws in either or both of the major fragments, the body and the head. Other helpful instruments include dental picks and a Freer elevator. The deformity involves some degree of rotation and angulation, and often this can be subtle. Reduction is achieved by utilizing both the medial and lateral fracture reads, working back and forth between them until the reduction is anatomic. For simple fractures, a pointed reduction clamp (Weber clamp) can aid in reduction. One tine is placed immediately posterior to the medial malleolus, avoiding the neurovascular structures, and the other is placed on the talar head. As an alternative, a clamp can be modified. The tines of a small Weber clamp can be straightened with pliers, and the tips placed into small drill holes in each fragment, through either incision. Provisional fixation is provided by multiple retrograde K-wires through both incisions (**Fig. 56.3**).

56.6.3 Intraoperative Reduction Assessment

Fluoroscopic imaging is essential to assess reduction and hardware placement. Evaluation of reduction is facilitated by knowledge of normal anatomy. The AP view of the talar neck is seen on the Canale view. This view is easily obtained by flexing the knee, placing the foot flat on the table by plantarflexing it, rotating the entire leg internally 15 to 20 degrees, and aiming the C-arm in the AP plane. The net effect of the rotation and plantarflexion is that the calcaneus is removed from behind the talus, thus ensuring that they are not superimposed. This allows you to see the true shape and dimension of the neck of the talus (**Fig. 56.4**). The medial border of the talus should be straight. The typical deformity involves varus.

On the lateral view, the typical deformity is extension. The axis of the talus and that of the first metatarsal should be parallel in the lateral image. In fact, the axis of the talar neck should be parallel to the first metatarsal in both the AP and lateral images. Other clues on the lateral view are the facets of the subtalar joint. The anterior and middle facets are part of the head fragment, while the posterior facet is on the body fragment.

When the reduction is accurate, the lateral view will show that the subtalar joint is congruent in its entirety, seen on the posterior and middle facets (**Fig. 56.5**). In cases of extreme comminution, this important landmark may be one of the best (and only) indicators of reduction (**Fig. 56.6**).

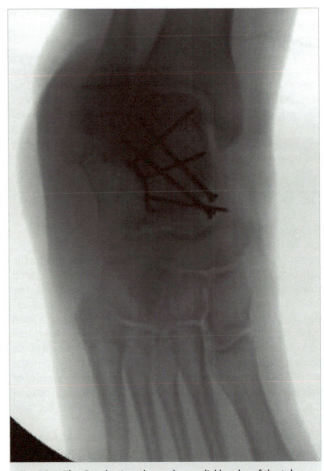

Fig. 56.4 The Canale view shows the medial border of the talar neck, as well as the axis of the talus. The axis of the talus should be collinear with the first metatarsal.

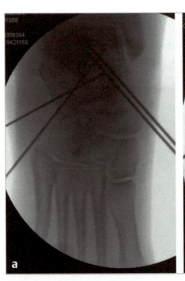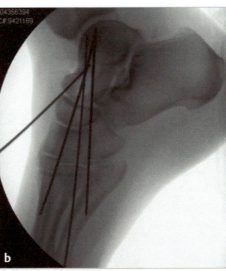

Fig. 56.3 (a,b) Provisional fixation is provided by multiple K-wires.

56.6.4 Internal Fixation

Despite the mechanical advantage of posterior to anterior screw fixation, multiple studies have documented the ability of minifragment fixation placed anteriorly to provide stable fixation. The advantages of anterior fixation include the ability to place it through the approaches done for reduction. In addition, the ability to mix screw and plate fixation is a significant advantage of anterior placement of implants.

After reduction and provisional fixation, the lateral fixation is usually placed first. Multiple screws have more torsional and angular control of deformity than a single screw. Choices for screw fixation include 4.0-, 3.5-, 2.7-, and 2.4-mm screws. While smaller implants are obviously weaker, the use of multiple smaller diameter gains more torsional and angular control. As an alternative to screws fixation, a minifragment plate can be contoured to the lateral cortex of the neck, from the articular cartilage of the head to the lateral gutter. The plate is typically a 2.0-mm plate, with 2.0- or 2.4-mm screws. For comminuted or very distal fractures, a 2.0-mm t-plate can be used, so that multiple points of fixation are placed in the head fragment.

Once the lateral side is fixed, the foot can be abducted at the talonavicular joint, allowing for the placement of multiple screws in the medial side of the talus. The same size screws can be used, from 4.0 to 2.4 mm. The screws should not be placed with a lag technique if there has been any comminution at all. Rather, a positioning screw is placed, to prevent the varus deformity that can occur if the medial neck shortens. If there is extensive medial comminution, then a medial plate can be placed. However, the placement of a medial plate is challenging. The placement of a plate in the ankle must be avoided. To help gain proximal fixation, and avoid intra-articular placement, a 2.0-mm t-plate can be used, with the transverse limb of the plate placed proximally. Voids created by missing bone can be dealt with by placing structural graft, or morselized graft, which can be locally obtained from the tuberosity of the calcaneus.

56.7 Tips and Pearls

I always use a sterile triangle positioning device to operate on the talar neck. Not only does this greatly facilitate the use of fluoroscopy, but also it positions the foot in a plantigrade orientation, which also seems to make it easier to judge the reduction and the correct orientation of the implants.

The best reduction aid seems to be the use of joysticks in each major fragment. The 2.5-mm Schanz screws, which are often found in a small (wrist) external fixator, are ideal. The threaded end will stay in place, and the shaft is stout enough to allow for manipulation in any plane.

The extruded talus body is a particularly difficult challenge. Although the extruded body is usually not reducible by closed means, closed manipulation should be attempted in the emergency room, as it is sometimes successful (**Fig. 56.7**). Adequate sedation and flexion at the knee can help. Failing this, a reduction in the operating room must be undertaken to avoid skin necrosis and neurovascular compromise. An external fixator can be placed between the tibia and the medial cuneiform, and a second frame placed laterally between the fibula and the base of the fifth and fourth metatarsal shafts. Together, these frames can sometimes open up the space needed to reduce the body. On occasion, the displaced body is entrapped by soft tissues, such as the posterior

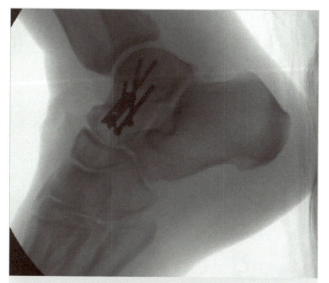

Fig. 56.5 The lateral view shows once again that the axis of the talar neck is collinear with the first metatarsal. In addition, the facets of the subtalar joint are seen to be congruent.

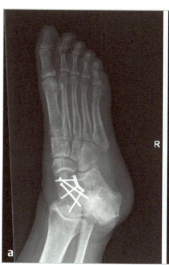
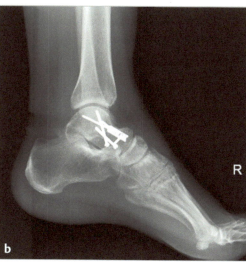

Fig. 56.6 (a,b) Four months postoperatively, the fracture is healed and the patient is recovering.

tibial tendon, and will require an open reduction. In these cases, the use of Schanz screw joysticks has proven to be invaluable.

Screws are best placed in a configuration that is spread apart. In the medial column, they invariably are placed through the head of the talus, where the heads can be countersunk in subchondral bone (**Fig. 56.8**). Sometimes, abduction of the foot does not adequately expose the head. This can be accomplished by using a small rongeur to remove the overhanging navicular which blocks access to the head of the talus in many patients.

56.8 Hazards and Pitfalls

Assume that a radiographic reduction is likely to yield malreduction. For this reason alone, the overwhelming majority of neck of talus fractures should be fixed with two simultaneous approaches.

The deformity that is likely to occur is most often a combination of varus and extension. Knowing that this is the case, it is important to avoid shortening of the dorsal medial neck.

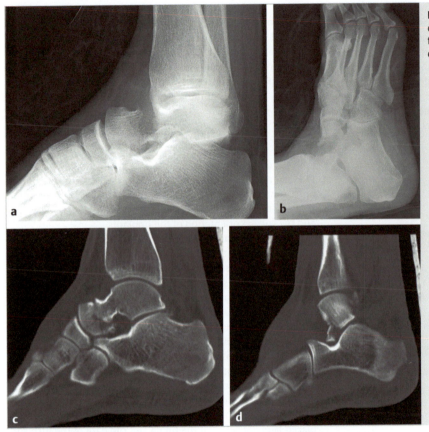

Fig. 56.7 (a,b) Injury films of talus fracture dislocation. **(c,d)** After closed reduction in the emergency room. Note the lateral process fracture in **d**.

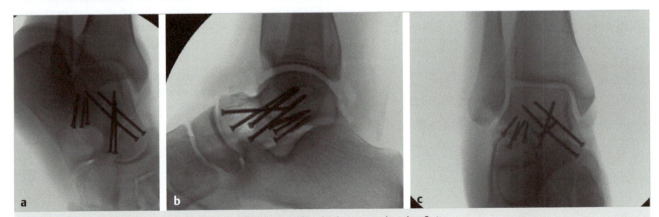

Fig. 56.8 (a–c) Intraoperative views showing the reduction and multiple screws placed to fix it.

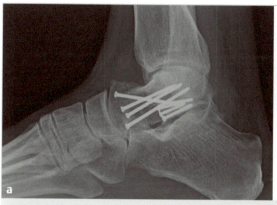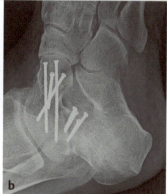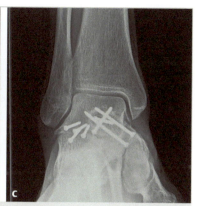

Fig. 56.9 (a–c) In spite of the comminution and displacement at injury, the fracture has healed 1 year postoperatively. The patient has early arthrosis of the subtalar and talonavicular joints.

56.9 Complications/Bailout/ Salvage

Fracture malunion and nonunion can compromise foot function significantly. Nonunion can be addressed with debridement of the fracture site, autogenous bone grafting, and plate fixation. Malunion can be addressed with a similar approach, using a structural tricortical iliac crest graft.

Subtalar arthrosis is the most likely reason for poor outcome, and is best addressed with subtalar arthrodesis.

AVN and collapse of the body is a particularly vexing problem, and while multiple strategies may exist for reconstruction, none are particularly gratifying.

56.10 Postoperative Care

Initially, the limb is immobilized with the ankle in neutral. After 2 weeks, patients can be changed to a lightweight resting splint, but are cautioned to maintain strict non-weight-bearing precautions. Active assisted range of motion of the ankle and subtalar joints is generally safe at this point, as is passive range of motion of toes, to minimize intrinsic stiffness. Weight-bearing is delayed until 12 weeks, or longer in cases of more significant comminution.

Radiographs taken at 6 to 10 weeks postsurgery should be scrutinized for evidence of a Hawkins sign. This can be seen as subchondral radiolucency at the talar dome and is a sign of revascularization of the talar body and the absence of osteonecrosis.

56.11 Outcomes

In spite of historical directives to operate on displaced talar neck fractures emergently, the literature supports urgent management, rather than viewing the injury as a surgical emergency.[2] With a more modern focus on anatomic reduction and

stable fixation, the union rates are generally high, and the risk of AVN is generally low.[3,4] The risk of varus malunion in comminuted fractures is still a concern. The injury was once considered likely to cause significant disability. Although it remains a definite concern, with the focus on getting the injury treated optimally, a distinct focus on quality of reduction, minimization of surgical morbidity, and the use of modern implants, the majority of talar neck fractures tend to do rather well; the problems they do encounter are often amenable to a reconstructive solution (**Fig. 56.9**).

A 2015 meta-analysis demonstrated the overall rate of osteonecrosis at 31%, with increasing rates with higher Hawkins types.[5] There is a significantly higher incidence of osteonecrosis in Vallier's Hawkins type IIB (subtalar joint dislocated) than type IIA (subtalar joint subluxed) fractures.[1]

The mean rate of subtalar arthritis was 49%, but this increased to 81% in studies with greater than 2-year follow-up.[5]

References

1. Vallier HA, Reichard SG, Boyd AJ, Moore TA. A new look at the Hawkins classification for talar neck fractures: which features of injury and treatment are predictive of osteonecrosis? J Bone Joint Surg Am 2014;96(3):192–197

2. Bellamy JL, Keeling JJ, Wenke J, Hsu JR. Does a longer delay in fixation of talus fractures cause osteonecrosis? J Surg Orthop Adv 2011;20(1):34–37

3. Lindvall E, Haidukewych G, DiPasquale T, Herscovici D Jr, Sanders R. Open reduction and stable fixation of isolated, displaced talar neck and body fractures. J Bone Joint Surg Am 2004;86-A(10):2229–2234

4. Vallier HA, Nork SE, Barei DP, Benirschke SK, Sangeorzan BJ. Talar neck fractures: results and outcomes. J Bone Joint Surg Am 2004;86-A(8):1616–1624

5. Dodd A, Lefaivre KA. Outcomes of talar neck fractures: a systematic review and meta-analysis. J Orthop Trauma 2015;29(5):210–215

57 Extensile Open Reduction and Internal Fixation of Intra-articular Joint Calcaneus Fractures

Brian S. Winters and Joseph N. Daniel

Abstract

Calcaneus fractures continue to be the most common fractures in the foot and challenging in its treatment. A number of studies have described improved functional outcomes and decreased risk of posttraumatic subtalar joint arthritis with open reduction and internal fixation using various techniques. If you adhere to certain indications and a meticulous surgical technique, you can expect your patients to achieve a good functional result when compared to nonoperative treatment. This chapter will help guide you to evaluate calcaneus fractures, determine the appropriate treatment, and successfully perform an open reduction and internal fixation when indicated.

Keywords: *calcaneus fracture, open reduction and internal fixation, extensile lateral, percutaneous, sinus tarsi approach*

57.1 Indications

- Calcaneus fractures are the most common fractures of the foot:
  - Closed fractures: 83%.
  - Open fractures: 17%.
- Anatomy:
  - Body/tuberosity:
    - ❖ Main attachment of the Achilles tendon.
  - Sustentaculum tali:
    - ❖ Acts as a fulcrum for the flexor hallucis longus tendon and supports the talar neck.
    - ❖ Attachment for the deltoid and talocalcaneal ligaments.
    - ❖ Contained in the anteromedial fragment in calcaneal fractures:
      - – Also referred to as the "constant" fragment.
  - Anterior process:
    - ❖ Articulates with the calcaneocuboid joint and head of the talus.
  - Posterior articular facet:
    - ❖ The largest facet that makes up the subtalar joint and is the major weight-bearing surface of the calcaneus.
  - Anterior and middle articular facets:
    - ❖ Usually confluent with each other.
    - ❖ The middle facet sits on top of the sustentaculum tali.
- Mechanisms of injury:
  - Intra-articular (70–75%):
    - ❖ Axial load to the hindfoot, such as what occurs during a motor vehicle accident (MVA) or a fall from height.
      - – Joint-depression-type (**Fig. 57.1**).
      - – Tongue-type (**Fig. 57.2**).
- Extra-articular (25–30%):
  - ❖ Calcaneal tuberosity (**Fig. 57.3**).
    - – Forceful contraction of the gastroc-soleus muscle, which leads to an avulsion of the calcaneal tuberosity at the Achilles tendon insertion.
  - ❖ Sustentaculum tali:
    - – Forceful avulsion of the deltoid and talocalcaneal ligaments.
  - ❖ Anterior process:
    - – Inversion and plantarflexion of the foot, which leads to an avulsion at the bifurcate ligament and violation of the calcaneocuboid joint.
    - – Also commonly seen with intra-articular fractures as well (~ 63%).
  - Associated injuries:
    - ❖ Lumbar vertebrae.
    - ❖ Ipsilateral lower extremity.
    - ❖ Contralateral calcaneus.

57.1.1 Clinical Evaluation

- The initial step in evaluating any patient involved in a trauma is to employ the advanced trauma life support (ATLS) protocol.
- A thorough history should be obtained to determine the mechanism of injury, the locations of pain, presence of loss of consciousness, and, in the setting of an MVA, whether the patient was a restrained driver/passenger and if air bags were deployed.

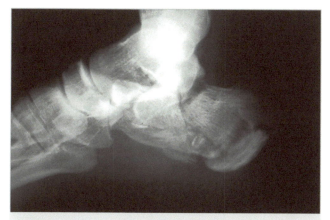

Fig. 57.1 Joint-depression-type calcaneus fracture.

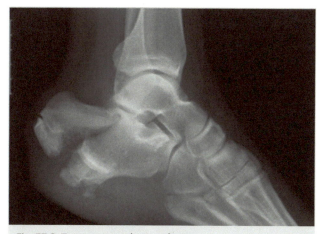

Fig. 57.2 Tongue-type calcaneus fracture.

- The physical examination of a patient with a presumed orthopaedic injury initially involves inspection of the skin integrity to determine if it is open or closed. The presence of any prior scars and skin quality should be carefully evaluated simultaneously.
- Palpate the distal pulses and obtain a vascular consultation if there is any concern about the arterial vascular supply to the limb.
- A thorough motor and sensory exam should then be obtained. It is not uncommon for weakness and numbness to be present after a foot and ankle injury and therefore one must have a high index of suspicion if a deficit is present.
- Once the above have been established, further evaluation of the foot and ankle can be performed. Findings consistent with a calcaneus fracture include diffuse tenderness to palpation, ecchymosis, swelling, and shortening/widening/varus alignment of the hindfoot. The ankle should always be included in the examination to rule out additional injuries, such as a peroneal tendon dislocation.
- The lumbar spine, pelvis, and bilateral lower extremities should always be evaluated in addition to the foot and ankle.

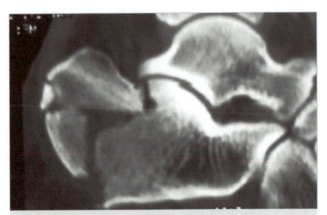

Fig. 57.3 Extra-articular calcaneal tuberosity fracture.

57.1.2 Radiographic Evaluation

- **X-rays:**
  - Mandatory views
    - ❖ Anteroposterior (AP), oblique, and lateral radiographs of the foot routinely provide sufficient information to make a definitive diagnosis of a calcaneus fracture.
    - ❖ AP, mortise, and lateral radiographs of the ankle should always be obtained as well.
      - A "fleck" sign at the lateral aspect of the distal fibula on the AP and mortise views suggests dislocation of the peroneal tendons.
      - AP and mortise views allow for assessment of subfibular impingement due to lateral wall blowout if present.
    - ❖ Harris' view (**Fig. 57.4a,b**):
      - Axial view of the calcaneus.
      - Allows for visualization of the tuberosity, hindfoot widening, varus alignment, and posterior facet involvement.
      - Foot is maximally dorsiflexed with the beam angled at 45 degrees.
  - Optional views
    - ❖ Broden's view:
      - Internal rotation views of the ankle in maximum dorsiflexion at 40, 30, 20, and 10 degrees
      - Useful intra-operatively to assess the reduction of the posterior facet.
  - Measurements:
    - ❖ Bohler's angle (**Fig. 57.5a**):
      - Determined on the lateral X-ray of the foot/ankle.
      - Angle is created between the intersection of a line drawn from the most superior aspect of the tuberosity to the posterior/superior aspect of the posterior facet and another drawn from the posterior/superior aspect of the posterior facet to the most superior aspect of the anterior process.

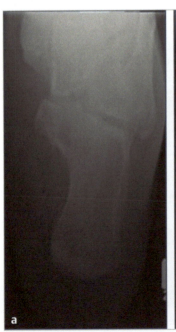
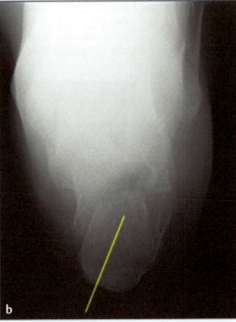

Fig. 57.4 (a) Harris' view of the calcaneus. **(b)** Harris' view of a calcaneus fracture illustrating the typical varus hindfoot alignment.

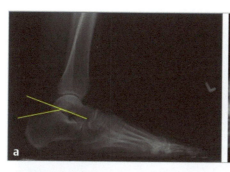
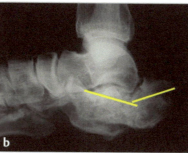

Fig. 57.5 (a) Normal Bohler's angle. (b) Abnormal Bohler's angle illustrating a depression-type calcaneus fracture.

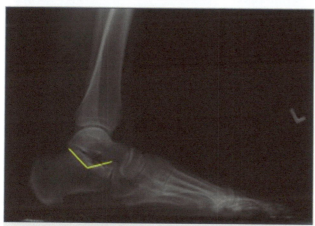

Fig. 57.6 The angle of Gissane.

- Normal is 20 to 40 degrees:
  i. If an angle is less than 20 degrees, this illustrates collapse of the posterior facet, which in turn causes a concomitant decrease in talar inclination (**Fig. 57.5b**):
    a. Decreases in talar inclination can subsequently lead to anterior ankle impingement and further disability.
  ❖ Crucial (critical) angle of Gissane (**Fig. 57.6**):
    - Determined on the lateral X-ray of the foot/ankle.
    - Angle is formed by the intersection of lines drawn at the downward and upward slopes of the calcaneal superior surface.
    - Follows the lateral process of the talus.
    - Normal is between 120 and 140 degrees.
    - If the angle is above 140 degrees, this illustrates collapse of the posterior facet.
  ○ The Essex-Lopresti classification differentiates joint-depression patterns and tongue-type fractures, based on the primary and secondary fracture lines:
    ❖ The primary fracture line is an oblique fracture line that divides the calcaneus into an anteromedial (constant fragment) and posterolateral fracture fragment, which routinely involves the posterior facet.
    ❖ In joint-depression fractures, the secondary fracture line exits posterior to the posterior facet.
    ❖ In tongue-type fractures, secondary fracture line exits at where the majority of the posterior facet remains in continuity with the tuberosity.

57.1.3 Nonoperative Options

- Initially immobilize in a non-weight-bearing splint in order to allow for swelling to subside with subsequent transition to a short leg non-weight-bearing cast at 2 weeks after injury:
  ○ Non-weight-bearing for 6 to 12 weeks:
    ❖ Sanders' type 1 fractures.
    ❖ Nondisplaced to minimally displaced Sanders' type 2 fractures (< 2 cm) with an intact Achilles mechanism.
    ❖ Nondisplaced avulsion extra-articular fractures:
      - Short leg plantarflexion cast due to the pull of the Achilles tendon.
    ❖ Nondisplaced anterior process fractures < 25% of the articular surface.
- Once union is obtained as demonstrated by office X-rays (AP, oblique, lateral, and Harris' views) and physical exam, transition to weight-bearing as tolerated in a CAM walker boot and start physical therapy, which should be performed in a sneaker for 6 weeks:
  ○ Wean out of the boot under the guidance of physical therapy.
  ○ Heel pain is common and can be controlled with either over-the-counter or custom-molded orthotics.
  ○ Additional physical therapy may be necessary to obtain optimal functional results.
- **Computed tomography (CT) scan:**
  ○ Gold standard for evaluating calcaneus fracture configurations and determining whether nonoperative or operative intervention is indicated.
  ○ Obtain 30-degree semicoronal, axial, sagittal, and three-dimensional reconstructions.
  ○ Sanders' classification (**Fig. 57.7a, b**):
    ❖ Based on evaluation of the posterior facet at its widest point on the 30-degree semicoronal views:
      - Type 1—nondisplaced fracture(s).
      - Type 2—one fracture line with two main fracture fragments.
      - Type 3—two fracture lines with three main fracture fragments.
      - Type 4—three or more fracture lines with four or more fracture fragments.
- **Magnetic resonance imaging (MRI) scan:**
  ○ Rarely indicated.
  ○ Only indication is to diagnose a calcaneal stress fracture in the setting of trauma and normal radiographs.

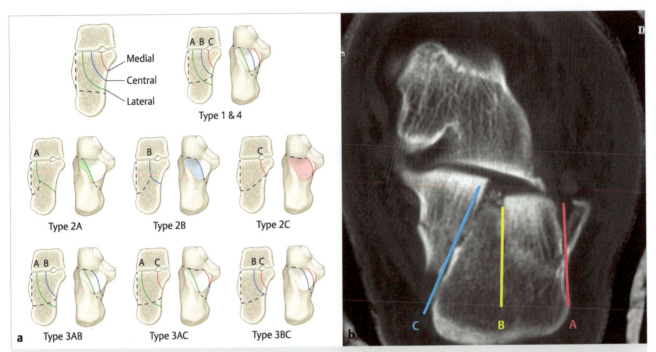

Fig. 57.7 (a) Sander's classification. (b) CT scan (semicoronal view) of a calcaneus fracture illustrating the fracture lines of a Sanders type 4.

57.1.4 Contraindications

- Uncontrolled psychiatric illness which may lead to poor patient compliance postoperatively.
- Uncontrolled diabetes.
- Severe peripheral vascular disease.
- Active smoking.
- Poor soft-tissue envelope.
- Low-demand patient.
- Comorbidities that can lead to wound complications (i.e., liver compromise).

57.2 Goals of Surgical Procedure

The ultimate goal is to achieve an anatomic reduction of the articular surfaces, restore calcaneal height/width/length/alignment, and early mobilization.

57.3 Advantages of Surgical Procedure

Open reduction and internal fixation can reduce the risk of developing posttraumatic arthritis with subsequent need for subtalar joint arthrodesis and postoperative stiffness by allowing early range of motion. The extensile open approach allows detailed anatomic assessment and visualization of the reduction and cartilaginous injury to the posterior facet of the subtalar joint, but can have a high wound complication rate without appropriate

procedure timing and soft-tissue handling. More limited surgical approaches and percutaneous procedures have been described with potentially lower wound complications, but these sacrifice full anatomic visualization of the reduction.

57.4 Key Principles

The key principles of an open reduction and internal fixation for a calcaneus fracture is to restore the articular surface of the posterior facet of the calcaneus, the height and width of the body, and the alignment of the calcaneus, while minimizing soft-tissue trauma.

57.5 Preoperative Preparation and Patient Positioning

57.5.1 Timing of the Surgery

Most calcaneal fractures requiring surgery are high-energy injuries with severe trauma to the soft tissue of the heel. Early surgery with the extensile approach, before the soft-tissue swelling has had a chance to resolve, can result in poor wound healing and complications. Prior to performing the surgery, the limb should be immobilized in a Jones bulky dressing or well-padded splint and the limb kept elevated until the swelling resolves. This is assessed through passively dorsiflexing and everting the hindfoot and looking for wrinkling of the lateral skin over the calcaneus where the surgical incision will be ("wrinkle test"). It is common for the surgery to be delayed for 7 to 14 days prior to adequate soft-tissue healing to allow for extensile surgical management.

57.5.2 Positioning

The patient positioning is based on the surgeon's preference. The supine position with a generous ipsilateral hip bump to enhance internal rotation is most commonly employed, although semilateral is preferred by some. Prone positioning is helpful for bilateral injuries.

57.6 Operative Technique

A variety of surgical approaches have been described including the extensile lateral (**Fig. 57.8**) and combined medial and lateral. If there are three or less fracture fragments, a straight approach at the level of the sinus tarsi can be utilized (**Fig. 57.9**). The visualization is limited with the sinus tarsi approach and manipulation of the fragments can be challenging; however, the incision is obviously smaller and soft-tissue healing is less of an issue.

The extensile lateral approach is more of the "workhorse" exposure permitting enhanced visualization and greater ease of identification and reduction of the fracture fragments. It begins with a vertical incision immediately lateral to the Achilles tendon and posterior to the peroneal tendon group extending plantarly to the level of the glabrous tissue. The incision then can be continued either gently curved or at a 90-degree angle with the horizontal limb extending to the level of the calcaneocuboid joint. The sural nerve is exposed and protected within the flap. A full-thickness flap is created beginning at the apex and dissecting sharply along the bone and including the peroneal tendons within the flap. Care must be taken to avoid injuring the peroneal tendons which may be entrapped in a fracture fragment or impinged between the widened calcaneus and the distal fibula. The entire lateral aspect of the calcaneus and the subtalar joint are exposed. The flap is retracted by driving smooth K-wires into the lateral fibula and the neck of the talus, holding the flap in a "no-touch" technique (**Fig. 57.10**). The primary and secondary fracture lines are identified and the soft tissue interposed is removed. It is important, however, to not strip the bone of overlying soft tissue given this can result in increased scarring and adhesions postoperatively. First, the fracture lines at the level of the anterior process of the calcaneus are reduced and held with temporary K-wires. The anterior process is then retracted in a plantar direction, using a lamina spreader held between the lateral aspect of the head of the talus and the stabilized anterior process of the calcaneus. The posterior facet is reduced from its plantarflexed position using a periosteal elevator and stabilized with a K-wire driven from the anterior process laterally to the posterior facet medially. There is usually some degree of varus misalignment, which can be challenging to correct with simple fracture mobilization. To that end, a threaded Steinmann pin can be placed within the tuberosity fragment to distract, and pull the fragment medially and finally plantarly (**Fig. 57.11**). This will aid in regaining the height of the calcaneal body and correcting the varus alignment. A C-arm Harris view will confirm medial wall alignment and this can be

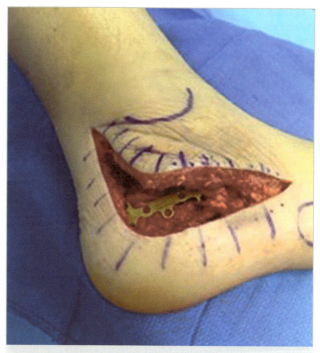

Fig. 57.8 Extensile lateral approach.

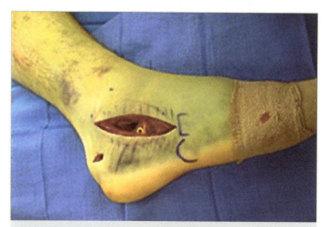

Fig. 57.9 Sinus tarsi "percutaneous" approach.

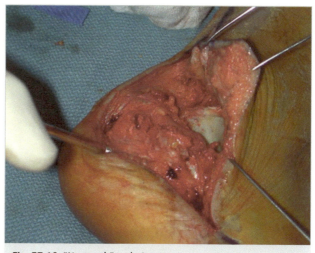

Fig. 57.10 "No-touch" technique.

held temporarily with K-wires driven from the posterior aspect of the tuberosity and into the sustentaculum tali, or constant fragment. The posterior facet is reduced lastly and stabilized with K-wires driven from medial to lateral, again into the sustentaculum tali (**Fig. 57.12**). Any step-off within the joint need to be carefully reduced to prevent the development of posttraumatic arthritis in the subtalar joint. Additionally, any nonviable joint fragments and intra-articular bone fragments should be removed. If the lateral wall of the calcaneus was removed to enhance initial visualization, it is then replaced. We prefer to use two 3.5-mm cortical screws just beneath the posterior facet in a lag mode fashion into the sustentaculum tali (stable fragment) to hold the joint surface reduced, followed by an appropriately selected plate. This is best achieved with an anatomic low-profile calcaneal plate utilizing locked or unlocked screws as per the surgeon's preference (**Fig. 57.13a, b**). The K-wires are then removed. If there were more than four fracture fragments involving the posterior facet of the calcaneus with significant comminution appreciated on the CT scan, consideration can be given for a primary subtalar arthrodesis (**Fig. 57.14a, b**). This is performed using at least two retrograde screws with a minimum of 5-mm diameter. We prefer cancellous screws to avoid loss of height, and we place them both within the body of the talus. In this situation, long or fully threaded screws should be used with threads crossing the fusion site to avoid compression and collapse/loss of calcaneal height.

We use a drain and have found fewer issues with the evolution of a postoperative hematoma and associated soft-tissue issues, as well as some decrease in narcotic demand. The wound is closed in layer with absorbable suture deep and nonabsorbable on the skin (**Fig. 57.15**). The closure must be performed without tension and with all suture knots placed on the vascular (outer side) side of the flap. Either horizontal mattress or an Allgöwer–Donati stitch is used.

57.7 Tips and Pearls

- Proper patient and incision placement allows for direct access to the joint, reduction of fracture lines, and easy use of intraoperative fluoroscopy.
- Respect the soft tissues from the initial incision until when the last stitch is placed. The tissues should always be "manipulated" and never "grabbed" to avoid tissue ischemia and subsequent necrosis. Maintain "no-touch" technique and consider using a drain when performing the extensile lateral approach.
- Ensure that the fracture lines are debrided of all soft tissue/hematoma/fracture fragments prior to placement of your internal fixation. This will help with your reduction.
- Critique your reduction and hindfoot alignment both clinically and radiographically prior to placing your internal fixation.

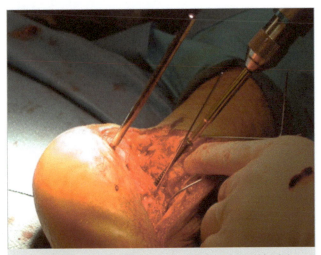

Fig. 57.11 Steinmann pin placement into the calcaneal body/tuberosity.

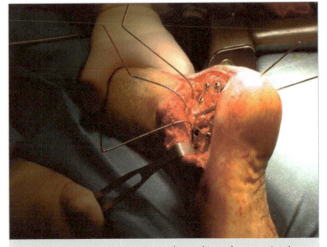

Fig. 57.12 K-wires were temporarily used in order to maintain reduction during final internal fixation placement.

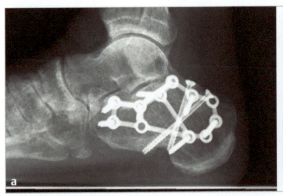

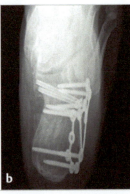

Fig. 57.13 (a) Open reduction and internal fixation (lateral X-ray). (b) Open reduction and internal fixation (Harris' view).

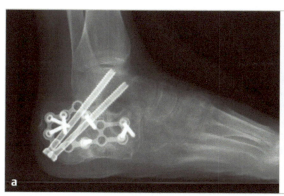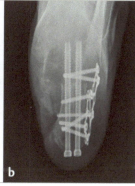

Fig. 57.14 **(a)** Open reduction and internal fixation of a calcaneus fracture with primary subtalar arthrodesis (lateral X-ray). **(b)** Open reduction and internal fixation of a calcaneus fracture with primary subtalar arthrodesis (Harris' view).

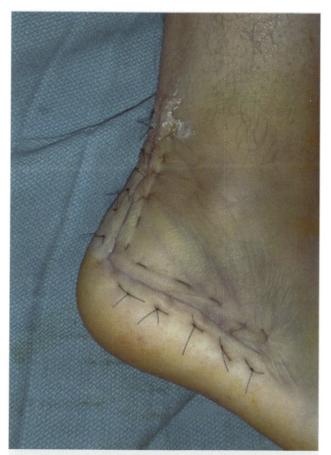

Fig. 57.15 Extensile lateral approach wound closure.

57.8 Hazards and Pitfalls

- A tongue-type and calcaneal tuberosity fractures may result in skin tenting and undue pressure over the posterior heel skin. This can result in rapid breakdown and skin necrosis, which is difficult to manage and has significant morbidity associated with it. This is a relative surgical emergency and the patient should be taken expeditiously to the operating room for reduction of the fracture, and not wait until the swelling resolves.
- The skin, sural nerve, and peroneal tendons are at risk of injury during the exposure and need to be protected accordingly.
- Obtain perfect lateral and Harris' views of the foot intraoperatively if placing a screw into the sustentaculum. Aberrant

placement can cause iatrogenic injury to the flexor hallucis longus tendon.
- Fracture/joint reduction can be difficult or impossible if the fracture lines are not adequately debrided.
- The reduction of the tuberosity fragment can be misleading on the lateral view of the foot. Ensure that a proper reduction was obtained using a Harris view.
- Always confirm that you are satisfied with your reduction (restore height, width, alignment, and articular congruity at the subtalar/calcaneocuboid joints) prior to placing your internal fixation. K-wires can be used to help accomplish this. In many situations, bone stock is limited and cannot tolerate several attempts.

57.9 Complications/Bailout/ Salvage

- If the peroneal tendons are inadvertently lacerated or injured, a repair should be performed.
- If the sural nerve is inadvertently injured, we recommend burying the proximal stump in the soft tissue or bone in an effort to avoid a painful stump neuroma. The sural nerve usually is most at risk at the distal aspect of the extensile lateral approach or with the sinus tarsi approach.
- Consider a bridge plate technique or hybrid external/internal fixation for severely comminuted fractures or tenuous fixation. These will need to be removed in a staged fashion once union is obtained.
- Improper screw placement (i.e., sustentacular screw): symptomatic hardware should be removed once fracture union is obtained or revised acutely if necessary.
- Nonunion: this is exceedingly rare, but if this were to occur, a bone stimulator can be considered at 3 months from surgery. Ensure no underlying metabolic conditions are present (i.e., low 25-hydroxy vitamin D level).
- Malunion: if symptomatic, attempt shoe-wear modification and/or custom orthotics.
- Infection: superficial infection can be treated with local wound care and oral antibiotics. Deep infection should be appropriately debrided and treated with intravenous antibiotics.
- Isolated posttraumatic subtalar/calcaneocuboid joint arthritis: if this develops, nonoperative treatment should be attempted, but if it fails, an in situ arthrodesis can be considered.
- Anterior ankle impingement with subtalar joint posttraumatic arthritis: if the height and articular congruity of the

posterior facet is not restored, this can occur. A distraction subtalar joint arthrodesis can be performed if nonoperative treatment fails.

57.10 Postoperative Care

The patient is maintained in a well-padded U and L splint for 2 weeks while maintaining absolute elevation of the limb above the level of the heart, except for toileting. We convert to a non-weight-bearing cast at 2 weeks, with a total of 6 weeks minimum of non-weight-bearing. At 6 weeks, we consider weight-bearing in a CAM boot, based on plain radiographs, but use discretion based on patient compliance. We usually discontinue immobilization at 12 weeks, again based on imaging. At the point at which we terminate immobilization, we initiate formal physical therapy.

57.11 Outcomes

Successful outcomes for open reduction and internal fixation of calcaneus fractures have been described. While this depends on the use of meticulous surgical technique and obtaining an anatomic reduction, it more importantly is related to patient selection. When all patients are taken into account, there is no significant difference in outcome between nonoperative and operative treatment at 1 year. When worker's compensation, smoking, peripheral vascular disease, and diabetes are appropriately excluded, operative intervention illustrates a significant decrease in the complication rate and subsequent need for a subtalar fusion with a concomitant improvement in pain and function. However, popularization of the percutaneous "sinus tarsi" approach in recent years has provided the orthopaedic surgeon with a means to address the operative calcaneus fracture, while minimizing the risk of complications in those patients possessing these medical comorbidities.

References

1. Agren PH, Wretenberg P, Sayed-Noor AS. Operative versus nonoperative treatment of displaced intra-articular calcaneal fractures: a prospective, randomized, controlled multicenter trial. J Bone Joint Surg Am 2013;95(15):1351–1357
2. Bèzes H, Massart P, Delvaux D, Fourquet JP, Tazi F. The operative treatment of intraarticular calcaneal fractures. Indications, technique, and results in 257 cases. Clin Orthop Relat Res 1993(290):55–59
3. Buch BD, Myerson MS, Miller SD. Primary subtaler arthrodesis for the treatment of comminuted calcaneal fractures. Foot Ankle Int 1996;17(2):61–70
4. Buckley R, Tough S, McCormack R, et al. Operative compared with nonoperative treatment of displaced intra-articular calcaneal fractures: a prospective, randomized, controlled multicenter trial. J Bone Joint Surg Am 2002;84-A(10):1733–1744
5. Ding L, He Z, Xiao H, Chai L, Xue F. Risk factors for postoperative wound complications of calcaneal fractures following plate fixation. Foot Ankle Int 2013;34(9):1238–1244
6. Pennal GF, Yadav MP. Operative treatment of comminuted fractures of the Os calcis. Orthop Clin North Am 1973;4(1):197–211
7. Sanders R, Fortin P, DiPasquale T, Walling A. Operative treatment in 120 displaced intraarticular calcaneal fractures. Results using a prognostic computed tomography scan classification. Clin Orthop Relat Res 1993(290):87–95
8. Sanders R, Gregory P. Operative treatment of intra-articular fractures of the calcaneus. Orthop Clin North Am 1995;26(2):203–214
9. Tomesen T, Biert J, Frölke JP. Treatment of displaced intra-articular calcaneal fractures with closed reduction and percutaneous screw fixation. J Bone Joint Surg Am 2011;93(10):920–928

Index

Note: Page numbers followed by *f* and *t* indicate figures and tables, respectively.

411

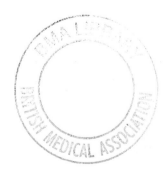